Jekel's

EPIDEMIOLOGY, BIOSTATISTICS, PREVENTIVE MEDICINE, and PUBLIC HEALTH

Jekel's
EPIDEMIOLOGY, BIOSTATISTICS, PREVENTIVE MEDICINE, and PUBLIC HEALTH

FIFTH EDITION

Joann G. Elmore, MD, MPH
Professor of Medicine
The Rosalinde and Arthur Gilbert Foundation Endowed
Chair in Health Care Delivery
David Geffen School of Medicine at UCLA
Professor of Health Policy and Management
UCLA Fielding School of Public Health
Director
UCLA National Clinician Scholars Program
Los Angeles, California

Dorothea M.G. Wild, MD, MPH
Research Affiliate
Institute of General Practice and Family Medicine
University of Bonn
Bonn, Germany

Heidi D. Nelson, MD, MPH, MACP, FRCP
Professor
Medical Informatics and Clinical Epidemiology
and Medicine
Director
Scholarly Projects
School of Medicine
Oregon Health & Science University
Portland, Oregon

David L. Katz, MD, MPH
President
True Health Initiative
Founding Director
Prevention Research Center
Yale University/Griffin Hospital
New Haven, Connecticut

ELSEVIER

Elsevier
3251 Riverport Lane
St. Louis, Missouri 63043

JEKEL'S EPIDEMIOLOGY, BIOSTATISTICS, PREVENTIVE MEDICINE,   ISBN: 978-0-323-64201-9
AND PUBLIC HEALTH, FIFTH EDITION

Notice

Practitioners and researchers must always rely on their own experience and knowledge in evaluating and
using any information, methods, compounds or experiments described herein. Because of rapid advances
in the medical sciences, in particular, independent verification of diagnoses and drug dosages should
be made. To the fullest extent of the law, no responsibility is assumed by Elsevier, authors, editors or
contributors for any injury and/or damage to persons or property as a matter of products liability,
negligence or otherwise, or from any use or operation of any methods, products, instructions, or ideas
contained in the material herein.

Previous edition copyrighted 2014, 2017, 2001.

Library of Congress Control Number: 2019950497

Content Strategist: Elyse O'Grady
Content Development Manager: Kathryn DeFrancesco
Content Development Specialist: Lisa Barnes
Publishing Services Manager: Deepthi Unni
Project Manager: Haritha Dharmarajan
Design Direction: Renee Duenow

Printed in India

Last digit is the print number: 9   8   7   6   5   4   3

 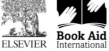

Working together
to grow libraries in
developing countries

www.elsevier.com • www.bookaid.org

Joann G. Elmore, MD, MPH is Professor of Medicine in the David Geffen School of Medicine at UCLA, Professor in the Department of Health Policy and Management at the UCLA Fielding School of Public Health, The Rosalinde and Arthur Gilbert Foundation Endowed Chair in Health Care Delivery, and Director of the UCLA National Clinical Scholars Program. Dr. Elmore's research has consistently addressed questions that push the boundaries of our scientific knowledge in a broad range of areas that include cancer screening, diagnostic accuracy, medical technology, statistical methods, medical education, computer image analyses and machine learning, health IT, and patient communication. For the past two decades, her research has been continuously well funded by the National Institutes of Health (NIH); she has to her credit more than 250 peer-reviewed publications in such journals as the *New England Journal of Medicine* and the *Journal of American Medical Association*. Dr. Elmore has served on national advisory committees for the Institute of Medicine/National Academy of Medicine, NIH, American Cancer Society, and the Robert Wood Johnson Foundation. Dr. Elmore received her medical degree from the Stanford University School of Medicine and completed residency training in internal medicine at Yale–New Haven Hospital, with advanced training in epidemiology from the Yale School of Epidemiology and Public Health and the Robert Wood Johnson Clinical Scholars Program at Yale.

Dorothea M.G. Wild, MD, MPH is a Research Affiliate at the Institute of General Practice and Family Medicine at the University of Bonn (Germany) and a primary care physician. In addition, Dr. Wild is President of the Planetree Germany office, an advocacy organization for more person centeredness in health care. She has a special interest in provider-patient communication, patient-centered care, and innovative care delivery models. Dr. Wild received residency training in internal medicine and preventive medicine at Griffin Hospital, Derby, Connecticut. She also received a Master of Public Health in Health Care Management from Yale University School of Public Health. After graduation, she worked first as a hospitalist, then as chief hospitalist at the Griffin Faculty Practice Plan.

Heidi D. Nelson, MD, MPH, MACP, FRCP is Professor of Medical Informatics and Clinical Epidemiology and Medicine, and Director of Scholarly Projects, a required 4-year curriculum supporting medical student research, at the Oregon Health & Science University in Portland, Oregon. Dr. Nelson has research expertise in clinical epidemiology and population health, women's health, systematic review methodology, clinical guideline development, and evidence-based health care. Dr. Nelson has led over 50 systematic reviews and meta-analyses for the US Preventive Services Task Force, National Institutes of Health, Agency for Healthcare Research and Quality, among other partners. This research has been used to determine clinical practice guidelines, health policy, and coverage decisions affecting millions of Americans.

David L. Katz, MD, MPH, FACPM, FACP, FACLM is Founding Director (1998–2019) of Yale University's Yale-Griffin Prevention Research Center, Past President of the American College of Lifestyle Medicine, Founder/President of True Health Initiative, and Founder/CEO of Diet ID, Inc. Dr. Katz earned his BA degree from Dartmouth College (1984), his MD from the Albert Einstein College of Medicine (1988), and his MPH from the Yale University School of Public Health (1993). The recipient of many awards for his contributions to public health, Dr. Katz has received three honorary doctorates.

ACKNOWLEDGMENTS

I acknowledge the important influence students have had in shaping our text and the meticulous and valuable editorial assistance that Raul Moreno and Annie Lee, PhD provided on this fifth edition. I also personally thank my son, Nicholas (Cole) R. Ransom, for his support and patience during the preparation of each new edition of this text. —**JE**

I gratefully acknowledge my chapter coauthors for their helpful comments and the influence of all the patients, families, and learners with whom I have interacted. Lastly, I thank my family for their never-ending patience and support. —**DW**

I gratefully acknowledge the contributions of previous and current authors of this remarkable textbook and feel honored to join their ranks with the fifth edition. Dr. Elmore has skillfully led us to an updated edition that builds on the past yet speaks to the future. I thank Martiniano J. Flores, PhD; Rochelle Fu, PhD; Amber Lin, MS; and David Yanez, MS, PhD for their advice and edits on the revised statistics chapters. Hopefully these updated chapters help readers understand how statistics link data to discovery. —**HN**

Casey Covarrubias, MPH
Program Administrator
National Clinician Scholars Program
    at UCLA
Los Angeles, California

**Linda C. Degutis, DrPH, MSN,
FRSPH (Hon.)**
Executive Director, *Defense Health
    Horizons*
Uniformed Services University of the
    Health Sciences
Bethesda, MD

Martiniano J. Flores, PhD
Biostatistician, Edwards Lifesciences
Irvine, California

Elizabeth C. Katz, PhD
Associate Professor
Department of Psychology
Towson University
Towson, Maryland

**Thiruvengadam Muniraj, MD,
PhD, MRCP(UK)**
Assistant Professor of Medicine
Yale University
New Haven, Connecticut

Haq Nawaz, MD, MPH
Internist
Griffin Hospital
Derby, Connecticut

Mark B. Russi, MD, MPH
Professor of Medicine (Occupational
    Medicine) and of Epidemiology
    (Environmental Health)
Director, Occupational Health Services,
    Yale-New Haven Hospital
New Haven, Connecticut

Patricia E. Wetherill, MD
Clinical Assistant Professor of Medicine
New York Medical College
Valhalla, New York

PREFACE (TO THE 5TH EDITION)

We are very pleased and proud to bring you this fifth edition of what proved to be in earlier editions a best-selling title in its content area of epidemiology, biostatistics, preventive medicine, and public health. This text is unique in that medical, dental, nursing, preventive, and public health students can purchase just one book to learn about the four key areas covered on their national boards and enhance their knowledge on areas relevant to their future careers. Our goal is to provide a comprehensive overview of these four key topics without getting bogged down in unnecessary details.

This text grew out of courses we taught to Yale medical students more than 20 years ago. Dr. James Jekel had a unique ability to summarize and clarify complex topics in a fun and easy manner. Handouts from his classes were kept by many of us for years (yes, stapled together pieces of paper that were frequently referred to, with our own added yellow highlighting and comments in the margins). It was only after much encouragement that Dr. Jekel finally agreed to turn these handouts into the first edition of this text and set this whole enterprise in motion. We gratefully acknowledge Dr. Jekel's influence on the first three editions and are pleased to report that he is spending well-earned time in true retirement with his large extended family.

Many individuals have told us that our book is more "readable" and interesting than other books because of our writing style and the wide variety of real data examples. Some have also told us that they had always found topics such as statistics baffling and boring until they read our book. For this, we thank Dr. Jekel for setting the high standards for the text.

In the fourth edition we added new chapters as we unbundled the treatment of preventive medicine and public health into separate sections. The expansion of our text allowed the inclusion of important new topics that were formerly neglected: from the epidemiology of mental health disorders, to disaster planning, to health care reform, to the One Health concept that highlights the indelible links among the health of people, other species, and the planet itself.

While most of our text has stood the test of time, in this fifth edition we added a new chapter on injury prevention and an infusion of updated figures, tables, and citations. We also added clinical vignettes to highlight the relevance of the topic to individuals pursuing clinical careers. Our hope is that the book feels fresh and current to new and returning readers, yet comfortably familiar to those who have read our previous editions.

As with any book that aims to cover four such large topics, there are predictable challenges regarding inclusions and exclusions, depth versus breadth. Thus we did our best to balance brevity, clarity, and helping readers obtain an understanding of key concepts, without adding extensive pages of information and unnecessary detail.

In the fifth edition, we also added new coauthors, including Dr. Heidi D. Nelson, Professor of Medical Informatics, Clinical Epidemiology and Medicine at Oregon Health and Science University. Dr. Nelson has led many of the evidence reviews for the US Preventive Services Task Force over the years. Dr. Nelson's keen eye for clarity in writing has infused the textbook with a reorganized—and much better-flowing—biostatistics section. Other contributing authors are noted in the contents list and on the title page of their respective chapters. We are most grateful to this group of experts for bringing our readers an authoritative treatment of important topics we could not have addressed on our own.

We are also grateful for the many encouraging comments and suggestions that we receive from our students and colleagues, both in the United States and elsewhere. Our book is now used internationally, and previous editions have been translated into several other languages.

For this fifth edition, we were cognizant of mandatory "board testing" and the many fields where health professional students need help to prepare. We therefore reviewed and addressed the core content covered in the many national boards: the US Medical Licensing Exam (USMLE) Step I, Public Health and General Preventive Medicine, Preventive Medicine Core, American Board of General Dentistry, and the nursing National Council Licensure Examination (NCLEX).

In addition to helping health professional students pass their national board tests, we want students to look back after reading our book and realize that they learned practical concepts that will serve them well for the rest of their lives. There are many careers in health and health care with unique challenges and approaches. In clinical practice we need to pay attention to the social determinants of health and also the interconnections of our global environment. As we review medical evidence we notice that assumptions are often not perfectly satisfied, statistical models are not exactly correct, distributions are not normally distributed, and there is an important difference between clinical significance and statistical significance. As we strive to integrate our clinical and scientific knowledge to improve health and health care, we also need to take into consideration all of the political, social, financial, and cultural factors.

The provision of health care and public health is an art as well as a science, and it is our goal to inspire a learning environment that is filled with the realistic applications that students find inviting and rewarding. We hope that instructors and students will experience a fulfilling introduction to these key topics in our fifth edition.

Joann G. Elmore, MD, MPH
For the authors

CONTENTS

ix

SECTION 1

Epidemiology

Basic Epidemiologic Concepts and Principles

"Medicine is a science of uncertainty and an art of probability."

William Osler, MD

1. WHAT IS EPIDEMIOLOGY?

Epidemiology is usually defined as the study of factors that determine the occurrence and distribution of disease in a population. As a scientific term, epidemiology was introduced in the 19th century, derived from three Greek roots: *epi,* meaning "upon"; *demos,* "people" or "population"; and *logos,* "discussion" or "study." Epidemiology deals with much more than the study of **epidemics,** in which a disease spreads quickly or extensively, leading to more cases than normally seen.

Epidemiology can best be understood as the basic science of public health and the practice of clinical medicine. The field of epidemiology provides methods to study disease, injury, and clinical practice. Whereas health care practitioners typically manage data concerning a single patient, **epidemiologists** deal with data from groups of patients or even entire populations. The scientific methods used to collect such data are described in the Epidemiology section of this text (Chapters 1–7), and the methods used to analyze the data are reviewed in the Biostatistics section (Chapters 8–13). Use of the data to guide clinical preventive health measures is then described (Chapters 14–23), followed by use of the epidemiologic data within the field of public health (Chapters 24–30).

The scientific study of disease can be approached at the following four levels:
1. Submolecular or molecular level (e.g., cell biology, genetics, biochemistry, and immunology)
2. Tissue or organ level (e.g., anatomic pathology)
3. Level of individual patients (e.g., clinical medicine)
4. Level of populations (e.g., epidemiology)

Perspectives gained from these four levels are related, thus the scientific understanding of disease can be maximized by coordinating research among the various levels and disciplines.

Some people distinguish between classical and clinical epidemiology. **Classical epidemiology** studies the distribution and determinants of disease in populations and the community origins of health problems, particularly those related to infectious agents; nutrition; the environment; human behavior; and the psychologic, social, economic, and spiritual state of a population. Classical epidemiologists are interested in discovering risk factors that might be altered in a population to prevent or delay disease, injury, and death.

Many illustrations from classical epidemiology concern infectious diseases, because these were the original impetus for the development of epidemiology and have often been its focus. Classical methods of surveillance and outbreak investigation remain relevant given the changing landscape of infections (e.g., resistant tuberculosis [TB], Ebola) and are relevant for such contemporary concerns as bioterrorism, with methods undergoing modification as they are marshaled against new challenges. One example of such an adapted approach is syndromic epidemiology, in which epidemiologists look for patterns of signs and symptoms that might indicate an origin in bioterrorism.

Clinical epidemiology is the application of principles of epidemiology to clinical medicine. Investigators involved in clinical epidemiology often use research designs and statistical tools similar to those used by classical epidemiologists. However, clinical epidemiologists often study patients in health care settings rather than in the community at large. Their goal is to improve the prevention, early detection, diagnosis, treatment, prognosis, and care of illness in individual patients who are at risk for, or already affected by, specific diseases.[1]

Epidemiology can also be divided into *infectious disease epidemiology* and *chronic disease epidemiology*. Historically, the first has depended more heavily on laboratory support (especially microbiology and serology), whereas the second has depended on complex sampling and statistical methods. However, this distinction is becoming less significant with the increasing use of molecular laboratory markers (genetic and other) in chronic disease epidemiology and complex statistical analyses in infectious disease epidemiology. Many illnesses, including TB and acquired immunodeficiency syndrome (AIDS), may be regarded as both infectious and chronic.

The name of a given medical discipline indicates both a method of research into health and disease and the body of knowledge acquired by using that method. For example, pathology is a field of medical research with its own goals and methods, but investigators and clinicians also speak of "the pathology of lung cancer." Similarly, epidemiology refers to a field of research that uses particular methods, but it can also be used to denote the resulting body of knowledge about the distribution and natural history of diseases—that is, the nutritional, behavioral, environmental, and genetic sources of disease as identified through epidemiologic studies.

2. ETIOLOGY AND NATURAL HISTORY OF DISEASE

Etiology is the cause or origin of a disease or abnormal condition. The way a disease progresses in the absence of medical or public health intervention is often called the **natural history** of the disease. Public health and medical personnel take advantage of available knowledge about the stages of disease, mechanisms and causes of disease, and risk factors to determine how and when to intervene. The goal of intervention, whether preventive or therapeutic, is to alter the natural history of a disease in a favorable way.

2.1 STAGES OF DISEASE

The development and expression of a disease occur over time and can be divided into three stages: predisease, latent, and symptomatic. During the **predisease** stage, before the disease process begins, early intervention may avert exposure to the agent of disease (e.g., lead, *trans*-fatty acids, microbes), preventing the disease process from starting; this is called **primary prevention**. During the **latent stage**, when the disease process has already begun but is still asymptomatic, screening for the disease and providing appropriate treatment may prevent progression to symptomatic disease; this is called **secondary prevention**. During the symptomatic stage, when disease manifestations are evident, intervention may slow, arrest, or reverse the progression of disease; this is called **tertiary prevention**. These concepts are discussed in more detail in Chapters 15 to 17.

2.2 MECHANISMS AND CAUSES OF DISEASE

When discussing the etiology of disease, epidemiologists distinguish between the biologic mechanisms and the social, behavioral, and environmental causes of disease. We often need to understand the causes of a disease. For example, osteomalacia is a bone disease (i.e., a weakening of the bone, often through a vitamin D deficiency) that may have both social and biologic causes. In the traditional and customary observance of purdah, women who have reached puberty avoid public display by spending most of their time indoors or by wearing clothing that covers virtually all of the body when they go outdoors. Because these practices block the action of the sun on bare skin, they prevent the irradiation of ergosterol in the skin. However, irradiated ergosterol is an important source of D vitamins, which are necessary for bone growth. If a woman's diet is also deficient in vitamin D during the rapid growth period of puberty, she may develop osteomalacia as a result of insufficient calcium absorption. Thus osteomalacia can adversely affect future pregnancies by causing the pelvis to become distorted (more pear shaped), making the pelvic opening too small for a fetus to pass through. In this example, the social, nutritional, and environmental causes set in motion the biochemical and other biologic mechanisms of osteomalacia, which may ultimately lead to maternal and infant mortality.

Likewise, excessive fat intake, smoking, and lack of exercise are behavioral factors that contribute to the biologic mechanisms of atherogenesis (i.e., formation of plaque in the arteries), including elevated blood levels of low-density lipoprotein (LDL) cholesterol or reduced blood levels of high-density lipoprotein (HDL) cholesterol. These behavioral risk factors may have different effects, depending on the genetic pattern of each individual and the interaction of genes with the environment and other risk factors.

Epidemiologists attempt to discover the social and behavioral causes of disease, which offer clues to methods of prevention. Epidemiologic hypotheses frequently guide laboratory scientists as they seek to understand biologic mechanisms of disease, which may suggest methods of treatment.

2.3 HOST, AGENT, ENVIRONMENT, AND VECTOR

The causes of a disease are often considered in terms of a triad of factors: the host, the agent, and the environment.

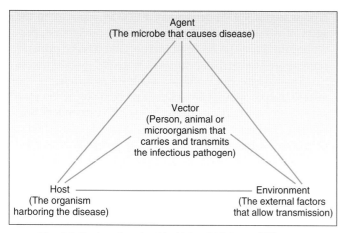

Fig. 1.1 Factors Involved in Natural History of Disease.

For many diseases, it is also useful to add a fourth factor, the vector (Fig. 1.1). In measles, the *host* is a human who is susceptible to measles infection; the *agent* is a highly infectious virus that can produce serious disease in humans; and the *environment* is a population of unvaccinated individuals, which enables unvaccinated susceptible individuals to be exposed to others who are infectious. The *vector* in this case is relatively unimportant. In malaria, however, the host, agent, and environment are all significant, but the vector, the *Anopheles* mosquito, assumes paramount importance in the spread of disease.

The **host** is the "who" of the triangle, the person or organism harboring the disease. Host factors are responsible for the degree to which the individual is able to adapt to the stressors produced by the agent. Host resistance is influenced by a person's genotype (e.g., dark skin reduces sunburn), nutritional status and body mass index (e.g., obesity increases susceptibility to many diseases), immune system (e.g., compromised immunity reduces resistance to cancer as well as microbial disease), and behavior (e.g., physical exercise enhances resistance to many diseases, including depression). Several factors can work synergistically, such as nutrition and immune status. Measles is seldom fatal in well-nourished children, even in the absence of measles immunization and modern medical care. By contrast, 25% of children with marasmus (starvation) or kwashiorkor (protein-calorie malnutrition related to weaning) may die from complications of measles.

The **agent** is the "what" of the triangle, whatever causes the disease. Agents of disease or illness can be divided into several categories. *Biologic agents* include allergens, infectious organisms (e.g., bacteria, viruses), biologic toxins (e.g., botulinum toxin), and foods (e.g., high-fat diet). *Chemical agents* include chemical toxins (e.g., lead) and dusts, which can cause acute or chronic illness. *Physical agents* include kinetic energy (e.g., involving bullet wounds, blunt trauma, and crash injuries), radiation, heat, cold, and noise. *Social and psychologic stressors* can also be considered agents in the development of health problems, including social disadvantage, abuse, and illiteracy, for example.

The "where" of the triangle is the **environment** and the external factors that cause or allow disease transmission. The environment influences the probability and circumstances of contact between the host and the agent. Poor restaurant sanitation increases the probability that patrons will be exposed to *Salmonella* infections. Bad roads and adverse weather conditions increase the number of automobile collisions. The environment also includes social, political, and economic factors. Crowded homes and schools make exposure to infectious diseases more likely, and the political structure and economic health of a society influence the nutritional and vaccine status of its members.

Vectors of disease are the "how" of the triangle and include insects (e.g., mosquitoes associated with spread of malaria), arachnids (e.g., ticks associated with Lyme disease), and mammals (e.g., raccoons associated with rabies in the eastern United States). The concept of the vector can be applied more widely, however, to include human groups (e.g., vendors of heroin, cocaine, and methamphetamine) and even inanimate objects that serve as vehicles to transmit disease (e.g., contaminated needles associated with hepatitis and AIDS). A vector may be considered part of the environment or it may be treated separately (see Fig. 1.1). To be an effective transmitter of disease, the vector must have a specific relationship to the agent, the environment, and the host.

In the case of human malaria, the vector is a mosquito of the genus *Anopheles,* the agent is a parasitic organism of the genus *Plasmodium,* the host is a human, and the environment includes standing water that enables the mosquito to breed and to come into contact with the host. Specifically, the plasmodium must complete part of its life cycle within the mosquito; the climate must be relatively warm and provide a wet environment in which the mosquito can breed; the mosquito must have the opportunity to bite humans (usually at night, in houses where sleeping people lack screens and mosquito nets) and thereby spread the disease; the host must be bitten by an infected mosquito; and the host must be susceptible to the disease.

2.4 RISK FACTORS AND PREVENTABLE CAUSES

Risk factors for disease and preventable causes of disease, particularly life-threatening diseases such as cancer, have been the subject of much epidemiologic research. In 1964 the US Surgeon General released a report indicating the risk of death from lung cancer in smokers was almost 11 times that in nonsmokers.[2] That same year a World Health Organization (WHO) expert committee estimated the majority of cancer cases were potentially preventable and were caused by "extrinsic factors." Advances in knowledge based on epidemiologic studies have consolidated the WHO findings to the point where few if any researchers now question its main conclusion.[3] Unfortunately, the phrase "extrinsic factors" (or its near-synonym, "environmental factors") has often been misinterpreted to mean only man-made chemicals, which was certainly not the intent of the WHO committee. In addition to man-made or naturally occurring carcinogens, the 1964 report included viral infections, nutritional deficiencies or excesses, reproductive activities, and a variety of other factors determined "wholly or partly by personal behavior."

The WHO conclusions are based on research using a variety of epidemiologic methods. Given the many different types of cancer cells and the large number of causal factors to be considered, how do epidemiologists estimate the percentage of deaths caused by preventable risk factors in a country such as the United States?

One method looks at each type of cancer and determines (from epidemiologic studies) the percentage of individuals in the country who have identifiable, preventable causes of that cancer. These percentages are added up in a weighted manner to determine the total percentage of all cancers having identifiable causes.

A second method examines annual age-specific and gender-specific cancer incidence rates in countries that maintain comparable effective infrastructure for disease detection and compares countries that have the lowest rates of a given type of cancer with countries that have the highest rates. For a particular cancer type, the low rate in a country presumably results, in part, from a low prevalence of the risk factors for that cancer. However, there are many other potential reasons that need to be considered in these analyses that we will describe in this text.

2.4.a. BEINGS Model

The acronym **BEINGS** can serve as a mnemonic device for the major categories of risk factors for disease, some of which are easier to change or eliminate than others (Box 1.1). Currently, genetic factors are among the most difficult to change, although this field is rapidly developing and becoming more important to epidemiology and prevention. Immunologic factors are usually the easiest to change, if effective vaccines are available.

"B"—Biologic and behavioral factors. The risk for particular diseases may be influenced by gender, age, weight, bone density, and other biologic factors. In addition, human behavior is a central factor in health and disease. Cigarette smoking, an obvious example of a behavioral risk factor, contributes to a variety of health problems, including myocardial infarction (MI); lung, esophageal, and nasopharyngeal cancer; and chronic obstructive pulmonary disease.

Much attention focuses on the rapid increase in the prevalence rates of overweight and obesity in the US population. Increasing rates of obesity are found worldwide as part of

a cultural transition related to the increased availability of calorie-dense foods and a simultaneous decline in physical activity, resulting in part from mechanized transportation and sedentary lifestyles.[4–9]

Obesity and overweight have negative health effects, particularly by reducing the age at onset of and increasing the prevalence of type 2 diabetes. Obesity is established as a major contributor to premature death in the United States,[10,11] although the exact magnitude of the association remains controversial, resulting in part from the complexities of the causal pathway involved (i.e., obesity leads to death indirectly, by contributing to the development of chronic disease).

Multiple behavioral factors are associated with the spread of some diseases. In the case of AIDS, the spread of human immunodeficiency virus (HIV) can result from unprotected sexual intercourse between men and from shared syringes among intravenous drug users, which are the two predominant routes of transmission in the United States. HIV infection can also result from unprotected vaginal intercourse, which is the predominant transmission route in Africa and other parts of the world. Other behaviors that can lead to disease, injury, or premature death (before age 65) are excessive intake of alcohol, abuse of both legal and illegal drugs, driving while intoxicated, and homicide and suicide attempts. In each of these cases, as in cigarette smoking and HIV infection, changes in behavior could prevent the untoward outcomes. Many efforts in health promotion depend heavily on modifying human behavior, as discussed in Chapter 15.

"E"—Environmental factors. Epidemiologists are frequently the first professionals to respond to an apparent outbreak of new health problems, such as legionnaires' disease and Lyme disease, which involve important environmental factors. In their investigations, epidemiologists describe the patterns of the disease in the affected population, develop and test hypotheses about causal factors, and introduce methods to prevent further cases of disease. Chapter 3 describes the standard approach to investigating an epidemic.

During an outbreak of severe pneumonia among individuals attending a 1976 American Legion conference in Philadelphia, Pennsylvania, epidemiologists conducted studies suggesting the epidemic was caused by an infectious agent distributed through the air-conditioning and ventilation systems of the primary conference hotels. Only later, after the identification of *Legionella pneumophila*, was it discovered that this small bacterium thrives in air-conditioning cooling towers and warm-water systems. It was also shown that respiratory therapy equipment that is merely rinsed with water can become a reservoir for *Legionella*, causing hospital-acquired legionnaires' disease.

An illness first reported in 1975 in Old Lyme, Connecticut, was the subject of epidemiologic research suggesting that the arthritis, rash, and other symptoms of the illness were caused by infection with an organism transmitted by a tick. This was enough information to initiate preventive measures. By 1977 it was clear that the disease, then known as Lyme disease, was spread by *Ixodes* ticks, opening the way for more specific

---

BOX 1.1   Beings Acronym for Categories of Preventable Cause of Disease

Biologic factors and **B**ehavioral factors
Environmental factors
Immunologic factors
Nutritional factors
Genetic factors
Services, **S**ocial factors, and **S**piritual factors

prevention and research. Not until 1982, however, was the causative agent, *Borrelia burgdorferi*, discovered.

"I"—Immunologic factors. Smallpox is the first infectious disease known to have been eradicated from the globe (although samples of the causative virus remain stored in US and Russian laboratories). Smallpox eradication was possible because vaccination against the disease conferred individual immunity and produced herd immunity. **Herd immunity** results when disease transmission is effectively reduced by immunizing enough individuals so that the disease does not spread in a population.

Immunodeficiency is a term that describes inadequate immune function that predisposes an individual to infections and other illnesses. Immunodeficiency may result from several causes, including genetic abnormalities, AIDS, and other factors. Transient immune deficiency has been noted after some infections (e.g., measles) and after the administration of certain vaccines (e.g., live measles vaccine). This result is potentially serious in malnourished children. The use of cancer chemotherapy and the long-term use of corticosteroids also produce immunodeficiency, which may often be severe.

"N"—Nutritional factors. In the 1950s it was shown that Japanese Americans living in Hawaii had a much higher rate of MI than people of the same age and gender in Japan, while Japanese Americans in California had a still higher rate of MI than similar individuals in Japan.[12–14] The investigators believed that dietary variations were the most important factors producing these differences in disease rates, as generally supported by subsequent research. The traditional Japanese diet, including more fish, vegetables, and fruit in smaller portions than the usual American diet, is healthier for the heart.

"G"—Genetic factors. It is well established that the genetic inheritance of individuals interacts with diet and environment in complex ways to promote or protect against a variety of illnesses, including heart disease and cancer. As a result, genetic epidemiology is a growing field of research that addresses, among other things, the distribution of normal and abnormal genes in a population, and whether these are in equilibrium. Considerable research examines the possible interaction of various genotypes with environmental, nutritional, and behavioral factors, as well as with pharmaceutic treatments. Ongoing research concerns the extent to which environmental adaptations can reduce the burden of diseases with a heavy genetic component.

Genetic disease now accounts for a higher proportion of illness than in the past, not because the incidence of genetic disease is increasing, but because the incidence of noninherited disease is decreasing and our ability to identify genetic diseases has improved.

Genetic screening is important for identifying problems in newborns, such as phenylketonuria and congenital hypothyroidism, for which therapy can be extremely beneficial if instituted early enough. Screening is also important for identifying other genetic disorders for which counseling can be beneficial. In the future, the most important health benefits from genetics may come from identifying individuals who are at high risk for specific problems, or who would respond particularly well (or poorly) to specific drugs. Examples might include individuals at high risk for MI; breast or ovarian cancer (e.g., carriers of *BRCA1* and *BRCA2* genetic mutations); environmental asthma; or reactions to certain foods, medicines, or behaviors. Screening for susceptibility genes undoubtedly will increase in the future, but there are concerns about potential problems, such as medical insurance carriers hesitating to insure individuals with known genetic risks, the challenges of communicating results to patients, and the lack of understanding about estimates of the risk itself.

"S"—Services, social factors, and spiritual factors. Medical care services may be beneficial to health but also can be dangerous. One of the important tasks of epidemiologists is to determine the benefits and hazards of medical care in different settings. **Iatrogenic disease** occurs when a disease is induced inadvertently by treatment or during a diagnostic procedure. A US Institute of Medicine report estimated that 2.9% to 3.7% of hospitalized patients experience "adverse events" during their hospitalization. Of these events, about 19% are caused by medication errors and 14% by wound infections.[15] This report estimated that about 44,000 deaths each year are associated with medical errors in hospitals. Other medical care–related causes of illness include unnecessary or inappropriate diagnostic or surgical procedures. For example, more than 50% of healthy women who undergo annual screening mammography over a 10-year period will have at least one mammogram interpreted as suspicious for breast cancer and will therefore be advised to undergo additional testing, even though they do not have cancer.[16]

The effects of social and spiritual factors on disease and health have been less intensively studied than have other causal factors. Evidence is accumulating, however, that personal beliefs concerning the meaning and purpose of life, perspectives on access to forgiveness, and support received from members of a social network are powerful influences on health. Studies have shown that experimental animals and humans are better able to resist noxious stressors when they are receiving social support from other members of the same species. Social support may be achieved through the family, friendship networks, and membership in various groups, such as clubs and churches. One study reviewed the literature concerning the association of religious faith with generally better health and found that strong religious faith was associated with better health and quality of life.[17]

Many investigators have explored factors related to health and disease in populations with similar behaviors. For example, Mormons and Seventh-Day Adventists are religious groups who have lower-than-average age-adjusted death rates from many common types of disease and specifically from heart disease, cancer, and respiratory disorders. This protection may be the result of their abstinence from alcohol and tobacco, although it is unclear that these behaviors are solely responsible for the health differences. As one study noted, "It is difficult . . . to separate the effects of health practices from other aspects of lifestyle common among those belonging to such religions, for example, differing social stresses and network systems."[18]

3. ECOLOGIC ISSUES IN EPIDEMIOLOGY

Classical epidemiologists have long regarded their field as "human ecology," "medical ecology," or "geographic medicine," because an important characteristic of epidemiology is its **ecologic perspective**.[19] People are seen not only as individual organisms, but also as members of communities, in a social context. The world is understood as a complex ecosystem in which disease patterns vary greatly from one country or region to another. The types and rates of diseases in an area are a form of "fingerprint" that indicates the standard of living, the lifestyle, the predominant occupations, and the climate, among other factors. Because of the tremendous growth in world population, now more than 7.6 billion, and rapid technologic developments, humans have had a profound impact on the global environment, often with deleterious effects. The existence of wide biodiversity, which helps to provide the planet with greater adaptive capacity, has become increasingly threatened. Every action that affects the ecosystem, even an action intended to promote human health and well-being, produces a reaction in the system, and the result is often not positive. (See http://www.cdc.gov and https://www.census.gov/popclock/.)

3.1 SOLUTION OF PUBLIC HEALTH PROBLEMS AND UNINTENDED CREATION OF NEW PROBLEMS

One of the most important insights of ecologic thinking is that as people change one part of a system, they inevitably change other parts. An epidemiologist is constantly alert for possible negative side effects that a medical or health intervention might produce. In the United States, the reduced mortality in infancy and childhood has increased the prevalence of chronic degenerative diseases because now most people experience the effects of aging. Table 1.1 summarizes some of the health and societal problems introduced by the solution of earlier health problems.

3.1.a. Vaccination and Patterns of Immunity

Understanding **herd immunity** is essential to any discussion of current ecologic problems in immunization. A vaccine provides herd immunity if it not only protects the immunized individual, but also prevents that person from transmitting the disease to others. This causes the prevalence of the disease organism in the population to decline. Herd immunity is illustrated in Fig. 1.2, where it is assumed that each infected person comes into sufficient contact with two other persons to expose both of them to the disease if they are susceptible. Under this assumption, if there is no herd immunity against the disease and everyone is susceptible, the number of cases doubles every disease generation (see Fig. 1.2A). However, if there is 50% herd immunity against the disease, the

TABLE 1.1 Examples of Unintended Consequences from Solution of Earlier Health Problems		
Initial Health Problem	**Solution**	**Unintended Consequences**
Childhood infections	Vaccination	Decrease in the level of immunity during adulthood, caused by a lack of repeated exposure to infection
High infant mortality rate	Improved sanitation	Increase in the population growth rate; appearance of epidemic paralytic poliomyelitis
Sleeping sickness in cattle	Control of tsetse fly (the disease vector)	Increase in the area of land subject to overgrazing and drought, caused by an increase in the cattle population
Malnutrition and need for larger areas of tillable land	Erection of large river dams (e.g., Aswan High Dam, Senegal River dams)	Increase in rates of some infectious diseases, caused by water system changes that favor the vectors of disease

number of cases is small and remains approximately constant (see Fig. 1.2B). In this model, if there is greater than 50% herd immunity, as would be true in a well-immunized population, the infection should die out eventually. The degree of immunity necessary to eliminate a disease from a population varies depending on the type of infectious organism, the time of year, and the density and social patterns of the population.

Immunization may seem simple: immunize every person in childhood and there will be no problems from the targeted diseases. Although there is some truth to this, in reality the control of diseases by immunization is more complex. The examples of diphtheria, smallpox, and poliomyelitis and human papillomavirus (HPV) are used here to illustrate issues concerning vaccination programs and population immunity, and syphilis is used to illustrate natural herd immunity to infection.

Diphtheria. Vaccine-produced immunity in humans tends to decrease over time. This phenomenon has a different impact at present, when infectious diseases such as diphtheria are less common, than it did in the past. When diphtheria was a more common disease, people who had been vaccinated against it were exposed more frequently to the causative agent, and this exposure could result in a mild reinfection. The reinfection would produce a **natural booster effect** and maintain a high level of immunity. As diphtheria became less common because of immunization programs, fewer people were exposed, resulting in fewer subclinical booster infections.

In Russia, despite the wide availability and use of diphtheria vaccine, many adults were found to be susceptible to *Corynebacterium diphtheria* during an epidemic in the early

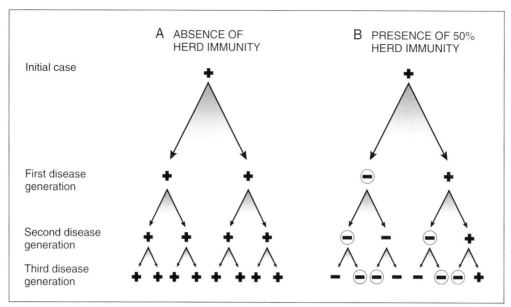

Fig. 1.2 Effect of Herd Immunity on Spread of Infection. Diagrams illustrate how an infectious disease such as measles could spread in a susceptible population if each infected person were exposed to two other persons. (A) In the absence of herd immunity, the number of cases doubles each disease generation. (B) In the presence of 50% herd immunity, the number of cases remains constant. The *plus sign* represents an infected person; the *minus sign* represents an uninfected person; the *circled minus sign* represents an immune person who will not pass the infection to others. The *arrows* represent significant exposure with transmission of infection (if the first person is infectious) or equivalent close contact without transmission of infection (if the first person is not infectious).

1990s. The majority of the reported cases were found among individuals older than 14 years. This was not caused by lack of initial immunization, because more than 90% of Russian adults had been fully immunized against diphtheria when they were children. The disease in older people was apparently caused by a decline in adult immunity levels. Before the epidemic was brought under control, it produced more than 125,000 cases of diphtheria and caused 4000 deaths.[20] An additional single vaccination is now recommended for adults to provide the booster effect.

Smallpox. The worldwide eradication of smallpox was accomplished by effective immunization. Early attempts at preventing smallpox included actions, reportedly by a Buddhist nun, who would grind scabs from patients with the mild form and blow them into the nose of nonimmune individuals; this was called variolation. The term vaccination comes from *vaca,* or "cow," a term related to observations that milkmaids developed the less severe form of smallpox transmitted from cows.

Attempts at eradication included some potential risks. The dominant form of smallpox in the 1970s was variola minor (alastrim). This was a relatively mild form of smallpox that, although often disfiguring, had a low mortality rate. However, alastrim provided individual and herd immunity against the much more disfiguring and often fatal variola major form of the disease (classic smallpox). To eliminate alastrim while increasing rates of variola major would have been a poor exchange. Fortunately the smallpox

vaccine was effective against both forms of smallpox, and the immunization program was successful in eradicating both variola minor and variola major.

Poliomyelitis. The need for herd immunity was also shown by poliomyelitis. Polio was officially eradicated in 36 Western Pacific countries in 2000 and Europe was declared polio free in 2002. Polio remains endemic in only three countries (Afghanistan, Pakistan, and Nigeria) at the time of writing this text, and the number of reported cases has been reduced from hundreds of thousands to less than 50 each year.

Human papillomavirus (HPV). The HPV vaccination protects against infection with human papillomaviruses. There are many different types of HPV, with several types thought to cause genital warts and cancer (e.g., cervical, anal, oropharyngeal, penile). Each year in the United States it is estimated that HPV causes 32,500 cancers in men and women, and HPV vaccination is thought to be able to prevent most of these cancers from developing.[21,22]

Syphilis. Syphilis is caused by infection with bacteria known as spirochetes and progresses in several stages. In the primary stage, syphilis produces a highly infectious skin lesion known as a chancre, which is filled with spirochete organisms. This lesion subsides spontaneously. In the secondary stage, a rash or other lesions may appear; these also subside spontaneously. A latent period follows, after which a tertiary stage may occur. Untreated infection typically results in immunity to future infection by the disease agent, but this immunity is not absolute. It does not protect individuals from progressive damage to their own body. It does provide some herd immunity, however, by making the infected individual unlikely to develop a new infection if reexposed to syphilis.[23] Ironically, when penicillin came into general use, syphilis infections were killed so quickly that chancre immunity did not develop, and high-risk individuals continued to repeatedly reacquire and spread the disease.

3.1.b. Effects of Sanitation

In the 19th century, diarrheal diseases were the primary killer of children and a leading cause of adult mortality. The sanitary revolution, which began in England about the middle of the century, was the most important factor in reducing infant mortality. Interestingly, the reduction of infant mortality contributed in a major way to increasing the effective birth rate and the overall rate of population growth. The sanitary revolution was therefore one of the causes of today's worldwide population problem.

Care must be taken, however, to avoid oversimplifying the factors that produce population growth. On the one hand, a reduction in infant mortality temporarily helps to produce a significant difference between the birth and death rates in a population, resulting in rapid population growth—the **demographic gap**. On the other hand, the control of infant mortality seems to be necessary before specific populations are willing to accept population control. When the infant mortality rate is high, a family may want to have a large number of children to have reasonable confidence that one or two will survive to adulthood.

In addition to affecting population growth, the sanitary revolution of the 19th century affected disease patterns in unanticipated ways. In fact, improvements in sanitation were a fundamental cause of the appearance of epidemic paralytic poliomyelitis late in the 19th century. This may seem counterintuitive, but it illustrates the importance of an ecologic perspective and offers an example of the so-called iceberg phenomenon, discussed later. The three polioviruses are enteric viruses transmitted by the fecal-oral route. People who have developed antibodies to all three types of poliovirus are immune to their potentially paralytic effects and show no symptoms or signs of clinical disease if exposed. Newborns receive passive antibodies from their mothers, and these maternal antibodies normally prevent polioviruses from invading the central nervous system in an infant's first year of life. As a result, exposure of a young infant to polioviruses rarely leads to paralytic disease, but instead produces a subclinical (largely asymptomatic) infection, which causes infants to produce their own active antibodies and cell-mediated immunity.

Although improved sanitation reduced the proportion of people who were infected with polioviruses, it also delayed the time when most infants and children were exposed to the polioviruses. Most were exposed after they were no longer protected by maternal immunity, with the result that a higher percentage developed the paralytic form of the disease. Epidemic paralytic poliomyelitis can therefore be seen as an unwanted side effect of the sanitary revolution. Further, because members of the upper socioeconomic groups had the best sanitation, they were hit first and most severely, until the polio vaccine became available.

3.1.c. Vector Control and Land Use Patterns

Sub-Saharan Africa provides a disturbing example of how negative side effects from vectors of disease can result from positive intentions of land use. A successful effort was made to control the tsetse fly, which is the vector of African sleeping sickness in cattle and sometimes in humans. Control of the vector enabled herders to keep larger numbers of cattle, and this led to overgrazing. Overgrazed areas were subject to frequent droughts, and some became dust bowls with little vegetation.[24] The results were often famine and starvation for cattle and humans.

3.1.d. River Dam Construction and Patterns of Disease

For a time, it was common to build large river dams in developing countries to produce electricity and increase the amount of available farmland by irrigation. During this period, the warnings of epidemiologists about potential negative effects of such dams went unheeded. The Aswan High Dam in Egypt provides a case in point. Directly after the dam was erected, the incidence of schistosomiasis increased in the areas supplied by the dam, just as epidemiologists predicted. Similar results followed the construction of the main dam and tributary dams for the Senegal River Project in West Africa. Before the dams were erected, the sea would move far inland during the dry season and mix with fresh river water, making the river water too salty to support the larvae of the blood flukes responsible for schistosomiasis or the mosquitoes that transmit malaria, Rift Valley fever, and dengue fever.[25] Once the dams were built, the incidence of these diseases increased until clean water, sanitation, and other health interventions were provided.

3.2 SYNERGISM OF FACTORS PREDISPOSING TO DISEASE

There may be a synergism between diseases or between factors predisposing to disease, such that each makes the other worse or more easily acquired. Sexually transmitted diseases, especially syphilis that produces open sores, facilitate the spread of HIV. In addition, the compromised immunity caused by AIDS permits the reactivation of previously latent infections, such as tuberculosis.

The relationship between malnutrition and infection is also synergistic. Not only does malnutrition make infections worse, but infections make malnutrition worse as well. A malnourished child has more difficulty producing antibodies and repairing tissue damage, which makes the child less resistant to infectious diseases and their complications. This scenario is observed in the case of measles. In isolated societies without medical care or measles vaccination, less than 1% of well-nourished children may die from measles or its complications, whereas 25% of malnourished children may die.

Infection can worsen malnutrition by imposing greater demands on the body, so the relative deficiency of nutrients becomes greater. Also, infection tends to reduce the appetite, so intake is reduced. In the presence of infection, the diet is frequently changed to emphasize bland foods, which often are deficient in proteins and vitamins. In patients with gastrointestinal infection, food rushes through the irritated bowel at a faster pace, causing diarrhea, and fewer nutrients are absorbed.

The combination of ecologic factors in a specific geographic region and genetic factors in a pathogen can interact to produce new strains of influenza virus. Many of the epidemic strains of influenza virus have names that refer to China (e.g., Hong Kong flu, Beijing flu) because of agricultural practices in these regions. In rural areas, domesticated pigs are in close contact with ducks and people. The duck and the human strains of influenza infect pigs, and the genetic material of the two influenza strains may mix in the pigs, producing a new variant of influenza. These new variants can then infect humans. If the genetic changes in the influenza virus are major, the result is called an **antigenic shift**, and the new virus may produce a **pandemic** (a widespread outbreak of influenza that could involve multiple continents). If the genetic changes in the influenza virus are minor, the phenomenon is called an **antigenic drift**, but this still can produce major regional outbreaks of influenza. The avian influenza (H5N1) virus from Southeast Asia differs greatly from human strains, and it has caused mortality in most people who contract the infection from birds. Should this strain of influenza acquire the capacity to spread from one human to another, the world is likely to see a **global pandemic** (worldwide epidemic).

The same principles apply to chronic diseases. Overeating and sedentary living interact so that each one worsens the impact of the other. As another example, the coexistence of cigarette smoking and pneumoconiosis (especially in coal workers) makes lung cancer more likely than a simple sum of the individual risks.

4. CONTRIBUTIONS OF EPIDEMIOLOGISTS

4.1 INVESTIGATING EPIDEMICS AND NEW DISEASES

Using the surveillance and investigative methods detailed in Chapter 3, epidemiologists have often provided the initial hypotheses about disease causation for other scientists to test in the laboratory. Epidemiologic methods have suggested the probable type of agent and modes of transmission for the diseases listed in Table 1.2 and others, usually within months of their recognition as new or emergent diseases. Knowledge of the modes of transmission led epidemiologists to suggest ways to prevent each of these diseases before the causative agents were determined or extensive laboratory results were available. Laboratory work to identify the causal agents, clarify the pathogenesis, and develop vaccines or treatments for most of these diseases continues many years after this basic epidemiologic work was done.

Concern about the many, more recently discovered and resurgent diseases[26] is currently at a peak, both because of a variety of newly emerging disease problems and because of the threat of bioterrorism.[27] The rapid growth in world population, increased travel and contact with new ecosystems (e.g., rain forests), declining effectiveness of antibiotics and

TABLE 1.2 Example of Early Hypotheses by Epidemiologists on Natural History and Prevention Methods for Diseases

Disease	Date of Appearance	EPIDEMIOLOGIC HYPOTHESES	
		Agent and Route of Spread	Methods of Prevention
Lyme disease	1975	Infectious agent, spread by ticks	Avoid ticks
Legionnaires' disease	1976	Small infectious agent, spread via air-conditioning systems	Treat water in air-conditioning systems
Toxic shock syndrome	1980	Staphylococcal toxin, associated with use of tampons (especially Rely brand)	Avoid using long-lasting tampons
Acquired immunodeficiency syndrome (AIDS)	1981	Viral agent, spread via sexual activity, especially male homosexual activity, and via sharing of needles and exchange of blood and blood products during intravenous drug use and transfusions	Use condoms Avoid sharing needles Institute programs to exchange needles and screen blood
Eosinophilia-myalgia syndrome	1989	Toxic contaminant, possibly associated with use of dietary supplements of L-tryptophan	Change methods of product manufacturing
Hantavirus pulmonary syndrome	1993	Hantavirus, spread via contact with contaminated droppings of deer mice	Avoid contact with excreta of deer mice
New-variant Creutzfeldt-Jakob disease	1996	Prions, spread via ingestion of beef infected with bovine spongiform encephalopathy	Avoid eating infected beef Avoid feeding animal remains to cattle
Severe acute respiratory syndrome (SARS)	2003	Animal coronavirus transferred to humans by handling and eating unusual food animals	Avoid handling, killing, and eating nonstandard food animals

insecticides, and many other factors encourage the development of new diseases or the resurgence of previous disorders. In addition, global climate change may extend the range of some diseases or help to create others.

4.2 STUDYING THE BIOLOGIC SPECTRUM OF DISEASE

The first identified cases of a new disease are often fatal or severe, leading observers to conclude that the disease is always severe. As more becomes known about the disease, however, less severe (and even asymptomatic) cases usually are discovered. With infectious diseases, asymptomatic infection may be uncovered either by finding elevated antibody titers to the organism in clinically well people or by culturing the organism from such people.

This variation in the severity of a disease process is known as the **biologic spectrum of disease**, or the *iceberg phenomenon*.[28] The latter term is appropriate because most of an iceberg remains unseen, below the surface, analogous to asymptomatic and mild cases of disease. An outbreak of diphtheria illustrates this point (Fig. 1.3).[29] The iceberg phenomenon is paramount to epidemiology, because studying only symptomatic individuals may produce a misleading picture of the disease pattern and severity.[30] The biologic spectrum also applies to viral disease.[31]

4.3 SURVEILLANCE OF COMMUNITY HEALTH INTERVENTIONS

Randomized trials of preventive measures in the field (i.e., **field trials**) are an important phase of evaluating a new

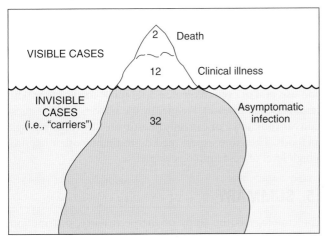

Fig. 1.3 Iceberg Phenomenon, as Illustrated by a Diphtheria Epidemic in Alabama. In epidemics, the number of people with severe forms of the disease (part of iceberg above water as shown here by 2 patients who died and 12 patients with symptoms of clinical illness) may be much smaller than the number of people with mild or asymptomatic clinical disease (part of iceberg below water as shown by the 32 "invisible" cases that would have remained invisible without extensive epidemiologic surveillance). (Data from Jekel JF, et al: *Corynebacterium diphtheriae* survives in a partly immunized group. *Public Health Rep* 85:310, 1970.)

vaccine before it is given to the community at large. Field trials, however, are only one phase in the evaluation of immunization programs. After a vaccine is introduced, ongoing surveillance of the disease and vaccine side effects is essential to ensure the vaccine's continued safety and effectiveness.

The importance of continued surveillance can be illustrated in the case of immunization against poliomyelitis. In 1954 large-scale field trials of the Salk inactivated polio vaccine were done, confirming the value and safety of the vaccine.[32] In 1955, however, the polio surveillance program of the Centers for Disease Control and Prevention (CDC) discovered an outbreak of vaccine-associated poliomyelitis, which was linked to vaccine from one specific laboratory.[33] Ultimately, 79 vaccinated individuals and 105 of their family members were found to have developed poliomyelitis. Apparently a slight change from the recommended procedure for producing the vaccine had allowed clumping of the poliovirus to occur, which shielded some of the virus particles in the center of the clumps so that they were not killed by formaldehyde during vaccine production. As a result, some people received a vaccine containing live virus. It was only through the vaccine surveillance program that the problem was detected quickly and the dangerous vaccine removed from use.

Routine smallpox vaccination among the entire American population stopped in 1972 after the eradication of the disease was announced. However, after the terrorist attacks on September 11, 2001, the United States developed a smallpox response plan in case of future bioterrorism events. Surveillance of the small number of persons vaccinated against smallpox since 2000 then revealed cases of vaccine-associated cardiomyopathy, and this outcome encouraged the CDC to curtail a large-scale vaccination program. As part of its response plan, the United States now has a stockpile of smallpox vaccines sufficient to vaccinate everyone at high risk in the country who would need it in the event of a smallpox emergency. Epidemiologists are thus contributing to national security by helping to establish new approaches to surveillance (i.e., **syndromic surveillance**) that identify not only changes in disease occurrence but also increases in potentially suspicious symptom patterns.

4.4 SETTING DISEASE CONTROL PRIORITIES

Disease control priorities should be based not only on the current size of the problem but also on the potential of a disease to spread to others; its likelihood of causing death and disability; and its cost to individuals, families, and the community. Disease control efforts are sometimes funded without considering these factors. In the 1950s a sharp drop in reported syphilis rates quickly led to declining support for syphilis control in the United States, which contributed to its subsequent rebound.[34] Sometimes health funding is influenced when powerful individuals or activists lobby for more money for research or control efforts for a particular disease or injury.

Although relatively few people in the United States were infected with HIV in the early 1980s, epidemiologists recognized that the potential threat to society posed by AIDS was far greater than the absolute numbers of infected individuals and associated costs suggested at that time. Accordingly, a much larger proportion of national resources was allocated to the study and control of AIDS than to efforts focused on other diseases affecting similar numbers of people. Special concerns with AIDS included the rapid increase in incidence over a very brief period, the high case fatality ratio during the initial outbreak and before therapy was developed and available, the substantial medical and social costs, the ready transmissibility of the disease, and known methods of prevention not being well applied.

In the 21st century a degree of control has been achieved over AIDS through antiretroviral drugs. However, new trends in other diseases have emerged. Most importantly, increased caloric intake and sedentary living have produced a rapid increase in overweight and obesity, leading to an increase in type 2 diabetes.

4.5 IMPROVING DIAGNOSIS, TREATMENT, AND PROGNOSIS OF CLINICAL DISEASE: SUPPORTING THE PRACTICE OF EVIDENCE-BASED MEDICINE

The application of epidemiologic methods to clinical questions helps us to improve clinical medicine, particularly in the diagnosis, therapy, and prognosis of disease. This is the domain of clinical epidemiology. The data gathered by epidemiologists can be used by clinicians to practice evidence-based medicine and guide the clinical care they provide.

Diagnosis is the process of identifying the nature and cause of a disease, illness, or problem through evaluation of the clinical history, review of symptoms, examination, or testing. Epidemiologic methods are used to improve disease diagnosis through selection of the best diagnostic tests, determination of the best cutoff points for such tests, and development of strategies to use in screening for disease. These issues are discussed in Chapters 7 and 13, as well as in the preventive medicine section of this book.

The methods of clinical epidemiology frequently are used to determine the most effective **treatment** in a given situation. Effectiveness is best studied using a randomized controlled trial comparing a treatment with a placebo, usual care, or another treatment.

Epidemiologic methods also help improve our understanding of a patient's **prognosis** (i.e., probable course and outcome of a disease).[35] Patients and families want to know the likely course of their illness, and investigators need accurate prognoses to stratify patients into groups with similar disease severity in research studies to evaluate treatments.

Epidemiologic methods permit **risk estimation**. These are perhaps best developed in various cardiac risk estimators using data from the Framingham Heart Study (see www.framinghamheartstudy.org) and in the Gail model for breast cancer risk (see http://www.cancer.gov).

4.6 IMPROVING HEALTH SERVICES RESEARCH

Health services research is a multidisciplinary scientific field that examines how people get access to health care and health care services, the costs of such services, and outcomes. The primary goals of health services research are to identify the most effective ways to manage, finance, and deliver high-quality care; to reduce medical errors; and to improve patient safety. Health services researchers use the same basic epidemiologic methods as covered in Chapters 1 to 7 and biostatistical methods as described in Chapters 8 to 13.

The principles and methods of epidemiology are used in planning and evaluating medical care and for quality improvement projects. In health planning, epidemiologic measures are employed to determine present and future community health needs. Demographic projection techniques can estimate the future size of different age groups. Analyses of patterns of disease frequency and use of services can estimate future service needs.[36] Additional epidemiologic methods can be used to determine the effects of medical care in health program evaluation as well as in the broader field of cost-benefit analysis (see Chapter 6).

4.7 PROVIDING EXPERT TESTIMONY IN COURTS OF LAW

Epidemiologists are often called on to testify regarding the state of knowledge about such topics as product hazards and the probable risks and effects of various environmental exposures, medications, or medical tests. The many types of lawsuits that may rely on epidemiologic data include those involving claims of damage from general environmental exposures (e.g., possible association of magnetic fields or cellular phone use and brain cancer), occupational illness claims (e.g., occupational lung damage from workplace asbestos), medical liability (e.g., adverse effects of vaccines or medications), and product liability (e.g., association of lung cancer with tobacco use, of toxic shock syndrome with tampon use, and of cyclooxygenase-1 inhibitor medications with cardiovascular disease). Frequently the answers to these questions are unknown or can only be estimated by epidemiologic methods. Therefore expert medical testimony often requires a high level of epidemiologic expertise.

5. SUMMARY

Epidemiology is the study of the occurrence, distribution, and determinants of diseases, injuries, and other health-related issues in specific populations. As such, it is concerned with all the biologic, social, behavioral, spiritual, economic, and psychologic factors that may increase the frequency of disease or offer opportunities for prevention. Epidemiologic methods are often the first scientific methods applied to a new health problem, to define its pattern in the population, and to develop hypotheses about its causes, methods of transmission, and prevention.

Epidemiologists generally describe the causes of a disease in terms of the host, agent, and environment, sometimes adding the vector as a fourth factor for consideration. In exploring the means to prevent a given disease, they look for possible behavioral, genetic, and immunologic causes in the host. They also look for biologic and nutritional causes, which are usually considered agents. Epidemiologists consider the physical, chemical, and social environment in which the disease occurs. Epidemiology is concerned with human ecology, particularly the impact of health interventions on disease patterns and on the environment. Knowing that the solution of one problem may create new problems, epidemiologists also evaluate possible unintended consequences of medical and public health interventions.

Contributions of epidemiologists to medical science include the following:

- Investigating epidemics and new diseases
- Studying the biologic spectrum of disease
- Instituting surveillance of community health interventions
- Suggesting disease control priorities
- Improving the diagnosis, treatment, and prognosis of clinical disease supporting the practice of evidence-based medicine
- Improving health services research
- Providing expert testimony in courts of law

REFERENCES

1. Haynes RB, Sackett DL, Guyatt GH, et al. *Clinical Epidemiology: How to Do Clinical Practice Research*. 3rd ed. Philadelphia, PA: Lippincott Williams & Wilkins; 2006.
2. US Surgeon General. *Smoking and Health*, Public Health Service Pub No 1103. Washington, DC: US Government Printing Office; 1964.
3. Doll R, Peto R. *The Causes of Cancer*. Oxford, UK: Oxford University Press; 1981.
4. Kimm SY, Glynn NW, Kriska AM, et al. Decline in physical activity in black girls and white girls during adolescence. *N Engl J Med*. 2002;347:709-715.
5. Swinburn BA, Sacks G, Hall KD, et al. The global obesity pandemic: shaped by global drivers and local environments. *Lancet*. 2011;378(9793):804-814.
6. Lakdawalla D, Philipson T. The growth of obesity and technological change. *Econ Hum Biol*. 2009;7:283-293.
7. Kumanyika SK. Global calorie counting: a fitting exercise for obese societies. *Annu Rev Public Health*. 2008;29:297-302.
8. Popkin BM. Global nutrition dynamics: the world is shifting rapidly toward a diet linked with noncommunicable diseases. *Am J Clin Nutr*. 2006;84:289-298.
9. Anderson PM, Butcher KE. Childhood obesity: trends and potential causes. *Future Child*. 2006;16:19-45.
10. Berenson GS, Bogalusa Heart Study Group. Health consequences of obesity. *Pediatr Blood Cancer*. 2012;58:117-121. doi: 10.1002/pbc.23373.
11. Mehta NK, Chang VW. Mortality attributable to obesity among middle-aged adults in the United States. *Demography*. 2009; 46:851-872.
12. Gordon T. Mortality experience among the Japanese in the United States, Hawaii, and Japan. *Public Health Rep*. 1957;72:543-553.
13. Keys A. The peripatetic nutritionist. *Nutr Today*. 1966;1(4): 19-24. Available at: https://journals.lww.com/nutritiontodayonline/Abstract/1966/12000/The_Peripatetic_Nutritionist.5.aspx#pdf-link.
14. Keys A. Coronary heart disease in seven countries. *Circulation*. 1970;41(suppl 1):I186-I195. Available at: https://doi.org/10.1016/S0899-9007(96)00410-8
15. Institute of Medicine. *To Err is Human*. Washington, DC: National Academies Press; 2000.
16. Elmore JG, Barton MB, Moceri VM, Polk S, Arena PJ, Fletcher SW. Ten-year risk of false positive screening mammograms and clinical breast examinations. *N Engl J Med*. 1998;338: 1089-1096.
17. Larson DB. *Scientific Research on Spirituality and Health: a Consensus Report*. Rockville, MD: National Institute for Healthcare Research; 1998.
18. Berkman LF, Breslow L. *Health and Ways of Living: the Alameda County Study*. New York, NY: Oxford University Press; 1983.
19. Kilbourne ED, Smillie WG. *Human Ecology and Public Health*. 4th ed. London, UK: Macmillan; 1969.
20. Centers for Disease Control and Prevention. Update: diphtheria epidemic—New Independent States of the Former Soviet Union, January 1995-March 1996. *MMWR*. 1996;45:693-697.
21. Centers for Disease Control and Prevention. HPV Vaccines: Vaccinating Your Preteen or Teen. Available at: https://www.cdc.gov/hpv/parents/vaccine.html. Updated August 23, 2018. Accessed June 6, 2019.
22. Center for Disease Control and Prevention. HPV and Cancer. Available at: https://www.cancer.gov/about-cancer/causes-prevention/risk/infectious-agents/hpv-fact-sheet. Updated May 28, 2019. Accessed June 6, 2019.
23. Jekel JF. Role of acquired immunity to T. pallidum in the control of syphilis. *Public Health Rep*. 1968;83:627-632.
24. Ormerod WE. Ecological effect of control of African trypanosomiasis. *Science*. 1976;191:815-821.
25. Jones, K. The silent scourge of development. *Yale Med*. 2005;39(3):18-23. Available at: https://medicine.yale.edu/news/yale-medicine-magazine/the-silent-scourge-of-development/
26. Jekel JF. Communicable disease control and public policy in the 1970s--hot war, cold war, or peaceful coexistence? *Am J Public Health*. 1972;62:1578-1585.
27. Institute of Medicine. Emerging Infections. Washington, DC: National Academic Press; 1992.
28. Morris JN. Uses of Epidemiology. Edinburgh and London: E&S Livingstone; 1957.
29. Jekel FJ, et al. Crynebacterium diptheriae survives in a partly immunized group. *Public Health Rep*. 1970;85(4):310-311. Available at: https://www.ncbi.nlm.nih.gov/pmc/articles/PMC2031618.
30. Evans AS. Subclinical Epidemiology. The first Harry A. Feldman Memorial lecture. *Am J Epidemiol*. 1987; 125:545-555.
31. Zerr DM, Meier AS, Selke SS, et al. A population based study of primary human herpesvirus 6 infection. *N Engl J Med*. 2005; 352:768-776.
32. Francis Jr T, Korns RF, Voight RB, et al. An evaluation of the 1954 poliomyelitis vaccine trials. *Am J Public Health Nations Health*. 1955;45(5 Pt2): 1-63.
33. Langmuir AD. The surveillance of communicable diseases of national importance. *N Engl J Med*. 1963; 268:182-192.
34. Berkman LF, Syme SL. Social networks, host resistance, and mortality: a nine-year follow-up study of Alameda County residents. *Am J Epidemiol*. 1979:109:186-204.

35. Horwitz RI, Cicchetti DV, Horwitz SM. A Comparison of the Norris and Killip coronary prognostic indices. *J Chronic Dis.* 1984;37:369-375.
36. Connecticut Hospital Association. Impact of an aging population on utilization and bed needs of Connecticut hospitals. *Conn Med.* 1978;42:775-781.

SELECT READINGS

Centers for Disease Control and Prevention. *Principles of Epidemiology.* 3rd ed. Washington, DC: Public Health Foundation; 2012.

Fletcher RH, Fletcher SW, Fletcher GS. *Clinical Epidemiology: the Essentials.* 5th ed. Philadelphia, PA: Wolters Kluwer; 2012.

Gordis L. *Epidemiology.* 5th ed. Philadelphia, PA: Saunders; 2013. [An excellent text.]

Institute of Medicine. *Emerging Infections.* Washington, DC: National Academies Press; 1992. [Medical ecology.]

Institute of Medicine. *To Err is Human.* Washington, DC: National Academies Press; 2000.

Kelsey JL, Whittemore AS, Evans AS, Thompson WD. *Methods in Observational Epidemiology.* 2nd ed. New York, NY: Oxford University Press; 1996. [Classical epidemiology.]

WEBSITES

Centers for Disease Control and Prevention: http://www.cdc.gov/
Global population: https://www.census.gov/popclock/
Morbidity and Mortality Weekly Report: http://www.cdc.gov/mmwr/

■ REVIEW QUESTIONS

1. Epidemiology is broadly defined as the study of factors that influence the health of populations. The application of epidemiologic findings to decisions in the care of individual patients is:
   A. Generally inappropriate
   B. Known as clinical epidemiology
   C. Limited to chronic disease epidemiology
   D. Limited to infectious disease epidemiology
   E. Limited to biologic mechanisms rather than social and environmental considerations

2. Tim has a severe heart attack at age 58. The near-death experience so scares Tim that he quits smoking. Tim's wife is also scared into quitting smoking even though she feels fine. Tim's son resolves never to start smoking, seeing what cigarettes have done to his dad. The act of not smoking for Tim, Tim's wife, and Tim's son represents:
   A. Host, vector, and agent effects, respectively
   B. Herd immunity
   C. Tertiary prevention for Tim's son
   D. Tertiary prevention, primary prevention, and secondary prevention, respectively
   E. Tertiary prevention, secondary prevention, and primary prevention, respectively

3. Before quitting smoking, Tim, his cigarettes, and his tobacco smoke represent:
   A. Agent, host, and environment, respectively
   B. Agent, environment, and vector, respectively
   C. Vector, agent, and vehicle, respectively
   D. Host, vehicle, and agent, respectively
   E. Vehicle, vector, and agent respectively

4. For an infectious disease to occur, there must be interaction between:
   A. Behavioral factors and genetic factors
   B. The agent and the vector
   C. The host and the agent
   D. The vector and the environment
   E. The vector and the host

5. An example of the iceberg phenomenon would be:
   A. The primary prevention of colon cancer
   B. Giving a medicine that only partially treats an illness
   C. Widely publicized fatalities caused by emerging swine flu
   D. Conducting field trials in northern latitudes
   E. When cold temperatures favor disease outbreaks

6. Which of the following is beyond the scope of activities undertaken by epidemiologists?
   A. Analyzing cost effectiveness
   B. Establishing modes of disease transmission
   C. Studying how to prevent disease
   D. Providing data for genetic counseling
   E. Rationing health care resources

7. Herd immunity refers to:
   A. Immunity acquired from vaccines developed in herd animals
   B. Immunity naturally acquired within confined herds of animals or within overcrowded human populations
   C. The high levels of antibody present in a population after an epidemic
   D. The prevention of disease transmission to susceptible individuals through acquired immunity in others
   E. The vaccination of domestic animals to prevent disease transmission to humans

8. Attempts to eradicate a disease through widespread immunization programs may be associated with potential adverse effects. Which of the following adverse effects is correlated with the effectiveness of a vaccine?
   A. The emergence of resistant strains of infectious agents to which the vaccine is targeted
   B. The loss of the natural booster effect
   C. The occurrence of infection in younger age groups
   D. The occurrence of allergic reactions
   E. The risk of disorders of the autism spectrum

9. Evaluation of which of the following potentially preventable causes of disease is most likely to raise ethical concerns?
   A. Dietary intake

B. Genetic susceptibility

C. Immunization status

D. Smoking status

E. Social support networks

10. While the pork industry lobbied aggressively against dubbing the novel H1N1 influenza virus "swine flu," substantial evidence supported that this wholly new genetic variant of influenza developed from confined animal feed operations associated with commercial pig farming. The novel H1N1 virus resulted from:

A. Antigenic shift

B. Antigenic drift

C. Antibody shift

D. Antibody drift

E. Antisocial rift

ANSWERS AND EXPLANATIONS

1. **B.** Clinical practice is devoted to the care of individual patients. Outcomes in individual patients in response to clinical interventions cannot be known, however, until after the interventions have been tried. The basis for choosing therapy (or for choosing diagnostic tests) is prior experience in similar patients, rather than knowledge of what would work best for the individual. The use of clinically applied statistics, probability, and population-based data to inform medical decisions is known as clinical epidemiology. Clinical epidemiology pertains to all clinical care. Its findings and applications are not limited to infectious diseases (D) or chronic diseases (C), or to biologic mechanisms (E). Social and environmental considerations are highly relevant to clinical decision making (E). Far from being inappropriate (A), the application of epidemiologic principles to patient care is fundamental to evidence-based practice and is supportive of robust clinical decisions.

2. **E.** Prevention means intervening to interrupt the natural history of disease. Primary prevention represents the earliest possible interventions to foil disease before it even begins (e.g., Tim's son never starting to smoke). Secondary prevention is thwarting the progression of established disease that has not yet declared itself with symptoms or outward signs (e.g., Tim's asymptomatic wife quitting smoking). Tertiary prevention is slowing, arresting, or even reversing obvious or symptomatic disease to prevent worsening symptoms and further deterioration (e.g., Tim quitting smoking after his heart attack). Answer choices C and D get distinctions between these stages of disease prevention wrong. Herd immunity (B) is the prevention of disease transmission to susceptible individuals through acquired immunity in others. Herd immunity does not apply to the scenario involving Tim and his family. Likewise, definitions for host (i.e., susceptible individual), vector (i.e., unaffected carrier), and

agent (i.e., medium of harm) (A) do not apply to the characterizations of Tim and his family.

3. **D.** A vehicle is an inanimate carrier of an agent of harm (e.g., the gun for a bullet, the syringe for heroin, the cigarette for tobacco smoke). Host, vector, and agent are defined in the explanation to question 2. Environment is the context and conditions in which the host, agent, and vehicle or vector interact. Given these explanations, answer choices A, B, C, and E miss the mark.

4. **C.** The minimum requirement for disease transmission to occur is the interaction of the agent and the host in an environment that enables them to come together. A vector of transmission (B, D, and E) may or may not be involved. Likewise, behavioral factors and genetic factors (A) may or may not be involved.

5. **C.** When a new disease (e.g., H1N1 swine flu) emerges, the first cases that are reported tend to be the most severe cases. Continued investigation reveals that these cases are merely the "tip of the iceberg." Many more cases that are generally less severe are hidden from view initially, just as the bulk of an iceberg lies below the water and is not seen initially. The primary prevention of colon cancer (A) may address only the "tip of the iceberg" for that disease; a medicine that treats only some of the symptoms of an illness (B) may address only the "tip of the iceberg" for that illness. However, such prevention and treatment describe different "iceberg" situations than that of the named epidemiologic phenomenon. Although cold temperatures (E) could favor certain disease outbreaks (e.g., by causing more people to spend more time indoors close to each other), such situations have little to do with the iceberg phenomenon. Conducting field trials in northern latitudes (D) could result in the sighting of icebergs, but such trials also have little to do with the iceberg phenomenon.

6. **E.** Although the responsibilities of epidemiologists may include analyzing cost effectiveness (A) and recommending allocation of health care resources, the rationing of these resources is a political task and falls outside the purview of epidemiologists. Establishing modes of disease transmission (B) and identifying means of preventing disease spread (C) are integral aspects of epidemiology. Genetic epidemiologists participate in genetic counseling (D).

7. **D.** Herd immunity not only prevents the immunized individuals in a population from contracting a disease, but it also prevents them from spreading the disease to nonimmunized individuals in the population. Herd immunity prevents disease transmission to susceptible individuals as a result of acquired immunity in others. The characteristics of a particular infection and a particular population determine the level of prevailing immunity required to limit the spread of a disease. The presence of a

highly infectious illness (e.g., measles) in a population with multiple exposures (e.g., college students) requires that nearly everyone be immunized to prevent transmission. Herd immunity does not refer to herd animals (A), herds of animals (B), or vaccinating animals to prevent disease transmission to humans (E). It likewise does not refer to overcrowded populations of humans (B) or the high levels of antibodies present in a population after an epidemic (C).

8. **B.** When an infectious disease is common, numerous individuals become infected and develop immunity to the causative agent. When their immunity begins to wane and they come into contact with infected individuals, they are reexposed to the causative agent. This environmental reexposure boosts their immune system so that their protective immunity is maintained. The phenomenon is called the natural booster effect. One of the potential adverse effects associated with a widespread immunization program is the loss of the natural booster effect. If a vaccine is highly efficacious, it markedly reduces the chances of exposure to the causative agent in the environment. If exposure does occur after the vaccine's effect in an individual has declined with time, the vaccinated individual is at risk for infection. This is why booster vaccines are given at specified intervals. Other potential adverse effects associated with widespread immunization, such as allergic reactions (D), are rare and idiosyncratic and are unlikely to be correlated with the effectiveness of the vaccine. Widespread vaccination tends to delay exposure to the wild-type pathogen and tends to shift the disease to older age groups, rather than younger ones (C). Similar to antibiotics, vaccines are ineffective in some individuals. In contrast to antibiotics, which act by killing or arresting the growth of pathogens, vaccines act by sensitizing the immune system to pathogens and do not promote the emergence of resistant strains (A). An enormous body of high-quality evidence now refutes that there is any link between vaccines and autism spectrum disorders (E), and previous studies and authors suggesting this association have been discredited.

9. **B.** Currently available technology permits the identification of genetic susceptibility to some diseases (e.g., breast cancer). Because the ability to modify genetic risk is not nearly as great as the ability to recognize it, ethical concerns have been raised. Little good may come from informing people about a risk that they cannot readily modify, whereas harm, such as anxiety or increased difficulty and expense involved in obtaining medical insurance, might result. In contrast, social support networks (E), immunization status (C), dietary intake (A), and smoking status (D) all are factors that can be modified to prevent disease and are therefore less ethically problematic.

10. **A.** The H1N1 virus represents a major genetic change from the predecessor influenza variants from which it evolved. Reassortment of surface antigens from several strains of influenza across several host species (including birds and pigs) likely contributed to the virus's development. Such novel admixture of surface antigens resulting from the combination of existing viral strains is known as antigenic shift. Antigenic drift (B) is a more minor alteration in surface antigens resulting from mutations within a single virus strain. Antibody shift (C) and antibody drift (D) are not defined phenomenon. Antisocial rift (E) might occur between competing researchers vying for the title of world's leading influenza epidemiologist.

Epidemiologic Data Measurements

"You can have data without information, but you cannot have information without data."

Daniel Keys Moran

We are in the era of "big data" in health and health care. Large repositories of patient data can be mined to help us evaluate trends in disease burden or health risks, improve how resources are allocated, or decide on health policy. To improve the health of the world's populations we need high-quality information on population health.

Clinical phenomena must be measured accurately to develop and test hypotheses. Because epidemiologists study phenomena in populations, they need measures that summarize what happens at the population level. The fundamental epidemiologic measure is the frequency with which an event of interest (e.g., disease, injury, or death) occurs in the population of interest.

1. FREQUENCY

The frequency of a disease, injury, or death can be measured in different ways, and it can be related to different denominators, depending on the purpose of the research and the availability of data. The concepts of incidence and prevalence are of fundamental importance to epidemiology.

1.1 INCIDENCE (INCIDENT CASES)

Incidence is the frequency of occurrences of disease, injury, or death—that is, the number of transitions from well to ill, from uninjured to injured, or from alive to dead—in the study population *during the time period of the study*. The term *incidence* is sometimes used incorrectly to mean incidence rate (defined in a later section). Therefore, to avoid confusion, it may be better to use the term *incident cases*, rather than *incidence*. Fig. 2.1 shows the annual number of incident cases of acquired immunodeficiency syndrome (AIDS) for the first 12 years of monitoring in the United States (1981–1992).

1.2 PREVALENCE (PREVALENT CASES)

Prevalence (sometimes called point prevalence) is the number of persons in a defined population who have a specified disease or condition *at a given point in time*, usually the time when a survey is conducted. The term *prevalence* is sometimes

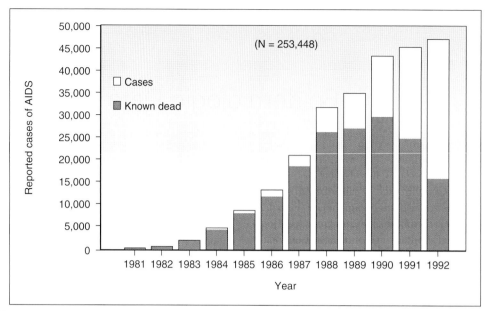

Fig. 2.1 Historical Data on Incident Cases of Acquired Immunodeficiency Syndrome in United States, by Year of Report, 1981–1992. The full height of a bar represents the number of incident cases of AIDS in a given year. The darkened portion of a bar represents the number of patients in whom AIDS was diagnosed in a given year, but who were known to be dead by the end of 1992. The clear portion represents the number of patients who had AIDS diagnosed in a given year and were still living at the end of 1992. (From Centers for Disease Control and Prevention: Summary of notifiable diseases—United States, 1992. *MMWR* 41:55, 1993.)

used incorrectly to mean prevalence rate (defined in a later section). Therefore, to avoid confusion, the awkward term *prevalent cases* is usually preferable to *prevalence*.

1.2.a Difference Between Point Prevalence and Period Prevalence

This text uses the term *prevalence* to mean **point prevalence**—that is, prevalence at a specific point in time. Some articles in the literature discuss **period prevalence,** which refers to the number of persons who had a given disease at any time during the specified time interval. Period prevalence is the sum of the point prevalence at the beginning of the interval plus the incidence during the interval. Because period prevalence is a mixed measure, composed of point prevalence and incidence, it is not recommended for scientific work.

1.3 ILLUSTRATION OF MORBIDITY CONCEPTS

The concepts of incidence (incident cases), point prevalence (prevalent cases), and period prevalence are illustrated in Fig. 2.2. This figure provides data concerning eight persons who have a given disease in a defined population in which there is no emigration or immigration. Each person is assigned a case number (case 1 through case 8). A line begins when a person becomes ill and ends when that person either recovers or dies. The symbol t_1 signifies the beginning of the study period (e.g., a calendar year) and t_2 signifies the end.

In case 1, the patient was already ill when the year began and was still alive and ill when it ended. In cases 2, 6, and 8, the patients were already ill when the year began, but recovered or died during the year. In cases 3 and 5, the patients

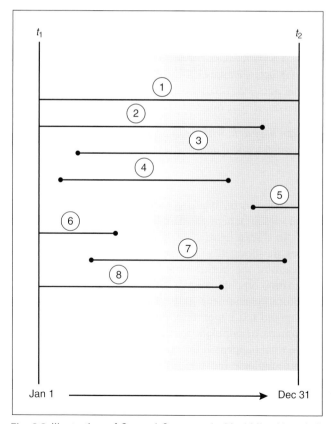

Fig. 2.2 Illustration of Several Concepts in Morbidity. Lines indicate when eight persons became ill *(start of a line)* and when they recovered or died *(end of a line)* between the beginning of a year (t_1) and the end of the same year $(\pm t_2)$. Each person is assigned a case number *(circled)*. Point prevalence: $t_1 = 4$ and $t_2 = 3$; period prevalence = 8. (Based on Dorn HF: A classification system for morbidity concepts. *Public Health Rep* 72:1043–1048, 1957.)

became ill during the year and were still alive and ill when the year ended. In cases 4 and 7, the patients became ill during the year and either recovered or died during the year. On the basis of Fig. 2.2, the following calculations can be made: There were four incident cases during the year (cases 3, 4, 5, and 7). The point prevalence at t_1 was 4 (the prevalent cases were 1, 2, 6, and 8). The point prevalence at t_2 was 3 (cases 1, 3, and 5). The period prevalence is equal to the point prevalence at t_1 plus the incidence between t_1 and t_2, or in this example, $4 + 4 = 8$. Although a person can be an incident case only once, the same person could be considered a prevalent case at many points in time, including the beginning and end of the study period (as with case 1).

1.4 RELATIONSHIP BETWEEN INCIDENCE AND PREVALENCE

Fig. 2.1 provides data from the U.S. Centers for Disease Control and Prevention (CDC) to illustrate the complex relationship between incidence and prevalence. It uses the historic example of AIDS in the United States during the first 12 years of reporting by the CDC: from 1981, when it was first recognized and defined, through 1992, after which the definition of AIDS underwent a major change. Because AIDS is a clinical syndrome (defined by being HIV positive and having either a CD4 cell count <200 cells/mm³ or having one or more opportunistic illnesses) the present discussion addresses the prevalence of AIDS rather than the prevalence of its causal agent, human immunodeficiency virus (HIV) infection.

In Fig. 2.1, the full height of each year's bar shows the total number of new AIDS cases reported to the CDC for that year. The darkened part of each bar shows the number of people

in whom AIDS was diagnosed in that year, and who were known to be dead by December 31, 1992. The clear space in each bar represents the number of people in whom AIDS was diagnosed in that year, and who presumably were still alive on December 31, 1992. The sum of the clear areas represents the **prevalent cases** of AIDS as of the last day of 1992. Of the people in whom AIDS was diagnosed between 1990 and 1992 and who had had the condition for a relatively short time, a fairly high proportion were still alive at the cutoff date. Their survival resulted from the recency of their infection and from improved treatment. However, almost all people in whom AIDS was diagnosed during the first 6 years of the epidemic had died by that date.

The total number of cases of an epidemic disease reported over time is its **cumulative incidence.** According to the CDC, the cumulative incidence of AIDS in the United States through December 31, 1991, was 206,392, and the number known to have died was 133,232.[2] At the close of 1991, there were 73,160 prevalent cases of AIDS (206,392 − 133,232). If these people with AIDS died in subsequent years, they would be removed from the category of prevalent cases.

Fig. 2.3 provides a vivid illustration of the importance of a consistent definition of a disease in making accurate comparisons of trends in rates over time. On January 1, 1993, the CDC made a major change in the criteria for defining AIDS. A backlog of patients whose disease manifestations met the new criteria was included in the counts for the first time in 1993, and this resulted in a sudden, huge spike in the number of reported AIDS cases (see Fig. 2.3).

Prevalence is the result of many factors: the periodic (annual) number of new cases; the immigration and emigration of persons with the disease; and the average duration of the disease, which is defined as the time from its onset until

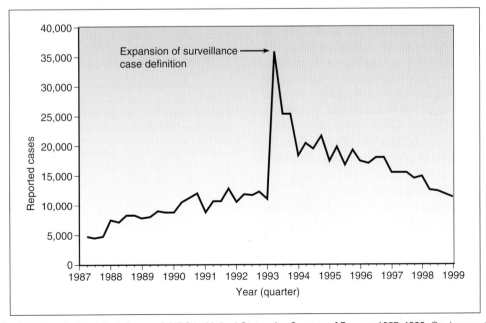

Fig. 2.3 Historical Incident Cases of AIDS in United States, by Quarter of Report, 1987–1999. On January 1, 1993, the CDC changed the criteria for defining AIDS. The expansion of the surveillance case definition resulted in a huge spike in the number of reported cases. (From Centers for Disease Control and Prevention: Summary of notifiable diseases—United States, 1998. *MMWR* 47:20, 1999.)

death or healing. The following is an approximate general formula for prevalence that cannot be used for detailed scientific estimation, but that is conceptually important for understanding and predicting the **burden of disease** on a society or population:

$$Prevalence = Incidence \times (average)Duration$$

This conceptual formula works only if the incidence of the disease and its duration in individuals are stable for an extended time. The formula implies that the prevalence of a disease can increase as a result of an increase in the following:
- Yearly numbers of new cases
  or
- Length of time that symptomatic patients survive before dying (or recovering, if that is possible)

In the specific case of AIDS, its incidence in the United States is declining, whereas the duration of life for people with AIDS is increasing as a result of antiviral agents and other methods of treatment and prophylaxis. These methods have increased the length of survival proportionately more than the decline in incidence, so that prevalent cases of AIDS continue to increase in the United States.

A similar situation exists in regard to cardiovascular disease. Its age-specific incidence has been declining in the United States in recent decades, but its prevalence has not. As advances in technology and pharmacotherapy forestall death, people live longer with disease.

2. RISK

2.1 DEFINITION

In epidemiology, **risk** is defined as the proportion of persons who are unaffected at the beginning of a study period, but who experience a **risk event** during the study period. The risk event may be death, disease, or injury, and the people at risk for the event at the beginning of the study period constitute a **cohort.** If an investigator follows everyone in a cohort for several years, the denominator for the risk of an event does not change (unless people are lost to follow-up). In a cohort, the denominator for a 5-year risk of death or disease is the same as for a 1-year risk, because in both situations the denominator is the number of persons counted at the beginning of the study.

Care is needed when applying actual risk estimates (which are derived from populations) to individuals. If death, disease, or injury occurs in an individual, the person's risk is 100%. As an example, the best way to approach patients' questions regarding the risk related to surgery is probably *not* to give them just numbers (e.g., "Your chances of survival are 99%"). They might then worry whether they would be in the 1% group or the 99% group. Rather, it is helpful to put the risk of surgery in the context of the many other risks they may take frequently, such as the risks involved in a long automobile trip.

2.2 LIMITATIONS OF THE CONCEPT OF RISK

Often it is difficult to be sure of the correct denominator for a measure of risk. Who is truly at risk? Only women are at risk for becoming pregnant, but even this statement must be modified, because for practical purposes, women aged 15 to 44 years are more likely to become pregnant than women outside of this age group. Even within this age group, some proportion are unlikely to become pregnant as they use birth control, do not engage in heterosexual relations, or have had a hysterectomy.

Ideally, for risk related to infectious disease, only the **susceptible population**—that is, people without antibody protection—would be counted in the denominator. However, antibody levels are usually unknown. As a practical compromise, the denominator usually consists of either the total population of an area or the people in an age group who probably lack antibodies.

Expressing the risk of death from an infectious disease, although seemingly simple, is quite complex. This is because such a risk is the product of many different proportions, as can be seen in Fig. 2.4. Numerous **subsets of the population**

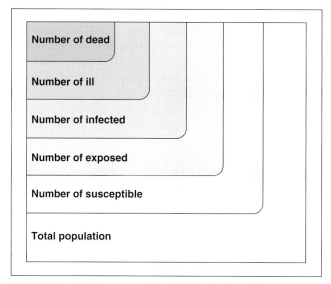

Fig. 2.4 Graphic Representation of Why the Death Rate From an Infectious Disease Is the Product of Many Proportions. If each of the five fractions to the right of the equal sign were 0.5, the persons who were dead would represent 50% of those who were ill, 25% of those who were infected, 12.5% of those who were exposed, 6.25% of those who were susceptible, and 3.125% of the total population. The formula may be viewed as below.

$$\frac{Number\ of\ dead}{Total\ population} = \frac{Number\ of\ dead}{Number\ of\ ill} \times \frac{Number\ of\ ill}{Number\ of\ infected} \times \frac{Number\ of\ infected}{Number\ of\ exposed}$$
$$\times \frac{Number\ of\ exposed}{Number\ of\ susceptible} \times \frac{Number\ of\ susceptible}{Total\ population}$$

must be considered. People who **die** of an infectious disease are a subset of people who are **ill** from the disease, who are a subset of the people who are **infected** by the disease agent, who are a subset of the people who are **exposed** to the infection, who are a subset of the people who are **susceptible** to the infection, who are a subset of the **total population.**

The proportion of clinically ill persons who die is the **case fatality ratio;** the higher this ratio, the more **virulent** the infection. The proportion of infected persons who are clinically ill is often called the **pathogenicity** of the organism. The proportion of exposed persons who become infected is sometimes called the **infectiousness** of the organism, but infectiousness is also influenced by the conditions of exposure. A full understanding of the epidemiology of an infectious disease would require knowledge of all the ratios shown in Fig. 2.4. Analogous characterizations may be applied to noninfectious disease.

The concept of risk has other limitations, which can be understood through the following thought experiment: assume that three different populations of the same size and age distribution (e.g., three nursing homes with no new patients during the study period) have the same overall risk of death (e.g., 10%) in the same year (e.g., from January 1 to December 31 in year X). Despite their similarity in risk, the deaths in the three populations may occur in very different patterns over time. Suppose that population A suffered a serious influenza epidemic in January (the beginning of the study year), and that most of those who died that year did so in the first month of the year. Suppose that the influenza epidemic did not hit population B until December (the end of the study year), so that most of the deaths in that population occurred during the last month of the year. Finally, suppose that population C did not experience the epidemic, and that its deaths occurred (as usual) evenly throughout the year. The 1-year risk of death (10%) would be the same in all three populations, but the **force of mortality** (described later) would not be the same. The force of mortality would be greatest in population A, least in population B, and intermediate in population C. Because the measure of risk cannot distinguish between these three patterns in the timing of deaths, a more precise measure—the rate—may be used instead.

3. RATES

3.1 DEFINITION

A *rate* is the number of events that occur in a defined time period, divided by the average number of people at risk for the event during the period under study. Because the population at the middle of the period can usually be considered a good estimate of the average number of people at risk during that period, the midperiod population is often used as the denominator of a rate. The formal structure of a rate is described in the following equation:

$$\text{Rate} = \frac{\text{Numerator}}{\text{Denominator}} \times \text{Constant multiplier}$$

Risks and rates usually have values less than 1 unless the event of interest can occur repeatedly, as with colds or asthma attacks. However, decimal fractions are awkward to think about and discuss, especially if we try to imagine fractions of a death (e.g., "one one-thousandth of a death per year"). Rates are usually multiplied by a **constant multiplier**—100, 1,000, 10,000, or 100,000—to make the numerator larger than 1 and thus easier to discuss (e.g., "one death per thousand people per year"). When a constant multiplier is used, the numerator and the denominator are multiplied by the same number, so the value of the ratio is not changed.

The **crude death rate** illustrates why a constant multiplier is used. In 2016 this rate for the United States was estimated as 0.00849 per year. However, most people find it easier to multiply this fraction by 1,000 and express it as 8.49 deaths per 1,000 individuals in the population per year (or multiply by 100,000 and then it would be 849 deaths). The general form for calculating the rate in this case is as follows:

$$\text{Crude death rate} = \frac{\text{No. deaths (same place and time period)}}{\text{Midperiod population (same place and time period)}} \times 1,000$$

Rates can be thought of in the same way as the velocity of a car. It is possible to talk about **average rates** or average velocity for a period of time. The average velocity is obtained by dividing the miles traveled (e.g., 55) by the time required (e.g., 1 hour), in which case the car averaged 55 miles per hour. This does not mean that the car was traveling at exactly 55 miles per hour for every instant during that hour. In a similar manner, the average rate of an event (e.g., death) is equal to the total number of events for a defined time (e.g., 1 year) divided by the average population exposed to that event (e.g., 12 deaths per 1000 persons per year).

A rate, as with a velocity, also can be understood as describing reality at an instant in time, in which case the death rate can be expressed as an **instantaneous death rate** or **hazard rate.** Because death is a discrete event rather than a continuous function, however, instantaneous rates cannot actually be measured; they can only be estimated. (Note that the rates discussed in this book are average rates unless otherwise stated.)

3.2 RELATIONSHIP BETWEEN RISK AND RATE

In an example presented earlier in section 2.2, populations A, B, and C were similar in size, and each had a 10% overall risk of death in the same year, but their patterns of death differed greatly. Fig. 2.5 shows the three different patterns and illustrates how, in this example, the concept of rate is superior to the concept of risk in showing differences in the force of mortality.

Because most of the deaths in population A occurred before July 1, the midyear population of this cohort would be the smallest of the three, and the resulting death rate would be the highest (because the denominator is the smallest and the

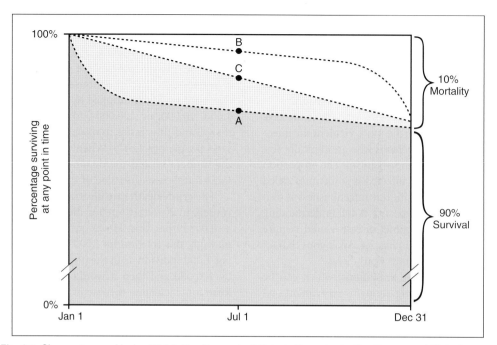

Fig. 2.5 Circumstances Under Which the Concept of Rate Is Superior to the Concept of Risk. Assume that populations A, B, and C are three different populations of the same size; that 10% of each population died in a given year; and that most of the deaths in population A occurred early in the year, most of the deaths in population B occurred late in the year, and the deaths in population C were evenly distributed throughout the year. In all three populations, the risk of death would be the same (10%) even though the patterns of death differed greatly. The rate of death, which is calculated using the midyear population as the denominator, would be the highest in population A, the lowest in population B, and intermediate in population C, reflecting the relative magnitude of the force of mortality in the three populations.

numerator is the same size for all three populations). In contrast, because most of the deaths in population B occurred at the end of the year, the midyear population of this cohort would be the largest of the three, and the death rate would be the lowest. For population C, both the number of deaths before July 1 and the death rate would be intermediate between those of A and B. Although the 1-year risk for these three populations did not show differences in the force of mortality, cohort-specific rates did so by reflecting more accurately the timing of the deaths in the three populations. This quantitative result agrees with the graph and with intuition, because if we assume that the quality of life was reasonably good, most people would prefer to be in population B. More days of life are lived by those in population B during the year, because of the lower force of mortality.

Rates are often used to estimate risk. A rate is a good approximation of risk if the:

- Event in the numerator occurs only once per individual during the study interval.
- Proportion of the population affected by the event is small (e.g., <5%).
- Time interval is relatively short.

If the time interval is long or the percentage of people who are affected is large, the rate is noticeably larger than the risk. If the event in the numerator occurs more than once during

the study—as can happen with colds, ear infections, or asthma attacks—a related statistic called **incidence density** (discussed later) should be used instead of rate.

In a cohort study, the denominator for a 5-year risk is the same as the denominator for a 1-year risk. However, the denominator for a rate is constantly changing. It decreases as some people die and others emigrate from the population, and it increases as some immigrate and others are born. In most real populations, all four of these changes—birth, death, immigration, and emigration—are occurring at the same time. The rate reflects these changes by using the midperiod population as an estimate of the average population at risk.

3.3 QUANTITATIVE RELATIONSHIP BETWEEN RISK AND RATE

As noted earlier, a rate may be a good approximation of a risk if the time interval under study is short. If the time interval is long, the rate is higher than the risk because the rate's denominator is progressively reduced by the number of risk events (e.g., deaths) that occur up to the midperiod. When the rate and risk are both small, the difference between the rate and the corresponding risk is also small. These principles can be shown by examining the relationship between the **mortality rate** and the **mortality risk** in population C in Fig. 2.5. Population C had an even mortality risk throughout the year and a total yearly mortality risk of 10%. By the middle of the year, death had occurred in 5%. The mortality rate would be $0.10/(1 - 0.05) = 0.10/0.95 = 0.1053 = 105.3$ per 1000 persons per year. In this example, the denominator is 0.95 because 95% of population C was still living at midyear to form the denominator. The yearly rate is higher than the yearly risk because the **average population at risk** is smaller than the **initial population at risk**.

What would be the **cumulative mortality risk** for population C at the end of 2 years, assuming a **constant yearly mortality rate** of 0.1053? It cannot be calculated by simply multiplying 2 years times the yearly risk of 10%, because the number still living and subject to the force of mortality by the beginning of the second year would be smaller (i.e., it would be 90% of the original population). Likewise, the cumulative risk of death over 10 years cannot be calculated by simply multiplying 10 years times 10%. This would mean that 100% of population C would be dead after one decade, yet intuition suggests that at least some of the population would live more than 10 years. In fact, if the mortality rate remained constant, the cumulative risks at 2 years, 5 years, 10 years, and 15 years would be 19%, 41%, 65%, and 79%.

3.4 CRITERIA FOR VALID USE OF THE TERM *RATE*

To be valid, a rate must meet certain criteria with respect to the correspondence between numerator and denominator. For example, all the events counted in the numerator must have happened to persons in the denominator. Also, all the persons counted in the denominator must have been at risk for the events in the numerator (e.g., the denominator of a cervical cancer rate should contain no men).

Before comparisons of rates can be made, the following must also be true: the numerators for all groups being compared must be defined or diagnosed in the same way; the constant multipliers being used must be the same; and the time intervals must be the same. These criteria may seem obvious, but it is easy to overlook them when making comparisons over time or between populations. For example, numerators may not be easy to compare if the quality of medical diagnosis differs over time. In the late 1800s, there was no diagnostic category called *myocardial infarction*, but many persons were dying of *acute indigestion*. By 1930, the situation was reversed: almost nobody died of acute indigestion, but many died of myocardial infarction. It might be tempting to say that the acute indigestion of the late 1800s was actually myocardial infarction, but there is no certainty that this is true.

Another example of the problems implicit in studying causes of disease over time relates to changes in commonly used classification systems. In 1948, there was a major revision in the **International Classification of Diseases** (ICD), the international coding manual for classifying diagnoses that helps clinicians, policy makers, and patients to navigate, understand, and compare health care systems and services. The World Health Organization (WHO) conducts and issues periodical revisions of the ICD. This revision of the ICD codes in 1948 was followed by sudden, major changes in the reported numbers and rates of many diseases. Subsequent ICD coding revisions (both between and within revisions) continue to cause changes in diagnoses. The current ICD consists of two parts: ICD-CM for clinical modification diagnosis coding (~68,000 codes) and the ICD-PCS for inpatient procedure classification system coding (~87,000 codes).

It is difficult not only to track changes in causes of death and disease over time, but also to make accurate comparisons of cause-specific rates of disease between populations, especially populations in different countries. Residents of different countries have different degrees of access to medical care, different levels in the quality of medical care available to them, and different styles of diagnosis. It is not easy to determine between how much of any apparent difference is real and how much is caused by variation in medical care and diagnostic styles.

3.5 SPECIFIC TYPES OF RATES

The concepts of incidence (incident cases) and prevalence (prevalent cases) were discussed earlier. With the concept of a rate now reviewed, it is appropriate to define different types of rates, which are usually developed for large populations and used for public health purposes.

3.5.a Incidence Rate

The incidence rate is calculated as the number of incident cases over a defined study period, divided by the population at risk at the midpoint of that study period. An incidence rate is usually expressed per 1,000, per 10,000, or per 100,000 population.

3.5.b Prevalence Rate

The so-called prevalence rate is actually a proportion and not a rate. The term is in common use, however, and is used here to indicate the proportion (usually expressed as a percentage) of persons with a defined disease or condition at the time they are studied. The 2015 Behavioral Risk Factor Survey reported that the prevalence rate for patients' self-report of physician-diagnosed arthritis varied from a low of 19% in California to a high of 38% in West Virginia.[1]

Prevalence rates can be applied to risk factors, to knowledge, and to diseases or other conditions. In selected states, the prevalence rate of rarely or never using seat belts among high school students varied from 5% in Kansas to 17.5% in Arkansas.[2] Likewise, the percentage of people recognizing stroke signs and symptoms in a 13-state study varied from 38% for some signs to 93% for others.[3]

3.5.c Incidence Density

Incidence density refers to the number of new events per *person-time* (e.g., per person-months or person-years). Suppose that three patients were followed after tonsillectomy and adenoidectomy for recurrent ear infections. If one patient was followed for 13 months, one for 20 months, and one for 17 months, and if 5 ear infections occurred in these 3 patients during this time, the incidence density would be 5 infections per 50 person-months of follow-up or 10 infections per 100 person-months. Incidence density is especially useful when the event of interest (e.g., colds, otitis media, myocardial infarction) can occur in a person more than once during the study period.

4. SPECIAL ISSUES ON USE OF RATES

Rates or risks are typically used to make one of three types of comparison. The first type is a comparison of an observed rate (or risk) with a target rate (or risk). For example, The United States set national health goals for 2020, including the expected rates of various types of death, such as the infant mortality rate. When the final 2020 statistics are published, the observed rates for the nation and for subgroups will be compared with the target objectives set by the government.

The second type is a comparison of two different populations *at the same time.* This is probably the most common type. One example involves comparing the rates of death or disease in two different countries, states, or ethnic groups for the same year. Another example involves comparing the results in treatment groups to the results in control groups participating in randomized clinical trials. A major research concern is to ensure that the two populations are not only similar but also measured in exactly the same way.

The third type is a comparison involving the same population *at different times.* This approach is used to study time trends. Because there also are trends over time in the composition of a population (e.g., increasing proportion of elderly people in the US population), adjustments must be made for such changes before concluding that there are real differences over time in the rates under study. Changes over time (usually improvement) in diagnostic capabilities must also be taken into account.

4.1 CRUDE RATES VERSUS SPECIFIC RATES

There are three broad categories of rates: crude, specific, and standardized. Rates that apply to an entire population, without reference to any characteristics of the individuals in it, are **crude rates.** The term *crude* simply means that the data are presented without any processing or adjustment. When a population is divided into more homogeneous subgroups based on a particular characteristic of interest (e.g., age, sex/gender, race, risk factors, or comorbidity), and rates are calculated within these groups, the result is **specific rates** (e.g., age-specific rates, gender-specific rates). Standardized rates are discussed in the next section.

Crude rates are valid, but they are often misleading. Here is a quick challenge: try to guess which of the following three countries—Sweden, Ecuador, or the United States—has the highest and lowest crude death rate. Those who guessed that Ecuador has the highest and Sweden the lowest have the sequence exactly reversed. Table 2.1 lists the estimated crude death rates and the corresponding life expectancy at birth.

TABLE 2.1   Crude Death Rate and Life Expectancy for Three Countries (2017 estimate)

Country	Crude Death Rate	Life Expectancy at Birth
Ecuador	5.1 per 1,000	77 years
United States	8.2 per 1,000	80 years
Sweden	9.4 per 1,000	82 years

Data from CIA, The World Factbook, under the name of the country. https://www.cia.gov/library/publications/resources/the-world-factbook/geos/us.html

For 2017, Ecuador had the lowest crude death rate and Sweden the highest, even though Ecuador had the highest age-specific mortality rates and the shortest life expectancy, and Sweden had just the reverse.

This apparent anomaly occurs primarily because the crude death rates do not take age into account. For a population with a young age distribution, such as Ecuador (median age 28 years), the birth rate is likely to be relatively high, and the crude death rate is likely to be relatively low, although the **age-specific death rates** (ASDRs) for each age group may be high. In contrast, for an older population, such as Sweden, a low crude birth rate and a high crude death rate would be expected. This is because age has such a profound influence on the force of mortality that an old population, even if it is relatively healthy, inevitably has a high overall death rate, and vice versa. The huge impact of age on death rates can be seen in Fig. 2.6, which shows data on probability of death at different ages in the United States in 2015. As a general principle, investigators should never make comparisons of the risk of death or disease between populations without controlling for age (and sometimes for other characteristics as well).

Why not avoid crude rates altogether and use specific rates? There are many circumstances when it is not possible to use specific rates, for example, if the:
- Frequency of the event of interest (i.e., the numerator) is unknown for the subgroups of a population
- Size of the subgroups (i.e., the denominator) is unknown
- Numbers of people at risk for the event are too small to provide stable estimates of the specific rates

If the number of people at risk is large in each of the subgroups of interest, however, specific rates provide the most information, and these should be sought whenever possible.

Although the biasing effect of age can be controlled for in several ways, the simplest (and usually the best) method is to calculate the ASDRs, so that the rates can be compared in similar age groups. The formula is as follows:

$$\text{Age-specific death rate} = \frac{\begin{array}{c}\text{No. deaths to people in a particular age group}\\ \left(\text{defined place and time period}\right)\end{array}}{\begin{array}{c}\text{Midperiod population}\\ \left(\text{same age group, place, and time period}\right)\end{array}} \times 1,000$$

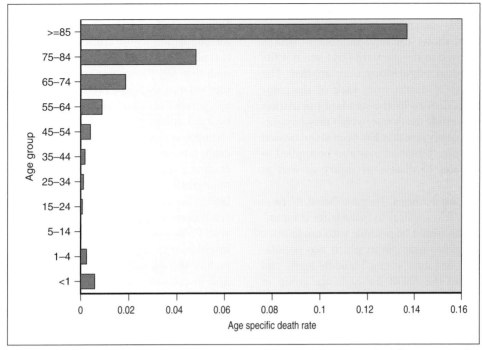

Fig. 2.6 Age-Specific Death Rates (ASDRs) for Deaths From All Causes—United States, 2015. Graph illustrates the profound impact of age on death rates. (Data from estimates of death rates for 2015 using the 2010 census data. From Sherry L, Murphy BS, Jiaquan Xu MD, et al: Division of vital statistics. *Natl Vital Stat Rep* 66:6, 2017.)

Crude death rates are the sum of the ASDRs in each of the age groups, weighted by the relative size of each age group. The underlying formula for any summary rate is as follows:

$$\text{Summary rate} = \sum w_i r_i$$

where w_i = the individual weights (proportions) of each age-specific group, and r_i = the rates for the corresponding age group. This formula is useful for understanding why crude rates can be misleading. In studies involving two age-specific populations, a difference in the relative weights (sizes) of the old and young populations will result in different weights for the high and low ASDRs, and no fair comparison can be made. This general principle applies not only to demography and population epidemiology, where investigators are interested in comparing the rates of large groups, but also to clinical epidemiology, where investigators may want to compare the risks or rates of two patient groups who have different proportions of severely ill, moderately ill, and mildly ill patients.[4]

A similar problem occurs when investigators want to compare death rates in different hospitals to measure the quality of care. To make fair comparisons among hospitals, investigators must make some adjustment for differences in the types and severity of illness and surgery in the patients who are treated. Otherwise, the hospitals that care for the sickest patients would be at an unfair disadvantage in such a comparison.

4.2 STANDARDIZATION OF DEATH RATES

Standardized rates, also known as **adjusted rates,** are crude rates that have been modified (adjusted) to control for the effects of age or other characteristics and allow valid comparisons of rates. To obtain a summary death rate that is free from age bias, investigators can age-standardize (age-adjust) the crude rates by a direct or indirect method. Standardization is usually applied to death rates, but it may be used to adjust any type of rate.

4.2.a Direct Standardization

Direct standardization is the most common method to remove the biasing effect of differing age structures in different populations. In direct standardization, the ASDRs of the populations to be compared are applied to a single, standard population. This is done by multiplying each ASDR from each population under comparison by the number of persons in the corresponding age group in the standard population. Because the age structure of the standard population is the same for all the death rates applied to it, the distorting effect of different age distributions in the real populations is eliminated. Overall death rates can then be compared without age bias.

The standard population may be any real (or realistic) population. In practice, it is often a larger population that contains the subpopulations to be compared. For example, the death rates of two cities in the same state can be compared by using the state's population as the standard population.

Likewise, the death rates of states may be compared by using the US population as the standard.

The direct method shows the total number of deaths that would have occurred in the standard population if the ASDRs of the individual populations were applied. The total expected number of deaths from each of the comparison populations is divided by the standard population to give a standardized crude death rate, which may be compared with any other death rate that has been standardized in the same way. The direct method may also be applied to compare incidence rates of disease or injury as well as death.

Standardized rates are fictitious. They are "what if" rates only, but they do allow investigators to make fairer comparisons of death rates than would be possible with crude rates. Box 2.1 shows a simplified example in which two populations, A and B, are divided into "young," "middle-aged," and "older" subgroups, and the ASDR for each age group in population B is twice as high as that for the corresponding age group in population A. In this example, the standard population is simply the sum of the two populations being compared. Population A has a higher overall crude death rate (4.51%) than population B (3.08%), despite the ASDRs in B being twice the ASDRs in A. After the death rates are standardized, the adjusted death rate for population B correctly reflects the fact that its ASDRs are twice as high as those of population A.

4.2.b Indirect Standardization

Indirect standardization is used if ASDRs are unavailable in the population whose crude death rate needs to be adjusted. It is also used if the population to be standardized is small, such that ASDRs become statistically unstable. The indirect method uses **standard rates** and applies them to the known age groups (or other specified groups) in the population to be standardized.

Suppose that an investigator wanted to see whether the death rates in a given year for male employees of a particular company, such as workers in an offshore oil rig, were similar to or greater than the death rates for all men in the US population. To start, the investigator would need the observed crude death rate and the ASDRs for all US men for a similar year. These would serve as the **standard death rates.** Next, the investigator would determine the number of male workers in each of the age categories used for the US male population. The investigator would then determine the observed total deaths for 1 year for all the male workers in the company.

The first step for indirect standardization is to multiply the standard death rate for each age group in the standard population by the number of workers in the corresponding age group in the company. This gives the number of deaths that would be *expected* in each age group of workers if they had the same death rates as the standard population. The expected numbers of worker deaths for the various age groups are then summed to obtain the total number of deaths that would be expected in the

---

BOX 2.1 Direct Standardization of Crude Death Rates of Two Populations, Using the Combined Weights as the Standard Population (Fictitious Data)

Part 1 Calculation of Crude Death Rates

Age Group	POPULATION A — Population Size		Age-Specific Death Rate		Expected No. Deaths	POPULATION B — Population Size		Age-Specific Death Rate		Expected No. Deaths
Young	1,000	×	0.001	=	1	4,000	×	0.002	=	8
Middle-aged	5,000	×	0.010	=	50	5,000	×	0.020	=	100
Older	4,000	×	0.100	=	400	1,000	×	0.200	=	200
Total	10,000				451	10,000				308
Crude death rate				$\frac{451}{10{,}000} = 4.51\%$					$\frac{308}{10{,}000} = 3.08\%$	

Part 2 Direct Standardization Rates of the Part 1 Crude Death Rates, With the Two Populations Combined to Form the Standard Weights

Age Group	POPULATION A — Population Size		Age-Specific Death Rate		Expected No. Deaths	POPULATION B — Population Size		Age-Specific Death Rate		Expected No. Deaths
Young	5,000	×	0.001	=	5	5,000	×	0.002	=	10
Middle-aged	10,000	×	0.010	=	100	10,000	×	0.020	=	200
Older	5,000	×	0.100	=	500	5,000	×	0.200	=	1,000
Total	20,000				605	20,000				1,210
Standardized death rate				$\frac{605}{20{,}000} = 3.03\%$					$\frac{1{,}210}{20{,}000} = 6.05\%$	

BOX 2.2 Indirect Standardization of Crude Death Rate for Men in a Company, Using the Age-Specific Death Rates for Men in a Standard Population (Fictitious Data)

Part 1 Beginning Data

Age Group	MEN IN STANDARD POPULATION				MEN IN COMPANY		
	Proportion of Standard Population	Age-Specific Death Rate		Observed Death Rate	No. Workers	Age-Specific Death Rate	Observed No. Deaths
Young	0.40	× 0.001	=	0.0004	2,000	× ? =	?
Middle-aged	0.30	× 0.010	=	0.0030	3,000	× ? =	?
Older	0.30	× 0.100	=	0.0300	5,000	× ? =	?
Total	1.00			0.0334	10,000		
Observed death rate	0.0334, or 334/10,000						480/10,000

Part 2 Calculation of Expected Death Rate, Using Indirect Standardization of Part 1 Rates and Applying Age-Specific Death Rates From the Standard Population to the Numbers of Workers in the Company

Age Group	MEN IN STANDARD POPULATION				MEN IN COMPANY		
	Proportion of Standard Population	Age-Specific Death Rate		Observed Death Rate	No. Workers	Age-Specific Death Rate	Expected No. Deaths
Young	0.40	× 0.001	=	0.0004	2,000	× 0.001 =	2
Middle-aged	0.30	× 0.010	=	0.0030	3,000	× 0.010 =	30
Older	0.30	× 0.100	=	0.0300	5,000	× 0.100 =	500
Total	1.00			0.0334	10,000		532
Expected death rate							532/10,000

Part 3 Calculation of Standardized Mortality Ratio (SMR)

$$\text{SMR} = \frac{\text{Observed death rate for men in the company}}{\text{Expected death rate for men in the company}} \times 100$$

$$= \frac{0.0480}{0.0532} \times 100$$

$$= (0.90)(100) = 90$$

= Men in the company actually had a death rate that was only 90% of the standard population

---

entire worker group, if the ASDRs for company workers were the same as the ASDRs for the standard population. Next, the total number of *observed* deaths among the workers is divided by the total number of *expected* deaths among the workers to obtain a value known as the **standardized mortality ratio** (SMR). Lastly, the SMR is multiplied by 100 to eliminate fractions, so that the expected mortality rate in the standard population equals 100. If the employees in this example had an SMR of 140, it would mean that their mortality was 40% greater than would be expected on the basis of the ASDRs of the standard population. Box 2.2 presents an example of indirect standardization.

4.3 CAUSE-SPECIFIC RATES

Remember that rates refer to events in the numerator, occurring to a population in the denominator. To compare the rates of events among comparable populations, the denominators must be made comparable. For example, making rates gender or age specific would allow a comparison of events among groups of men or women or among people in a certain age bracket. Because the numerator describes the specific events that are occurring, the numerators are comparable when rates are cause specific. A particular event (e.g., gunshot wound, myocardial infarction) could be compared among differing populations. Comparing cause-specific death rates over time or between countries is often risky, however, because of possible differences in diagnostic standards or availability of health care. In countries with inadequate medical care, 10% to 20% of deaths may be diagnosed as "symptoms, signs, and ill-defined conditions." Similar uncertainties may also apply to people who die without adequate medical care in more developed countries.[5]

Cause-specific death rates have the following general form:

$$\text{Cause-specific death rate} = \frac{\begin{pmatrix} \text{No. deaths due to a particular cause} \\ \text{(defined place and time period)} \end{pmatrix}}{\begin{pmatrix} \text{Midperiod population} \\ \text{(same place and time period)} \end{pmatrix}} \times 100{,}000$$

Table 2.2 provides data on the leading causes of death in the United States for 1950, 2000, and 2015, as reported by the National Center for Health Statistics (NCHS) and based on

TABLE 2.2 Age-Adjusted (Age-Standardized) Death Rates for Select Causes of Death in the United States, 1950, 2000 and 2015

Cause of Death	AGE-ADJUSTED DEATH RATE PER 100,000 PER YEAR[a]		
	1950	2000	2015
Cardiac diseases	586.8	257.6	168.5
Malignant neoplasms	193.9	199.6	158.5
Cerebrovascular disease	180.7	60.9	37.6
Unintentional injuries	78.0	34.9	43.2
Influenza and pneumonia	48.1	23.7	15.2
Diabetes	23.1	25.0	21.3
Suicide	13.2	10.4	13.3
Chronic liver disease and cirrhosis	11.3	9.5	10.8
Homicide	5.1	5.9	5.7
HIV disease	—	5.2	1.9
All causes	*1446*	*869*	*733*

HIV, Human immunodeficiency virus.
[a]The age-adjusted death rates for 1950 reflect the National Center for Health Statistics switch to the US population as shown by the year 2000 census (NCHS previously used the 1940 US census). This emphasizes that adjusted (standardized) rates are not actual rates, but relative rates based on the standard population chosen. From National Center for Health Statistics: *Health, United States, 2016,* Hyattsville, MD, 2016, https://data.cdc.gov/NCHS/NCHS-Age-adjusted-Death-Rates-for-Selected-Major-C/6rkc-nb2q.

the underlying cause of death indicated on death certificates. These data are rarely accurate enough for epidemiologic studies of causal factors,[6] but are useful for understanding the relative importance of different disease groups and for studying trends in causes of death over time. For example, the table shows that age-specific rates for deaths caused by cardiac disease and cerebrovascular disease are less than half of what they were in 1950, whereas rates for deaths caused by malignant neoplasms have remained almost steady between 1950 and 2000, before dropping slightly in 2015.

5. COMMONLY USED RATES THAT REFLECT MATERNAL AND INFANT HEALTH

Many of the rates used in public health, especially the infant mortality rate, reflect the health of mothers and infants. The terms relating to the reproductive process are especially important to understand.

5.1 DEFINITIONS OF TERMS

The international definition of a **live birth** is the delivery of a product of conception that shows any sign of life after complete removal from the mother. A **sign of life** may consist of a breath or a cry, any spontaneous movement, a pulse or a heartbeat, or pulsation of the umbilical cord.

Fetal deaths are categorized as early, intermediate, or late. An **early fetal death,** commonly known as a **miscarriage,** occurs when a dead fetus is delivered within the first 20 weeks of gestation. According to international agreements, an **intermediate fetal death** is one in which a dead fetus is delivered between 20 and 28 weeks of gestation. A fetus born dead at 28 weeks of gestation or later is a **late fetal death,** commonly known as a **stillbirth.** An **infant death** is the death of a live-born infant before the infant's first birthday. A **neonatal death** is the death of a live-born infant before the completion of the infant's 28th day of life. A **postneonatal death** is the death of an infant after the 28th day of life but before the first birthday.

5.2 DEFINITIONS OF SPECIFIC TYPES OF RATES

5.2.a Crude Birth Rate

The crude birth rate is the number of live births divided by the midperiod population, as follows:

$$\text{Crude birth rate} = \frac{\text{No. live births} \left(\substack{\text{defined place} \\ \text{and time period}}\right)}{\text{Midperiod population} \left(\substack{\text{same place} \\ \text{and time period}}\right)} \times 1,000$$

5.2.b Infant Mortality Rate

Because the health of infants is unusually sensitive to maternal health (especially maternal nutrition and use of tobacco, alcohol, and drugs), environmental factors, and the quality of health services, the infant mortality rate (IMR) is often used as an overall index of the health status of a nation. This rate has the added advantage of being both age specific and available for most countries. The numerator and the denominator of the IMR are obtained from the same type of data collection system (i.e., vital statistics reporting), so in areas where infant deaths are reported, births are also likely to be reported, and in areas where reporting is poor, births and deaths are equally likely to be affected. The formula for the IMR is as follows:

$$\text{IMR} = \frac{\text{No. deaths to infants} < 1 \text{ year of age} \left(\substack{\text{defined place} \\ \text{and time period}}\right)}{\text{No. live births} \left(\substack{\text{same place} \\ \text{and time period}}\right)} \times 1,000$$

Most infant deaths occur in the first week of life and are caused by prematurity or intrauterine growth retardation. Both conditions often lead to respiratory failure. Some infant deaths in the first month are caused by congenital anomalies.

A subtle point, which is seldom of concern in large populations, is that for any given year, there is not an exact correspondence between the numerator and denominator of the IMR. This is because some of the infants born in a given calendar year will not die until the following year, whereas some of the infants who die in a given year were born in the previous year. Although this lack of exact correspondence does not usually influence the IMR of a large population, it might do so in a small population. To study infant mortality in small populations, it is best to accumulate data over 3 to 5 years. For detailed epidemiologic studies of the causes of infant mortality, it is best to link each infant death with the corresponding birth.

5.2.c Neonatal and Postneonatal Mortality Rates

Epidemiologists distinguish between neonatal and postneonatal mortality. The formulas for the rates are as follows:

$$\text{Neonatal mortality rate} = \frac{\left(\begin{array}{c}\text{No. deaths to infants} <28 \text{ days old} \\ \text{(defined place and time period)}\end{array}\right)}{\left(\begin{array}{c}\text{No. live births} \\ \text{(same place and time period)}\end{array}\right)} \times 1{,}000$$

$$\text{Postneonatal mortality rate} = \frac{\left(\begin{array}{c}\text{No. deaths to infants} \\ 28\text{-}365 \text{ days old} \\ \text{(defined place and time period)}\end{array}\right)}{\left(\begin{array}{c}\text{No. live births} \\ \text{(same place and} \\ \text{time period)}\end{array}\right) - \left(\begin{array}{c}\text{No. neonatal deaths} \\ \text{(same place and} \\ \text{time period)}\end{array}\right)} \times 1{,}000$$

The formula for the neonatal mortality rate is obvious, because it closely resembles the formula for the IMR. For the postneonatal mortality rate, however, investigators must keep in mind the criteria for a valid rate, especially the condition that all those counted in the denominator must be at risk for the numerator. Infants born alive are not at risk for dying in the postneonatal period if they die during the neonatal period. The correct denominator for the postneonatal mortality rate is the number of live births *minus* the number of neonatal deaths. When the number of neonatal deaths is small, however, as in the United States, with less than 5 per 1000 live births, the following approximate formula is adequate for most purposes:

$$\text{Approximate postneonatal mortality rate} = $$
$$\text{Infant mortality rate} - \text{Neonatal mortality rate}$$

As a general rule, the neonatal mortality rate reflects the quality of medical services and of maternal prenatal health (e.g., medical conditions, nutrition, smoking, alcohol, drugs), whereas the postneonatal mortality rate reflects the quality of the infant's environment.

5.2.d Perinatal Mortality Rate and Ratio

The use of the IMR has its limitations, not only because the probable causes of death change rapidly as the time since birth increases, but also because the number of infants born alive is influenced by the effectiveness of prenatal care. It is conceivable that an improvement in medical care could actually increase the IMR. This would occur, for example, if the improvement in care kept very sick fetuses viable long enough to be born alive, so that they die after birth and are counted

as infant deaths rather than as stillbirths. To avoid this problem, the **perinatal mortality rate** was developed. The term *perinatal* means "around the time of birth." This rate is defined slightly differently from country to country. In the United States, it is defined as follows:

$$\text{Perinatal mortality rate} =$$
$$\frac{\left(\begin{array}{c}\text{No. stillbirths} \\ \text{(defined place and} \\ \text{time period)}\end{array}\right) + \left(\begin{array}{c}\text{No. deaths to} \\ \text{infants} <7 \text{ days old} \\ \text{(same place and time period)}\end{array}\right)}{\left(\begin{array}{c}\text{No. stillbirths} \\ \text{(same place and} \\ \text{time period)}\end{array}\right) + \left(\begin{array}{c}\text{No. live births} \\ \text{(same place and} \\ \text{time period)}\end{array}\right)} \times 1{,}000$$

In this formula, stillbirths are included in the numerator to capture deaths that occur around the time of birth. Stillbirths are also included in the denominator because of the criteria for a valid rate. Specifically, all fetuses that reach the 28th week of gestation are at risk for late fetal death or live birth.

An approximation of the perinatal mortality rate is the **perinatal mortality ratio,** in which the denominator does not include stillbirths. In another variation, the numerator uses neonatal deaths instead of deaths at less than 7 days of life (also called *hebdomadal* deaths). The primary use of the perinatal mortality rate is to evaluate the care of pregnant women before and during delivery, as well as the care of mothers and their infants in the immediate postpartum period.

The concept of **perinatal periods of risk** focuses on perinatal deaths and their excess over the deaths expected in low-risk populations. Fetuses born dead with a birth weight of 500 to 1499 g constitute one group, for which *maternal health* would be investigated. Such cases are followed up to examine community and environmental factors that predispose to immaturity. Fetuses born dead with a birth weight of 1500 g or more constitute another group, for which *maternal care* is examined. For neonatal deaths involving birth weights of 1500 g or more, *care during labor and delivery* is studied. For postneonatal deaths of 1500 g or more, *infant care* is studied. Although this is a promising approach to community analysis, its ultimate value has yet to be fully established.

5.2.e Maternal Mortality Rate

Although generally considered a normal biologic process, pregnancy unquestionably puts considerable strain on women and places them at risk for numerous hazards they would not usually face otherwise, such as hemorrhage, infection, and toxemia of pregnancy. Pregnancy also complicates the course of other conditions, such as heart disease, diabetes, and tuberculosis. A useful measure of the progress of a nation in providing adequate nutrition and medical care for pregnant women is the **maternal mortality rate,** calculated as follows:

$$\text{Maternal mortality rate} =$$
$$\frac{\left(\begin{array}{c}\text{No. pregnancy-related deaths} \\ \text{(defined place and time period)}\end{array}\right)}{\left(\begin{array}{c}\text{No. live births} \\ \text{(same place and time period)}\end{array}\right)} \times 100{,}000$$

The equation is based on the number of **pregnancy-related** (puerperal) deaths. In cases of accidental injury or homicide, however, the death of a woman who is pregnant or has recently delivered is not usually considered "pregnancy related." Technically, the denominator of the equation should be the number of pregnancies rather than live births, but for simplicity, the number of live births is used to estimate the number of pregnancies. The constant multiplier used is typically 100,000, because in recent decades the maternal mortality rate in many developed countries has declined to less than 1 per 10,000 live births. Nevertheless, the US maternal mortality rate in 2014 was 18 per 100,000 live births, higher than 1 per 10,000. Of note, the 2011-2014 rate was lower for white Americans (12.4) than for all other races, with African American women experiencing a much higher maternal mortality rate of 40.0 per 100,000 live births.[7]

6. SUMMARY

Much of the data for epidemiologic studies of public health are collected routinely by various levels of government and made available to local, state, federal, and international groups. The United States and most other countries undertake a complete population census on a periodic basis, with the US census occurring every 10 years. Community-wide epidemiologic measurement depends on accurate determination and reporting of the following:

- Numerator data, especially events such as births, deaths, becoming ill (incident cases), and recovering from illness
- Denominator data, especially the population census

Prevalence data are determined by surveys. These types of data are used to create community rates and ratios for planning and evaluating health progress. The collection of such data is the responsibility of individual countries. Most countries report their data to the United Nations, which publishes large compendia online.

To be valid, a rate must meet certain criteria with respect to the denominator and numerator. First, all the people counted in the denominator must have been at risk for the events counted in the numerator. Second, all the events counted in the numerator must have happened to people included in the denominator. Before rates can be compared, the numerators for all groups in the comparison must be defined or diagnosed in the same way; the constant multipliers in use must be the same; and the time intervals under study must be the same.

Box 2.3 provides definitions of the basic epidemiologic concepts and measurements discussed in this chapter. Box 2.4 lists the equations for the most commonly used population rates.

BOX 2.3 Definitions of Basic Epidemiologic Concepts and Measurements

Incidence (incident cases): The frequency (number) of new occurrences of disease, injury, or death—that is, the number of transitions from well to ill, from uninjured to injured, or from alive to dead—in the study population during the time period being examined.

Point prevalence (prevalent cases): The number of persons in a defined population who had a specified disease or condition at a particular point in time, usually the time a survey was done.

Period prevalence: The number of persons who had a specified disease at any time during a specified time interval. Period prevalence is the sum of the point prevalence at the beginning of the interval plus the incidence during the interval. Because period prevalence combines incidence and prevalence, it must be used with extreme care.

Incidence density: The frequency (density) of new events per person-time (e.g., person-months or person-years). Incidence density is especially useful when the event of interest (e.g., colds, otitis media, myocardial infarction) can occur in a person more than once during the period of study.

Cohort: A clearly defined group of persons studied over a period of time to determine the incidence of death, disease, or injury.

Risk: The proportion of persons who are unaffected at the beginning of a study period, but who undergo the risk event (death, disease, or injury) during the study period.

Rate: The frequency (number) of new events that occur in a defined time period, divided by the average population at risk. Often, the midperiod population is used as the average number of persons at risk (see *Incidence rate*). Because a rate is almost always less than 1.0 (unless everybody dies or has the risk event), a constant multiplier is used to increase the numerator and the denominator to make the rate easier to think about and discuss.

Incidence rate: A rate calculated as the number of incident cases (see *Rate*) over a defined study period, divided by the population at risk at the midpoint of that study period. Rates of the occurrence of births, deaths, and new diseases all are forms of an incidence rate.

Prevalence rate: The proportion (usually expressed as a percentage) of a population that has a defined disease or condition at a particular point in time. Although usually called a rate, it is truly a proportion.

Crude rates: Rates that apply to an entire population, with no reference to characteristics of the individuals in the population. Crude rates are generally not useful for comparisons because populations may differ greatly in composition, particularly with respect to age.

Specific rates: Rates that are calculated after a population has been categorized into groups with a particular characteristic. Examples include age-specific rates and gender-specific rates. Specific rates generally are needed for valid comparisons.

BOX 2.3 Definitions of Basic Epidemiologic Concepts and Measurements—cont'd

Standardized (adjusted) rates: Crude rates that have been modified (adjusted) to control for the effects of age or other characteristics and allow for more valid comparisons of rates.

Direct standardization: The preferred method of standardization if the specific rates come from large populations and the needed data are available. The direct method of standardizing death rates, for example, applies the age distribution of some population—the standard population—to the actual age-specific death rates of the different populations to be compared. This removes the bias that occurs if an old population is compared with a young population.

Indirect standardization: The method of standardization used when the populations to be compared are small (so that age-specific death rates are unstable) or when age-specific death rates are unavailable from one or more populations but data

concerning the age distribution and the crude death rate are available. Here standard death rates (from the standard population) are applied to the corresponding age groups in the different population or populations to be studied. The result is an "expected" (standardized crude) death rate for each population under study. These expected values are those that would have been expected if the standard death rates had been true for the populations under study. Then the standardized mortality ratio is calculated.

Standardized mortality ratio (SMR): The observed crude death rate divided by the expected crude death rate. The SMR generally is multiplied by 100, with the standard population having a value of 100. If the SMR is greater than 100, the **force of mortality** is higher in the study population than in the standard population. If the SMR is less than 100, the force of mortality is lower in the study population than in the standard population.

BOX 2.4 Equations[a] for the Most Commonly Used Rates From Population Data

(1) $\text{Crude birth rate} = \dfrac{\text{No. live births (defined place and time period)}}{\text{Midperiod population (same place and time period)}} \times 1{,}000$

(2) $\text{Crude death rate} = \dfrac{\text{No. deaths (defined place and time period)}}{\text{Midperiod population (same place and time period)}} \times 1{,}000$

(3) $\text{Age-specific death rate} = \dfrac{\text{No deaths to people in a particular age group (defined place and time period)}}{\text{Midperiod population (same age group, place, and time period)}} \times 1{,}000$

(4) $\text{Cause-specific death rate} = \dfrac{\text{No deaths due to a particular cause (defined place and time period)}}{\text{Midperiod population (same place and time period)}} \times 100{,}000$

(5) $\text{Infant mortality rate} = \dfrac{\text{No. deaths to infants} <1 \text{ year old (defined place and time period)}}{\text{No. live births (same place and time period)}} \times 1{,}000$

(6) $\text{Neonatal mortality rate} = \dfrac{\text{No. deaths to infants} <28 \text{ days old (defined place and time period)}}{\text{No. live births (same place and time period)}} \times 1{,}000$

(7) $\text{Postneonatal mortality rate} = \dfrac{\text{No. deaths to infants } 28-365 \text{ days old (defined place and time period)}}{\text{No. live births (same place and time period)} - \text{No. neonatal deaths (same place and time period)}} \times 1{,}000$

(8) Approximate postneonatal mortality rate = Infant mortality rate − Neonatal mortality rate

(9) $\text{Perinatal mortality rate}^{a} = \dfrac{\text{No. stillbirths (defined place and time period)} + \text{No deaths to infants} <7 \text{ days old (same place and time period)}}{\text{No. stillbirths (same place and time period)} + \text{No. live births (same place and time period)}} \times 1{,}000$

(10) $\text{Maternal mortality rate} = \dfrac{\text{No. pregnancy-related deaths (defined place and time period)}}{\text{No. live births (same place and time period)}} \times 100{,}000$

[a]Several similar formulas are in use around the world.

REFERENCES

1. *State Statistics: State-specific 2015 BRFSS Arthritis Prevalence Estimates.* Available at: https://www.cdc.gov/arthritis/data_statistics/state-data-current.htm. Accessed on May 18, 2019.
2. Kann L, McManus T, Harris WA, et al. Youth risk behavior surveillance—United States, 2017. *MMWR Surveill Summ.* 2018;67:S1-S114. doi:10.15585/mmwr.ss6708a1.
3. Fang J, Keenan NL, Ayala C, et al. Awareness of stroke warning symptoms—13 states and the District of Columbia, 2005. *MMWR.* 2008;57:481-485.
4. Chan CK, Feinstein AR, Jekel JF, Wells CK. The value and hazards of standardization in clinical epidemiologic research. *J Clin Epidemiol.* 1988;41:1125-1134.
5. Becker TM, Wiggins CL, Key CR, Samet JM. Symptoms, signs, and ill-defined conditions: a leading cause of death among minorities. *Am J Epidemiol.* 1990;131:664-668.
6. Burnand B, Feinstein AR. The role of diagnostic inconsistency in changing rates of occurrence for coronary heart disease. *J Clin Epidemiol.* 1992;45:929-940.
7. *Pregnancy Mortality Surveillance System.* Available at: https://www.cdc.gov/reproductivehealth/maternalinfanthealth/pregnancy-mortality-surveillance-system.htm?CDC_AA_refVal=https%3A%2F%2Fwww.cdc.gov%2Freproductivehealth%2Fmaternalinfanthealth%2Fpmss.html. Accessed May 18, 2019.

SELECT READINGS

Brookmeyer R, Stroup DF. *Monitoring the Health of Populations: Statistical Principles and Methods for Public Health Surveillance.* New York, NY: Oxford University Press; 2004.
Elandt-Johnson RC. Definition of rates: some remarks on their use and misuse. *Am J Epidemiol.* 1975;102:267-271. [Risks, rates, and ratios.]

REVIEW QUESTIONS

1. A study involves tracking a condition that can recur in individuals over time (e.g., "heartburn" or dyspepsia). Which of the following measures would allow the authors of the study to make full use of their collected data?
   A. Attributable risk
   B. Incidence density
   C. Period prevalence
   D. Point prevalence
   E. Proportional hazards

2. During a given year, 12 cases of disease X are detected in a population of 70,000 college students when those 12 students present for medical attention. Many more students have mild symptoms of the disease and do not seek care. Of the 12 detected cases, 7 result in death. The ratio of 7/12 represents:
   A. The case fatality ratio
   B. The crude death rate
   C. The pathogenicity
   D. The standardized mortality ratio
   E. 1–prevalence

3. In regard to question 2, to report the incidence rate of disease X, it would be necessary to know:
   A. Nothing more than the data provided
   B. The pathogenicity
   C. The infectiousness of the disease
   D. The duration of the clinical illness
   E. The midyear population at risk

4. In regard to question 2, to report the prevalence of disease X, it would be necessary to know:
   A. The cure rate
   B. The duration of illness
   C. The number of cases at a given time
   D. The number of losses to follow-up
   E. The rate at which new cases developed

5. This is calculated after the two populations to be compared are "given" the same age distribution, which is applied to the observed age-specific death rates of each population.
   A. Age-specific death rate
   B. Case fatality ratio
   C. Cause-specific death rate
   D. Crude birth rate
   E. Direct standardization of death rate
   F. Incidence rate
   G. Indirect standardization of death rate
   H. Infant mortality rate
   I. Prevalence rate
   J. Standardized mortality ratio
   K. Standardized rate

6. This is the number of new cases over a defined study period, divided by the midperiod population at risk.
   A. Age-specific death rate
   B. Case fatality ratio
   C. Cause-specific death rate
   D. Crude birth rate
   E. Direct standardization of death rate
   F. Incidence rate
   G. Indirect standardization of death rate
   H. Infant mortality rate
   I. Prevalence rate
   J. Standardized mortality ratio
   K. Standardized rate

7. This is used if age-specific death rates are unavailable in the population whose crude death rate is to be adjusted.
   A. Age-specific death rate
   B. Case fatality ratio
   C. Cause-specific death rate
   D. Crude birth rate
   E. Direct standardization of death rate
   F. Incidence rate
   G. Indirect standardization of death rate
   H. Infant mortality rate
   I. Prevalence rate

J. Standardized mortality ratio

K. Standardized rate

8. This is the observed total deaths in a population, divided by the expected deaths in that population, multiplied by 100.
   A. Age-specific death rate
   B. Case fatality ratio
   C. Cause-specific death rate
   D. Crude birth rate
   E. Direct standardization of death rate
   F. Incidence rate
   G. Indirect standardization of death rate
   H. Infant mortality rate
   I. Prevalence rate
   J. Standardized mortality ratio
   K. Standardized rate

9. This is useful for studying trends in the causes of death over time.
   A. Age-specific death rate
   B. Case fatality ratio
   C. Cause-specific death rate
   D. Crude birth rate
   E. Direct standardization of death rate
   F. Incidence rate
   G. Indirect standardization of death rate
   H. Infant mortality rate
   I. Prevalence rate
   J. Standardized mortality ratio
   K. Standardized rate

10. This is often used as an overall index of the health status of a country.
    A. Age-specific death rate
    B. Case fatality ratio
    C. Cause-specific death rate
    D. Crude birth rate
    E. Direct standardization of death rate
    F. Incidence rate
    G. Indirect standardization of death rate
    H. Infant mortality rate
    I. Prevalence rate
    J. Standardized mortality ratio
    K. Standardized rate

ANSWERS AND EXPLANATIONS

1. **B.** Incidence density is a measure reported in terms of the frequency (density) of a condition per person-time (e.g., person-days, person-months, or person-years). It is a composite measure of the number of individuals observed and the period of observation contributed by each. For example, 10 individuals observed for 1 year each would represent 10 person-years of observation. One individual observed for 10 years would also represent 10 person-years of observation. Incidence density allows all data to be captured and reported, even when some individuals are lost to follow-up before the end of the observation period. Thus the measure allows investigators to make full use of their data without losses of information inevitable with less-inclusive metrics. Incident density is particularly useful when an event can recur in an individual during the observation period. In contrast, period prevalence (C) and point prevalence (D) fail to capture recurrent events over time because they describe events only during a given period (period prevalence) or at a given point in time (point prevalence). An individual with multiple recurrences of a condition would be indistinguishable from an individual having only a single occurrence with these metrics. Proportional hazards (E) is a statistical method used to characterize the effects of multiple variables on the risk of a binary outcome, such as survival. Attributable risk (A) expresses the extent to which a single factor is responsible for a particular outcome in a population.

2. **A.** The case fatality ratio for a particular condition is the number of deaths caused by the condition, divided by the total number of identified cases of the condition in a specified population. In this example, the case fatality ratio is 7/12, which, expressed as a percentage, is 58.3%. The crude death rate (B) is the number of deaths caused by the condition, divided by the midperiod population. Pathogenicity (C) is indicated by the proportion of infected persons with clinical illness. The standardized mortality ratio (D) is the number of observed deaths in a population subgroup, divided by the expected deaths based on a reference population. The term (1−prevalence) is not meaningful (D).

3. **E.** The incidence rate is the number of new cases in a specified population, during a specified period, divided by the midperiod population at risk. In the information provided in question 2, it does not say whether 70,000 represents the population at the midpoint or at the beginning of the observation period, and it does not say whether the entire population is at risk for disease X. Sometimes, incidence rates are based on the total population, although not everyone is at risk, because there is no convenient way to distinguish the susceptible from the immune population. An example would be incidence rates of hepatitis B in the United States; only the unimmunized population would truly be at risk, but the rate might be reported with the total population in the denominator.

4. **C.** By definition, the prevalence of a condition is the number of cases in a specified population at a particular time. If this information is known, nothing else is required to report the prevalence. The prevalence is influenced by the duration of illness (B), the cure or recovery rate (A), the cause-specific death rate, and by immigration and emigration. These are

factors that influence the number of cases in the study population at any particular time. The number of losses to follow-up (D) and the rate at which new cases develop (E) are not needed to report a prevalence; these have more to do with incidence metrics.

5. **E.** In direct standardization the age-specific death rates (ASDRs) are available for the populations to be compared. The age distribution of a hypothetical "standard" population (often consisting of the sum of the populations under comparison) is derived. The ASDRs from each of the populations are applied to the hypothetical age distribution, and these summary rates may be compared because they are free of age bias. Crude death rates may be low in developing countries because the population is relatively young; standardization helps correct age bias to better represent the data.

6. **F.** Incidence, or incident cases, is merely the number of new cases. To generate a rate, the number of new cases over a specified period is divided by the population at risk at the midpoint of the study period (recall the differences between risks and rates) and multiplied by a constant, such as 1,000 or 100,000, to facilitate expression.

7. **G.** When the age-specific death rates are unknown for the populations to be compared, direct standardization of rates is not feasible. Indirect standardization applies the death rates from a reference (e.g., US) population to the study populations. The reference rates are applied to the age distribution of the study populations, and the number of deaths expected in each group is calculated by assigning the reference

population mortality rates to the study population. The actual number of deaths in the study groups is compared with the expected number of deaths if they had the same age-specific death rates as the reference population.

8. **J.** The standardized mortality ratio is often derived from indirect standardization methods. The observed number of deaths in a population is divided by the expected number of deaths in that population, based on the reference population. The numerator and denominator usually are multiplied by 100 to avoid describing the ratio as a fraction.

9. **C.** For rates to be compared, the denominators (or populations) must be comparable. To compare events that are similar, the numerators must be defined in the same way. Cause-specific rates provide numerator data based on comparable diagnosis. Death rates may be similar in two populations, but the deaths may be caused by different conditions, with differing implications for public health management. Cause-specific rates would be useful in attempting to set priorities for funding of public health resources.

10. **H.** The infant mortality rate (IMR) is influenced by various aspects of maternal and fetal care, including nutrition, access to prenatal medical care, maternal substance abuse, the home environment, and social support networks; it is often used as an overall index of a country's health status. If infants are able to thrive, the overall health of a nation is thought to be adequate, whereas if infants are failing, and the resulting IMR is high, and the overall health of a nation is thought to be poor.

Epidemiologic Surveillance and Epidemic Outbreak Investigation

"Vaccines and antibiotics have made diseases a thing of the past; we've come to expect that public health and modern science can conquer all microbes. But nature is a formidable adversary."

Tom Frieden

This chapter describes the importance of disease surveillance and early identification of epidemics. Epidemics, or disease outbreaks, are defined as the occurrence of disease at an unusual or unexpected, elevated frequency. Reliable surveillance to define the usual rates of disease in an area is necessary before rates that are considerably elevated can be identified.

1. SURVEILLANCE OF DISEASE

1.1 RESPONSIBILITY FOR SURVEILLANCE

Surveillance is the entire process of collecting, analyzing, interpreting, and reporting data on the incidence of death, diseases, and injuries and the prevalence of certain conditions. Knowledge gained by surveillance is important for promoting and safeguarding public health. Surveillance is generally considered the foundation of disease control efforts. In the United States the Centers for Disease Control and Prevention (CDC) is the federal agency responsible for the surveillance of most types of acute diseases and the investigation of outbreaks. The CDC conducts surveillance if requested by a state or if an outbreak has the potential to affect more than one state. Data for disease surveillance are passed from local and state governments to the CDC, which evaluates the data and works with the state and local agencies regarding further investigation and control of any problems discovered.

According to the US Constitution, the federal government has jurisdiction over matters concerning interstate commerce, including disease outbreaks with interstate implications (outbreaks that originated in one state and have spread to other states or have the potential to do so). Each state government has jurisdiction over disease outbreaks with intrastate implications (outbreaks confined within one state's borders). If a disease outbreak has interstate implications, the CDC is a first responder and takes immediate action, rather than waiting for a request for assistance from a state government.

The World Health Organization (WHO) is a specialized agency of the United Nations concerned with international public health. Since its creation in 1948, the WHO has played a leading role in the eradication of smallpox. Its current priorities include communicable diseases such as human immunodeficiency virus (HIV)/acquired immunodeficiency syndrome (AIDS), Ebola, malaria, and tuberculosis.

1.2　CREATING A SURVEILLANCE SYSTEM

The development of a surveillance system requires clear objectives regarding the diseases or conditions to be covered (e.g., infectious diseases, side effects of vaccines, elevated lead levels, pneumonia-related deaths in patients with influenza). Also the objectives for each surveillance item should be clear, including surveillance of an infectious disease to determine whether a vaccine program is effective, the search for possible side effects of new vaccines or vaccine programs, and the determination of progress toward meeting health objectives for a particular disease.

The criteria for defining a case of a reportable disease or condition must be known to develop standardized reporting procedures and reporting forms. As discussed later, the case definition usually is based on clinical findings, laboratory results, and epidemiologic data on the time, place, and characteristics of affected persons. The intensity of the planned surveillance (active vs. passive) and duration of the surveillance (ongoing vs. time limited) must be known in advance.

The types of analysis needed (e.g., incidence, prevalence, case fatality ratio, years of potential life lost, quality-adjusted life years, costs) should be stated in advance. In addition, plans should be made for disseminating the findings on the Internet and in other publication venues.

These objectives and methods should be developed with the aid of the investigators charged with collecting, reporting, and using the data. A pilot test should be performed and evaluated in the field, perhaps in one or more demonstration areas, before the full system is attempted. When it is operational, the full system also should be continually evaluated. The CDC has extensive information on surveillance at its website, www.cdc.gov.

1.3　METHODS AND FUNCTIONS OF DISEASE SURVEILLANCE

Surveillance may be either passive or active. Most surveillance conducted on a routine basis is passive surveillance. In passive surveillance, physicians, clinics, laboratories, and hospitals required to report disease are given the appropriate forms and instructions, with the expectation that they will record all cases of reportable disease that come to their attention. Active surveillance, on the other hand, requires periodic (usually weekly) telephone calls, electronic contact, or personal visits to the reporting individuals and institutions to obtain the required data. Active surveillance is more labor intensive and costly, so it is seldom done routinely.

The percentage of patients with reportable diseases that are actually reported to public health authorities varies considerably.[1] One group estimated that the percentage reported to state-based passive reporting systems in the United States varied from 30% to 62% of cases.

Sometimes a change in medical care practice uncovers a previously invisible disease surveillance issue. For example, a hospital in Connecticut began reporting many cases of pharyngeal gonorrhea in young children. This apparently localized outbreak in one hospital was investigated by a rapid response team, which included Dr. Jekel, an original author of this textbook, who discovered that the cases began to appear only after the hospital started examining all throat cultures in children for gonococci and beta-hemolytic streptococci.[2]

In contrast to infectious diseases, the reporting of most other diseases, injuries, and conditions is less likely to be rapid or nationwide, and the associated surveillance systems tend to develop on a problem-by-problem basis. As discussed in Chapter 24, several states and regions have cancer registries, but the United States has no national cancer registry. Fatal diseases can be monitored to some extent by death certificates, but such diagnoses are often inaccurate, and reporting is seldom rapid enough for the detection of disease outbreaks. (The reporting systems for occupational and environmental diseases and injuries are discussed in Section 3 of this book.)

1.3.a.　Establishment of Baseline Data

Usual (baseline) rates and patterns of diseases can be known only if there is a regular reporting and surveillance system. Epidemiologists study the patterns of diseases by the time and geographic location of cases and the characteristics of the persons involved. Continued surveillance allows epidemiologists to detect deviations from the usual pattern of data, which prompt them to explore whether an epidemic (i.e., an unusual incidence of disease) is occurring or whether other factors (e.g., alterations in reporting practices) are responsible for the observed changes.

1.3.b.　Evaluation of Time Trends

The implications of secular (or long-term) trends in disease are usually different from those of outbreaks or epidemics and often carry greater significance. Fig. 3.1 shows that the number of reported cases of salmonellosis serotype Agona in the United Sates increased during the 1970s followed by a decrease over time with one brief increase in the late 1990s. The first question to ask about secular trends is whether the trend can be explained by changes in disease detection, disease reporting, or both, as is frequently the case when an apparent outbreak of a disease is reported. The announcement of a real or suspected outbreak may increase suspicion among physicians practicing in the community and thus lead to increased diagnosis and increased reporting of diagnosed cases. A long-term increase in a disease in one US region, particularly when it is related to a single serotype, is usually of greater public health significance than a localized outbreak, because it suggests the existence of a more widespread problem.

Fig. 3.2 shows a rise in the reported incidence and mortality from an Ebola outbreak in 2014. The data in this figure are presented in a semilogarithmic graph, with a logarithmic scale used for the (vertical) y-axis and an arithmetic scale for the (horizontal) x-axis. The figure illustrates one advantage of using a logarithmic scale: the lines showing incidence and mortality trace an approximately parallel rise. On a logarithmic scale, this means that the rise in rates is proportional, so the percentage of cases resulting in death—that is, the case fatality ratio—remains relatively constant over the time shown.

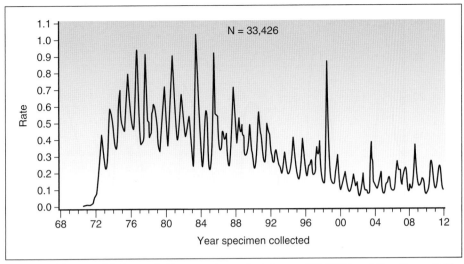

Fig. 3.1 Rate of Reported Salmonella Serotype Agona Isolates per 100,000 Population, 3-month Moving Average, by Month and Year, 1968–2011 (N=33,426). (Data from Centers for Disease Control and Prevention: *An atlas of salmonella in the United States, 1968–2011: laboratory-based enteric disease surveillance*, Atlanta, 2013, US Department of Health and Human Services. https://www.cdc.gov/salmonella/pdf/salmonella-atlas-508c.pdf.)

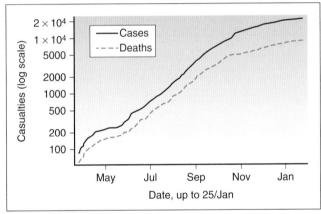

Fig. 3.2 Incidence Rates and Mortality Rates for Ebola Outbreak in 2014. (Data from https://www.sciencedaily.com/releases/2015/02/150206111704.htm.)

Seasonal variation. Many infectious diseases show a strong seasonal variation, with periods of highest incidence usually depending on the route of spread. To determine the usual number of cases or rates of disease, epidemiologists must therefore incorporate any expected seasonal variation into their calculations.

Infectious diseases that are spread by the respiratory route, such as influenza, colds, measles, and varicella (chickenpox), have a much higher incidence in the winter and early spring in the Northern Hemisphere. Fig. 3.3 shows historical data on the seasonal variation for varicella in the United States, by month, over a 6-year period. Notice the peaks after January and before summer of each year. Such a pattern was thought to occur during these months because people spent most of their time close together indoors, where the air changes slowly. The drying of mucous membranes, which occurs in winter because of low humidity and indoor heating, may also play a role in promoting respiratory infections. Since the

introduction of varicella vaccine, this seasonal pattern has been largely eliminated.

Diseases that are spread by insect or arthropod vectors (e.g., viral encephalitis from mosquitoes) have a strong predilection for the summer or early autumn. Lyme disease, spread by *Ixodes* ticks, is usually acquired in the late spring or summer, a pattern explained by the seasonally related life cycle of the ticks and the outdoor activity of people wearing less protective clothing during warmer months.

Infectious diseases that are spread by the fecal-oral route are most common in the summer, partly because of the ability of the organisms to multiply more rapidly in food and water during warm weather. The peak frequency of outbreaks attributable to drinking water occurs from May to August, whereas the peak for outbreaks attributable to recreational water (e.g., lakes, rivers, swimming pools) occurs from June to October. Fig. 3.4 shows a late-summer peak for aseptic meningitis, which is usually caused by viral infection spread by the fecal-oral route or by insects.

Because the peaks of different disease patterns occur at different times, the CDC sometimes illustrates the incidence of diseases by using an "epidemiologic year." In contrast to the calendar year, which runs from January 1 of one year to December 31 of the same year, the epidemiologic year for a given disease runs from the month of lowest incidence in one year to the same month in the next year. The advantage of using the epidemiologic year when plotting the incidence of a disease is that it puts the high-incidence months near the center of a graph and avoids having the high-incidence peak split between the two ends of the graph, as would occur with many respiratory diseases if they were graphed for a calendar year.

Other types of variation. Health problems can vary by the day of the week; Fig. 3.5 shows that recreational drowning

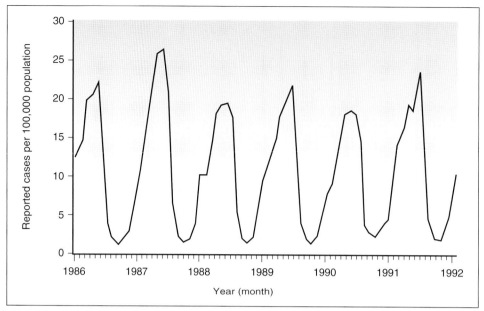

Fig. 3.3 Historical Incidence Rates of Varicella (Chickenpox) in the United States, by Month of Report, **1986–1992.** (Data from Centers for Disease Control and Prevention: Summary of notifiable diseases, United States, 1992. *MMWR* 41:53, 1992.)

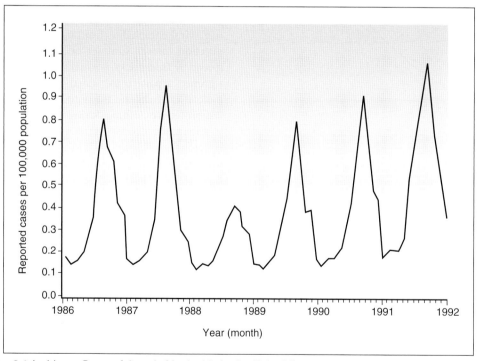

Fig. 3.4 Incidence Rates of Aseptic Meningitis in the United States, by Month of Report, 1986–1992. (Data from Centers for Disease Control and Prevention: Summary of notifiable diseases, United States, 1992. *MMWR* 41:20, 1992.)

occurs more frequently on weekends than on weekdays, presumably because more people engage in water recreation on weekends.

1.3.c. Identification and Documentation of Outbreaks

An epidemic, or disease outbreak, is the occurrence of disease at an unusual (or unexpected) frequency. Because the word

epidemic tends to create fear in a population, that term usually is reserved for a problem of wider than local implications, and the term *outbreak* typically is used for a localized epidemic. Nevertheless, the two terms often are used interchangeably.

It is possible to determine that the level of a disease is unusual only if the usual rates of the disease are known and

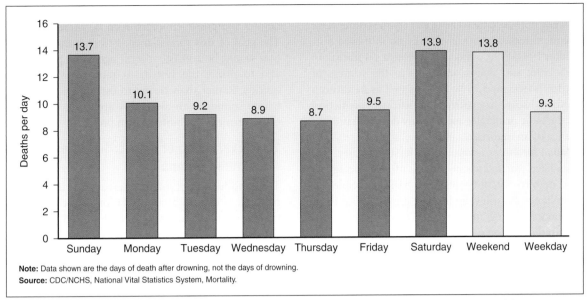

Note: Data shown are the days of death after drowning, not the days of drowning.
Source: CDC/NCHS, National Vital Statistics System, Mortality.

Fig. 3.5 Average Number of Deaths per Day from Unintentional Drowning, by Day of Week: United States, 1999–2010. (Data from https://www.cdc.gov/nchs/products/databriefs/db149.htm.)

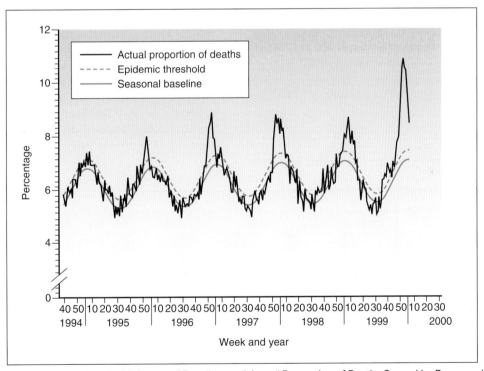

Fig. 3.6 Epidemic Threshold, Seasonal Baseline, and Actual Proportion of Deaths Caused by Pneumonia and Influenza in 122 Us Cities, 1994–2000. The epidemic threshold is 1.645 standard deviations above the seasonal baseline. The expected seasonal baseline is projected using a robust regression procedure in which a periodic regression model is applied to observed percentages of deaths from pneumonia and influenza since 1983. (Data from Centers for Disease Control and Prevention: Update: influenza activity—United States and worldwide, 1999–2000. *MMWR* 49:174, 2000.)

reliable surveillance shows that current rates are considerably elevated. For example, to determine when and where influenza and pneumonia outbreaks occur, the CDC uses a seasonally adjusted *expected* percentage of influenza and pneumonia deaths in the United States and a number called the epidemic threshold to compare with the reported percentage. (Pneumonias are included because influenza-induced pneumonias may be signed out on the death certificate as "pneumonia," with no mention of influenza.)

Fig. 3.6 provides data concerning the expected percentage of deaths caused by pneumonia and influenza in 122 US cities. The lower *(solid)* sine wave is the seasonal baseline, which is the expected percentage of pneumonia and influenza deaths per week in these cities. The upper *(dashed)* sine wave is the epidemic threshold, with essentially no influenza outbreak in winter 1994-1995, a moderate influenza outbreak in winter 1995-1996, and major outbreaks in the winters of 1996-1997, 1997-1998, and 1998-1999, as well as in autumn 1999. No other disease has such a sophisticated prediction model, but the basic principles apply to any determination of the occurrence of an outbreak.

Surveillance for bioterrorism. For at least a century, epidemiologists have worried about the use of biologic agents for military or terrorist purposes. The basic principles of disease surveillance are still valid in these domains, but there are special concerns worth mentioning. The most important need is for rapid detection of a problem. With regard to bioterrorism, special surveillance techniques are being developed to enable rapid detection of major increases in the most likely biologic agents[3] (Box 3.1). Detection is made more difficult if the disease is scattered over a wide geographic area, as with the anthrax outbreak in the United States after terrorist attacks in late 2001.

BOX 3.1   Example Diseases Considered Major Threats for Bioterrorism

Anthrax
Botulism
Brucellosis
Plague
Smallpox
Tularemia (inhalational)
Viral hemorrhagic fevers

A technique developed for more rapid detection of epidemics and possible bioterrorism is syndromic surveillance.[3] The goal of this surveillance is to characterize "syndromes" that would be consistent with agents of particular concern and to prime the system to report any such syndromes quickly. Rather than trying to establish a specific diagnosis before sounding an alert, this approach might provide an early warning of a bioterrorism problem.

1.3.d. Evaluation of Public Health and Disease Interventions

The introduction of major interventions intended to change patterns of disease in a population, especially the introduction of new vaccines, should be followed by surveillance to determine if the intended changes were achieved. Fig. 3.7 shows historical data on the impact of the two types of polio vaccine—the inactivated (Salk) vaccine and the oral (Sabin) vaccine—on the reported incident cases of poliomyelitis. The large graph in this figure has a logarithmic scale on the *y*-axis. It is used here because the decline in the poliomyelitis incidence rate was so steep that on an arithmetic scale, no detail would be visible at the bottom after the early 1960s. A logarithmic scale compresses the high rates on a graph compared with the lower rates, so that the detail of the latter can be seen.

Fig. 3.7 shows that after the inactivated vaccine was introduced in 1955, the rates of paralytic disease declined quickly. The public tended to think the problem had gone away, and many parents became less concerned about immunizing newborns. Because the inactivated vaccine did not provide herd immunity, however, the unimmunized infants were at great risk. A recurrent poliomyelitis spike occurred in 1958

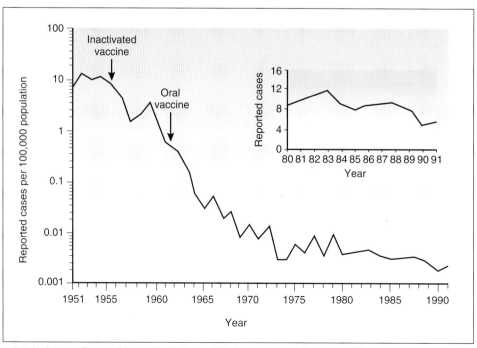

Fig. 3.7 Incidence Rates of Paralytic Poliomyelitis in the United States, by Year of Report, 1951–1991. (Data from Centers for Disease Control and Prevention: Summary of notifiable diseases, United States, 1991. *MMWR* 40:37, 1991.)

and 1959, when most of the new cases of paralytic poliomyelitis were in young children who had not been immunized. The rates declined again in 1960 and thereafter because the public was shaken out of its complacency to obtain vaccine and because a newer oral vaccine was introduced. This live, attenuated oral vaccine provided both herd immunity and individual immunity (see Fig. 1.2).

The failure of a vaccine to produce satisfactory immunity or the failure of people to use the vaccine can be detected by one of the following:

- A lack of change in disease rates
- An increase in disease rates after an initial decrease, as in the previous example of the polio vaccine
- An increase in disease rates in a recently vaccinated group, as occurred after the use of defective lots of inactivated polio vaccine in the 1950s

The importance of postmarketing surveillance was underscored through continued evaluation and close surveillance of measles rates in the United States. Investigators were able to detect the failure of the initial measles vaccines and vaccination schedules to provide long-lasting protection (see Chapter 1). Research into this problem led to a new set of recommendations for immunization against measles. According to CDC recommendations, two doses of measles vaccine should be administered to young children. The first dose should be given when the child is 12 to 15 months old (to avoid a higher failure rate if given earlier) and the second dose when the child is 4 to 6 years old, before school entry.[4] A third dose at about age 18 is also recommended.

With regard to medications, the importance of postmarketing surveillance was affirmed by the discovery of an increased incidence of cardiovascular events in people who took newly introduced cyclooxygenase-2 (COX-2) inhibitors. The discovery resulted in some COX-2 inhibitors being removed from the market.

1.3.e. Setting of Disease Control Priorities

Data on the patterns of diseases for the current time and recent past can help government and volunteer agencies establish priorities for disease control efforts. This is not a simple counting procedure. A disease is of more concern if its rates increase rapidly, as with AIDS in the 1980s or Ebola in 2014-2015, than if its rates are steady or declining. The severity of the disease is a critical feature, which usually can be established by good surveillance. AIDS received high priority because surveillance demonstrated its severity and its potential for epidemic spread.

1.3.f. Study of Changing Patterns of Disease

By studying the patterns of occurrence of a particular disease over time in populations and subpopulations, epidemiologists can better understand the changing patterns of the disease. Data derived from the surveillance of syphilis cases in New York City during the 1980s, when crack cocaine came into common use, proved valuable in suggesting the source of changing patterns of acquired and congenital syphilis. As shown in Fig. 3.8, the reported number of cases of primary

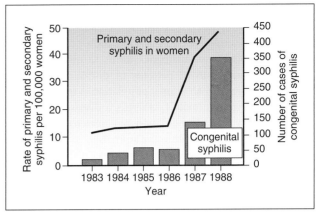

Fig. 3.8 Incidence of Congenital Syphilis in Infants Younger than 1 Year *(Bars)* and Incidence of Primary and Secondary Syphilis in Women *(Line)* in New York City, by Year of Report, 1983–1988. (Data from Centers for Disease Control and Prevention: Congenital syphilis, New York City, 1983–1988. *MMWR* 38:825, 1989.)

and secondary syphilis among women increased substantially beginning in 1987. Both this trend and the concurrent increase in congenital syphilis were strongly associated with women's use of crack (trading sex for drugs) and with their lack of prenatal care (a situation that allowed their syphilis to go undetected and untreated).

A new pattern of occurrence may be more ominous than a mere increase in the incidence of a disease. In the case of tuberculosis in the United States, yearly incidence decreased steadily from 1953 (when reporting began) until 1985, when 22,201 cases were reported. Thereafter, yearly incidence began to rise again. Of special concern was the association of this rise with the increasing impact of the AIDS epidemic and the increasing resistance of *Mycobacterium tuberculosis* to antimicrobial agents. This concern led to greater efforts to detect tuberculosis in people with AIDS and to use directly observed therapy to prevent antimicrobial resistance. Tuberculosis rates peaked in 1992, when 26,673 cases were reported, and then began declining again.

2. INVESTIGATION OF EPIDEMICS

2.1 NATURE OF EPIDEMICS

The common definition of epidemic is the unusual occurrence of a disease; the term is derived from Greek roots meaning "upon the population." Although people usually think of an epidemic as something that involves large numbers of people, it is possible to name circumstances under which just one case of a disease could be considered an epidemic. Because smallpox has been eliminated worldwide, a single case would represent a smallpox epidemic. Similarly, if a disease has been eradicated from a particular region (e.g., paralytic poliomyelitis in the Western Hemisphere) or if a disease is approaching elimination from an area and has the potential for spread (as with measles in the United States), the report of even one case in the geographic region might be considered unexpected and become a cause for concern.

When a disease in a population occurs regularly and at a relatively constant level, it is said to be endemic, based on Greek roots meaning "within the population."

Epidemiologists use analogous terms to distinguish between usual and unusual patterns of diseases in animals. A disease outbreak in an animal population is said to be epizootic ("upon the animals"), whereas a disease deeply entrenched in an animal population but not changing much is said to be enzootic ("within the animals").

Investigators of acute disease outbreaks ordinarily use a measure of disease frequency called the attack rate, particularly when the period of exposure is short (i.e., considerably <1 year). Rather than being a true rate, the attack rate is really the proportion of exposed persons that becomes ill. It is calculated as follows:

$$\text{Attack rate} = \text{Number of new cases of a disease}/$$
$$\text{Number of persons exposed in a particular outbreak} \times 100$$

In this equation, 100 is used as the constant multiplier so the rate can be expressed as a percentage. (For a discussion of other measures of disease frequency, see Chapter 2.)

2.2 PROCEDURES FOR INVESTIGATING AN EPIDEMIC

The forces for and against the occurrence of disease are usually in equilibrium. If an epidemic occurs, this equilibrium has been disrupted. The goal of investigation is to discover and correct recent changes so the balance can be restored and the epidemic controlled. The physician who is alert to possible epidemics not only would be concerned to give the correct treatment to individual patients, but also would ask, "Why did this patient become sick with this disease at this time and place?"

Outbreak investigation resembles crime investigation; both require "a lot of shoe leather."[5] Although there is no simple way to teach imagination and creativity in the investigation of disease outbreaks, there is an organized way of approaching and interpreting the data that assist in solving problems. This section outlines the series of steps to follow in investigating a disease outbreak, and Box 3.2 provides an example.[6]

2.2.a. Establish the Diagnosis

Establishing the diagnosis may seem obvious, but it is surprising how many people start investigating an outbreak without taking this first step. Many cases are solved just by making the correct diagnosis and showing that the disease occurrence was not unusual after all. A health department in North Carolina received panic calls from several people who were concerned about the occurrence of smallpox in their community. A physician assigned to investigate quickly discovered that the reported case of smallpox was actually a typical case of chickenpox in a young child. The child's mother did not speak English well, and the neighbors heard the word "pox" and panicked. The outbreak was stopped by a correct diagnosis.

2.2.b. Establish Epidemiologic Case Definition

The epidemiologic case definition is the list of specific criteria used to decide whether a person has the disease of concern.

BOX 3.2 Example of an Investigation of an Outbreak by Dr. Jekel, an Original Author of This Textbook

In January 1991 a liberal arts college in New England with a population of about 400 students reported 82 cases of acute gastrointestinal illness, mostly among students, over 102 hours. The college president sought help from local and state health authorities to determine whether the college cafeteria should be closed or the entire college should be closed and the students sent home—an option that would have disrupted the entire academic year.

Initial investigation focused on making a diagnosis. Clinical data suggested that the illness was of short duration, with most students found to be essentially well in 24 hours. The data also suggested that the illness was relatively mild. Only one student was hospitalized, and the need for hospitalization in this case was uncertain. In most cases the symptoms consisted of nausea and vomiting, with minimal or no diarrhea and only mild systemic symptoms, such as headache and malaise. Examination revealed only a low-grade fever. Initial food and stool cultures for pathogenic bacteria yielded negative results.

Based on this information, the investigating team developed a case definition. A case was defined as any person in the college who complained of diarrhea or vomiting between Monday, January 28, and Thursday, January 31. The large percentage of cases over this short time made it clear that the situation was unusual, and that the problem could be considered a disease outbreak.

The people who met the criteria of the case definition included resident students, commuter students, and employees. When the investigating team interviewed some of the affected people, they found that most, but not all, of the resident students had eaten only at the campus cafeteria. The epidemic time curve suggested that if cafeteria food were the source, one or more meals on 2 days in January could have been responsible, although a few cases had occurred before and after the peak of the outbreak (box figure). Near the beginning of the outbreak, two food handlers had worked while feeling ill with gastrointestinal symptoms. Health department records revealed, however, that the school cafeteria had always received high scores for sanitation, and officials who conducted an emergency reinspection of the facilities and equipment during the outbreak found no change. They detected no problem with sanitary procedures, except that the food handlers had worked while not feeling well.

Most of the commuter students with symptoms had brought food from home during the time in question. Almost none of them had eaten at the college cafeteria, although a few had eaten at an independently run snack bar on campus. Further

BOX 3.2 Example of an Investigation of an Outbreak by Dr. Jekel, an Original Author of This Textbook—cont'd

questioning revealed that the family members of several of the affected commuter students also reported a similar illness, either during the weeks preceding the outbreak or concurrent with it. One public school in a nearby town had closed briefly because of a similar illness in most of the students and staff members.

Although a college-wide questionnaire was distributed and analyzed, this process took several days, and the president wanted answers as soon as possible. Within 2 days of being summoned, the investigating team was able to make the following recommendations: the college, including the cafeteria, should remain open; college-wide assemblies and indoor sports events should be canceled for 2 weeks; and no person should be allowed to work as a food handler while ill. To show their confidence in the cafeteria, the members of the investigating team ate lunch there while sitting in a prominent place. The outbreak quickly faded away, and the college schedule was able to proceed more or less normally.

How was the investigating team able to make these recommendations so quickly? Although the epidemic time curve and information gathered from interviews offered numerous clues, past knowledge gained from similar outbreaks, from disease surveillance, and from research on the natural history of diseases all helped the investigators make their recommendations with confidence. In particular, the following observations made the diagnosis of bacterial infection unlikely: the self-limiting, mild course of disease; the lack of reported diarrhea, even though it was in the original case definition; and the fact that no bacterial pathogens could be cultured from the food and stool samples that had been collected. A staphylococcal toxin was considered initially, but the consistent story of a low-grade fever made a toxin unlikely; fever is a sign of infection, but not of an external (ingested) toxin.

The clinical and epidemiologic pattern was most consistent with an outbreak caused by a norovirus (the laboratory demonstration of a norovirus at that time was exceedingly difficult and costly, but we can now use real-time polymerase chain reaction testing). For noroviruses, the fecal-oral route of spread had been demonstrated for food and water, but many outbreaks revealed a pattern that also suggested a respiratory (propagated) route of spread, even though that possibility had not been confirmed. The latter possibility was the reason for suggesting the cancellation of assemblies and indoor sports events.

The outbreak investigation team was comfortable in recommending that the cafeteria remain open, because the commuters who had become ill had not eaten at the cafeteria, and because a similar illness was reported in the surrounding community. These factors made it unlikely that the cafeteria was the only source of infection, although there was a chance that infected food handlers had spread their illness to some people. The short duration and mild nature of the illness meant that there was no need to close the college, although a certain amount of disruption and class absenteeism would likely continue for a few more days.

Continued surveillance was established at the college, and this confirmed that the outbreak was waning. Cultures continued to yield negative results for bacterial pathogens, and analysis of the college-wide questionnaire did not change any conclusions. This outbreak illustrates that even without a definitive diagnosis, epidemiologic analysis enabled the investigators to rule out bacterial food contamination with a high degree of probability. This case also illustrates another principle: the ability of epidemiologic methods, even in the early phase of an outbreak, to guide control methods. In this outbreak, negative evidence (i.e., evidence that showed what the problem was not) permitted epidemiologists to calm a nervous population.

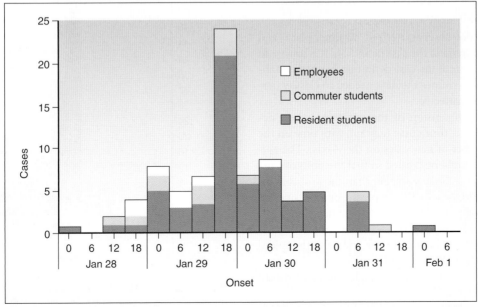

Epidemic Time Curve Showing Onset of Cases of Gastroenteritis at a Small College in New England from January 28 to February 1. The onset is shown in 6-hour periods for dates in January and February.

The case definition is not the same as a clinical diagnosis. Rather, it establishes consistent criteria that enable epidemiologic investigations to proceed before definitive diagnoses are available. Establishing a case definition is especially important if the disease is unknown, as was the case in the early investigations of legionnaires' disease, AIDS, hantavirus pulmonary syndrome, eosinophilia-myalgia syndrome, and severe acute respiratory syndrome. The CDC case definition for eosinophilia-myalgia syndrome included the following:

- A total eosinophil count greater than 1000 cells/μL
- Generalized myalgia (muscle pain) at some point during the course of the illness, of sufficient severity to limit the ability to pursue normal activities
- Exclusion of other neoplastic or infectious conditions that could account for the syndrome

The use of these epidemiologic and clinical criteria assisted in the outbreak investigation. No case definition is perfect because there are always some false positives (i.e., individuals without the disease who are wrongly included in the group considered to have the disease) and false negatives (i.e., diseased individuals wrongly considered to be disease free). Nevertheless, the case definition should be developed carefully and adhered to in the collection and analysis of data. The case definition also permits epidemiologists to make comparisons among the findings from different outbreak investigations.

2.2.c. Is an Epidemic Occurring?

Even if proven, cases must occur in sufficient numbers to constitute an epidemic. As emphasized previously, it is difficult to assess whether the number of cases is high unless the *usual* number is known by ongoing surveillance. It may be assumed, however, that a completely new disease or syndrome meets the criteria for an epidemic.

2.2.d. Characterize Epidemic by Time, Place, and Person

The epidemic should be characterized by time, place, and person, using the criteria in the case definition. It is unwise to start data collection until the case definition has been established, because it determines the data needed to classify persons as affected or unaffected.

Time. The time dimension of the outbreak is best described by an epidemic time curve (a graph with time on the *x*-axis and the number of new cases on the *y*-axis). The epidemic time curve should be created so that the units of time on the *x*-axis are considerably smaller than the probable incubation period, and the *y*-axis is simply the number of cases that became symptomatic during each time unit.

The epidemic time curve provides several important clues about what is happening in an outbreak and helps the epidemiologist answer the following questions:

- What was the type of exposure (single source or spread from person to person)?
- What was the probable route of spread (respiratory, fecal-oral, skin-to-skin contact, exchange of blood or body fluids, or via insect or animal vectors)?

- When were the affected persons exposed? What was the incubation period?
- In addition to primary cases (persons infected initially by a common source), were there secondary cases (person-to-person transmission of disease from primary cases to other persons, often members of the same household)?

In a common source exposure, many people come into contact with the same source, such as contaminated water or food, usually over a short time. If an outbreak is caused by this type of exposure, the epidemic curve usually has a sudden onset, a peak, and a rapid decline. If the outbreak is caused by person-to-person spread, however, the epidemic curve usually has a prolonged, irregular pattern, often known as a propagated outbreak.

Fig. 3.9 shows the epidemic time curve from an outbreak of gastrointestinal disease caused by a common source exposure to *Shigella boydii* at Fort Bliss, Texas. In this outbreak, spaghetti was contaminated by a food handler. The time scale in this figure is 12-hour periods. Note the rapid increase and rapid disappearance of the outbreak.

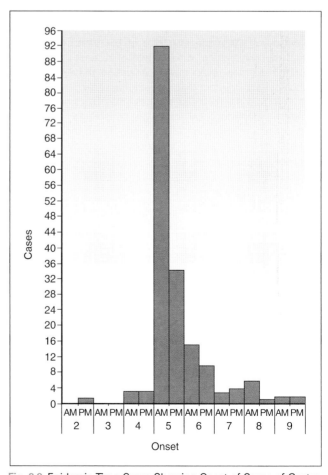

Fig. 3.9 Epidemic Time Curve Showing Onset of Cases of Gastrointestinal Disease Caused by *Shigella boydii* in Fort Bliss, Texas. The onset is shown in 12-hour periods for dates in November. (Data from Centers for Disease Control and Prevention: *Food and waterborne disease outbreaks: annual summary, 1976*, Atlanta, 1977, CDC.)

Fig. 3.10 shows the epidemic time curve from a propagated outbreak of bacillary dysentery caused by *Shigella sonnei*, which was transmitted from person to person at a training school for developmentally disabled individuals in Vermont. In this outbreak, the disease spread when persons, clothing, bedding, and other elements of the school environment were contaminated with feces. The time scale is shown in 5-day periods. Note the prolonged appearance of the outbreak.

Under certain conditions, a respiratory disease spread by the person-to-person route may produce an epidemic time curve that closely resembles that of a common-source epidemic. Fig. 3.11 shows the spread of measles in an elementary school. A widespread exposure apparently occurred at a school assembly, so the air in the school auditorium can almost be regarded as a common source. The first person infected in this situation is called the index case—the case that introduced the organism into the population. Sequential individual cases, however, can be seen every 12 days or so during the prior 2 months. The first of these measles cases should have warned school and public health officials to immunize all students immediately. If that had happened, the outbreak probably would have been avoided.

Sometimes an epidemic has more than one peak, either because of multiple common-source exposures or because of secondary cases. Fig. 3.12 shows the epidemic time curve for an outbreak of shigellosis among students who attended a summer camp in the eastern United States. The campers who drank contaminated water on the trip were infected with *Shigella* organisms. After they returned home, they infected others with shigellosis.

Epidemiologists occasionally encounter situations in which two different common-source outbreaks have the same time and place of exposure, but different incubation periods. Suppose that a group of people is exposed to contaminated shellfish in a restaurant. The exposure might cause an outbreak of shigellosis in 24 to 72 hours and an outbreak of hepatitis A about 2 to 4 weeks later in the same population.

The epidemic time curve is useful to ascertain the type of exposure and the time when the affected persons were exposed. If the causative organism is known, and the exposure seems to be a common source, epidemiologists can use knowledge about that organism's usual incubation period to determine the probable time of exposure. Two methods typically are used for this purpose. The data in Fig. 3.12,

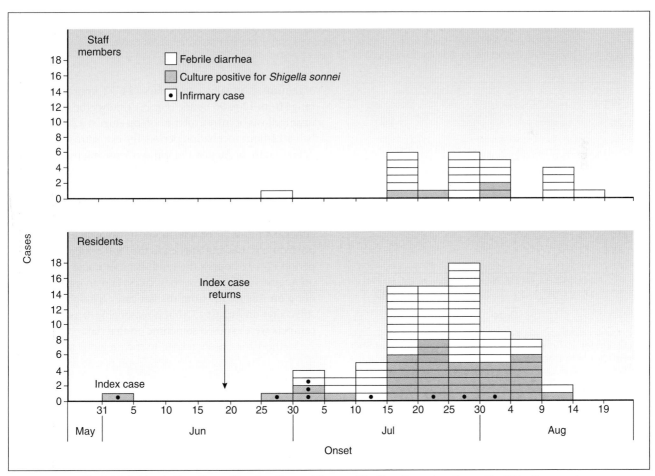

Fig. 3.10 Epidemic Time Curve Showing Onset of Cases of Bacillary Dysentery Caused by *Shigella sonnei* at a Training School in Brandon, Vermont, from May to August. The onset is shown in 5-day periods for dates in May, June, July, and August. (Data from Centers for Disease Control and Prevention: *Shigella* surveillance, Report No 37, Atlanta, 1976, CDC.)

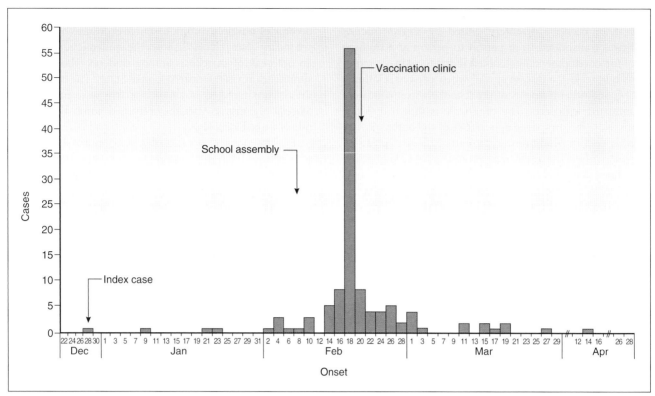

Fig. 3.11 Epidemic Time Curve Showing Onset of Cases of Measles at an Elementary School From December to April. The onset is shown in 2-day periods for dates in December 1975 and in January, February, March, and April 1976. (Data from Centers for Disease Control and Prevention: Measles surveillance, 1973–1976, Report No 10, Atlanta, 1977, CDC.)

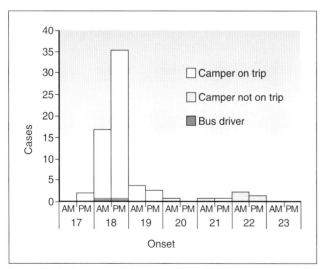

Fig. 3.12 Epidemic Time Curve Showing Onset of Cases of Shigellosis in Campers from New Jersey and New York in August. The onset is shown in 12-hour periods for dates in August 1971. (Data from Centers for Disease Control and Prevention: Shigella surveillance: annual summary, 1971, Atlanta, 1972, CDC.)

which pertain to *Shigella* infection among campers, assist in illustrating each method.

Method 1 involves taking the shortest and longest known incubation period for the causative organism and calculating backward in time from the first and last cases. If reasonably close together, these estimates bracket the probable time of exposure. For example, the incubation period for *Shigella*

organisms is usually 1 to 3 days (24–72 hours), but it may range from 12 to 96 hours.[7] Fig. 3.12 shows the first two cases of shigellosis occurred after noon on August 17. If these cases had a 12-hour incubation period, the exposure was sometime before noon on August 17 (without knowing the exact hours, it is not possible to be more specific). The longest known incubation period for *Shigella* is 96 hours, and the last camper case was August 21 after noon; 96 hours before that would be August 17 after noon. The most probable exposure time was either before noon or after noon on August 17. If the same procedure is used but applied to the *most common* incubation period (24–72 hours), the result is an estimate of after noon on August 16 (from the earliest cases) and an estimate of after noon on August 18 (from the last case). These two estimates still center on August 17, so it is reasonable to assume that the campers were exposed sometime on that date.

Method 2 is closely related to the previous method, but it involves taking the average incubation period and measuring backward from the epidemic peak, if that is clear. In Fig. 3.12, the peak is after noon on August 18. An average of 48 hours (2 days) earlier would be after noon on August 16, slightly earlier than the previous estimates. The most probable time of exposure was either after noon on August 16 or at any time on August 17.

Place. The accurate characterization of an epidemic involves defining the location of all cases, because a geographic clustering of cases may provide important clues. Usually, however, the geographic picture is not sufficient by itself, and other data are needed to complete the interpretation.

Sometimes a spot map that shows where each affected person lives, works, or attends school is helpful in solving an epidemic puzzle. The most famous of all public health spot maps was prepared in 1855 in London by John Snow. By mapping the location of cholera deaths in the epidemic of 1854, Snow found that they centered on the Broad Street water pump in London's Soho district (Fig. 3.13). His map showed that most of the persons killed by the outbreak lived in the blocks immediately surrounding the Broad Street pump. Based on this information, Snow had the pump handle removed to prevent anyone from drinking the water (although by the time he did this, the epidemic was already waning).

The use of spot maps currently is limited in outbreak investigations because these maps show only the numerator (number of cases) and do not provide information on the denominator (number of persons in the area). Epidemiologists usually prefer to show incidence rates by location, such as by hospital ward (in a hospital infection outbreak), by work area or classroom (in an occupational or school outbreak), or by block or section of a city (in a community outbreak).

When epidemiologists want to determine the general location of a disease and how it is spreading, they may compare trends in incidence rates in different regions. Fig. 3.14 shows the rates of reported *Salmonella enteritidis* infections by region in the United States over a 15-year period. There was an unusually high rate for the New England region during this time period shown. Beginning about halfway through the

time period, the mid-Atlantic states also began to show an excessive rate of salmonellosis from the same serotype, suggesting that the problem was spreading down the East Coast.

Cholera, caused by Vibrio cholerae, is an acute intestinal infection that can cause rapid and severe dehydrating diarrhea. In 1991 and again in 2010, Latin America experienced two of the largest cholera epidemics in modern history. The relationship between globally circulating pandemic Vibrio cholerae clones and local bacterial populations was initially not clear. However, whole-genome sequencing has since allowed scientists to understand the relationships. Both epidemics are now thought to be the result of intercontinental introductions of seventh pandemic El Tor Vibrio cholerae (See Fig. 3.15) and the genetic lineages local to Latin America are associated with disease that differs epidemiologically from epidemic cholera. This integrated view that takes into consideration local and global genetic lineages is important to the design of future disease control strategies.

A special problem in recent years has involved reports of clusters of cancer or other types of disease in neighborhoods or other small areas. From the theory of random sampling, epidemiologists would expect clusters of disease to happen by chance alone, but that does not comfort the people involved.

Distinguishing "chance" clusters from "real" clusters is often difficult, but identifying the types of cancer in a cluster may help epidemiologists decide fairly quickly whether the cluster represents an environmental problem. If the types of cancer in the cluster vary considerably and belong to the more common cell types (e.g., lung, breast, colon, prostate), the cluster probably is not caused by a hazardous local exposure.[8-10] However, if most of the cases represent only one type or a small number of related types of cancers, a more intensive investigation may be indicated.

The next step is to begin at the time the cluster is reported and observe the situation prospectively. The null hypothesis is that the unusual number of cases will not continue. Because this is a prospective hypothesis (see Chapter 9), an appropriate statistical test can be used to decide whether the number of cases continues to be excessive. If the answer is yes, there may be a true environmental problem in the area.

Person. Knowing the characteristics of persons affected by an outbreak may help clarify the problem and its cause. Important characteristics include age; gender; race; ethnicity; religion; source of water, milk, and food; immunization status; type of work or schooling; and travel and contacts with other affected persons.

Figs. 3.16 and 3.17 illustrate the value of analyzing personal characteristics of affected individuals for clues regarding the cause of the outbreak. Fig. 3.16 shows the age distribution of measles cases among children in the Navajo Nation; Fig. 3.17 shows the age distribution of measles cases among residents of Cuyahoga County, Ohio. The fact that measles in the Navajo Nation tended to occur in very young children is consistent with the hypothesis that the outbreak was caused by lack of immunization of preschool-age children. In contrast, the fact that very young children in Cuyahoga County were almost exempt from measles, while school-age children tended to be infected, suggests that the younger

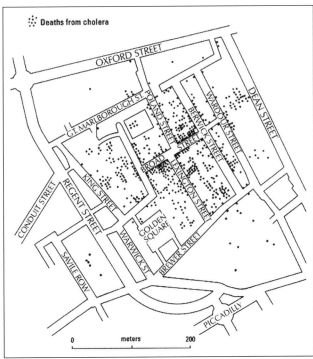

Fig. 3.13 Spot Map of Cholera Deaths in the Soho District of London, 1854, Based on a Map Prepared by John Snow in 1855. The deaths centered on the intersection of Broad and Lexington streets, where there was a popular community well (near the "L" of Lexington Street in the map). This well apparently was the source of the contamination. The present name of Broad Street is "Broadwick Street," and the John Snow Pub is on the southwest corner of Broadwick and Lexington streets. (Modified from http://www.doe.k12.de.us/infosuites/staff/ci/content_areas/files/ss/Cholera_in_19thc_London.pdf.)

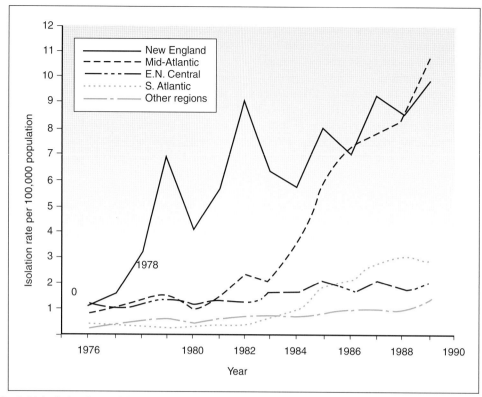

Fig. 3.14 Isolation Rate of *Salmonella Enteritidis* Infections per 100,000 Population in Various Regions of the United States, by Year of Report, 1976–1989. (Data from Centers for Disease Control and Prevention: Update: *Salmonella enteritidis* infections and shell eggs, United States, 1990. *MMWR* 39:909, 1990.)

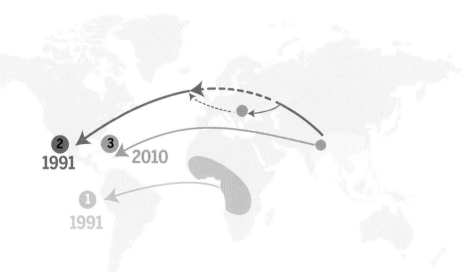

Fig. 3.15 Whole-Genome Sequencing to Characterize Cholera Across the Americas Over a 40-Year Time Span. (Intercontinental introductions of seventh pandemic V. cholerae El Tor into Latin America in 1991 and 2010. The direct introduction of the Latin American transmission #2 sublineage from South Asia or China or introduction via Eastern Europe in 1991 is uncertain and denoted by dashed lines. (Data from http://science.sciencemag.org/content/358/6364/789/tab-figures-data)

children had been immunized, and that the outbreak in this situation resulted from the failure of measles vaccine to produce long-lasting immunity. If they were not immunized early, the children of Cuyahoga County probably would have had measles earlier in life and would have been immune by the time they entered school. Fortunately, this type of outbreak has been almost eliminated by the requirement that children receive a second dose of measles vaccine before entering school.

2.2.e. Develop Hypotheses Regarding Source, Patterns of Spread, and Mode of Transmission

The source of infection is the person (the index case) or vehicle (e.g., food, water) that initially brought the infection into the affected community. The source of infection in the outbreak of gastrointestinal illness at Fort Bliss was an infected food handler who contaminated spaghetti that was eaten by many people more or less simultaneously (see Fig. 3.9).

The pattern of spread is the pattern by which infection can be carried from the source to the individuals infected. The primary distinction is between a common-source pattern, such as occurs when contaminated water is consumed by many people in the same time period, and a propagated pattern, in which the infection disseminates itself by spreading directly from person to person over an extended period. There is also a mixed pattern, in which persons acquire a disease through a common source and spread it to family members or others (secondary cases) by personal contact (see Fig. 3.12).

Affected persons in common-source outbreaks may have only one brief point-source exposure, or they may have a continuous common-source exposure. In the Fort Bliss outbreak, the infected spaghetti was the point source. In another example from Milwaukee, an epidemic of *Cryptosporidium* infection was caused by contamination of the public water supply for the southern part of the city over a several-day period; this was a continuous common-source exposure.[11]

Many types of infections have more than one pattern of spread. *Shigella* infection can be spread through contaminated water (continuous common source) or through person-to-person contact (propagated spread). HIV can be spread to several intravenous drug users through the sharing of a single infected syringe (continuous common source), and HIV can be passed from one person to another through sexual contact (propagated spread).

The mode of transmission of epidemic disease may be respiratory, fecal-oral, vectorborne, skin to skin, or through exchange of serum or other body fluids. In some cases, transmission is through contact with fomites—objects that can passively carry

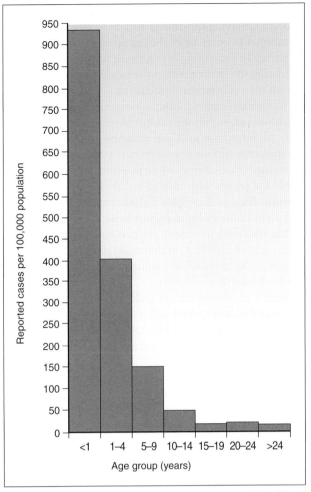

Fig. 3.16 Incidence Rates of Measles in Members of the Navajo Nation, by Age Group, 1972–1975. (Data from Centers for Disease Control and Prevention: Measles surveillance, 1973–1976, Report No 10, Atlanta, CDC, 1977.)

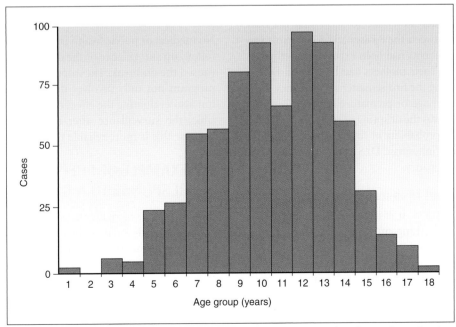

Fig. 3.17 Incidence of Measles in Residents of Cuyahoga County, Ohio, by Age Group, from October 1973 to February 1974. (Data from Centers for Disease Control and Prevention: Measles surveillance, 1973–1976, Report No 10, Atlanta, 1977, CDC.)

organisms from one person to another, such as soiled sheets or doorknobs. Some organisms can live for days on fomites.

2.2.f. Test Hypotheses

Laboratory studies are important in testing epidemiologic hypotheses and may include one or more of the following:

- Cultures from patients and, if appropriate, from possible vehicles, such as food or water
- Stool examinations for ova and parasites
- Serum tests for antibodies to the organism suspected of causing the disease (e.g., tests of acute and convalescent serum samples to determine if there has been an increase in antibodies to the organism over time)
- Tests for nonmicrobiologic agents, such as toxins or drugs

A common, efficient way of testing hypotheses is to conduct case control studies (see Chapter 5). For a foodborne outbreak of disease, the investigator assembles the persons who have the disease (cases) and a sample of the persons who ate at the same place at the suspected time of exposure but do not have the disease (controls). The investigator looks for possible risk factors (e.g., food items eaten) that were considerably more common in the cases than in the controls. Both groups are questioned regarding the specific foods they did or did not eat before the outbreak. For each item of food and drink, the percentage of controls who consumed it is subtracted from the percentage of cases who consumed it. The food item showing the greatest difference in consumption percentage between cases and controls is the most likely risk factor.

The case control method also can be used in an epidemic of noninfectious disease. In 1971 it was noted that eight young women with adenocarcinoma of the vagina were treated at one hospital over a 4-year period.[12] Because of the rarity of this type of cancer, the number of cases would qualify as an outbreak. When the investigators performed a case control study, they used 32 controls (4 matched control women for every case of adenocarcinoma). They were able to show that the only significant difference between the 8 cases and 32 controls was that 7 of the 8 cancer patients had been exposed to diethylstilbestrol (DES) in utero. Their mothers had been given DES, a synthetic estrogen, during the first semester of pregnancy in an effort to prevent miscarriage or premature labor. In contrast, none of the 32 controls was the offspring of mothers given DES during pregnancy. The probability of finding this distribution by chance alone was infinitesimal. DES is no longer used for any purpose during pregnancy.

2.2.g. Initiate Control Measures

When an outbreak is noted, it is usually accompanied by a general outcry that something must be done immediately. Therefore it may be necessary to start taking control measures before the source of the outbreak and the route of spread are known for certain. If possible, control measures should be initiated in such a way as not to interfere with the investigation of the outbreak. Four common types of intervention are used to control an outbreak, as follows:

1. Sanitation often involves modification of the environment. Sanitation efforts may consist of removing the pathogenic agent from the sources of infection (e.g., water, food); removing the human source of infection from environments where he or she can spread it to others (quarantine); or preventing contact with the source, perhaps by cleaning the environment or removing susceptible people from the environment (evacuation).

2. Prophylaxis implies putting a barrier to the infection, such as a vaccine, within the susceptible hosts. Although a variety of immunizations are recommended for the entire population and usually are initiated during infancy, other measures that offer short-term protection are also available for people who plan to travel to countries with endemic diseases. Examples include antimalarial drugs and hyperimmune globulin against hepatitis A.

3. Diagnosis and treatment are performed for the persons who are infected (e.g., in outbreaks of tuberculosis, syphilis, and meningococcal meningitis) so that they do not spread the disease to others.

4. Control of disease vectors includes mosquitoes (involved in malaria, dengue, and yellow fever) and *Ixodes* ticks (involved in Lyme disease). Examples include use of mosquito nets around bedding to genetically engineered mosquitoes.

Although a disease outbreak may require one or more of these interventions, some outbreaks simply fade away when the number of infected people is so high that few susceptible individuals remain.

One important aspect of the control effort is the written and oral communication of findings to the appropriate authorities, the appropriate health professionals, and the public. This communication (1) enables other agencies to assist in disease control, (2) contributes to the professional fund of knowledge about the causes and control of outbreaks, and (3) adds to the available information on prevention.

2.2.h. Initiate Specific Follow-up Surveillance to Evaluate Control Measures

No medical or public health intervention is adequate without follow-up surveillance of the disease or problem that initially caused the outbreak. The importance of a sound surveillance program not only involves detecting subsequent outbreaks but also evaluating the effect of the control measures. If possible, the surveillance after an outbreak should be *active* because this is more reliable than passive surveillance.

2.3 EXAMPLE OF PREPAREDNESS AND RESPONSE TO A GLOBAL HEALTH THREAT

In addition to severe illness, pandemic diseases cause numerous adverse effects, including fear, economic instability, and premature deaths.[13] Over time, epidemiologists have improved their ability to detect and respond to new pandemic threats. These improvements are attributable to increased communication among countries through the Internet, media, and organized public health systems and to advances in laboratory and diagnostic testing. Also innovative surveillance systems monitor indirect signals of disease activity, such as influenza surveillance based on tracking call volume to telephone triage advice lines, over-the-counter drug sales, and health information–seeking behavior in the form of queries to online search engines.[14–17] The WHO and the CDC Global Disease Detection Operations Center have implemented epidemic alert and rapid response systems to help control international outbreaks and strengthen international public health security.

A representative example of improved preparedness for global health threats is the rapid, effective global response to the 2009 influenza A (H1N1) pandemic that affected more than 200 countries and territories. Ongoing disease surveillance detected the increased number of cases of patients with influenza-like signs and symptoms, allowing epidemiologists to identify and characterize the pandemic virus quickly. Epidemiologic investigations and surveillance characterized the severity, risk groups, and burden of disease; within 20 weeks of virus detection, diagnostic testing was made available to 146 countries, and through an international donation program, a vaccine was developed and made available to 86 countries.

3. SUMMARY

Surveillance of disease activity is the foundation of public health control of disease. It may be active or passive. Its functions include determining the baseline rates of disease, detecting outbreaks, and evaluating control measures. Surveillance data are used for setting disease control policy. The investigation of disease outbreaks is a primary function of public health agencies, but the practicing physician makes important contributions in detecting and reporting acute outbreaks. A standard approach to the investigation of disease outbreaks was developed in the 20th century. This procedure involves making a diagnosis, establishing a case definition, and determining whether there is a definite outbreak.

If an outbreak is occurring, the cases of disease are characterized by time (especially using an epidemic time curve), place (usually determining rates in people who live and work in different locations), and person (determining the personal characteristics and patterns of the people involved in the outbreak and ascertaining how they differ from those of people not involved). This characterization is followed by the development and testing of hypotheses regarding the source of infection, the pattern of spread, and the mode of transmission. These hypotheses are then tested using laboratory data (e.g., cultures, paired sera, analysis for toxins) or research methods (e.g., case control studies), depending on the hypotheses. Control measures and follow-up surveillance are initiated as soon as is practical.

REFERENCES

1. Harkess JR, Gildon BA, Archer PW, Istre GR. Is passive surveillance always insensitive? An evaluation of shigellosis surveillance in Oklahoma. *Am J Epidemiol*. 1988;128(4):878-881.
2. Helgerson SD, Jekel JF, Hadler JL. Training public health students to investigate disease outbreaks: examples of community service. *Public Health Rep*. 1988;103:72-76.
3. Centers for Disease Control and Prevention. *Emergency Preparedness and Response*. Updated March 2, 2018. Available at: www.emergency.cdc.gov. Accessed March 15, 2019.
4. Centers for Disease Control and Prevention. *Measles Mumps, and Rubella (MMR) Vaccination: Information for Healthcare Professionals*. Updated January 11, 2018. Available at: https://www.cdc.gov/vaccines/vpd/mmr/hcp/index.html. Accessed March 15, 2019.
5. Roueché B. *The Medical Detectives*. New York, NY: Truman Talley Books; 1981.
6. Centers for Disease Control and Prevention. *Epidemiology Training & Resources*. Available at: www.cdc.gov/eis/request-services/epiresources.html. Updated: March 13, 2019. Accessed: Jue 7, 2019.
7. Heymann DL, ed. *Control of Communicable Diseases Manual*. 20th ed. Washington, DC: American Public Health Association; 2014.
8. Brooks-Robinson S, Helgerson SD, Jekel JF. An epidemiologic investigation of putative cancer clusters in two Connecticut towns. *J Environ Health*. 1987;50:161-164.
9. Jacquez GM, Grimson, RR, Kheifets, L, Wartenberg, DE, eds. Papers from the Workshop on statistics and computing in disease clustering. Port Jefferson, New York, 23-24 July 1992. *Stat Med*. 1993;12(19-20):1751-1968.
10. National Conference on Clustering of Health Events. Atlanta, Georgia, February 16-17, 1989. *Am J Epidemiol*. 1990;132 (1 Suppl):S1-S202.
11. Mac Kenzie WR, Hoxie NJ, Proctor ME, et al. A massive outbreak in Milwaukee of Cryptosporidium infection transmitted through the public water supply. *N Engl J Med*. 1994;331:161-167.
12. Herbst AL, Ulfelder H, Poskanzer DC. Adenocarcinoma of the vagina: association of maternal stilbestrol therapy with tumor appearance in young women. *N Engl J Med*. 1971;284:878-881.
13. Centers for Disease Control and Prevention. Ten great public health achievements—worldwide, 2001-2010. *JAMA*. 2011;306 (5):484-487.
14. Espino JU, Hogan WR, Wagner MM. Telephone triage: a timely data source for surveillance of influenza-like diseases. *AMIA Annu Symp Proc*. 2003:215-219.
15. Magruder SF. Evaluation of over-the-counter pharmaceutical sales as a possible early warning indicator of human disease. *Johns Hopkins Univ Appl Phys Lab Tech Dig*. 2003;24:349-353.
16. Eysenbach G. Infodemiology: tracking flu-related searches on the web for syndromic surveillance. *AMIA Annu Symp Proc*. 2006:244-248.
17. Ginsberg J, Mohebbi MH, Patel RS, Brammer L, Smolinski MS, Brilliant L. Detecting influenza epidemics using search engine query data. *Nature*. 2009;457(7232):1012-1014.

SELECT READINGS

Brookmeyer R, Stroup DF. *Monitoring the Health of Populations: Statistical Principles and Methods for Public Health Surveillance*. New York, NY: Oxford University Press; 2004.

WEBSITES

Updated guidelines for evaluating public health surveillance systems: recommendations from the Guidelines Working Group: http://www.cdc.gov/mmwr/preview/mmwrhtml/rr5013a1.htm

CDC case definitions for infectious conditions under public health surveillance: https://www.cdc.gov/mmwr/preview/mmwrhtml/00047449.htm

REVIEW QUESTIONS

1. An outbreak of disease should be reported to the local or state health department:
   A. Only if the diagnosis is certain
   B. Only if the disease is infectious
   C. Only if the disease is serious
   D. Only if the outbreak involves at least 10 people
   E. Always

2. Arizona, Colorado, and New Mexico report cases of an unexplained respiratory tract illness with a high case fatality ratio. Which of the following is most reliably true regarding this event?
   A. The cases represent an epidemic.
   B. The identification of the cases is an example of active surveillance.
   C. It is appropriate for the CDC to investigate the cases.
   D. The seemingly new cases may be an artifact of improved health department surveillance.
   E. If the illnesses represent an endemic disease, the cases do not constitute an outbreak.

3. Cases of "flesh-eating" group A streptococcal disease are reported in a defined population. Which of the following types of information would be most helpful for determining whether these cases represent a disease outbreak?
   A. The clinical features and methods of diagnosing the disease
   B. The disease vector and reservoir
   C. The exact location and timing of disease onset
   D. The incubation period and pattern of disease transmission
   E. The usual disease patterns and reporting practices

4. An official from the state department of public health visits outpatient clinics and emergency departments to determine the number of cases of postexposure prophylaxis for rabies. The official's action is an example of:
   A. Active surveillance
   B. Case finding
   C. Outbreak investigation
   D. Screening
   E. Secondary prevention

5. An article highlighting the long-term consequences of inadequately treated Lyme disease is published in a medical journal. After a summary of the article appears in popular newspapers and magazines, patients with vague joint pains begin insisting that their physicians test them for Lyme disease. Cases in which the test results are positive are reported as cases of Lyme borreliosis. This represents:
   A. Outbreak investigation
   B. An epidemic of Lyme borreliosis
   C. A change in reporting that would underestimate incidence
   D. A change in surveillance that would overestimate the prevalence

   E. A change in screening that would underestimate the likelihood of an outbreak

6. The US President invites a group of legislators to a formal luncheon at the White House. Within 24 hours, 11 of the 17 diners experience abdominal pain, vomiting, and diarrhea. The President does not eat the salmon and feels fine. Of the 11 symptomatic guests, 4 have fever and 7 do not; 5 have an elevated white blood cell count and 6 do not; 6 ate shrimp bisque and 5 did not; 9 ate salmon mousse and 2 did not; and 1 goes on to have surgery for acute cholecystitis resulting from an impacted calculus (stone) in the common bile duct. Of the 11 symptomatic guests, 10 recover within 3 days; the exception is the senator who underwent surgery and recovered over a longer period. The guests at this luncheon had shared no other meals at any time recently. The fact that 11 of 17 diners become sick:
   A. Is a coincidence until proven otherwise
   B. Represents a disease outbreak
   C. Is attributable to bacterial infection
   D. Is not an outbreak because the usual pattern of disease is unknown
   E. Should be investigated by the CDC

7. Considering all the details from question 6, the attack rate is:
   A. 4/11
   B. 5/11
   C. 9/11
   D. 1/17
   E. 11/17

8. Considering all the details from question 6, the earliest priority in investigating the phenomenon would be to:
   A. Close the kitchen temporarily
   B. Define a case
   C. Perform a case control study
   D. Perform stool tests
   E. Submit food samples to the laboratory

9. Considering all the details from question 6, the best case definition for the guests' disease would be:
   A. Abdominal pain, vomiting, and diarrhea within 24 hours of the luncheon
   B. Acute viral gastroenteritis
   C. Staphylococcal food poisoning
   D. The onset of abdominal pain and fever after the luncheon
   E. An elevated white blood cell count

10. Considering all the details from question 6, and suspecting that the disease may be the result of a common-source exposure involving contaminated food, the investigators attempt to determine which food is responsible. Their initial task is to:
    A. Analyze food specimens from the luncheon in the laboratory
    B. Close the kitchen

C. Examine the kitchen and interview the food preparers about their techniques
D. Interview luncheon attendees to find out what they ate
E. Perform a case control study

ANSWERS AND EXPLANATIONS

1. **E.** By definition, an outbreak represents a deviation from the expected pattern of health and disease in a population. Any outbreak may reveal a new health threat or point to the breakdown of some aspect of the system designed to protect health in the population. Any seeming deviation from the expected pattern of disease (i.e., any apparent outbreak) should always be reported, regardless of whether the diagnosis is certain (A). Waiting for definitive diagnoses to confirm suspicion may cause dangerous delay; initial suspicions will suffice to initiate the appropriate investigations toward characterization and control of the threat. Outbreaks of infectious (B) and noninfectious disease may be equally dangerous and important, and a seemingly mild disease may represent a serious health threat to certain vulnerable populations. Thus all unusual disease patterns should be reported, even if the disease does not seem serious (C) and even if only a few people are affected. Indeed, for rare diseases, even a single case might be cause enough for alarm (e.g., smallpox). Having at least 10 affected individuals (D) is not necessary.

2. **C.** The respiratory tract illness described in the question was the hantavirus pulmonary syndrome. Because fatalities were reported from more than one state, the investigation of the illness would fall within the jurisdiction of the Centers for Disease Control and Prevention. The question implies that the case reports were unsolicited (this was an "unexplained" illness that people happened to notice, not a well-established illness that people were looking for). Thus the cases would be an example of passive surveillance rather than active surveillance (B), as through improved monitoring by a health department (D). The question does not provide enough information to determine whether the reported cases constitute an epidemic (A) or an outbreak. To make this determination, the illness would need to be characterized sufficiently to ascertain whether a sudden change in the pattern of disease had occurred. Even if the condition were endemic (E), this would not exclude the possibility of an outbreak (i.e., unexpected increase in disease activity).

3. **E.** Steps in the evaluation of an outbreak include establishing a diagnosis; developing a case definition; determining whether an outbreak exists; characterizing the outbreak by time, place, and person; developing and testing hypotheses; initiating control measures; and initiating follow-up surveillance. To complete all these steps, considerable information about the disease in question is required. An early determination about the probability of an outbreak depends most, however, on knowing the usual disease patterns and knowing the reporting practices that bring the disease to attention. In this case, if group A streptococcal fasciitis generally does not occur at all in the population, the occurrence of even one correctly reported case might represent an outbreak. Because the disease is severe, the regular occurrence of unreported cases would be unlikely, so even without active surveillance, reporting probably would be fairly reliable and complete. Although the information provided is extremely limited, this scenario would strongly suggest the occurrence of an outbreak. The clinical features and methods of diagnosing the disease (A) and exact location and timing of disease onset (C) are important for establishing the case definition and may contribute to the degree of confidence with which one determines "cases." The disease vector and reservoir (B) and the incubation period and pattern of disease transmission (D) are important in understanding a disease process and may contribute to the case definition and hypotheses about causes.

4. **A.** Whenever a public health official visits health care delivery sites to assess the pattern of a disease or condition, the assessment constitutes active surveillance. The question does not provide enough information to determine whether an "outbreak" (C) of rabies exposure is under consideration. Case finding (B) refers to testing a group of patients for a disease that is not yet clinically apparent; an example is taking chest x-ray films or electrocardiograms in a group of patients being admitted to the hospital without cough or chest pain, perhaps before surgery. Screening (C) is an effort to identify occult (asymptomatic) disease or risk factors in a population. Secondary prevention (E) is an effort to prevent clinical consequences of a disease after the disease is identified. The administration of postexposure rabies vaccines might qualify as secondary prevention, but a public health official's review of cases in which the vaccines were given would not qualify as secondary prevention.

5. **D.** Whenever public attention is focused on a particular health problem, an increase in the number of reported cases of the problem is likely. However, even when available diagnostic tests are almost perfect (with sensitivities and specificities approaching 100%; not the case for Lyme disease tests), if the prevalence of the actual disease in the tested population is low, the majority of positive test results will be false positive (see Chapter 13, Bayes theorem). Thus the number of false-positive cases of Lyme disease will necessarily increase as more people with vaguely characterized clinical syndromes are tested. This increase in "Lyme disease" reporting represents an epidemic of Lyme disease testing, not an epidemic of the disease itself (B). The increased testing does not represent an outbreak investigation (A), because the question does not specify what the expected patterns of the disease are or suggest that the increased testing is being performed to investigate new and unusual patterns in disease. Increased testing would tend to overestimate the

likelihood of an outbreak (E) and overestimate prevalence, not underestimate incidence (C).

6. **B.** Although there is no formal surveillance of these lun-
cheons, clearly the situation described represents the
unexpected occurrence of disease; almost two-thirds
of diners becoming sick after a meal does not represent a usual pattern (D). The usual pattern of disease
in this case does not derive from surveillance but
from common experience. Nobody expects so many
people to sicken simultaneously after lunch; this
"attack rate" clearly represents more than coincidence
(A). The CDC would not investigate so small and
localized an outbreak unless requested to do so by
local public health officials (E). The illness presented
here could have been caused by bacterial infection
(C), but other microorganisms, toxins, and even de-
liberate poisoning are also on the list of possibilities.

7. **E.** The attack rate is the proportion (yes, it is called a
"rate" but is actually a ratio or proportion) of exposed
persons who become ill. Given the information in
question 6, the exposure at this stage (before the investigation) is most inclusively and best defined as "participation in the luncheon." As the outbreak investigation proceeds, the definition of exposure could change,
for instance, if a particular food, such as the salmon
mousse, were implicated. The denominator used to
calculate the attack rate would then change to represent only the persons exposed to the contaminated
food. There were 17 diners, so 17 is the attack rate denominator. The numerator is the number of people
who became ill. The question suggests that the illness is
abdominal pain, vomiting, and diarrhea, and that 11
people had these symptoms. Thus the attack rate is
11/17. However, if the case definition is further restricted to include only those affected individuals who
additionally had fever, or only those who had an elevated white blood cell count, the numerator would
change, and the attack rate would be 4/17 or 5/17,
respectively. The proportion of ill individuals having
fever was 4/11 (A). The proportion of ill individuals
having an elevated white blood cell count was 5/11 (B).
The proportion of ill individuals eating the salmon
mousse was 9/11 (C). The proportion of all diners
(ill and not ill) requiring surgery was 1/17 (D).

8. **B.** Establishing a diagnosis or a case definition is the earliest priority in an outbreak investigation. Investigators
cannot investigate the origin of a problem until they
precisely define the problem. Laboratory tests (D and
E), control measures (A), and case control studies (C)
are usually performed later in an investigation, after
hypotheses have been generated regarding transmission and cause.

9. **A.** The case definition is required to distinguish between
cases and noncases of the disease under investigation (i.e.,
to distinguish who is "ill" and who is "not ill" by strict criteria). The ideal case definition would permit the inclusion
of all cases and the exclusion of all noncases, providing

perfect sensitivity and specificity (see Chapter 7). The
case definition should include salient features about
time, place, and person. The relevant time is "within
24 hours of the luncheon" (not before the luncheon, not
days later). The relevant place is "the luncheon" (i.e., all
cases must have been in attendance at the event). The
relevant person is an attendee at the lunch event (implied), and someone having symptoms—in this case
"abdominal pain, vomiting, and diarrhea." The onset of
abdominal pain and fever after the luncheon (D) could
also be a case definition, but this definition is not as
specific as to symptoms or time and therefore is not as
good; it will necessarily be less specific and tend to produce more false-positives (i.e., it will tend to label more
"noncases" as "cases"; see specificity and positive predictive value in Chapter 7). An elevated white blood cell
count (E) could be part of a case definition, but without
additional criteria for place and time and other associated symptoms, this single criterion would be quite poor
as a case definition. Acute viral gastroenteritis (B) and
staphylococcal food poisoning (C) are on the differential
(list of possible diagnoses) for the affected guests' illness,
but these are clinical syndromes with highly variable
presentations and symptoms. A good case definition
needs to specify precise symptoms explicitly; neither
acute viral gastroenteritis nor staphylococcal food poisoning does this.

10. **D.** Even before developing hypotheses about the source
of infection, investigators would have to characterize
this outbreak by time, place, and person. In this fairly
simple example, virtually all this information is in the
case definition. The time and place of exposure were
the lunch hour at the White House, and the cases were
the symptomatic guests. With sufficient information
to generate the hypothesis that this outbreak is caused
by contaminated food, the investigators can begin to
determine what food to implicate. To do so, they must
find out what foods were eaten preferentially by the
symptomatic guests. A simple interview of all attendees would be an initial step. It is also possible, however, that the outbreak of "abdominal pain, vomiting,
and diarrhea" is unrelated to the food served at the
luncheon. For example, the symptoms might relate to
a problem with a lavatory, with only guests who used
the restroom during the luncheon affected. Until a
specific food cause is firmly suspected, analyzing food
specimens from the luncheon in the laboratory (A),
closing the kitchen (B), and examining the kitchen
and interviewing the food preparers about their techniques (C) would be premature. A case control study
(E) would be useful to help establish an association
between the symptoms and the presumed exposure,
but before such a study can be performed, the illness
(i.e., specific symptoms) and the exposure (i.e., specific foods or other sources) must be established.
Finding out what everyone ate is the logical starting
point to see if any food cause can be implicated.

The Study of Risk Factors and Causation

"Your age is your No. 1 risk factor for almost every disease, but it's not a disease itself."

Craig Venter

Epidemiologists are frequently involved in studies to determine causation—that is, to find the specific cause(s) of a disease. For example, large amounts of data are now available for investigators to perform observational studies where they examine the association between what is known in epidemiologic jargon as an exposure (e.g., a behavior, exposure to something in the environment, a procedure) and an outcome (e.g., a disease or death). However, because there are so many exposures occurring simultaneously in the lives of humans that can never be completely accounted for, observational studies cannot provide evidence of cause and effect: they can only provide evidence of a relationship or "association." An association does not prove causation.

Proving cause and effect is a more difficult and elusive task than might be supposed, and it leaves considerable room for obfuscation, as shown in a newspaper article on cigarette smoking.[1] The article quoted a spokesperson for the Tobacco Institute (a trade association for cigarette manufacturers) as saying that "smoking was a risk factor, though not a cause, of a variety of diseases."

Is a risk factor a cause, or is it not? To answer this question, we begin this chapter with a review of the basic concepts concerning causation. Studies can yield statistical associations between a disease and an exposure; epidemiologists need to interpret the meaning of these relationships and decide if the associations are artifactual, noncausal, or causal. When studies find an association between two things, it does not necessarily mean one thing "caused" the other one to happen. There are important steps in the determination of cause and effect, and many potential sources of bias and pitfalls in casual research need to be considered.

1. TYPES OF CAUSAL RELATIONSHIPS

Most scientific research seeks to identify causal relationships. The three fundamental types of causes, as discussed here in order of decreasing strength, are sufficient cause, necessary cause, and risk factor (Box 4.1).

1.1 SUFFICIENT CAUSE

A sufficient cause precedes a disease and has the following relationship with the disease: if the cause is present, the disease will always occur. However, examples in which this proposition holds true are surprisingly rare, apart from certain genetic abnormalities that, if homozygous, inevitably lead to a fatal disease (e.g., Tay-Sachs disease).

Smoking is not a sufficient cause of bronchogenic lung cancer, because many people who smoke do not acquire lung cancer before they die of something else. It is unknown whether all smokers would eventually develop lung cancer if

---

BOX 4.1 Types of Causal Relationships

Sufficient cause: If the factor (cause) is present, the effect (disease) will always occur.

Necessary cause: The factor (cause) must be present for the effect (disease) to occur; however, a necessary cause may be present without the disease occurring.

Risk factor: If the factor is present, the probability that the effect will occur is increased.

Directly causal association: The factor exerts its effect in the absence of intermediary factors (intervening variables).

Indirectly causal association: The factor exerts its effect through intermediary factors.

Noncausal association: The relationship between two variables is statistically significant, but no causal relationship exists because the temporal relationship is incorrect (the presumed cause comes after, rather than before, the effect of interest) or because another factor is responsible for the presumed cause and the presumed effect.

---

they continued smoking and lived long enough, but within the human life span, smoking cannot be considered a sufficient cause of lung cancer.

1.2 NECESSARY CAUSE

A necessary cause precedes a disease and has the following relationship with the disease: the cause must be present for the disease to occur, although it does not always result in disease. In the absence of the organism *Mycobacterium tuberculosis,* tuberculosis cannot occur. *M. tuberculosis* can thus be called a necessary cause, or prerequisite, of tuberculosis. It cannot be called a sufficient cause of tuberculosis, however, because it is possible for people to harbor the *M. tuberculosis* organisms all their lives and yet have no symptoms of the disease.

Cigarette smoking is not a necessary cause of bronchogenic lung cancer because lung cancer can and does occur in the absence of cigarette smoke. Exposure to other agents, such as radioactive materials (e.g., radon gas), arsenic, asbestos, chromium, nickel, coal tar, and some organic chemicals, has been shown to be associated with lung cancer, even in the absence of active or passive cigarette smoking.[2]

1.3 RISK FACTOR

A risk factor is an exposure, behavior, or attribute that, if present and active, clearly increases the probability of a particular disease occurring in a group of people compared with an otherwise similar group of people who lack the risk factor. A risk factor, however, is neither a necessary nor a sufficient cause of disease. Although smoking is the most important risk factor for bronchogenic carcinoma, producing 20 times as high a risk of lung cancer in men who are heavy smokers as in men who are nonsmokers, smoking is neither a sufficient nor a necessary cause of lung cancer.

What about the previously cited quotation, in which the spokesperson from the Tobacco Institute suggested

"smoking was a risk factor, though not a cause, of a variety of diseases"?[1] If by "cause" the speaker included only necessary and sufficient causes, he was correct. However, if he included situations in which the presence of the risk factor clearly increased the probability of the disease, he was wrong. An overwhelming proportion of scientists who have studied the question of smoking and lung cancer believe the evidence shows not only that cigarette smoking is a cause of lung cancer, but also that it is the most important cause, even though it is neither a necessary nor a sufficient cause of the disease.

1.4 CAUSAL AND NONCAUSAL ASSOCIATIONS

The first and most basic requirement for a causal relationship to exist is an **association** between the outcome of interest (e.g., a disease or death) and the presumed cause. The outcome must occur either significantly more often or significantly less often in individuals who are exposed to the presumed cause than in individuals who are not exposed. In other words, exposure to the presumed cause must make a difference, or it is not a cause. Because some differences would probably occur as a result of random variation, an association must be **statistically significant,** meaning that the difference must be large enough to be unlikely if the exposure really had no effect. As discussed in Chapter 9, "unlikely" is usually defined as likely to occur no more than 1 time in 20 opportunities (i.e., 5% of the time, or 0.05) by chance alone.

If an association is causal, the causal pathway may be direct or indirect. The classification depends on the absence or presence of **intermediary factors,** which are often called **intervening variables, mediating variables,** or **mediators.**

A **directly causal association** occurs when the factor under consideration exerts its effect without intermediary factors. A severe blow to the head could cause brain damage and death without other external causes being required.

An **indirectly causal association** occurs when one factor influences one or more other factors through intermediary variables. Poverty itself may not cause disease and death, but by preventing adequate nutrition, housing, and medical care, poverty may lead to poor health and premature death. In this case, the nutrition, housing, and medical care would be called intervening variables. Education seems to lead to better health indirectly, presumably because it increases the amount of knowledge about health, the level of motivation to maintain health, and the ability to earn an adequate income.

A statistical association may be strong but may not be causal. In such a case, it would be a **noncausal association.** An important principle of data analysis is that association does not prove causation. If a statistically significant association is found between two variables, but the presumed cause occurs **after** the effect (rather than before it), the association is not causal. For example, quitting smoking is associated with an increased incidence of lung cancer. However, it is unlikely that quitting causes lung cancer or that continuing to smoke would be protective. What is much more likely is that smokers having early, undetectable or undiagnosed lung cancer start to feel sick because of their growing malignant disease. This sick feeling prompts them to stop smoking and thus, temporarily, they may feel a little better. When cancer is diagnosed shortly thereafter, it appears that there is a causal association, but this is false. The cancer started before the quitting was even considered. The temporality of the association precludes causation.

Likewise, if a statistically significant association is found between two variables, but some other factor is responsible for both the presumed cause and the presumed effect, the association is not causal. For example, baldness may be associated with the risk of coronary artery disease (CAD), but baldness itself probably does not cause CAD. Both baldness and CAD are probably functions of age, gender, and dihydrotestosterone level.

Finally, there is always the possibility of **bidirectional causation.** In other words, each of two variables may reciprocally influence the other. For example, there is an association between the density of fast-food outlets in neighborhoods and people's purchase and consumption of fast foods. It is possible that people living in neighborhoods dense with sources of fast food consume more of it because fast food is so accessible and available. It is also possible that fast-food outlets choose to locate in neighborhoods where people's purchasing and consumption patterns reflect high demand. In fact, the association is probably true to some extent in both directions. This bidirectionality creates somewhat of a feedback loop, reinforcing the placement of new outlets (and potentially the movement of new consumers) into neighborhoods already dense with fast food.

2. STEPS IN DETERMINATION OF CAUSE AND EFFECT

Investigators must have a model of causation to guide their thinking. The scientific method for determining causation can be summarized as having three steps, which should be considered in the following order[3]:
1. Investigation of the statistical association.
2. Investigation of the temporal relationship.
3. Elimination of all known alternative explanations.

These steps in epidemiologic investigation are similar in many ways to the steps followed in an investigation of murder, as discussed next.

2.1 INVESTIGATION OF STATISTICAL ASSOCIATION

Investigations may test hypotheses about risk factors or protective factors. For causation to be identified, the presumed **risk factor** must be present significantly more often in persons with the disease of interest than in persons without the disease. To eliminate chance associations, this difference must be large enough to be considered statistically significant. Conversely, the presumed **protective factor** (e.g., a vaccine) must be present significantly less often in persons with the disease than in persons without it. When the presumed factor (either a risk factor or a protective factor) is not associated with a statistically different frequency of disease, the factor cannot be considered causal. It might be argued that an additional, unidentified factor, a **"negative" confounder** (see later), could be obscuring a real association between the factor and the disease. Even in that case, however, the principle is not violated, because proper research design and statistical analysis would show the real association.

The first step in an epidemiologic study is to show a statistical association between the presumed risk or protective factor and the disease. The equivalent early step in a murder investigation is to show a geographic and temporal association between the murderer and the victim—that is, to show that both were in the same place at the same time, or that the murderer was in a place from which he or she could have caused the murder.

The relationship between smoking and lung cancer provides an example of how an association can lead to an understanding of causation. The earliest epidemiologic studies showed that smokers had an average overall death rate approximately two times that of nonsmokers; the same studies also indicated that the death rate for lung cancer among all smokers was approximately 10 times that of nonsmokers.[4] These studies led to further research efforts, which clarified the role of cigarette smoking as a risk factor for lung cancer and for many other diseases as well.

In epidemiologic studies the research design must allow a statistical association to be shown, if it exists. This usually means comparing the rate of disease before and after exposure to an intervention that is designed to reduce the disease of interest, or comparing groups with and without exposure to risk factors for the disease, or comparing groups with and without treatment for the disease of interest. Statistical analysis is needed to show that the difference associated with the intervention or exposure is greater than would be expected by chance alone, and to estimate how large this difference is. Research design and statistical analysis work closely together (see Chapter 5).

If a statistically significant difference in risk of disease is observed, the investigator must first consider the direction and extent of the difference. Did therapy make patients better or worse, on average? Was the difference large enough to be etiologically or clinically important? Even if the observed difference is real and large, **statistical association does not prove causation.** It may seem initially that an association is causal, when in fact it is not. For example, in the era before antibiotics were developed, syphilis was treated with arsenical compounds (e.g., salvarsan), despite their toxicity. An outbreak of fever and jaundice occurred in many of the patients treated with arsenicals.[5] At the time, it seemed obvious that the outbreak was caused by the arsenic. Many years later, however, medical experts realized that such outbreaks were most likely caused by an infectious agent, probably hepatitis B or C virus, spread by inadequately sterilized needles during administration of the arsenical compounds. Any statistically significant association can only be caused by one of four possibilities: true causal association, chance, random error, or systematic error (bias or its special case, confounding, as addressed later).

Several criteria, if met, increase the probability that a statistical association is true and causal[6] (Box 4.2). (These criteria often can be attributed to the 19th-century philosopher John Stuart Mill.) In general, a statistical association is more likely to be **causal** if the criteria in Box 4.2 are true.

Fig. 4.1 provides an example of a statistical association showing a dose-response relationship based on an early investigation of cigarette smoking and lung cancer.[7] The investigators found the following rates of lung cancer deaths, expressed as the number of deaths per 100,000 population per year: 7 deaths in men who did not smoke, 47 deaths in men who smoked about one-half pack of cigarettes a day, 86 deaths in men who smoked about one pack a day, and 166 deaths in men who smoked two or more packs a day.

Even if all the previously cited criteria for a statistically significant association hold true, the proof of a causal relationship also depends on the demonstration of the necessary temporal relationship and the elimination of alternative explanations, which are the next two steps discussed.

2.2 INVESTIGATION OF TEMPORAL RELATIONSHIP

Although some philosophical traditions consider time as circular, Western science assumes that time runs only one way. To show causation, the suspected causal factor must have occurred or been present before the effect (e.g., the disease) developed. Proving the time relationship is more complex than it might seem unless **experimental control** is possible— that is, randomization followed by measurement of the risk factor and disease in both groups before and after the experimental intervention.

With chronic diseases, the timing of the exposure to the risk factor and onset of the effect on the chronic disease is often unclear. When did atherosclerosis begin? When did the first bronchial cell become cancerous? Likewise, the onset of the risk factor may be unclear. When did the blood pressure begin to increase? When did the diet first become unhealthy? Because of long but varying **latent periods** between the onset of risk factors and the onset of the resulting diseases, the temporal relationships may be obscured. These associations can be complex and can form vicious cycles. A chronic disease such as obesity can cause osteoarthritis, which can lead to inactivity that makes the obesity worse. Research design has an important role in determining the temporal sequence of cause and effect (see Chapter 5). If information on the cause and the effect is obtained simultaneously, it is difficult to decide whether the presumed cause or the presumed effect began first. On the one hand, basic demographic variables such as gender and race—internal factors that are present from birth—presumably would have begun to have an effect before diseases caused by any external factors began. On the other hand, it is often impossible in a survey or in a single medical visit to determine which variables occurred first.

With respect to temporal relationships in the case of a murder, the guilty party must have been in the presence of the victim immediately before the victim's death (unless some remote technique was used). In fictional murder mysteries, an innocent but suspect individual often stumbles onto the crime scene immediately after the murder has taken place and is discovered bending over the body. The task of a defense attorney in such a case would be to show that the accused individual actually appeared *after* the murder, and that someone *else* was there at the time of the murder.

> ## BOX 4.2 Statistical Association and Causality: Factors That Increase Likelihood of Statistical Association Being Causal
>
> - The association shows **strength**; the difference in rates of disease between those with the risk factor and those without the risk factor is large.
> - The association shows **consistency**; the difference is always observed if the risk factor is present.
> - The association shows **specificity**; the difference does not appear if the risk factor is absent.
> - The association has **biologic plausibility**; the association makes sense, based on what is known about the natural history of the disease.
> - The association exhibits a **dose-response relationship**; the risk of disease is greater with stronger exposure to the risk factor.

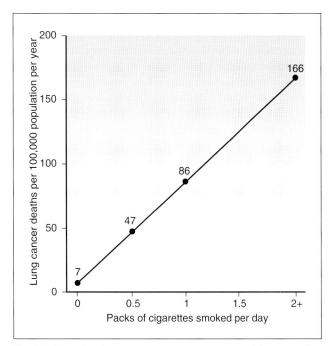

Fig. 4.1 Example of dose-response relationship in epidemiology. The *x*-axis is the approximate *dose* of cigarettes per day, and the *y*-axis is the rate of deaths from lung cancer. (Data from Doll R, Hill AB: Lung cancer and other causes of death in relation to smoking: a second report on the mortality of British doctors. *BMJ* 2:1071–1081, 1956. doi:10.1136/bmj.2.5001.1071).

2.3 ELIMINATION OF ALL KNOWN ALTERNATIVE EXPLANATIONS

In a murder case, the verdict of "not guilty" (i.e., "not proved beyond a reasonable doubt") usually can be obtained for the defendant if his or her attorney can show that there are other possible scenarios to explain what happened, and that one of them is at least as likely as the scenario that implicates the defendant. Evidence that another person was at the scene of the crime and had a motive for murder as strong as or stronger than the motive of the accused person would cast sufficient doubt on the guilt of the accused to result in an acquittal.

In the case of an epidemiologic investigation concerning the causation of disease, even if the presumed causal factor is associated statistically with the disease and occurs before the disease appears, it is necessary to show that there are no other likely explanations for the association.

On the one hand, proper research design can reduce the likelihood of competing causal explanations. *Randomization,* if done correctly, ensures that neither self-selection nor investigator bias influences the allocation of participants into treatment (or experimental) group and control group. Randomization also means that the treatment and control groups should be reasonably comparable with regard to disease susceptibility and severity. The investigator can work to reduce measurement bias (discussed later) and other potential problems, such as a difference between the number of participants lost to follow-up.

On the other hand, the criterion that all alternative explanations be eliminated can *never* be met fully because it is violated as soon as someone proposes a new explanation that fits the data and cannot be ruled out. For example, the classic theory of the origin of peptic ulcers (stress and hypersecretion) was challenged by the theory that *Helicobacter pylori* infection is an important cause of these ulcers.[8] The fact that scientific explanations are always tentative—even when they seem perfectly satisfactory and meet the criteria for statistical association, timing, and elimination of known alternatives—is shown in the following example on the causation of cholera.

2.3.a Alternative Explanation for Cholera in 1849

In 1849, there was an almost exact correspondence between the predicted cholera death rates in London based on the miasma theory and the observed cholera rates at various levels of elevation above the Thames River (Fig. 4.2). At the time, the accuracy of this prediction was hailed as an impressive confirmation of miasma theory.[9] According to this theory, cholera was caused by *miasmas* (noxious vapors), which have their highest and most dangerous concentrations at low elevations. The true reason for the association between cholera infection and elevation was that the higher the elevation, the less likely that wells would be infected by water from the Thames (which was polluted by pathogens that cause cholera) and the less likely that people would use river water for drinking. In later decades the *germ theory* of cholera became popular, and this theory has held to the present. Although nobody accepts miasma theory now, it would be difficult to

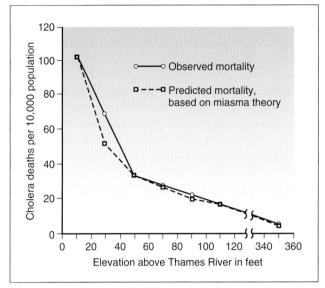

Fig. 4.2 Predicted and observed cholera rates at various elevations above Thames River, London, 1849. (From Langmuir AD: Epidemiology of airborne infection. *Bacteriol Rev* 25:173–181, 1961. PubMed PMID: 14462173; PubMed Central PMCID: PMC441089.)

improve on the 1849 prediction of cholera rates that were based on that theory.

3. BIAS IN CAUSAL RESEARCH

Bias, also known as **differential error,** is a dangerous source of inaccuracy in epidemiologic research. Bias usually produces deviations or distortions that tend to go in one direction. Bias becomes a problem when it weakens a true association, produces a false association, or distorts the apparent direction of the association between variables.

So many sources of bias in research have been identified that to list them can be overwhelming. It is easiest to think of the chronologic sequence of a clinical trial (see Chapter 5) and categorize biases in terms of assembly bias or detection bias.

3.1 ASSEMBLY BIAS

The first step in a clinical trial involves assembling the groups of participants to be studied. If the characteristics of the intervention group and those of the control group are not comparable at the start, any differences between the two groups that appear in results (outcomes) might be caused by assembly bias instead of the intervention itself. Assembly bias in turn may take the form of selection bias or allocation bias.

3.1.a Selection Bias

Selection bias results when *participants* are allowed to select the study group they want to join. If subjects are allowed to choose, those who are more educated, more adventuresome, or more health conscious may want to try a new therapy or preventive measure. Any differences subsequently noted may be partly or entirely caused by differences among subjects rather than to the effect of the intervention. Almost any non-random method of allocation of subjects to study groups may produce bias.

Selection bias may be found in studies of treatment methods for terminal diseases. The most severely ill patients are often those most willing to try a new treatment, despite its known or unknown dangers, presumably because these patients believe that they have little to lose. Because of self-selection, a new treatment might be given to the patients who are sickest, with relatively poor results. These results could not be fairly compared with the results among patients who were not as sick.

3.1.b Allocation Bias

Allocation bias may occur if *investigators* choose a nonrandom method of assigning participants to study groups. It also may occur if a random method is chosen, but not followed, by staff involved in conducting a clinical trial. In one study the investigators thought that patients were being randomly assigned to receive care from either the teaching service or the nonteaching service of a university-affiliated hospital. When early data were analyzed, however, it was clear that the randomization process tended to be bypassed, particularly during the hospital's night shift, to ensure that *interesting* patients were allocated to the teaching service.[10] In clinical trials, maintaining the integrity of the randomization process also requires resisting the pressures of study participants who prefer to be placed in a group who will receive a new form of treatment or preventive care.[11]

3.2 INTERNAL VALIDITY, EXTERNAL VALIDITY, AND GENERALIZABILITY

According to the ethics of scientific research, randomized clinical trials must allow potential study subjects to participate or not, as they choose. This requirement introduces an element of self-selection into the participant pool before randomization into individual study groups even takes place. Because of the subsequent randomization process, study results are presumed to have **internal** validity (i.e., validity for participants in the study). However, the degree to which results may be generalized to people who did not participate in the study may be unclear, because a self-selected study group is not truly representative of any population. In other words, such a study may lack **external** validity (i.e., validity for the general population).

Questions of **generalizability** (i.e., external validity) have arisen in regard to the Physicians' Health Study, a costly but well-performed field trial involving the use of aspirin to reduce cardiovascular events and beta carotene to prevent cancer.[12] All the approximately 22,000 participants in the study were male US physicians, age 40 to 75, who met the exclusion criteria (also known as *baseline criteria*) of never having had heart disease, cancer, gastrointestinal disease, a bleeding tendency, or an allergy to aspirin. Early participants agreed to take part in the study, but after a trial period, the investigators dropped participants with poor compliance from the study

group. To what group of people in the US population can investigators generalize results obtained from a study of predominantly white, exclusively male, compliant, middle-aged or older physicians who were in good health at the start? Specifically, such results may not be generalizable to women or young men, and are probably not generalizable to people of color, those of lower socioeconomic status, or those with the excluded health problems. The unusually healthy character of these highly select research participants became evident only when their mortality rate, at one point in the study, was shown to be just 16% of the rate expected for men the same age in the United States. As a result, the investigators were forced to extend the study to obtain sufficient outcome events.

As another example of generalizability, while randomized trials have shown that primary prevention of diabetes is possible, population-level approaches are needed for widespread benefit. The Diabetes Prevention Program (DPP) showed that a lifestyle intervention was associated with a markedly reduced incidence of type 2 diabetes,[13] yet translating and adapting this program into the general community requires careful consideration. Significant effort has gone into translation and implementation into diverse settings, which require adaptations to the intervention to enhance the feasibility of program delivery and participant engagement.

3.3 DETECTION BIAS

When a clinical study is underway, the investigators focus on detecting and measuring possibly causal factors (e.g., high-fat diet or smoking) and outcomes of interest (e.g., disease or death) in the study groups. Care must be taken to ensure that the differences observed in the groups are not attributable to *measurement bias* or *recall bias* or other forms of detection bias.

Detection bias may be the result of failure to detect a case of disease, a possible causal factor, or an outcome of interest. In a study of a certain type of lung disease, if the case group consists of individuals receiving care in the pulmonary service of a hospital, whereas the control group consists of individuals in the community, early disease among the controls may be missed because they did not receive the intensive medical evaluation that the hospitalized patients received. The true difference between the cases and controls might be less than the apparent difference.

Detection bias may also occur if two groups of study subjects have large differences in their rates of loss to follow-up. In some clinical trials, the subjects who are lost to follow-up may be responding more poorly than the subjects who remain under observation, and they may leave to try other therapies. In other clinical trials, the subjects who are lost to follow-up may be those who respond the best, and they may feel well and thus lose interest in the trial.

3.3.a Measurement Bias

Measurement bias may occur during the collection of baseline or follow-up data. Bias may result from something as simple as measuring the height of patients with their shoes on, in which case all heights would be too large, or measuring their weight with their clothes on, in which case all weights would be too large. Even this situation is rather complicated, because the heels of men's shoes may differ systematically in height from those of women's shoes, while further variation in heel size may occur within each gendered group.

In the case of blood pressure values, bias can occur if some investigators or some study sites have blood pressure cuffs that measure incorrectly and cause the measurements to be higher or lower than the true values. Data from specific medical laboratories can also be subject to measurement bias. Some laboratories consistently report higher or lower values than others because they use different methods. Clinical investigators who collect laboratory data over time in the same institution or who compare laboratory data from different institutions must obtain the normal standards for each laboratory and adjust their analyses accordingly.

3.3.b Recall Bias

Recall bias takes many forms. It may occur if people who have experienced an adverse event, such as a disease, are more likely to recall previous risk factors than people who have never experienced that event. Although all study subjects may forget some information, bias results if members of one study group are collectively more likely to remember events than are members of the other study group. Recall bias is a major problem in research into causes of congenital anomalies. Mothers who give birth to abnormal infants tend to think more about their pregnancy and are more likely to remember infections, medications, and injuries. This attentiveness may produce a *spurious* (falsely positive) association between a risk factor (e.g., respiratory infections) and the outcome (congenital abnormality).

4. OTHER COMMON PITFALLS IN CAUSAL RESEARCH

In addition to the challenges of bias, among the most frequently encountered other pitfalls in causal research are random error, confounding, synergism, and effect modification (Box 4.3).

BOX 4.3   Common Pitfalls in Causal Research

Bias: A differential error that produces findings consistently distorted in one direction as a result of nonrandom factors.

Random error: A nondifferential error that produces findings that are too high and too low in approximately equal frequency because of random factors.

Confounding: The confusion of two supposedly causal variables, so that part or all of the purported effect of one variable is actually caused by the other.

Synergism: The interaction of two or more presumably causal variables, so that the total effect is greater than the sum of the individual effects.

Effect modification (interaction): A phenomenon in which a third variable alters the direction or strength of association between two other variables.

4.1 RANDOM ERROR

Random (chance) error, also known as **nondifferential error,** produces findings that are too high and too low in approximately equal amounts. Although a serious problem, random error is usually less damaging than bias because it is less likely to distort findings by reversing their overall direction. Nonetheless, random error decreases the probability of finding a real association by reducing the statistical power of a study.[14]

4.2 CONFOUNDING

Confounding (from Latin roots meaning "to pour together") is the confusion of two supposedly causal variables, so that part or all of the purported effect of one variable is actually caused by the other. For example, the percentage of gray hairs on the heads of adults is associated with the risk of myocardial infarction, but presumably that association is not causal. Age itself increases both the proportion of gray hairs and the risk of myocardial infarction.

By convention, when a third variable masks or weakens a true association between two variables, this is **negative confounding.** When a third variable produces an association that does not actually exist, this is **positive confounding.** To be clear, neither type of confounding is a "good thing" (i.e., neither is a positive factor); both are "bad" (i.e., negative in terms of effect).

4.3 SYNERGISM

Synergism (from Greek roots meaning "work together") is the interaction of two or more presumably causal variables, so that the combined effect is clearly greater than the sum of the individual effects. This is the type of situation when one plus one is greater than two effect. For example, the risk of lung cancer is greater when a person has exposure to both asbestos and cigarette smoking than would be expected on the basis of summing the observed risks from each factor alone.[15]

4.4 EFFECT MODIFICATION (INTERACTION)

Sometimes the direction or strength of an association between two variables differs according to the value of a third variable. This is usually called **effect modification** by epidemiologists and **interaction** by biostatisticians.

A biologic example of effect modification can be seen in the ways in which Epstein-Barr virus (EBV) infection manifests in different geographic areas. Although EBV usually results in infectious mononucleosis in the United States, it often produces Burkitt lymphoma in African regions where malaria is endemic. In the 1980s, to test whether malaria modifies the effects of EBV, investigators instituted a malaria suppression program in an African region where Burkitt lymphoma was usually found and followed the number of new cases. They reported that the incidence of Burkitt lymphoma decreased after malaria was suppressed, although other factors seemed to be involved as well.[16]

An example of effect modification can be seen in the reported rates of hypertension among white men and women surveyed in the United States.[17] In both men and women, the probability of hypertension increased with age. In those 30 to 44 years, however, men were more likely than women to have hypertension, whereas in older groups, the reverse was true. In the age group 45 to 64, women were more likely than men to have hypertension; in those 65 and older, women were much more likely to have hypertension. Gender did not reverse the trend of increasing rates of hypertension with increasing age, but the rate of increase did depend on gender. Thus we can say that gender modified the effect of age on blood pressure. Statistically there was an interaction between age and gender as predictors of blood pressure.

5. IMPORTANT REMINDERS ABOUT RISK FACTORS AND DISEASE

Although it is essential to avoid the pitfalls described previously, it is also necessary to keep two important concepts in mind. First, *one causal factor may increase the risk for several different diseases.* Cigarette smoking is a risk factor for cancer of the lung, larynx, mouth, and esophagus, as well as for chronic bronchitis and chronic obstructive pulmonary disease (COPD). Second, *one disease may have several different causal factors.* Although a strong risk factor for COPD, smoking may be only one of several contributing factors in a given case. Other factors may include occupational exposure to dust (e.g., coal dust, silicon) and genetic factors (e.g., α_1-antitrypsin deficiency). Similarly, the risk of myocardial infarction is influenced not only by a person's genes, diet, exercise, and smoking habits, but also by other medical conditions, such as high blood pressure and diabetes. A key task for epidemiologists is to determine the relative contribution of each causal factor to a given disease. This contribution, called the **attributable risk,** is discussed in Chapter 6.

The possibility of confounding and effect modification often makes the interpretation of epidemiologic studies difficult. Age, whether young or old, may be a confounder because it has a direct effect on the risk of death and of many diseases, so its impact must be removed before the causal effect of other variables can be known. Advancing age may also be an effect modifier, because it can change the magnitude of the risk of other variables.[18] The risk of myocardial infarction (MI) increases with age and with increasing levels of cholesterol and blood pressure—yet cholesterol and blood pressure also increase with age. To determine whether an association exists between cholesterol levels and MI, the effects of age and blood pressure must be controlled. Likewise, to determine the association between blood pressure and MI, the effects of age and cholesterol levels must be controlled. Although control can sometimes be achieved by research design and sample selection (e.g., by selecting study subjects in a narrow range of age and blood pressure), it is usually accomplished through statistical analysis (see Chapter 11).

6. SUMMARY

Epidemiologists are concerned with discovering the causes of disease in the environment, nutrition, lifestyle, and genes of individuals and populations. Causes are factors that, if removed or modified, would be followed by a change in disease burden. In a given population, smoking and obesity would increase the disease burden, whereas vaccines would increase health by reducing the disease burden. Research to determine causation is complicated, particularly because epidemiologists often do not have experimental control and must rely on observational methods.

When studies find an association between two things, it does not mean one thing caused the other one to happen. Writers for the lay media often describe the results of medical publications using active tense, yet there is a big difference in meaning between saying "A was associated with reduced risk of B" and saying "A reduces risk of B." The difference may seem subtle, but it is important.[19]

Several criteria must be met to establish a causal relationship between a factor and a disease. First, a statistical association must be shown, and the association becomes more impressive if it is strong and consistent. Second, the factor must precede the disease. Third, there should be no alternative explanations that fit the data equally well. Demonstrating that these criteria are met is complicated by the hazards of bias, random error, confounding, synergism, and effect modification. Internal validity defines whether a study's results may be trusted, whereas external validity defines the degree to which the results may be considered relevant to individuals other than the study participants themselves.

REFERENCES

1. No split seen over tobacco. *New York Times.* September 24, 1991:C3. Available at: https://nyti.ms/2z27vi9.
2. Doll R, Peto R. *The Causes of Cancer.* New York, NY: Oxford University Press; 1981.
3. Bauman KE. *Research Methods for Community Health and Welfare.* New York, NY: Oxford University Press; 1980.
4. US Surgeon General. *Smoking and Health.* Public Health Service Pub No. 1103. Washington, DC: US Government Printing Office; 1964.
5. Anderson GW, Arnstein MG, Lester MR. Chapter 17. In: *Communicable Disease Control.* 4th ed. New York, NY: Macmillan; 1962.
6. Susser M. *Causal Thinking in the Health Sciences.* New York, NY: Oxford University Press; 1973.
7. Doll R, Hill AB. Lung cancer and other causes of death in relation to smoking; a second report on the mortality of British doctors. *Br Med J.* 1956;2:1071-1081.
8. Suerbaum S, Michetti P. *Helicobacter pylori* infection. *N Engl J Med.* 2002;347:1175-1186.
9. Langmuir AD. Epidemiology of airborne infection. *Bacteriol Rev.* 1961;24:173-181.
10. Garrell M, Jekel JF. A comparison of quality of care on a teaching and non-teaching service in a university affiliated community hospital. *Conn Med.* 1979;43:659-663.

11. Lam JA, Hartwell SW, Jekel JF. "I prayed real hard, so I know I'll get in": living with randomization in social research. *New Dir Program Eval.* 1994;63:55-66.

12. Physicians' Health Study Steering Committee: Final report on the aspirin component of the ongoing Physicians' Health Study. *N Engl J Med* 321:129–135, 1989.

13. Diabetes Prevention Program (DPP) Research Group. The Diabetes Prevention Program (DPP): description of lifestyle intervention. *Diabetes Care.* 2002;25:2165-2171.

14. Kelsey JL, Whittemore AS, Evans AS, Thompson WD. Ch. 9 Case-control Studies: II. Further Design Considerations and Analysis. In: *Methods in Observational Epidemiology.* 2nd ed. New York, NY: Oxford University Press; 1996.

15. Hammond EC, Selikoff IJ, Seidman H. Asbestos exposure, cigarette smoking, and death rates. *Ann N Y Acad Sci.* 1979;330: 473-490.

16. Geser A, Brubaker G, Draper CC. Effect of a malaria suppression program on the incidence of African Burkitt's lymphoma. *Am J Epidemiol.* 1989;129:740-752.

17. National Center for Health Statistics. *Health Promotion and Disease Prevention: United States, 1990.* Vital and Health Statistics, Series 10, No. 185. Atlanta, GA: Centers for Disease Control and Prevention; 1993.

18. Jacobsen SJ, Freedman DS, Hoffmann RG, Gruchow HW, Anderson AJ, Barboriak JJ. Cholesterol and coronary artery disease: age as an effect modifier. *J Clin Epidemiol.* 1992;45: 1053-1059.

19. Zweig MD, DeVoto E. Observational studies: Does the language fit the evidence? Association vs. causation. *Health News Review.* Available at: https://www.healthnewsreview.org/toolkit/tips-for-understanding-studies/does-the-language-fit-the-evidence-association-versus-causation/. Accessed May 2019.

SELECT READINGS

Last JM. *A Dictionary of Epidemiology* (Miquel Porta ed.). 5th ed. New York, NY: Oxford University Press; 2008.

REVIEW QUESTIONS

1. This must be associated with the exposure and the outcome.
   A. Biologic plausibility
   B. Confounder
   C. Effect modifier
   D. External validity
   E. Internal validity
   F. Intervening variable
   G. Measurement bias
   H. Necessary cause
   I. Recall bias
   J. Sufficient cause
   K. Synergism

2. This alters the nature of a true relationship between an exposure and an outcome.
   A. Biologic plausibility
   B. Confounder
   C. Effect modifier

3. An example of this type of systematic distortion of study data is weighing subjects while they are fully dressed.
   A. Biologic plausibility
   B. Confounder
   C. Effect modifier
   D. External validity
   E. Internal validity
   F. Intervening variable
   G. Measurement bias
   H. Necessary cause
   I. Recall bias
   J. Sufficient cause
   K. Synergism

4. This is a multiplicative effect between exposure variables.
   A. Biologic plausibility
   B. Confounder
   C. Effect modifier
   D. External validity
   E. Internal validity
   F. Intervening variable
   G. Measurement bias
   H. Necessary cause
   I. Recall bias
   J. Sufficient cause
   K. Synergism

5. When the study sample adequately resembles the larger population from which it was drawn, the study is said to have this.
   A. Biologic plausibility
   B. Confounder
   C. Effect modifier
   D. External validity
   E. Internal validity
   F. Intervening variable
   G. Measurement bias
   H. Necessary cause
   I. Recall bias
   J. Sufficient cause
   K. Synergism

6. This is present if it is possible to conceive of an underlying mechanism by which an apparent cause could induce an apparent effect.
   A. Biologic plausibility
   B. Confounder

C. Effect modifier
D. External validity
E. Internal validity
F. Intervening variable
G. Measurement bias
H. Necessary cause
I. Recall bias
J. Sufficient cause
K. Synergism

7. This is *a* means or *the* means by which the causal factor leads to the outcome.
   A. Biologic plausibility
   B. Confounder
   C. Effect modifier
   D. External validity
   E. Internal validity
   F. Intervening variable
   G. Measurement bias
   H. Necessary cause
   I. Recall bias
   J. Sufficient cause
   K. Synergism

8. This is absolutely required for a disease to occur, but it will not necessarily produce the disease.
   A. Biologic plausibility
   B. Confounder
   C. Effect modifier
   D. External validity
   E. Internal validity
   F. Intervening variable
   G. Measurement bias
   H. Necessary cause
   I. Recall bias
   J. Sufficient cause
   K. Synergism

9. This is a systematic distortion in outcome assessments in retrospective studies; it is eliminated by a prospective design.
   A. Biologic plausibility
   B. Confounder
   C. Effect modifier
   D. External validity
   E. Internal validity
   F. Intervening variable
   G. Measurement bias
   H. Necessary cause
   I. Recall bias
   J. Sufficient cause
   K. Synergism

10. This is sufficient to produce disease.
    A. Biologic plausibility
    B. Confounder
    C. Effect modifier

D. External validity
E. Internal validity
F. Intervening variable
G. Measurement bias
H. Necessary cause
I. Recall bias
J. Sufficient cause
K. Synergism

11. This is present when study results are obtained in an unbiased manner.
    A. Biologic plausibility
    B. Confounder
    C. Effect modifier
    D. External validity
    E. Internal validity
    F. Intervening variable
    G. Measurement bias
    H. Necessary cause
    I. Recall bias
    J. Sufficient cause
    K. Synergism

ANSWERS AND EXPLANATIONS

1. **B.** A confounder is a third variable that is associated with the exposure variable and the outcome variable in question but is not in the causal pathway between the two. Cigarette smoking is a confounder of the relationship between alcohol consumption and lung cancer. Cigarette smoking is associated with the outcome, lung cancer, and with the exposure, alcohol consumption, but is not thought to be involved in the pathway through which alcohol could lead to lung cancer. If an investigator were to assess the relationship between alcohol consumption and lung cancer and not take smoking into account, alcohol would be found to be associated with an increased risk of lung cancer. When the study has controls in place to account for smoking (i.e., when varying degrees of alcohol consumption are compared in participants with comparable cigarette consumption), the association between alcohol and lung cancer essentially disappears. Almost all the increased risk that seemed to be attributable to alcohol is actually caused by cigarettes. In other words, heavy drinkers might develop lung cancer, but not because they consume a lot of alcohol. They have lung cancer because they tend to smoke. The alcohol is relatively innocent when it comes to lung cancer, and the apparent association is caused by confounding. Note that if cigarette consumption did not vary with alcohol exposure, there would be no apparent relationship and no confounding.

2. **C.** In contrast to a confounder, an effect modifier does not obscure the nature of a relationship between two other variables; rather, it changes the relationship. Consider the effect of age on the pharmacologic action of the drug methylphenidate. In children the

drug is used to treat hyperactivity and attention-deficit disorder, both of which are conditions in which there is too much activity. In adults the same drug is used to treat narcolepsy, a condition characterized by extreme daytime somnolence and, in essence, a paucity of energy and activity. There are true, measurable, and different effects of methylphenidate on energy and activity levels in children and in adults. The effects are not confounded by age but altered by it. This is effect modification. In contrast to confounders, which must be controlled, effect modifiers should not be controlled. Instead, effect modifiers should be analyzed to enhance understanding of the causal relationship in question.

3. **G.** In contrast to random error, measurement bias is a systematic distortion of study data. Random error produces some measurements that are too large, some that are too small, and perhaps some that are correct. Such error would contribute to variability within groups, limiting an investigator's ability to detect a significant difference between groups. Random error reduces the power of a study to show a true difference in outcome. When error is systematic, rather than random, statistical power may be preserved, but the study's validity (i.e., its most critical attribute) is threatened. Consider a study of weight loss in which the control participants and the intervention participants were weighed fully clothed and with shoes on at enrollment. After a weight loss intervention, the control participants were again weighed fully dressed, but the intervention participants were weighed after disrobing. This would be a biased and invalid measure of the intervention and resultant weight loss. Bias may threaten internal validity, external validity, or both.

4. **K.** When the combined effect of two or more variables on an outcome is greater than the sum of the separate effects of the variables, their interaction is called *synergy* or *synergism*. Cigarette smoking and asbestos exposure have a synergistic effect on the risk of lung cancer. If the relative risk or risk ratio for lung cancer in smokers is X and if the relative risk for lung cancer in asbestos workers is Y, the relative risk in those with both exposures is closer to $X \times Y$ than to $X + Y$.

5. **D.** The external validity of a study is determined by the resemblance of the study population to the larger population from which it was drawn. In a well-designed study of antihypertensive therapy in the prevention of stroke in middle-class white men, the validity of the findings for middle-class white women and for men and women of other socioeconomic and ethnic groups is uncertain. Although internal validity defines whether a study's results may be trusted, external validity defines the degree to which the results may be considered relevant to individuals other than the study participants themselves. Another term used to discuss external validity is generalizability. The greater a study's external validity, the more applicable or generalizable it is to populations outside of the study population.

6. **A.** Before one variable (a "cause" or "exposure") can be thought to induce another variable (the "effect" or "outcome"), the relationship must pass the test of biologic plausibility (i.e., the relationship must make sense biologically and mechanistically). In determining biologic plausibility, an open mind is essential because what is implausible now may become plausible as the science of medicine advances.

7. **F.** An intervening variable, or *mediator* or *mediating variable*, often represents an important mechanism by which an initial causal variable leads ultimately to a particular outcome. High-fructose corn syrup is related to obesity, but the connection between the two is largely indirect. For example, studies find fructose blunts levels of leptin, a hormone that regulates appetite, which can lead to overeating and weight gain. In this case, leptin is an intervening or mediating variable in one causal pathway between fructose and weight gain. Fructose also is shuttled directly to the liver, where it is converted to triglycerides (fat), ultimately driving insulin resistance, hyperinsulinemia (high insulin in the blood), and weight gain. Triglycerides and insulin are intervening or mediating variables in another causal pathway between fructose and weight gain.

8. **H.** A necessary cause is a factor that is required for a disease to occur. A necessary cause does not invariably lead to the disease, but the disease will certainly not occur unless the necessary cause is present. In the case of an infectious disease, exposure to a pathogen is always a necessary cause. Some people exposed to the pathogen may fail to acquire the disease, however, because of robust immunity, limited exposure, or other factors. Thus exposure to a pathogen is necessary but not sufficient. Necessary cause can be applied more broadly than disease scenarios. For example, impact between two vehicles is necessary to have a fatal head-on collision but is not necessarily sufficient to produce the fatal result. The speed of the crash, the angle of the collision, whether the drivers were restrained, and whether air bags deployed, all influence the ultimate result.

9. **I.** Recall bias is a systematic distortion found especially in retrospective studies. For example, in a case control study of congenital anomalies, the mothers of children born with any congenital anomaly might be more likely to recall being exposed during pregnancy to toxic substances (e.g., medications) than would the mothers of children born without congenital anomalies. This differential recall produces systematic error. In a prospective study, exposure is established at enrollment, before the subjects are distinguished on the basis of outcome (indeed, before the outcomes have occurred). Any differences in recall between groups would therefore likely be random, not systematic. Recall bias is minimized in a prospective study.

10. **J.** A sufficient cause is one that, if present, is all that is necessary to cause a particular disease or condition. However, a sufficient cause need not be necessary. For example, menopause is sufficient to cause infertility, but is not necessary to cause infertility. Hysterectomies, genetic disorders, and anatomic abnormalities are also sufficient to cause infertility but likewise not necessary.

11. **E.** The most important criterion on which a study is judged is its internal validity. If study results are obtained in an unbiased manner, the study is said to have internal validity. If the study is biased, it lacks internal validity, and its results are unreliable and meaningless. Consider, hypothetically, that in a study of prostate cancer, the outcome in men treated with orchiectomy (surgical removal of testes) is found to be worse than the outcome in men treated with orange juice. If men debilitated by illness had been assigned to orchiectomy, whereas men with no overt signs of illness had been assigned to orange juice therapy, the better outcome seen with orange juice therapy would be invalid because of the biased design of the study. Internal validity can be present only if bias is eliminated. Even if results are internally valid, however, it may not be possible to generalize results. To generalize, the investigator must have externally valid results, as discussed in answer 5.

5

Common Research Designs and Issues in Epidemiology

CHAPTER OUTLINE

"If we knew what we were doing it would not be called research, would it?"

Albert Einstein

1. FUNCTIONS OF RESEARCH DESIGN

Research is the process of answering a question that can be answered with appropriately collected data. The question may simply be, "What is (or was) the frequency of a disease in a certain place at a certain time?" The answer to this question is descriptive, but contrary to a common misperception, this does not mean that obtaining the answer (descriptive research) is a simple task. All research, whether quantitative or qualitative, is descriptive, and no research is better than the quality of the data obtained. To answer a research question correctly, the data must be obtained and described appropriately. The rules that govern the process of collecting and arranging the data for analysis are called research designs.

Another research question may be, "What caused this disease?" **Hypothesis generation** is the process of developing a list of possible candidates for the causes of the disease and obtaining initial evidence that supports one or more of these candidates. When one or more hypotheses are generated, the hypothesis must be tested (**hypothesis testing**) by making predictions from the hypotheses and examining new data to determine if the predictions are correct. If a hypothesis is not supported, it should be discarded or modified and tested again. Some research designs are appropriate for hypothesis generation, and some are appropriate for hypothesis testing. Some designs can be used for either, depending on the circumstances. No research design is perfect, however, because each has its advantages and disadvantages.

The basic function of most epidemiologic research designs is either to describe the pattern of health problems accurately or to enable a fair, unbiased comparison to be made between a group with and a group without a risk factor, disease, or preventive or therapeutic intervention. A good epidemiologic research design should perform the following functions:

- Enable a comparison of a variable (e.g., disease frequency) between two or more groups at one point in time or, in some cases, within one group before and after receiving an intervention or being exposed to a risk factor
- Allow the comparison to be quantified in absolute terms (as with a risk difference or rate difference) or in relative terms (as with a relative risk or odds ratio; see Chapter 6)
- Permit the investigators to determine when the risk factor and the disease occurred, to determine the temporal sequence
- Minimize biases, confounding and other problems that would complicate interpretation of the data

The research designs discussed in this chapter are the primary designs used in epidemiology. Depending on design choice, research designs can assist in developing hypotheses, testing hypotheses, or both. All designs can be used to generate hypotheses; and a few designs can be used to test them—with the caveat that hypothesis development and testing of the same hypothesis can never occur in a single study. Randomized clinical trials or randomized field trials are usually the best designs for testing hypotheses when feasible to perform.

2. TYPES OF RESEARCH DESIGN

Because some research questions can be answered by more than one type of research design, the choice of design depends on a variety of considerations, including the clinical topic (e.g., whether the disease or condition is rare or common) and the cost and availability of data. Research designs are often described as either observational or experimental.

In observational studies the investigators simply observe groups of study participants to learn about the possible effects of a treatment or risk factor; the assignment of participants to a treatment group or a control group remains outside the investigators' control. Observational studies can be either descriptive or analytic. In descriptive observational studies, no hypotheses are specified in advance, preexisting data are often used, and associations may or may not be causal. In analytic observational studies, hypotheses are specified in advance, new data are often collected, and differences between groups are measured.

In an experimental study design the investigator has more control over the assignment of participants, often placing them in treatment and control groups (e.g., by using a randomization method before the start of any treatment). Each type of research design has advantages and disadvantages, as discussed subsequently and summarized in Table 5.1 and Fig. 5.1.

TABLE 5.1 Advantages and Disadvantages of Common Types of Studies Used in Epidemiology

Studies	Advantages	Disadvantages
Qualitative research	Generates hypotheses and initial exploration of issues in participants' own language without bias of investigator	Cannot test study hypotheses Can explore only what is presented or stated Has potential for bias
Cross-sectional surveys	Are fairly quick and easy to perform Are useful for hypothesis generation	Do not offer evidence of a temporal relationship between risk factors and disease Are subject to late-look bias Are not good for hypothesis testing
Ecologic studies	Are fairly quick and easy to perform Are useful for hypothesis generation	Do not allow for causal conclusions to be drawn because the data are not associated with individual persons Are subject to ecologic fallacy Are not good for hypothesis testing
Cohort studies	Can be performed retrospectively or prospectively Can be used to obtain a true (absolute) measure of risk Can study many disease outcomes Are good for studying rare risk factors	Are time consuming and costly (especially prospective studies) Can study only the risk factors measured at the beginning Can be used only for common diseases May have losses to follow up
Case control studies	Are fairly quick and easy to perform Can study many risk factors Are good for studying rare diseases	Can obtain only a relative measure of risk Are subject to recall bias Selection of controls may be difficult Temporal relationships may be unclear Can study only one disease outcome at a time
Randomized controlled trials	Are the gold standard for evaluating treatment interventions (clinical trials) or preventive interventions (field trials) Allow investigator to have extensive control over research process	Are time consuming and usually costly Can study only interventions or exposures that are controlled by investigator May have problems related to therapy changes and dropouts May be limited in generalizability Are often unethical to perform at all
Systematic reviews and meta-analysis	Decrease subjective element of literature review Increase statistical power Allow exploration of subgroups Provide quantitative estimates of effect	Mixing poor quality studies together in a review or meta-analysis does not improve the underlying quality of studies
Cost-effectiveness analysis	Clinically important	Difficult to identify costs and payments in many health care systems

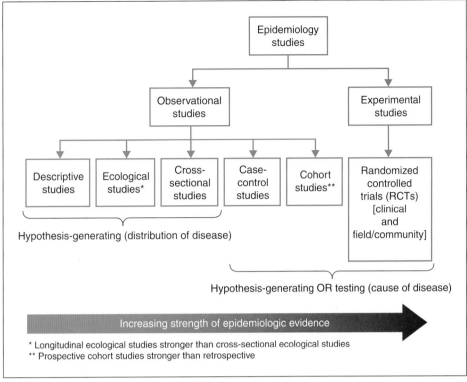

Fig. 5.1 Epidemiologic Study Designs and Increasing Strength of Evidence.

2.1 OBSERVATIONAL DESIGNS FOR GENERATING HYPOTHESES

2.1.a. Qualitative Studies

Qualitative research involves an investigation of clinical issues by using anthropologic techniques such as ethnographic observation, open-ended semistructured interviews, focus groups, and key informant interviews. The investigators attempt to listen to the participants without introducing their own bias as they gather data. They then review the results and identify patterns in the data in a structured and sometimes quantitative form. Results from qualitative research are often invaluable for informing and making sense of quantitative results and providing greater insights into clinical questions and public health problems. The two approaches (quantitative and qualitative) are complementary, with qualitative research providing rich, narrative information that tells a story beyond what reductionist statistics alone might reveal.

2.1.b. Cross-Sectional Surveys

A cross-sectional survey is a survey of a population at a single point in time. Surveys may be performed by trained interviewers in people's homes, by telephone interviewers using random-digit dialing, or by mailed, emailed, or web-based questionnaires. Telephone surveys or email questionnaires are often the quickest, but they typically have many nonresponders and refusals, and some people do not have telephones or email access, or they may block calls or emails even if they do. Mailed surveys are also relatively inexpensive, but they usually have poor response rates, often 50% or less, except in the case of the US census, where response is required by law, and follow-up of all nonresponders is standard.

Cross-sectional surveys have the advantage of being fairly quick and easy to perform. They are useful for determining the prevalence of risk factors and the frequency of prevalent cases of certain diseases for a defined population. They also are useful for measuring current health status and planning for some health services, including setting priorities for disease control. Many surveys have been undertaken to determine the knowledge, attitudes, and health practices of various populations, with the resulting data increasingly being made available to the general public (e.g., www.healthyamericans.org). A major disadvantage of using cross-sectional surveys is that data on the exposure to risk factors and the presence or absence of disease are collected simultaneously, creating difficulties in determining the temporal relationship of a presumed cause and effect. Another disadvantage is that cross-sectional surveys are biased in favor of longer-lasting and more indolent (mild) cases of diseases. Such cases are more likely to be found by a survey because people live longer with mild cases, enabling larger numbers of affected people to survive and to be interviewed. Severe diseases that tend to be rapidly fatal are less likely to be found by a survey. This phenomenon is often called **Neyman bias** or **late-look bias**. It is known as **length bias** in screening programs, which tend to find (and select for) less aggressive illnesses because patients are more likely to be found by screening (see Chapter 16).

Repeated cross-sectional surveys may be used to determine changes in risk factors and disease frequency in populations over time (but not the nature of the association between risk factors and diseases). Although the data derived from these surveys can be examined for such associations to generate hypotheses, cross-sectional surveys are not appropriate for testing the effectiveness of interventions. In such surveys, investigators may find that participants who reported immunization against a disease had fewer cases of the disease. The investigators would not know, however, whether this finding actually meant that people who sought immunization were more concerned about their health and less likely to expose themselves to the disease, known as **healthy participant bias**. If the investigators randomized the participants into two groups, as in a randomized clinical trial, and immunized only one of the groups, this would exclude self-selection as a possible explanation for the association.

Cross-sectional surveys are of particular value in infectious disease epidemiology, in which the prevalence of antibodies against infectious agents, when analyzed according to age or other variables, may provide evidence about when and in whom an infection has occurred. Proof of a recent acute infection can be obtained by two serum samples separated by a short interval. The first samples, the acute sera, are collected soon after symptoms appear. The second samples, the convalescent sera, are collected many days to weeks later. A significant increase in the serum titer of antibodies to a particular infectious agent is regarded as proof of recent infection.

2.1.c. Cross-Sectional Ecologic Studies

Cross-sectional ecologic studies relate the frequency with which some characteristic (e.g., smoking) and some outcome of interest (e.g., lung cancer) occur in the same geographic area (e.g., a city, state, or country). In contrast to all other epidemiologic studies, the unit of analysis in ecologic studies is *populations,* not individuals. These studies are often useful for suggesting hypotheses but cannot be used to draw causal conclusions. Ecologic studies provide no information as to whether the people who were exposed to the characteristic were the same people who developed the disease, whether the exposure or the onset of disease came first, or whether there are other explanations for the observed association. Concerned citizens are sometimes unaware of these study design weaknesses (sometimes called the **ecologic fallacy**) and use findings from cross-sectional ecologic surveys to make such statements as, "There are high levels of both toxic pollution and cancer in northern New Jersey, so the toxins are causing the cancer." Although superficially plausible, this conclusion may or may not be correct. For example, what if the individuals in the population who are exposed to the toxins are universally the people not developing cancer? Therefore the toxic pollutants would be exerting a protective effect for individuals despite the ecologic evidence that may suggest the opposite conclusion.

In many cases, nevertheless, important hypotheses initially suggested by cross-sectional ecologic studies were later supported by other types of studies. The rate of dental caries in children was found to be much higher in areas with low levels of natural fluoridation in the water than in areas with high levels of natural fluoridation.[1] Subsequent research established that this association was causal, and the introduction of water fluoridation and fluoride treatment of teeth has been followed by striking reductions in the rate of dental caries.[2]

2.1.d. Longitudinal Ecologic Studies

Longitudinal ecologic studies use ongoing surveillance or frequent repeated cross-sectional survey data to measure trends in disease rates over many years in a defined population. By comparing the trends in disease rates with other changes in the society (e.g., wars, immigration, introduction of a vaccine or antibiotics), epidemiologists attempt to determine the impact of these changes on disease rates.

For example, the introduction of the polio vaccine resulted in a precipitous decrease in the rate of paralytic poliomyelitis in the US population (see Chapter 3 and Fig. 3.7). In this case, because of the large number of people involved in the immunization program and the relatively slow rate of change for other factors in the population, longitudinal ecologic studies were useful for determining the impact of this public health intervention. Nevertheless, confounding with other factors can distort the conclusions drawn from ecologic studies, so if time is available (i.e., it is not an epidemic situation), investigators should perform field studies, such as randomized controlled field trials (see upcoming discussion; also see Section 2.3.b), before pursuing a new, large-scale public health intervention.

Another example of longitudinal ecologic research is the study of rates of malaria in the US population since 1930. As shown in Fig. 5.2, the peaks in malaria rates can be readily related to social events such as wars and immigration. The use of a logarithmic scale in the figure for the *y*-axis data visually minimizes the relative decrease in disease frequency, making it less impressive to the eye, but this scale enables readers to see in detail the changes occurring when rates are low.

Important causal associations have been suggested by longitudinal ecologic studies. About 20 years after an increase in the smoking rates in men, the lung cancer rate in the male population began increasing rapidly. Similarly, about 20 years after women began to smoke in large numbers, the lung cancer rate in the female population began to increase. The studies in this example were longitudinal ecologic studies in the sense that they used only national data on smoking and lung cancer rates, which did not relate the individual cases of lung cancer to individual smokers. The task of establishing a causal relationship was left to cohort and case control studies.

2.2 OBSERVATIONAL DESIGNS FOR GENERATING OR TESTING HYPOTHESES

2.2.a. Cohort Studies

A cohort is a clearly identified group of people to be studied. In cohort studies, investigators begin by assembling one or more cohorts, either by choosing persons specifically because they were or were not exposed to one or more risk factors of

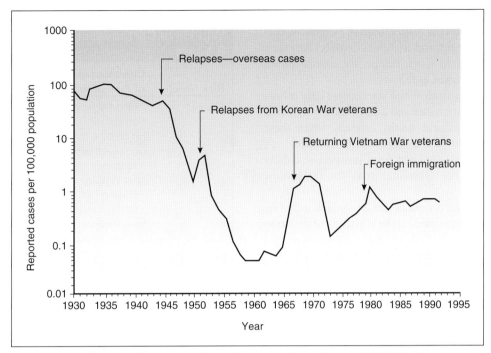

Fig. 5.2 Incidence Rates of Malaria in the United States, by Year of Report, 1930–1992. (From Centers for Disease Control and Prevention: Summary of notifiable diseases, United States, 1992. *MMWR* 41:38, 1992.)

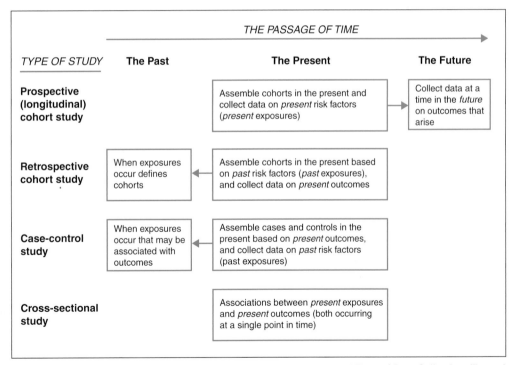

Fig. 5.3 Relationship between Time of Assembling Study Participants and Time of Data Collection. Illustration shows prospective cohort study, retrospective cohort study, case control study, and cross-sectional study.

interest, or by taking a random sample of a given population. Participants are assessed to determine whether they develop the diseases of interest, and whether the risk factors predict the diseases that occur. The defining characteristic of cohort studies is that groups are typically defined on the basis of exposure and are followed for outcomes. This is in contrast to case control studies (see upcoming discussion; also see Section 2.2.b), in which groups are assembled on the basis of outcome status and are queried for exposure status. There are two general types of cohort studies, prospective and retrospective; Fig. 5.3 shows the time relationships of these two types.

Prospective cohort studies. In a prospective cohort study, the investigator assembles the study groups in the present, collects baseline data on them, and continues to collect data for a period that can last many years. Prospective cohort studies offer three main advantages, as follows:

1. The investigator can control and standardize data collection as the study progresses and can check the outcome events (e.g., diseases and death) carefully when these occur, ensuring the outcomes are correctly classified.

2. The estimates of risk obtained from prospective cohort studies represent true (absolute) risks for the groups studied.

3. Many different disease outcomes can be studied, including some that were not anticipated at the beginning of the study.

However, any disease outcomes that were not pre-planned—or supported by evidence that was available a priori (before the start of the study)—would be hypothesis generating only. Sometimes studies have secondary outcomes that are determined a priori, but for which the study is not adequately powered and thus can only be hypothesis generating.

Cohort studies also have disadvantages. In such studies, only the risk factors defined and measured at the beginning of the study can be used. Other disadvantages of cohort studies are their high costs, the possible loss of study participants to follow-up, and the long wait until results are obtained.

The classic cohort study is the Framingham Heart Study, initiated in 1950 and continuing today.[3] Table 5.2 shows the 8-year risk of heart disease as calculated from the early Framingham Study's equations.[4] These risk ratios have been updated with more recent data that provide longer length of follow-up and the clarity of the message makes them useful for sharing with patients. Examples of other large cohort studies are the Nurses' Health Study, begun in 1976 and continuing to track more than 120,000 nurses in the United States (www.nhs3.org), and the National Child Development Study, initiated after the Second World War and continuing to follow a large birth cohort in the United Kingdom.[5]

Retrospective cohort studies. The time and cost limitations of prospective cohort studies can be mitigated in part by conducting retrospective cohort studies. In this approach the investigator uses historical data to define a risk group (e.g., people exposed to the Hiroshima atomic bomb in August 1945) and follows group members up to the present to see what outcomes (e.g., cancer and death) have occurred. This type of study has many of the advantages of a prospective cohort study, including the ability to calculate an absolute risk. However, it lacks the ability to monitor and control data collection that characterizes a prospective cohort study.

A retrospective cohort study in 1962 investigated the effects of prenatal x-ray exposure.[6] In prior decades, radiographs were often used to measure the size of the pelvic outlet of pregnant women, thus exposing fetuses to x-rays in utero. The investigators identified one group of participants

TABLE 5.2 Risk That 45-Year-Old Man Will Have Cardiovascular Disease Within 8 Years

Risk Group	Characteristics of Risk Group	Risk (%)	Ratio
Lowest	All the following factors: Nonsmoker No glucose intolerance No hypertrophy of left ventricle Low systolic blood pressure (≤105 mm Hg) Low cholesterol level (≤185 mg/dL)	2.2	—
Intermediate	One of the following factors:		
	Smoker	3.8	1.7
	Glucose intolerance	3.9	1.8
	Hypertrophy of left ventricle	6	2.7
	Severe hypertension (systolic blood pressure ≥195 mm Hg)	8.4	3.8
	High cholesterol level (≥335 mg/dL)	8.5	3.8
Highest	All the factors listed under Intermediate	77.8	35.4

http://hp2010.nhlbihin.net/atpiii/calculator.asp
Data from Pearson T, Becker D: Cardiovascular risk: computer program for IBM-compatible systems, using the Framingham Study 8-year risk equations, Johns Hopkins University; and Breslow L: *Science* 200: 908–912, 1978.

who had been exposed in utero and another group who had not. They determined how many participants from each group had developed cancer during childhood or early adulthood (up to the time of data collection). The individuals who had been exposed to x-rays in utero had a 40% increase in the risk of childhood cancers, or a risk ratio of 1.4, after adjustments for other factors.

2.2.b. Case Control Studies

The investigator in a case control study selects the case group and the control group on the basis of a defined outcome (e.g., having a disease of interest vs. not having a disease of interest) and compares the groups in terms of their frequency of past exposure to possible risk factors (see Fig. 5.3). This strategy can be understood as comparing "the risk of having the risk factor" in the two groups. However, the actual risk of the outcome cannot be determined from such studies because the underlying population remains unknown. Instead, case control studies can estimate the relative risk of the outcome, known as the **odds ratio**.

In the case control study the cases and controls are assembled and then questioned (or their relatives or medical records are consulted) regarding past exposure to risk factors.

For this reason, case control studies were often called "retrospective studies" in the past; this term does not distinguish them from retrospective cohort studies and thus is no longer preferred. The time relationships in a case control study are similar to those in a cross-sectional study in that investigators learn simultaneously about the current disease state and any past risk factors. In terms of assembling the participants, however, a case control study differs from a cross-sectional study because the sample for the case control study is chosen specifically from groups with and without the disease of interest. Often, everyone with the disease of interest in a given geographic area and time period can be selected as cases. This strategy reduces bias in case selection.

Case control studies are especially useful when a study must be performed quickly and inexpensively or when the disease under study is rare (e.g., prevalence <1%). In a cohort study a huge number of study participants would need to be followed to find even a few cases of a rare disease, and the search might take a long time even if funds were available. If a new cancer were found in 1 of 1000 people screened per year (a rate that does occur with many cancers), an investigator would have to study 50,000 people to find just 50 cases over a typical follow-up time of 1 year. Although case control studies can consider only one outcome (one disease) per study, many risk factors may be considered, a characteristic that makes such studies useful for generating hypotheses about the causes of a disease. Methodologic standards have been developed so that the quality of information obtained from case control studies can approximate that obtained from much more difficult, costly, and time-consuming randomized clinical trials.

Despite these advantages, the use of case control studies has several drawbacks. In determining risk factors, a major problem is the potential for recall bias (see Chapter 4). Also, it is not easy to know the correct control group for cases. Members of a control group are usually matched individually to members of the case group on the basis of age, gender, and often race. If possible, the investigator obtains controls from the same diagnostic setting in which cases were found, to avoid potential bias (e.g., if the disease is more likely to be detected in one setting than in another). If the controls were drawn from the same hospital and were examined for a disease of the same organ system (e.g., pulmonary disease), presumably a similar workup (including chest radiograph and spirometry) would be performed, so that asymptomatic cases of the disease would be less likely to be missed and incorrectly classified as controls. Similarly, in a study of birth defects, the control for each case might be the next infant who was born at the same hospital, of the same gender and race, with a mother of similar age from the same location. This strategy would control for season, location, gender, race, and age of mother. Given the difficulties of selecting a control group with no bias whatsoever, investigators often assemble two or more control groups, one of which is drawn from the general population.

A potential danger of studies that use matching is **overmatching**. If cases and controls were inadvertently matched on some characteristic that is potentially causal, that *cause* would be missed. For example, if cases and controls in early studies of the causes of lung cancer had been matched on smoking status, smoking would not appear as a potentially causal factor.

A case control study was successful in identifying the risk associated with taking a synthetic hormone, diethylstilbestrol (DES), during pregnancy. In 1971 the mothers of seven of eight teenage girls diagnosed with clear cell adenocarcinoma of the vagina in Boston claimed to have taken DES while the child was in utero.[7] For controls, the authors identified girls without vaginal adenocarcinoma who were born in the same hospital and same date of birth as the cases. The authors identified 4 controls for each case. None of the mothers of the 32 (control) girls without vaginal adenocarcinoma had taken DES during the corresponding pregnancy.

2.2.c. Nested Case Control Studies

In a cohort study with a nested case control study design, a cohort of participants is first defined, and the baseline characteristics of the participants are obtained by interview, physical examination, and pertinent laboratory or imaging studies. The participants are then followed to determine the outcome. Participants who develop the condition of interest become cases in the nested case control study; participants who do not develop the condition become eligible for the control group of the nested case control study. The cases and a representative (or matched) sample of controls are studied, and data from the two groups are compared by using analytic methods appropriate for case control studies.

A nested case control design was used in a study of meningitis. Participants were drawn from a large, prospective cohort study of patients admitted to the emergency department because of suspected meningitis.[8,9] In the nested case control study the cases were all the patients with a diagnosis of nonbacterial meningitis, and the controls represented a sample of patients not diagnosed with meningitis. The goal was to determine whether there was an association between the prior use of nonsteroidal antiinflammatory drugs and the frequency of nonbacterial meningitis. Using patients from the larger cohort study, for whom data had already been obtained, made the nested case control study simpler and less costly.

A variant of the nested case control design is the case cohort study.[10] In this approach the study also begins with a cohort study, and the controls are similarly drawn from the cohort study but are identified *before* any cases develop, so some may later become cases. The analysis for case cohort studies is more complex than for other case control studies.

2.3 EXPERIMENTAL DESIGNS FOR TESTING HYPOTHESES

Two types of randomized controlled trials (RCTs) are discussed here: randomized controlled clinical trials (RCCTs) and randomized controlled field trials (RCFTs). Both designs follow the same series of steps shown in Fig. 5.4 and have

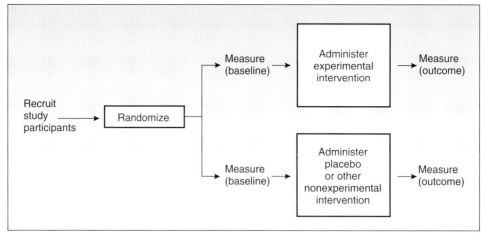

Fig. 5.4 Relationship between Time of Recruiting Study Participants and Time of Data Collection in Randomized Controlled Trial (RCT; Clinical or Field).

many of the same advantages and disadvantages. The major difference between the two is that clinical trials are typically used to test therapeutic interventions in ill persons, whereas field trials are typically used to test preventive interventions in well persons in the community.

2.3.a. Randomized Controlled Clinical Trials

In an RCCT, often referred to simply as an RCT, patients are enrolled in a study and randomly assigned to one of the following two groups:

- Intervention or treatment group, who receives the experimental treatment
- Control group, who receives the nonexperimental treatment, consisting of either a placebo (inert substance) or a standard treatment method

The RCCT is considered the gold standard for studying interventions because of the ability to minimize bias in the information obtained from participants. Nevertheless, RCCTs do not eliminate bias completely, so these trials pose some challenges and ethical dilemmas for investigators.

To be enrolled in an RCCT, patients must agree to participate without knowing whether they will receive the experimental or the nonexperimental treatment. When this condition is met, and patients are kept unaware of which treatment they receive during the trial, it establishes a **single-blind study** (or single blinded; i.e., the participant is blind to the treatment). If possible, the observers who collect the data and those who are doing the analyses are also prevented from knowing which type of treatment each patient is given. When both participants and investigators are blinded, the trial is said to be a **double-blind study** (or double blinded). Unfortunately, there is some ambiguity in the way blinding is described in the literature, thus we recommend including descriptions that clearly communicate which of the relevant groups were unaware of allocation.[11]

Ideally trials should have a third level of blinding, sometimes known as **allocation concealment**. This third type of blinding means that the investigators delivering the intervention are also blinded as to whether they are providing experimental or control treatment (i.e., they are blinded to the allocation of participants to the experimental or control group). When participants, investigators who gather the data, and analysts are all blinded, this is functionally a triple-blind study (or triple blinded), which is optimal. To have true blinding, the nonexperimental treatment must appear identical (e.g., in size, shape, color, taste) to the experimental treatment.

Fig. 5.5 shows the pill packet from a trial of two preventive measures from a famous RCT, the Physicians' Health Study (see Chapter 4). The round tablets were either aspirin or a placebo, but the study participants (and investigators) could not tell which based on size, shape, and color. The elongated capsules were either betacarotene or a placebo, but again the study participants (and investigators) could not distinguish between them.

It is usually impossible and unethical to have patients participate blindly in a study involving a surgical intervention, because blinding would require a sham operation (although sometimes this is done). In studies involving nonsurgical interventions, investigators often can develop an effective placebo. For example, when investigators designed a computer game to teach asthmatic children how to care for themselves, with the goal of reducing hospitalizations, they distributed similar-looking computer games to children in the intervention group and the control group, but the games for the control group were without asthma content.[12]

Undertaking an RCCT is difficult, and potentially unethical, if the intervention is already well established in practice and strongly believed to be the best available, whether that belief had been confirmed scientifically by carefully designed and controlled studies. Because no RCCTs have compared prenatal care versus no prenatal care, there is no conclusive proof that prenatal care is valuable, and questions about its value are raised from time to time. The standard of practice might preclude a RCCT in which one arm involved no prenatal care. However, studies in which variations in the frequency, duration, and content of prenatal care were compared would likely avoid the ethical dilemma, while

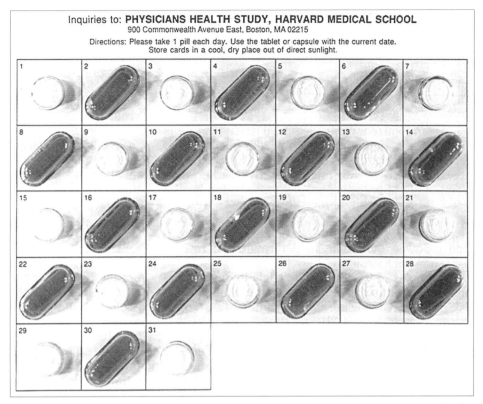

Inquiries to: PHYSICIANS HEALTH STUDY, HARVARD MEDICAL SCHOOL
900 Commonwealth Avenue East, Boston, MA 02215
Directions: Please take 1 pill each day. Use the tablet or capsule with the current date.
Store cards in a cool, dry place out of direct sunlight.

Fig. 5.5 "Bubble" Pill Packet Provided Monthly to 22,000 Physicians in Physicians' Health Study. In this simultaneous trial of aspirin to reduce cardiovascular disease and betacarotene to prevent cancer, the round white tablets contained either aspirin or placebo and the elongated capsules either betacarotene or placebo. The participants did not know which substances they were taking. (Courtesy Dr. Charles Hennekens, Director, Physicians' Health Study, Boston.)

generating useful information. At a time when both medical ethics and evidence-based practice are salient concerns, there are new challenges involved in putting time-honored practices to the rigorous test of randomized trials.

In RCCTs, many biases remain possible, although some biases have been minimized by the randomized, prospective design and by blinding of participants and investigators. For example, two groups under comparison may exhibit different rates at which patients drop out of the study or become lost to follow-up, and this difference could produce a greater change in the characteristics of the remaining study participants in one group than in the other.

Therapy changes and dropouts are special problems in RCCTs involving severe diseases, such as advanced cancer. The patients receiving the new treatment may continue to fail to respond, and either they or their physicians may decide to try a different treatment, which they must be allowed to do. Patients also may leave a study if the new treatment has unpleasant side effects, even though the treatment may be effective. In the past, some medications for hypertension reduced male potency, and many men discontinued their medication when this happened, despite its beneficial effect on their hypertension.

An apparent selection bias, called **publication bias**, makes it difficult to arrive at an overall interpretation of the results of clinical trials reported in the literature. For various reasons, pharmaceutical companies or investigators, or both, may not want to publish RCTs with negative results (i.e., results that do not favor the intervention being tested). Even journal editors may not be enthusiastic about publishing negative trials because they may not be interesting to their readers (i.e., unless they contradict established dogma and would be paradigm challenging and news generating). Published RCCTs on a new intervention, as a group, may therefore give a more favorable impression of the intervention than would be likely if all trials of that intervention (including trials that returned negative results) had been published.

To reduce this problem, a group of editors collaborated to create a policy whereby their journals would consider publication only of results of RCCTs that had been registered with a clinical trial registry "before the onset of patient enrollment."[13] This requirement that all trials be registered before they begin is important if the sponsors and investigators want to be eligible to publish in a major medical journal. It is now possible to explore the clinical trial registry to find out what studies remain unpublished (http://clinicaltrials.gov).

2.3.b. Randomized Controlled Field Trials

An RCFT is similar to an RCCT (see Fig. 5.4), except that the intervention in an RCFT is usually preventive rather than therapeutic and conducted in the community. Appropriate participants are randomly allocated to receive the preventive measure (e.g., vaccine, oral drug) or to receive the placebo (e.g., injection of sterile saline, inert pill). They are followed over time to determine the rate of disease in each group. Examples of RCFTs include trials of vaccines to prevent paralytic poliomyelitis[14] and aspirin to reduce cardiovascular disease.[15]

The RCFTs and the RCCTs have similar advantages and disadvantages. One disadvantage is that results may take a long time to obtain, unless the effect of the treatment or preventive measure occurs quickly. The Physicians' Health Study cited earlier illustrates this problem. Although its trial of the preventive benefits of aspirin began in 1982, the final report on the aspirin component of the trial was not released until 7 years later.

Another disadvantage of RCFTs and RCCTs involves **external validity**, or the ability to generalize findings to other groups in the population (vs. **internal validity**, or the validity of results for study participants). After the study groups for an RCT have been assembled and various potential participants excluded according to the study's exclusion criteria, it may be unclear which population is actually represented by the remaining people in the trial.

2.4 TECHNIQUES FOR DATA SUMMARY, COST-EFFECTIVENESS ANALYSIS, AND POST-APPROVAL SURVEILLANCE

Meta-analysis, decision analysis, and cost-effectiveness analysis are important techniques for examining and using data collected in clinical research. Meta-analysis is used to summarize the information obtained in many single studies on one topic. Decision analysis and cost-effectiveness analysis are used to summarize data and show how data can inform clinical or policy decisions. All three techniques are discussed in more detail in Chapter 13. One of the most important uses of summary techniques has been to develop recommendations for clinical preventive services (e.g., by the US Preventive Services Task Force) and community preventive services (e.g., by the US Community Services Task Force). These task forces have used a hierarchy to indicate the quality of evidence, such that RCTs are at the apex (best internal validity), followed by designs with fewer protections against bias (see Chapter 18).

The usual drug approvals by the US Food and Drug Administration (FDA) are based on RCTs of limited size and duration. Longer term post-approval surveillance (now called Phase 4 clinical testing) is increasingly exhibiting its importance.[16] Such post-approval surveillance permits a much larger study sample and a longer observation time, so that side effects not seen in the earlier studies may become obvious. A much-publicized example of such findings was the removal from the market of some cyclooxygenase-2 (COX-2) inhibitor medications (a type of nonsteroidal antiinflammatory drug [NSAID]), because of an increase in cardiovascular events in these patients.[17,18]

3. RESEARCH ISSUES IN EPIDEMIOLOGY

3.1 DANGERS OF DATA DREDGING

The common research designs described in this chapter are frequently used by investigators to gather and summarize data. Looking for messages in data carries the potential danger of finding those that do not really exist. In studies with large amounts of data, there is a temptation to use modern computer techniques to see which variables are related to which other variables and to make many associations. This process is sometimes referred to as "data dredging" and is often used in medical research, although this is sometimes not clarified in the published literature. Readers of medical literature should be aware of the special dangers in this activity.

The search for associations can be appropriate as long as the investigator keeps two points in mind. First, the scientific process requires that hypothesis development and hypothesis testing be based on *different* data sets. One data set is used to develop the hypothesis or model, which is used to make predictions, which are then tested on a new data set. Second, a correlational study (e.g., using Pearson correlation coefficient or chi-square test) is useful only for developing hypotheses, not for testing them. Stated in slightly different terms, a correlational study is only a form of a screening method, to identify possible associations that might (or might not) be real. Investigators who keep these points in mind are unlikely to make the mistake of thinking every association found in a data set represents a true association.

One example of the problem of data dredging was seen in the report of an association between coffee consumption and pancreatic cancer, obtained by looking at many associations in a large data set, without repeating the analysis on another data set to determine if it was consistent.[19] This approach was severely criticized at the time, and several subsequent studies failed to find a true association between coffee consumption and pancreatic cancer.[20]

How does this problem arise? Suppose there were 10 variables in a descriptive study, and the investigator wanted to associate each one with every other one. There would be 10×10 possible cells (Fig. 5.6). Ten of these would be each variable times itself, however, which is always a perfect correlation. That leaves 90 possible associations, but half of these would be "$x \times y$" and the other half "$y \times x$." Because the p values for bivariate tests are the same regardless of which is considered the independent variable and which the dependent variable, there are only half as many truly independent associations, or 45. If the $p = 0.05$ cutoff point is used for defining a significant finding (alpha level) (see Chapter 9), then 5 of 100 independent associations would be expected to occur by chance alone.[21] In the example, it means that slightly more than two "statistically significant" associations would be expected to occur just by chance.

The problem with multiple hypotheses is similar to that with multiple associations: the greater the number of hypotheses tested, the more likely that at least one of them will

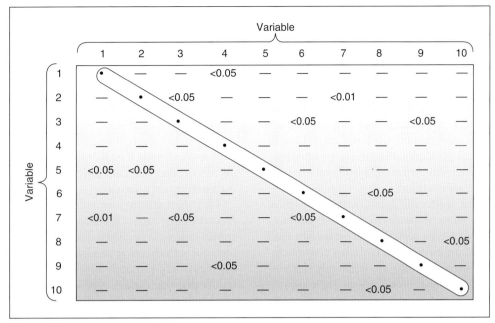

Fig. 5.6 **Matrix of Possible Statistical Associations between 10 Different Variables from Same Research Study.** Perfect correlations of one variable with itself are shown by dots; nonstatistically significant relationships are shown by dashes; and statistically significant associations are shown by the *p* values. (Redrawn from Jekel JF: Should we stop using the *p*-value in descriptive studies? *Pediatrics* 60:124–126, 1977.)

be found "statistically significant" by chance alone. One possible way to handle this problem is to lower the *p* value required before rejecting the null hypothesis. This was done in a study testing the same medical educational hypothesis at five different hospitals.[21] If the alpha level in the study had been set at 0.05, there would have been an almost 25% probability of finding a statistically significant difference by chance alone in at least one of the five hospitals, because each hospital had a 5% (alpha = 0.05) probability of showing a difference from chance alone. To keep the risk of a false-positive finding in the entire study to no more than 0.05, the alpha level chosen for rejecting the null hypothesis was made more stringent by dividing alpha by 5 (number of hospitals) to make it 0.01. This method of adjusting for multiple hypotheses is called the **Bonferroni correction** to alpha, and it is quite stringent. Other possible adjustments are less stringent, but are more complicated statistically and used in different situations (e.g., Tukey, Scheffe, and Newman-Keuls procedures).[22]

3.2 COMMUNITY-BASED PARTICIPATORY RESEARCH

Community-based participatory research (CBPR) is an equitable, partnered approach to research that involves community members and organizational representatives, in addition to researchers in all aspects of the research process.[23,24] All partners contribute expertise and share decision making and ownership of the research. The goal of CBPR is to increase knowledge and understanding of a given phenomenon and integrate the knowledge gained to promote policy and social change to improve the health and quality of life of community members. CBPR projects often start with the community and use an iterative process, incorporating research, reflection, and action in a cyclical process.

3.3 ETHICAL ISSUES

Most research institutions have a committee specifically charged with the responsibility of reviewing all proposed research and ensuring that it is ethical. This type of committee is often called an **institutional review board** (IRB). IRBs have their foundation in the World Medical Association's Declaration of Helsinki, originally drafted in the 1960s. The primary goals of IRBs are to ensure the following:

- All research involving human subjects is of high quality so that any risks involved are justified
- The potential benefits to the study participants or to society in general are greater than the potential harm from the research
- Researchers obtain documented informed consent from study participants or their guardians
- Researchers protect the confidentiality of their research data
- Study participants are allowed to withdraw from the research at any time, without this action adversely affecting their care

Most universities and hospitals now require that all human research protocols be approved by an IRB, regardless if the research is externally funded.

All scientists are bound by the obligations of honesty and integrity in their research. Investigators have a responsibility to protect human subjects, implement privacy and confidentiality protections, register clinical trials, interpret their data objectively, and disclose all potential conflicts of interest in any reports and publications.[25] Industry-sponsored research is at greatest risk for conflicts of interest, and thus safeguards are helpful. With industry-sponsored research, ideally all the research data are available and analyzed independently of the sponsor.

Scientists have a professional responsibility to describe their study design and methods accurately and in sufficient detail and to assure readers that the work was carried out in accordance with ethical principles. Plagiarism, ghostwriting, and taking credit or payment for authorship of work written by another individual are unethical.

In this era of intense media and public interest in medical news, investigators need to be careful in the presentation of their research findings. Media coverage can be fraught with misinterpretation and unjustified extrapolation and conclusions.[26] Preliminary research results are frequently reported by the media as a critical new "breakthrough." Investigators therefore need to avoid raising false public expectations or providing misleading information.

4. SUMMARY

Research is the attempt to answer questions with valid data. Epidemiologic research seeks to answer questions about the distribution of health, disease, or risk factors; to develop hypotheses about the causes of ill health and the effectiveness of preventive and curative interventions; and to test these hypotheses. Observational research designs suitable for generating hypotheses include qualitative studies, cross-sectional surveys, cross-sectional ecologic studies, and longitudinal ecologic studies. A cross-sectional study collects data about a population at one point in time, whereas a longitudinal study is conducted over a period of time. Cross-sectional surveys are useful in determining the prevalence of risk factors and diseases in the population but are weak in determining the temporal relationship between variables. Ecologic studies obtain the rate of a disease and the frequency of exposure to a risk factor for an entire population, but the unit of study is the population, not the individuals within it, so exposure and disease cannot be linked in individual participants.

Observational research designs suitable for generating or testing hypotheses include prospective cohort studies, retrospective cohort studies, and case control studies. In cohort studies, one study group consists of persons exposed to risk factors, and another group consists of persons not exposed. These groups are studied to determine and compare their rates of disease. Fig. 5.3 illustrates the difference between a prospective and a retrospective cohort study. In case control studies the case group consists of persons who have a particular disease, and the control group consists of persons who do not have the disease but are matched individually to the cases (e.g., in terms of age, gender, and type of medical workup). Each group is studied to determine the frequency of past exposure to possible risk factors. Based on this information, the relative odds that a disease is linked with a particular risk factor (odds ratio) can be calculated. The use of a

cohort study with a nested case control design may enable some hypotheses to be tested quickly and cost effectively.

The experimental designs suitable for testing hypotheses are randomized controlled clinical trials (RCCTs, or RCTs) and randomized controlled field trials (RCFTs). Both types of trials follow the steps shown in Fig. 5.4. The major difference between these two types is that RCTs are generally used to test therapeutic interventions, whereas RCFTs are usually conducted to test preventive interventions. A trial is called a double-blind study if neither the participants nor the observers who collect the data know which type of intervention each participant receives.

Large data sets may contain associations by chance alone. Data dredging carries the greatest risk with analyses of large cohort data sets (i.e., when questions not part of the original basis for a study are appended). Institutional review boards evaluate study protocols before projects are undertaken to ensure that the research is of high quality with minimal and acceptable risk to study participants (human subjects).

REFERENCES

1. Arnim SS, Aberle SD, Pitney EH. A study of dental changes in a group of Pueblo Indian children. *J Am Dent Assoc.* 1937;24: 478-480.
2. Centers for Disease Control and Prevention. Achievements in public health, 1900–1999: fluoridation of drinking water to prevent dental caries. *MMWR.* 1999;48:933-940.
3. Dawber TR, Meadors GF, Moore Jr FE. Epidemiological approaches to heart disease: the Framingham Study. *Am J Public Health Nations Health.* 1951;41:279-281.
4. Breslow L. Risk factor intervention for health maintenance. *Science.* 1978;200:908-912.
5. Institute of Education. *Centre for Longitudinal Studies.* Available at: http://www.cls.ioe.ac.uk/page.aspx?&sitesectionid=724&site sectiontitle=National+Child+Development+Study. Accessed March 15, 2019.
6. MacMahon B. Prenatal x-ray exposure and childhood cancer. *J Natl Cancer Inst.* 1962;28:1173-1191.
7. Herbst AL, Ulfelder H, Poskanzer DC. Adenocarcinoma of the vagina: association of maternal stilbestrol therapy with tumor appearance in young women. *N Engl J Med.* 1971;284: 878-881.
8. Hasbun R, Abrahams J, Jekel J, Quagliarello VJ. Computed tomography of the head before lumbar puncture in adults with suspected meningitis. *N Engl J Med.* 2001;345:1727-1733.
9. Quagliarello VJ. Personal communication. 1999.
10. Last JM, Spasoff RA, Harris SS, eds. *A Dictionary of Epidemiology.* 4th ed. New York, NY: Oxford University Press; 2001.
11. Devereaux PJ, Manns BJ, Ghali WA, et al. Physician interpretations and textbook definitions of blinding terminology in randomized controlled trials. *JAMA.* 2001;285:2000-2003.
12. Rubin DH, Leventhal JM, Sadock RT, et al. Educational intervention by computer in childhood asthma: a randomized clinical trial testing the use of a new teaching intervention in childhood asthma. *Pediatrics.* 1986;77(1):1-10.
13. DeAngelis CD, Drazen JM, Frizelle FA, et al. Clinical trial registration: a statement from the International Committee of Medical Journal Editors. *JAMA.* 2004;292:1363-1364.

14. Francis Jr T, Korns RF, Voight RB, et al. An evaluation of the 1954 poliomyelitis vaccine trials. *Am J Public Health Nations Health*. 1955;45(5 Pt 2):1-63.

15. Steering Committee of the Physicians' Health Study Research Group. Final report on the aspirin component of the ongoing Physicians' Health Study. *N Engl J Med*. 1989;321:129-135.

16. Vlahakes GJ. The value of phase 4 clinical testing. *N Engl J Med*. 2006;354:413-415.

17. Antman EM, Bennett JS, Daugherty A, et al. Use of nonsteroidal antiinflammatory drugs: an update for clinicians: a scientific statement from the American Heart Association. *Circulation*. 2007;115(12):1634-1642. doi:10.1161/CIRCULATIONAHA.106.181424.

18. Kearney PM, Baigent C, Godwin J, Halls H, Emberson JR, Patrono C. Do selective cyclo-oxygenase-2 inhibitors and traditional non-steroidal anti-inflammatory drugs increase the risk of atherothrombosis? Meta-analysis of randomised trials. *BMJ*. 2006;332(7553):1302-1308. doi:10.1136/bmj.332.7553.1302.

19. MacMahon B, Yen S, Trichopoulos D, Warren K, Nardi G. Coffee and cancer of the pancreas. *N Engl J Med*. 1981;304:630-633.

20. Feinstein AR, Horwitz RI, Spitzer WO, Battista RN. Coffee and pancreatic cancer. The problems of etiologic science and epidemiologic case-control research. *JAMA*. 1981;246:957-961.

21. Jekel JF. Should we stop using the P value in descriptive studies? *Pediatrics*. 1977;60:124-126.

22. Dawson B, Trapp RG. *Basic & Clinical Biostatistics*. 4th ed. New York, NY: Lange Medical Books/McGraw-Hill; 2004.

23. Minkler M, Wallerstein N. *Community-Based Participatory Research for Health*. New York, NY: John Wiley & Sons; 2011.

24. Israel BA, Eng E, Schulz AJ, Parker EA. *Methods for Community-Based Participatory Research for Health*. New York, NY: John Wiley & Sons; 2012.

25. American College of Physicians. *ACP Ethics Manual Seventh Edition*. Available at: http://www.acponline.org/running_practice/ethics/manual/manual6th.htm#research. Accessed March 15, 2019.

26. Health News Review. Available at: https://www.healthnewsreview.org/. Accessed March 15, 2019.

SELECT READINGS

Fletcher RH, Fletcher SW, Fletcher GS. Clinical *Epidemiology: the Essentials*. 5th ed. Philadelphia, PA: Wolters Kluwer; 2012.

Gordis L. *Epidemiology*. 4th ed. Philadelphia, PA: Saunders-Elsevier; 2009.

Koepsell TD, Weiss NS. *Epidemiologic Methods*. New York, NY: Oxford University Press; 2003.

Schlesselman JJ. *Case-Control Studies: Design, Conduct, Analysis*. New York, NY: Oxford University Press; 1982. [A classic.]

WEBSITES

Healthy Americans: http://healthyamericans.org/

REVIEW QUESTIONS

1. The basic goal of epidemiologic research, especially with observational data, is to:
   A. Describe associations between exposures and outcomes
   B. Identify sources of measurement error and bias
   C. Establish direct causality
   D. Maximize external validity
   E. Reject the alternative hypothesis

2. Studies may be conducted to generate or test hypotheses. The best design for testing a hypothesis is a:
   A. Case control study
   B. Cross-sectional survey
   C. Longitudinal ecologic study
   D. Randomized controlled trial
   E. Retrospective cohort study

3. The members of a public health team have a continuing interest in controlling measles infection through vaccination. To estimate the level of immunity in a particular population in a quick and efficient manner, what type of study should they conduct?
   A. Case control study of measles infection
   B. Cross-sectional survey of vaccination status
   C. Randomized trial of measles vaccination
   D. Retrospective cohort study of measles vaccination
   E. Ecologic study of measles in the population

4. A published study purported to show that a variety of symptoms were more common among participants with a history of suboptimally treated Lyme disease than among controls who had no history of Lyme disease. The data were obtained largely by a survey of the participants. The study is most likely subject to which of the following distortions?
   A. Ecologic fallacy, length bias, and lead-time bias
   B. Intervention bias, random error, and length bias
   C. Late-look bias, measurement bias, and length bias
   D. Lead-time bias, late-look bias, and selection bias
   E. Selection bias, recall bias, and random error

5. Cross-sectional surveys are subject to the Neyman bias, or late-look bias. This may be explained as the tendency to:
   A. Detect only the late stages of a disease, when manifestations are more severe
   B. Detect only the cases of a disease that are asymptomatic
   C. Find more disease in older cohorts
   D. Detect fatalities preferentially
   E. Detect the more indolent cases of a disease preferentially

6. A potential bias in screening programs that is analogous to the late-look bias is:
   A. Spectrum bias, because the cases are clustered at one end of the disease spectrum
   B. Retrospective bias, because the severity of illness can only be appreciated in retrospect
   C. Length bias, because cases lasting longer are more apt to be detected
   D. Selection bias, because the program selects out severe cases
   E. Selection bias, because the program selects out asymptomatic illness

7. Which of the following measures the chance of having a risk factor?
   A. Kappa
   B. Odds ratio
   C. *p* value
   D. Relative risk
   E. Risk ratio

8. A case control study may have a particular advantage over a cohort study when the disease in question is:
   A. Fatal
   B. Indolent
   C. Infectious
   D. Virulent
   E. Rare

9. In a case control study that is being planned to study possible causes of myocardial infarction (MI), patients with MI serve as the cases. Which of the following would be a good choice to serve as the controls?
   A. Patients whose cardiac risk factors are similar to those of the cases and who have never had an MI in the past
   B. Patients whose cardiac risk factors are similar to those of the cases and who have had an MI in the past
   C. Patients who have never had an MI in the past
   D. Patients whose cardiac risk factors are dissimilar to those of the cases and who have had an MI in the past
   E. Patients whose cardiac risk factors are unknown and who have had an MI in the past

ANSWERS AND EXPLANATIONS

1. **A.** Virtually all epidemiologic research involves the study of two or more groups of participants who differ in terms of their exposure to risk factors or some defined outcome. The basic goal of the research is to compare the frequency of different exposures and outcomes between groups to look for associations. Most epidemiologic studies are not sufficient to determine causality (C). Identifying sources of measurement error and bias (B) and having external validity (D) are desirable but are not basic goals of doing the research. All research sets out to reject the null hypothesis, looking for evidence in support of the alternative hypothesis (E).

2. **D.** Randomized controlled trials (including RCFTs and RCCTs) are experimental studies and represent the gold standard for hypothesis testing. These studies are costly in time and money, however. They are best reserved for testing hypotheses that already are supported by the results of prior studies of less rigorous design (i.e., observational studies). Often the RCT is the final hurdle before a hypothesis is sufficiently supported to become incorporated into clinical practice. (Unfortunately though, RCTs sometimes produce results opposite what would be expected given observational evidence.) Observational studies such as case control studies (A), cross-sectional surveys (B), longitudinal ecologic studies (C), and retrospective cohort studies (E) are appropriate for hypothesis generation and, sometimes (depending on their design and purpose) for testing certain hypotheses. For none of these designs, however, is it ever appropriate both to generate and to test the same hypotheses in any single study.

3. **B.** Clarifying the research question lays the foundation for selecting a specific and useful study design. In this example, the study should answer the following questions: Is there adequate immunity to measles in the population? If immunity is inadequate, how should vaccination policy be directed to optimize protection of the community? A cross-sectional survey of vaccination status (or antibody titers, or both) of community members would be the most expedient, cost-effective means to obtain answers to questions concerning the allocation of public health resources to prevent the spread of measles through vaccination. Cross-sectional surveys are often useful in setting disease control priorities. Answer choices A, C, and E are about studies investigating measles infection, not immunity. A retrospective cohort study of measles vaccination (D) might be appropriate for looking at the effectiveness of vaccination in the community (i.e., comparing measles incidence in those vaccinated and those not) but would not be appropriate to estimate the level of immunity in a particular population.

4. **E.** In testing study hypotheses, bias must be diligently avoided. Although participants often can be randomized in a prospective study, they cannot usually be randomized in a retrospective study, such as the study on Lyme disease described in the question. In almost any retrospective study, there is a risk of selection bias (i.e., if participants are allowed to choose, those who most believe their symptoms are related to the exposure in question may want to participate). In the quantification of symptoms, many of which are subjective, measurement bias is possible (i.e., the firm believers in the cause of their symptoms may report their symptoms as being more severe). Additionally, in any retrospective study in which participants are surveyed, the category that defines their role in the study (as a member of the "exposed" group or member of the "nonexposed" group) may influence their recall of relevant events. In the study described, the participants with a history of Lyme disease might be more likely to recall symptoms suggestive of the disease or its late complications than would the controls, who have no history of disease and might dismiss or fail to remember episodes of minor joint pain. Recall bias is one of the most important limitations of case control studies. Random error is possible in any study and is never completely avoided. Lead-time bias is germane only to screening programs and the study of

the time course of a disease, such as the time between the diagnosis and the outcome (e.g., death). Lead-time bias is the tendency for early detection to increase the interval between detection and the outcome without altering the natural history of the disease. Length bias refers to the tendency to detect preferentially more indolent cases of disease in a population screening program; it is not germane to the study in question. Similarly, late-look bias, the tendency to detect preferentially less severe cases of disease in a population after patients with severe disease have been removed from consideration (e.g., through death), is also not germane to the study question. The ecologic fallacy refers to the tendency to presume that an association found in a population (e.g., frequency of an exposure and frequency of a disease) is operative in individuals. Because the study in question is a study of individuals, the ecologic fallacy is irrelevant. The study is not an intervention study, however, and "intervention bias" is not an established form of bias. Any form of bias can invalidate the findings of a study. Thus investigators must be vigilant in preventing bias (which can generally only be addressed prospectively—i.e., *before* a study is done). Given the explanations here, answers A, B, C, and D are incorrect.

5. **E.** At any given moment, the prevalence of disease in a population is influenced by the incidence of disease (the frequency with which new cases arise) and the duration. Diseases of long duration are more apt to accumulate in a population than are diseases that run a short course (resulting in either full recovery or death). Even within the categories of a particular illness, such as prostate cancer, the prevalence of the more indolent cases (i.e., the slowly progressive cases) is likely to be higher than the prevalence of the aggressive cases. This is because the indolent cases accumulate, whereas the aggressive cases result in a rapid demise (and death removes people who would otherwise be considered from investigator consideration). A cross-sectional survey preferentially detects the indolent cases that tend to accumulate and misses the cases that have recently occurred but already resulted in death. This is the late-look bias: One is looking too late to find aggressive cases that already have led to death. Thus because of late-look or Neyman bias, investigators will preferentially miss (not detect) fatalities (D) and severe, late-stage disease (A). The age of the cohorts (C) or symptoms of disease (B) are not relevant concerns.

6. **C.** Length bias, the tendency to detect preferentially long-lasting cases of subclinical illness whenever screening is conducted, is analogous to late-look bias. Length bias occurs for the same reasons as late-look bias (see the answer to question 5). A screening program usually is prospective and would not be subject to any type of "retrospective bias" (B). The intent of any disease screening program is to detect asymptomatic and unrecognized cases. Selection bias (D and E) refers to the selection of individuals to participate, and screening programs may be subject to selection bias. This would limit external validity but is not a comparable effect to the late-look bias. Spectrum bias (A) is said to occur if the clinical spectrum (variety) of the patients used to measure the sensitivity and specificity of a diagnostic test differs from the clinical spectrum of the patients to whom the test would be applied, so that the values obtained are inaccurate in the test's actual use.

7. **B.** The odds ratio, usually derived from a case control study, indicates the relative frequency of a particular risk factor in the cases (i.e., participants with the outcome in question) and in the controls (i.e., participants without the outcome in question). The outcome already has occurred; the risk for developing the outcome cannot be measured directly. What is measured is exposure, which is presumably the exposure that preceded the outcome and represented a risk factor for it. The odds ratio may be considered the risk of having been exposed in the past, given the presence or absence of the outcome now. The odds ratio may be considered the risk of having the risk factor. The odds ratio approximates the risk ratio (E) when the disease in question is rare. The relative risk (D) and the risk ratio are the same measurement (the terms are interchangeable). Kappa (A) is a measure of interrater agreement. The *p* value (C) is a measure of statistical significance, the probability of finding an effect as great or greater by chance alone (the smaller the *p* value, the greater the statistical significance).

8. **E.** The groups in a case control study are assembled on the basis of the outcome. If the outcome is rare, this design is particularly advantageous. Risk factors in a defined group with the rare outcome can be assessed and compared with risk factors in a group without the outcome. Two potential problems of conducting a cohort study for a rare disease are that too few cases would arise to permit meaningful interpretation of the data and that a very large sample size would be required, resulting in great (often prohibitive) expense. Considerations of fatality (A), indolence (B), infectiousness (C), and virulence (D) are not relevant.

9. **C.** The usual goal of a case control study is to determine differences in the risk factors seen in the participants with a particular outcome (which in this example is myocardial infarction) and the participants without the outcome. If the two groups of participants were matched on the basis of risk factors for the outcome (i.e., had similar cardiac risk factors, as in answer choices A and B), the potentially different influences of these factors would be eliminated by design. Matching on the basis of known (established) risk factors to isolate differences in unknown (as yet unrecognized) risk factors is often appropriate.

However, if the cases and controls resemble one another too closely, there is a risk of overmatching, with the result that no differences are detectable, and the study becomes useless. If the case control study is used to measure the effectiveness of a treatment, it would be appropriate for the cases and controls to be similar in risk factors for the disease. In trying to elucidate possible causes (i.e., possible risk factors) for MI, however, participants should be dissimilar in risk factors so that differences can be explored in association with the outcome. Recruiting patients with unknown (and thus potentially similar) risk factors (E) would be undesirable for this reason. Likewise, it would be undesirable to include people who have ever had an MI in the past (B, D, and E), because they have the outcome of interest; it is impossible to see what factors are associated with having an MI versus not having an MI when everyone has had an MI.

6

Assessment of Risk and Benefit in Epidemiologic Studies

"Knowing only the relative data is like having a 50% off coupon for selected items at a department store. But you don't know if the coupon applies to a diamond necklace or to a pack of chewing gum. Only by knowing what the coupon's true value is–the absolute data–does the 50% have any meaning."

Steve Woloshin and Lisa Schwartz

CASE INTRODUCTION

Imagine you are the Director of the Public Health Department and are given $1 million to spend on a new breast cancer screening program for your community. You are asked to choose between the following three options. Which would you select?

1. Reduces death rate by 34% compared with no screening program
2. Produces an absolute reduction in deaths from cancer of 0.06%
3. Prevents 1 death for every 1588 patients screened over 10 years. (See Section 5.1 for discussion of this case.)

The practice of medicine requires information on the benefits of medical and public health procedures. Providers and

patients want to know how much benefit will be gained. As very few things in life are without risk, we also need to know about potential harms of these interventions. Epidemiology research can help to provide this critical data on benefits versus risks. However, there are many different ways of describing benefit and risks. If you hear that a new drug "reduces heart attack risk by 50%," this sounds impressive until you dig deeper and consider more than this "relative risk" information. If you consider the "absolute risk" information about this new drug, you might find that it reduces heart attacks from 2 per 100 to 1 per 100 (the risk halved from 2% to 1%); this absolute risk method of describing the data sounds far less impressive but more useful at conveying the true impact of a medical intervention. In this chapter we review basic concepts related to assessment of risk and benefit and describe use of these estimates in health policy and communication with patients.

1. DEFINITION OF STUDY GROUPS

Causal research in epidemiology requires that two fundamental distinctions be made. The first distinction is between people who have and people who do not have exposure to the risk factor (or protective factor) under study (the **independent variable**). The second distinction is between people who have and people who do not have the disease (or other outcome) under study (the **dependent variable**). These distinctions are seldom simple, and their measurements are subject to random errors and biases.

In addition, epidemiologic research may be complicated by other requirements. It may be necessary to analyze several independent (possibly causal) variables at the same time, including how they interact. For example, the frequency of hypertension is related to age and gender, and these variables interact in the following manner: Before about age 50, men are more likely to be hypertensive; but after age 50, women are more likely to be hypertensive. Another complication involves the need to measure different degrees of *strength of exposure* to the risk factor, the *duration of exposure* to the risk factor, or both. Investigators study strength and duration in combination, for example, when they measure exposure to cigarettes in terms of pack-years, which is the average number of packs smoked per day times the number of years of smoking. Depending on the risk factor, it may be difficult to determine the time of onset of exposure. This is true for risk factors such as sedentary lifestyle and excess intake of dietary sodium. Another complication of analysis is the need to measure different levels of *disease severity*. Exposure and outcome may vary across a range of values, rather than simply be present or absent.

Despite these complexities, much epidemiologic research still relies on the dichotomies of exposed/unexposed and diseased/nondiseased, which are often presented in the form of a **standard 2 × 2 table** (Table 6.1).

Causal research depends on the measurement of differences. In cohort studies the difference is between the frequency of disease in **persons exposed** to a risk factor and the frequency of disease in **persons not exposed** to the same risk factor. In case control studies the difference is between the frequency of the risk factor in **case participants** (persons with the disease) and the frequency of the risk factor in **control participants** (persons without the disease).

The exposure may be to a *nutritional* factor (e.g., high–saturated fat diet), an *environmental* factor (e.g., radiation after Chernobyl disaster), a *behavioral* factor (e.g., cigarette smoking), a *physiologic* characteristic (e.g., high serum total cholesterol level), a *medical* intervention (e.g., antibiotic), or a *public health* intervention (e.g., vaccine). Other factors also play a role, and the categorization may vary (e.g., nutritional choices are often regarded as behavioral factors).

2. COMPARISON OF RISKS IN DIFFERENT STUDY GROUPS

Although differences in risk can be measured in absolute terms or in relative terms, the method used depends on the type of study performed. For reasons discussed in Chapter 5, case control studies allow investigators to obtain only a relative measure of risk, whereas cohort studies and randomized controlled trials allow investigators to obtain absolute and relative measures of risk. When possible, it is important to examine absolute and relative risks because they provide different information.

After the differences in risk are calculated (by the methods outlined in detail subsequently), the level of statistical significance must be determined to ensure that any observed difference is probably real (i.e., not caused by chance; significance testing is discussed in detail in Chapter 9). When the difference is statistically significant, but not clinically important, it is real but trivial. When the difference appears to be clinically important, but is not statistically significant, it may be a false-negative (beta) error if the sample size is small (see Chapter 12), or it may be a chance finding.

2.1 ABSOLUTE DIFFERENCES IN RISK

Disease frequency usually is measured as a risk in cohort studies and clinical trials and as a rate when the disease and death data come from population-based reporting systems. An absolute difference in risks or rates can be expressed as a risk difference or as a rate difference. The **risk difference** is the risk in the exposed group minus the risk in the unexposed group. The **rate difference** is the rate in the exposed group minus the rate in the unexposed group (rates are defined in Chapter 2). The discussion in this chapter focuses on risks, which are used more often than rates in cohort studies.

When the level of risk in the exposed group is the same as the level of risk in the unexposed group, the risk difference is 0, and the conclusion is that the exposure makes no difference to the disease risk being studied. If an exposure is harmful (as in the case of cigarette smoking), the risk difference is expected to be greater than 0. If an exposure is protective (as in the case of a vaccine), the risk difference is expected to be less than 0 (i.e., a negative number, which in this case indicates a reduction in disease risk in the group exposed to the vaccine). The risk difference also is known as the **attributable risk** because it is an estimate of the amount of risk that *can*

TABLE 6.1 Standard 2 × 2 Table for Showing Association Between a Risk Factor and a Disease

RISK FACTOR	DISEASE STATUS Present	DISEASE STATUS Absent	Total
Positive	a	b	a + b
Negative	c	d	c + d
TOTAL	a + c	b + d	a + b + c + d

Interpretation of the Cells

a = Participants with both the risk factor and the disease
b = Participants with the risk factor, but not the disease
c = Participants with the disease, but not the risk factor
d = Participants with neither the risk factor nor the disease
a + b = All participants with the risk factor
c + d = All participants without the risk factor
a + c = All participants with the disease
b + d = All participants without the disease
a + b + c + d = All study participants

be attributed to, or is attributable to (is caused by), the risk factor.

In Table 6.1 the risk of disease in the exposed individuals is $a/(a + b)$, and the risk of disease in the unexposed individuals is $c/(c + d)$. When these symbols are used, the attributable risk (AR) can be expressed as the difference between the two:

$$AR = \text{Risk}_{(exposed)} - \text{Risk}_{(unexposed)}$$
$$= [a/(a+b)] - [c/(c+d)]$$

Fig. 6.1 provides historical data on age-adjusted death rates for lung cancer among adult male smokers and non-smokers in the US population and in the United Kingdom (UK) population.[1,2] For the United States, the lung cancer death rate in smokers was 191 per 100,000 population per year, whereas the rate in nonsmokers was 8.7 per 100,000 per year. Because the death rates for lung cancer in the population were low (<1% per year) in the year for which data are shown, the rate and the risk for lung cancer death would be essentially the same. The risk difference (attributable risk) in the United States can be calculated as follows:

$$191/100,000 - 8.7/100,000 = 182.3/100,000$$

Similarly, the attributable risk in the United Kingdom can be calculated as follows:

$$166/100,000 - 7/100,000 = 159/100,000$$

2.2 RELATIVE DIFFERENCES IN RISK

Relative risk (RR) can be expressed in terms of a risk ratio (also abbreviated as RR) or estimated by an odds ratio (OR).

2.2.a Relative Risk (Risk Ratio)

The **relative risk**, which is also known as the risk ratio (both abbreviated as RR), is the ratio of the risk in the exposed group to the risk in the unexposed group. If the risks in the exposed group and unexposed group are the same, RR = 1. If the risks in the two groups are not the same, calculating RR provides a straightforward way of showing in relative terms how much different (greater or smaller) the risks in the exposed group are compared with the risks in the unexposed group. The risk for the disease in the exposed group usually is greater if an exposure is harmful (as with cigarette smoking) or smaller if an exposure is protective (as with a vaccine). In terms of the groups and symbols defined in Table 6.1, relative risk (RR) would be calculated as follows:

$$RR = \text{Risk}_{(exposed)} / \text{Risk}_{(unexposed)}$$
$$= [a/(a+b)] / [c/(c+d)]$$

The data on lung cancer deaths in Fig. 6.1 are used to determine the **attributable risk** (AR). The same data can be used to calculate the RR. For men in the United States, 191/100,000 divided by 8.7/100,000 yields an RR of 22. Fig. 6.2 shows the conversion from absolute to relative risks. Absolute risk is shown on the left axis and relative risk on the right axis. In relative risk terms the value of the risk for lung

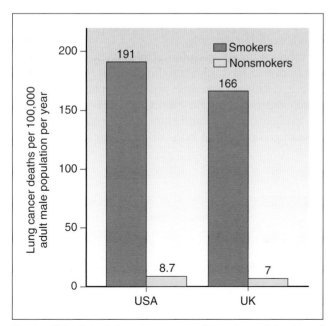

Fig. 6.1 Risk of death from lung cancer. Comparison of the risks of death from lung cancer per 100,000 adult male population per year for smokers and nonsmokers in the United States (USA) and United Kingdom (UK). (Data from US Centers for Disease Control: Chronic disease reports: deaths from lung cancer—United States, 1986. *MMWR* 38:501–505, 1989; Doll R, Hill AB: Lung cancer and other causes of death in relation to smoking; a second report on the mortality of British doctors. *BMJ* 2:1071–1081, 1956.)

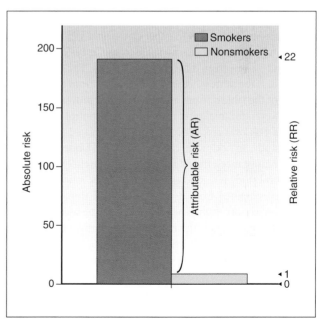

Fig. 6.2 Risk of death from lung cancer. Diagram shows the risks of death from lung cancer per 100,000 adult male population per year for smokers and nonsmokers in the United States, expressed in absolute terms *(left axis)* and in relative terms *(right axis)*. (Data from US Centers for Disease Control: Chronic disease reports: deaths from lung cancer—United States, 1986. *MMWR* 38:501–505, 1989.)

cancer death in the unexposed group is 1. Compared with that, the risk for lung cancer death in the exposed group is 22 times as great, and the attributable risk is the difference, which is 182.3/100,000 in absolute risk terms and 21 in relative risk terms.

It also is important to consider the number of people to whom the relative risk applies. A large relative risk that applies to a small number of people may produce few excess deaths or cases of disease, whereas a small relative risk that applies to a large number of people may produce many excess deaths or cases of disease.

2.2.b Odds Ratio

People may be unfamiliar with the concept of odds and the difference between "risk" and "odds." Based on the symbols used in Table 6.1, the **risk** of disease in the exposed group is $a/(a + b)$, whereas the **odds** of disease in the exposed group is simply a/b. If a is small compared with b, the odds would be similar to the risk. If a particular disease occurs in 1 person among a group of 100 persons in a given year, the risk of that disease is 1 in 100 (0.0100), and the odds of that disease are 1 to 99 (0.0101). If the risk of the disease is relatively large (>5%), the odds ratio is not a good estimate of the risk ratio. The odds ratio can be calculated by dividing the odds of exposure in the diseased group by the odds of exposure in the nondiseased group. In the terms used in Table 6.1, the formula for the OR is as follows:

$$OR = (a/c)/(b/d)$$
$$= ad/bc$$

In mathematical terms, it would make no difference whether the odds ratio was calculated as $(a/c)/(b/d)$ or as $(a/b)/(c/d)$ because cross-multiplication in either case would yield ad/bc. In a case control study, it makes no sense to use $(a/b)/(c/d)$ because cells a and b come from different study groups. The fact that the odds ratio is the same whether it is developed from a horizontal analysis of the table or from a vertical analysis proves to be valuable, however, for analyzing data from case control studies. Although a risk or a risk ratio cannot be calculated from a case control study, an odds ratio can be calculated. Under most real-world circumstances, the odds ratio from a carefully performed case control study is a good estimate of the risk ratio that would have been obtained from a more costly and time-consuming prospective cohort study. The odds ratio may be used as an estimate of the risk ratio if the risk of disease in the population is low. (It can be used if the risk ratio is <1%, and probably if <5%.) The odds ratio also is used in logistic methods of statistical analysis (logistic regression, log-linear models, Cox regression analyses), discussed briefly in Chapter 11.

2.2.c Which Side Is Up in the Risk Ratio and Odds Ratio?

If the risk for a disease is the same in the group exposed to a particular risk factor or protective factor as it is in the group not exposed to the factor, the risk ratio is expressed simply as 1.0. Hypothetically, the risk ratio could be 0 (i.e.,

if the individuals exposed to a protective factor have no risk, and the unexposed individuals have some risk), or it may be infinity (i.e., if the individuals exposed to a risk factor have some risk, and the unexposed individuals have no risk). In practical terms, however, because there usually is some disease in every large group, these extremes of the risk ratio are rare.

When risk factors are discussed, placing the exposed group in the numerator is a convention that makes intuitive sense (because the number becomes larger as the risk factor has a greater impact), and this convention is followed in the literature. However, the risk ratio also can be expressed with the exposed group in the denominator. Consider the case of cigarette smoking and myocardial infarction (MI), in which the risk of MI for smokers is greater than for nonsmokers. On the one hand, it is acceptable to put the smokers in the numerator and express the risk ratio as 2/1 (i.e., 2), meaning that the risk of MI is about twice as high for smokers as for nonsmokers of otherwise similar age, gender, and health status. On the other hand, it also is acceptable to put the smokers in the denominator and express the risk ratio as 1/2 (i.e., 0.5), meaning that nonsmokers have half the risk of smokers. Clarity simply requires that the nature of the comparison be explicit.

Another risk factor might produce 4 times the risk of a disease, in which case the ratio could be expressed as 4 or as 1/4, depending on how the risks are being compared. When the risk ratio is plotted on a logarithmic scale (Fig. 6.3), it is easy to see that, regardless of which way the ratio is expressed, the distance to the risk ratio of 1 is the same. Mathematically, it does not matter whether the risk for the exposed group or the unexposed group is in the numerator. Either way the risk ratio is easily interpretable.

Although the equation for calculating the odds ratio differs from that for calculating the risk ratio, when the odds ratio is calculated, the same principle applies: The ratio is usually expressed with the exposed group in the numerator, but mathematically it can be interpreted equally well if the exposed group is placed in the denominator.

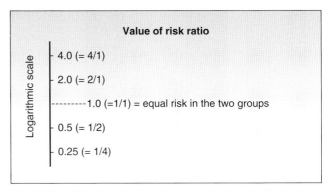

Fig. 6.3 Possible risk ratios plotted on logarithmic scale. Scale shows that reciprocal risks are equidistant from the neutral point, where the risk ratio is equal to 1.0.

When two risks or two rates are being compared, if there is no difference (i.e., the risks or rates are equal), the risk (rate) difference is expressed as 0. When the same two rates are compared by a relative risk or an odds ratio, however, the condition of no difference is represented by 1.0 because the numerator and denominator are equal.

3. ATTRIBUTABLE RISK MEASURES

One of the most useful applications of epidemiology is to estimate how much disease burden is caused by certain modifiable risk factors. This is useful for policy development because the impact of risk factors or interventions to reduce risk factors can be compared with costs in cost-benefit and cost-effectiveness analyses (see Chapter 14). Also, health education is often more effective when educators can show how much impact a given risk factor has on individual risks. In addition to the risk difference, relative risk, and odds ratio, the three most common measures of the impact of exposures are as follows (Box 6.1):

1. Attributable risk percent in the exposed
2. Population attributable risk
3. Population attributable risk percent

In the discussion of these measures, historical data on smoking and lung cancer are used as the examples of risk factor and disease, and the calculations are based on rates for the United States shown in Fig. 6.1.

3.1 ATTRIBUTABLE RISK PERCENT IN THE EXPOSED

If an investigator wanted to answer the question, "Among smokers, what percentage of the total risk for fatal lung cancer is caused by smoking?" it would be necessary to calculate the attributable risk percent in the exposed, which is abbreviated as $AR\%_{(exposed)}$. There are two methods of calculation, one based on absolute differences in risk and the other based on relative differences in risk. The following equation is based on absolute differences:

$$AR\%_{(exposed)} = \frac{Risk_{(exposed)} - Risk_{(unexposed)}}{Risk_{(exposed)}} \times 100$$

If the US data on the lung cancer death rates (expressed as deaths per 100,000/year) in adult male smokers and non-smokers are used, the calculation is as follows:

$$AR\%_{(exposed)} = \frac{(191 - 8.7)}{191} \times 100 = \frac{182.3}{191} \times 100 = 95.4\%$$

BOX 6.1 Equations for Comparing Risks in Different Groups and Measuring Impact of Risk Factors

(1) Risk difference	= Attributable risk (AR)
	= $Risk_{(exposed)} - Risk_{(unexposed)}$
	= $(a/[a + b]) - (c/[c + d])$
	where a represents subjects with both the risk factor and the disease; b represents subjects with the risk factor, but not the disease; c represents subjects with the disease, but not the risk factor; d represents subjects with neither the risk factor nor the disease
(2) Relative risk (RR)	= Risk ratio (RR)
	= $Risk_{(exposed)}/Risk_{(unexposed)}$
	= $(a/[a + b])/(c/[c + d])$
(3) Odds ratio (OR)	= $(a/b)/(c/d)$
	= $(a/c)/(b/d)$
	= ad/bc
(4) Attributable risk percent in the exposed ($AR\%_{[exposed]}$)	= $\dfrac{Risk_{(exposed)} - Risk_{(unexposed)}}{Risk_{(exposed)}} \times 100$
	= $\dfrac{RR - 1}{RR} \times 100$
	$\simeq \dfrac{OR - 1}{OR} \times 100$
(5) Population attributable risk (PAR)	= $Risk_{(total)} - Risk_{(unexposed)}$
(6) Population attributable risk percent (PAR%)	= $\dfrac{Risk_{(total)} - Risk_{(unexposed)}}{Risk_{(total)}} \times 100$
	= $\dfrac{(Pe)(RR - 1)}{1 + (Pe)(RR - 1)} \times 100$
	where Pe stands for the effective proportion of the population exposed to the risk factor

If the absolute risk is unknown, the relative risk (RR) can be used instead to calculate the $AR\%_{(exposed)}$, with the following formula:

$$AR\%_{(exposed)} \frac{(RR-1)}{RR} \times 100$$

Earlier in this chapter, the RR for the US data was calculated as 22, so this figure can be used in the equation:

$$AR\%_{(exposed)} \frac{(22-1)}{22} \times 100 = 95.5\%$$

The percentage based on the formula using relative risk is the same as the percentage based on the formula using absolute risk (except for rounding errors). Why does this work? The important point to remember is that the relative risk for the unexposed group is always 1 because that is the group to whom the exposed group is compared. The attributable risk, which is the amount of risk in excess of the risk in the unexposed group, is RR = 1 (see Fig. 6.2). Because the odds ratio may be used to estimate the risk ratio if the risk of disease in the population is small, the $AR\%_{(exposed)}$ also can be estimated by using odds ratios obtained from case control studies and substituting them for the RR in the previous formula.

3.2 POPULATION ATTRIBUTABLE RISK

The population attributable risk (PAR) allows an investigator to answer the question, "Among the general population, how much of the total risk for fatal disease X is caused by exposure to Y?" PAR is defined as the risk in the total population minus the risk in the unexposed population:

$$PAR = Risk_{(total)} - Risk_{(unexposed)}$$

Answers to this type of question are not as useful to know for counseling patients but are of considerable value to policy makers. Using the US data shown in Fig. 6.1, the investigator would subtract the risk in the adult male nonsmokers (8.7/100,000/year) from the risk in the total adult male population (72.5/100,000/year) to find the population attributable risk (63.8/100,000/year). It can be presumed that if there had never been any smokers in the United States, the total US lung cancer death rate in men would be much lower, perhaps close to 8.7/100,000 per year. The excess over this figure—63.8/100,000 per year based on these data—could be attributed to smoking.

3.3 POPULATION ATTRIBUTABLE RISK PERCENT

The population attributable risk percent (PAR%) answers the question, "Among the general population, what percentage of

the total risk for X (e.g., fatal lung cancer) is caused by the exposure Y (e.g., smoking)?" As with the $AR\%_{(exposed)}$, the PAR% can be calculated using either absolute or relative differences in risk. The following equation is based on absolute differences:

$$PAR\% = \frac{Risk_{(total)} - Risk_{(unexposed)}}{Risk_{(total)}} \times 100$$

When the US data discussed earlier for men are used, the calculation is as follows:

$$PAR\% = \frac{(72.5 - 8.7)}{72.5} \times 100 = \frac{63.8}{72.5} \times 100 = 88\%$$

The PAR% instead could be calculated using the risk ratio (or the odds ratio if the data come from a case control study). First, it is necessary to incorporate another measure into the formula—the proportion exposed, which is abbreviated as Pe and is defined as the effective proportion of the population exposed to the risk factor. The equation is as follows:

$$PAR\% = \frac{(Pe)(RR-1)}{1 + (Pe)(RR-1)} \times 100$$

In the case of smoking, the Pe would be the *effective* proportion of the adult population who smoked. This figure must be estimated, rather than being obtained directly, because of the long latent period from the start of smoking until the onset of lung cancer and the occurrence of death. The proportion of smokers has generally been decreasing over time in the United States, with recent prevalence at the time of publication of this text at less than 25% of the population. Here, the Pe is assumed to be 0.35, or 35%.

As calculated earlier, the relative risk (RR) for lung cancer in the United States was 22. If this number is used, the calculation can be completed as follows:

$$PAR\% = \frac{(0.35)(22-1)}{1 + (0.35)(22-1)} \times 100 = \frac{7.35}{1 + 7.35} = 88\%$$

Fig. 6.4 shows diagrammatically how the formula for PAR% works.

4. APPLICATION OF RISK ASSESSMENT DATA TO POLICY ANALYSIS

4.1 ESTIMATING BENEFIT OF INTERVENTIONS IN POPULATIONS

Population attributable risk (PAR) data often can be used to estimate the benefit of a proposed intervention, such as the

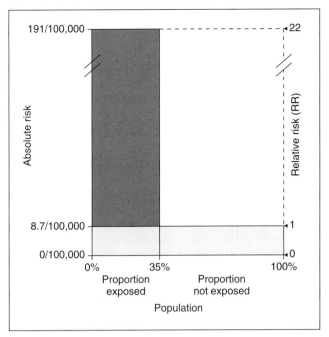

Fig. 6.4 Population attributable risk percent (PAR%). Diagram shows how the equation for PAR% works. The x-axis shows the population, divided into two groups: the 35% of the population representing the proportion exposed (Pe) to the risk factor (i.e., the effective population of smokers), and the remaining 65% of the population, who are nonsmokers. The right side of the y-axis shows the relative risk (RR) of lung cancer death. For reference, the left side of the y-axis shows the absolute risk of lung cancer death. Dark-gray shading, light-gray shading, and a light blue are used to show the relationship between the risk factor (smoking) and the disease outcome (lung cancer death) in the smokers and nonsmokers. The light blue part represents outcomes that are not attributable to the risk factor in nonsmokers. The dark gray part represents the outcomes that are attributable to the risk factor in smokers. The light gray part represents the outcomes that are not attributable to the risk factor in smokers (i.e., lung cancer deaths that are not attributable to smoking, although the deaths occurred in smokers). The equation is as follows:

$$PAR\% = \frac{(Pe)(RR - 1)}{1 + (Pe)(RR - 1)} \times 100$$

$$= \frac{(0.35)(22 - 1)}{1 + (0.35)(22 - 1)} \times 100$$

$$= \frac{7.35}{1 + 7.35} \times 100 = 88\%$$

number of lung cancer deaths that would be prevented by instituting a smoking reduction program in a large population. For example, assume that in the United States the proportion of men who smoke has averaged about 25% for more than two decades (as it did during much of the 1990s). Also assume that the amount of smoking has been constant among men who smoke, and that the lung cancer death rate in this group remains constant (represented by lung cancer death rate in Table 6.2, which is 191/100,000/year for smokers vs 8.7/100,000/year for nonsmokers). Given these assumptions,

the rate of lung cancer deaths in the total adult male population would be a weighted average of the rates in smokers and nonsmokers:

$$
\begin{aligned}
\text{Rate per 100,000 male} \\
\text{population per year} &= \left(\text{Weight}_{\text{smokers}}\right)\left(\text{Rate}_{\text{smokers}}\right) + \\
&\quad \left(\text{Weight}_{\text{nonsmokers}}\right)\left(\text{Rate}_{\text{nonsmokers}}\right) \\
&= (0.25)(191) + (0.75)(8.7) \\
&= 47.8 + 6.5 = 54.3
\end{aligned}
$$

The PAR, also expressed as a rate per 100,000 male population, would be calculated as follows:

$$PAR = 54.3 - 8.7 = 45.6$$

If a major smoking reduction program (possibly financed by the tobacco settlement money) were to reduce the proportion of adult male smokers from 25% to 20% for an extended period, and if the lung cancer death rates for male smokers and nonsmokers remained constant, the revised rate of lung

TABLE 6.2 Measures of Smoking and Lung Cancer Deaths in Men, United States, 1986	
Measure	Amount
Lung cancer deaths among smokers[a]	191/100,000/year
Lung cancer deaths among nonsmokers[a]	8.7/100,000/year
Proportion exposed (Pe) to the risk factor (effective population of smokers, averaged over time)	35%, or 0.35
Population risk of lung cancer death[b]	72.5/100,000/year
Relative risk (RR)[b]	22 (191/8.7 = 22)
Attributable risk (AR)[b]	182.3/100,000/year (191 − 8.7 = 182.3)
Attributable risk percent in the exposed (AR%[exposed])[b]	95.4% (182.3/191 × 100 = 95.4)
Population attributable risk (PAR)[b]	63.8/100,000/year (72.5 − 8.7 = 63.8)
Population attributable risk percent (PAR%)[b]	88% (63.8/72.5 × 100 = 88)

[a]Data from US Centers for Disease Control: Chronic disease reports: deaths from lung cancer—United States, 1986. *MMWR* 38:501–505, 1989.
[b]These rates were calculated from the data with note "a" and the assumption that an average of 35% of the adult male population smoked. The text describes measures obtained when smoking rates are 25% and 20%.

cancer deaths in the total adult male population would be calculated as follows:

$$\text{Rate per 100,000 male}$$
$$\text{population per year} = \left(\text{Weight}_{\text{smokers}}\right)\left(\text{Rate}_{\text{smokers}}\right) +$$
$$\left(\text{Weight}_{\text{nonsmokers}}\right)\left(\text{Rate}_{\text{nonsmokers}}\right)$$
$$= (0.20)(191) + (0.80)(8.7)$$
$$= 38.2 + 7.0 = 45.2$$

Under these conditions, per 100,000 male population:

$$\text{PAR} = 45.2 - 8.7 = 36.5$$

The difference between the first PAR (45.6) and the second PAR (36.5) is 9.1/100,000 adult men. This means that a smoking reduction program that was able to reduce the proportion of adult male smokers from 25% to 20% eventually would be expected to prevent about 9 lung cancer deaths per 100,000 men per year. If there were 100 million men, the intervention would be responsible for preventing 9,100 deaths per year. If there were a similar number of women, and they had a similar reduction in smoking rate and lung cancer death rate, 9,100 deaths per year would be prevented in women, bringing the total to 18,200 deaths prevented in the adult population per year.

4.2 COST-EFFECTIVENESS ANALYSIS

In cost-effectiveness analysis, investigators estimate the costs in dollars of an intervention along with the corresponding effects of that intervention. For health interventions, the *effects* are usually measured in terms of the number of injuries, illnesses, or deaths prevented. Although external factors may complicate the calculation of costs and effects, it is generally more difficult to measure effects, partly because many costs are known quickly, whereas effects may take a long time to measure.

In the previous example of a smoking reduction program, if the costs of the program were $1 billion per year, and if 18,200 lung cancer deaths were prevented per year, it would have cost about $54,945 to prevent each death. If the costs of the program were assigned to a hypothetical population of 200 million adults, instead of to the individuals whose deaths the program prevented, it would have cost $5 per adult per year. If the costs of the program were assigned to the adults who quit smoking (5%), it would have cost about $100 per *quitter* per year.

These amounts may seem high, but it is important to keep in mind that the cost estimates here are fictitious, and that the adult population size estimates are crude. It also is important to remember that in addition to preventing lung cancer deaths, a smoking reduction program would offer other benefits. These would include reductions in the rates of various nonfatal and fatal illnesses among smokers, including heart attacks, chronic obstructive pulmonary disease, and other cancers (nasopharyngeal, esophageal, bladder). If the assumptions were accurate, and if all the positive effects of

smoking cessation were included in the analysis, the costs per health benefit would be much less than those shown previously. The cost effectiveness of the program would vary depending on which segment of the population were assigned to pay the costs and how the outcomes of interest were defined.

4.3 COST-BENEFIT ANALYSIS

In cost-benefit analysis, costs and benefits are measured in dollars. To calculate the benefits of a smoking reduction program, investigators would have to convert the positive effects (e.g., reduction in lung cancer deaths) into dollar amounts before making the comparison with costs. In their calculation of benefits, they would consider a variety of factors, including the savings in medical care and the increased productivity from added years of life. This approach would require them to estimate the average costs of care for one case of lung cancer, the dollar value (in terms of productivity) of adding 1 year of life, and the average number of productive years of life gained by preventing lung cancer. Investigators also would include the time value of money in their analysis by discounting benefits that would occur only in the future. (For more details on cost-effectiveness analysis and cost-benefit analysis, see Chapter 14.)

4.4 OTHER METHODS OF DESCRIBING THE VALUE OF INTERVENTIONS

The anticipated value of an intervention—whether it is a vaccine, a type of treatment, or a change in nutrition or behavior—is frequently expressed in absolute terms (absolute risk reduction), in relative terms (relative risk reduction), or as the reduction in incidence density (e.g., reduction in risk per 100 person-years). These epidemiologic expressions, however, may not give patients or their physicians a clear sense of the impact of a particular intervention. Each method tends to communicate different factors, so a variety of measures are needed (Box 6.2).

4.4.a Absolute and Relative Risk Reduction

The **absolute risk reduction** (ARR) and the **relative risk reduction** (RRR) are descriptive measures that are easy to calculate and understand.[3] For example, assume that the yearly risk of a certain disease is 0.010 in the presence of the risk factor and 0.004 in the absence of the risk factor. The ARR and RRR would be calculated as follows:

$$\text{ARR} = \text{Risk}_{\text{(exposed)}} - \text{Risk}_{\text{(unexposed)}} = 0.010 - 0.004$$
$$= 0.006$$

$$\text{RRR} = \frac{\text{Risk}_{\text{(exposed)}} - \text{Risk}_{\text{(unexposed)}}}{\text{Risk}_{\text{(exposed)}}} = \frac{0.010 - 0.004}{0.010}$$
$$= \frac{0.006}{0.010} = 0.6 = 60\%$$

BOX 6.2 Calculation of Risk Reduction and Other Measures to Describe the Practical Value of Treatment

PART 1 Beginning Data and Assumptions

(a) Treatment-Derived Benefit

Various studies have shown that the risk of stroke in patients with atrial fibrillation can be prevented by long-term treatment with warfarin, an anticoagulant. Baker[5] reviewed the results of five of these studies and reported the following:

Average number of strokes *without* warfarin treatment 　**= 5.1 per 100 patient-years**
= 0.051/patient/year

Average number of strokes *with* warfarin treatment 　**= 1.8 per 100 patient-years**
= 0.018/patient/year

(b) Treatment-Induced Harm

Patients who are treated with drugs are always at some risk of harm. Averages are not available for serious adverse events, such as cerebral and gastrointestinal hemorrhage, in the five studies analyzed by Baker.[5] Assume here that the average number of serious adverse events in patients with atrial fibrillation treated with warfarin is 1 per 100 patient-years = 0.01 per patient per year (fictitious data).

PART 2 Measures of Treatment-Derived Benefit

Risk difference
$$= Risk_{(exposed)} - Risk_{(unexposed)}$$
$$= 5.1 - 1.8 = \textbf{3.3/100 patient-years}$$

Absolute risk reduction (ARR)
$$= Risk_{(exposed)} - Risk_{(unexposed)}$$
$$= 0.051 - 0.018 = \textbf{0.033}$$

Relative risk reduction (RRR)
$$= \frac{Risk_{(exposed)} - Risk_{(unexposed)}}{Risk_{(exposed)}}$$

$$= \frac{0.051 - 0.018}{0.051} = \frac{0.033}{0.051} = 0.65 = \textbf{65\%}$$

PART 3 Measures of Treatment-Induced Harm (Fictitious Data)

$$\text{Absolute risk increase}\left(ARI\right) = Risk_{(exposed)} - Risk_{(unexposed)} = 0.01$$

PART 4 Calculation of NNT and NNH

(a) NNT is the number of patients with atrial fibrillation who would need to be treated with warfarin for 1 year each to prevent one stroke.

$$NNT = 1/ARR = 1/0.033 = 30.3 = \sim 31 \text{ patients}$$

(b) NNH is the number of patients with atrial fibrillation who would need to be treated with warfarin for 1 year each to cause serious harm.

$$NNH = 1/ARI = 1/0.01 = 100 \text{ patients}$$

(c) Whenever the ARR is larger than the ARI (i.e., the NNH is larger than the NNT), more patients would be helped than would be harmed by the treatment. The ratio can be calculated in two different ways:

$$ARR/ARI = 0.033/0.01 = 3.3$$

$$NNH/NNT = 100/30.3 = 3.3$$

This means that the number of patients who would be helped is three times as large as the number who would be harmed. This result and the calculations on which it is based may be oversimplifications because the amount of benefit may be quantitatively and qualitatively different from the amount of harm derived from a treatment.

Data for the average number of strokes with and without warfarin treatment from Baker D: Anticoagulation for atrial fibrillation. White Institute for Health Services Research. *Health Failure Quality Improvement Newsletter* 4(Sept 15):1997.

In this example, an intervention that removed the risk factor would reduce the risk of disease by 0.006 in absolute terms (ARR) or produce a 60% reduction of risk in relative terms (RRR). When the RRR is applied to the effectiveness of vaccines, it is called the **vaccine effectiveness** or the **protective efficacy** (see Chapter 15).

4.4.b Reduction in Incidence Density

In estimating the effects of treatment methods used to eradicate or prevent a disease, it is important to incorporate the length of time that treatment is needed to obtain one **unit of benefit,** usually defined as the eradication or prevention of disease in one person.[4] The simplest way to incorporate length of time is to use incidence density, expressed in terms of the **number of person-years** of treatment. When anticoagulant treatment with warfarin was given on a long-term basis to prevent cerebrovascular accidents (strokes) in patients who had atrial fibrillation, its benefits were reported in terms of the reduction in strokes per 100 patient-years. When one investigator reviewed five studies of warfarin versus placebo treatment in patients with atrial fibrillation, the average number of strokes that occurred per 100 patient-years was 1.8 in patients treated with warfarin and 5.1 in patients treated with placebo.[5] As shown in Box 6.2, the risk difference between these groups is 3.3 per 100 patient-years, the ARR is 0.033 per patient-year, and the RRR is 65%.

4.4.c Number Needed to Treat or Harm

An increasingly popular measure used to describe the practical value of treatment is called the **number needed to treat** (NNT), meaning the number of patients who would need to receive a specific type of treatment for one patient to benefit from the treatment.[6] The NNT is calculated as the number 1 divided by the ARR. In its simplest form, this is expressed as a proportion: NNT = 1/ARR. For example, a new therapy healed leg ulcers in one-third of patients whose ulcers were resistant to all other forms of treatment. In this case the ARR is 0.333, and the NNT is 1/0.333 = 3. These results suggest that, on average, it would be necessary to give this new therapy to three patients with resistant leg ulcers to benefit one patient. The NNT is helpful for making comparisons of the effectiveness of different types of interventions.[6–8]

The basis for the **number needed to harm** (NNH) is similar to that for the NNT, but it is applied to the negative effects of treatment. In the NNH the fundamental item of data is the **absolute risk increase** (ARI), which is analogous to the ARR in the NNT. The NNH formula is similar to that of the NNT: NNH = 1/ARI. The results of one clinical trial can be used to illustrate the calculation of the NNH.[9] In this trial, infants in the intervention group were given iron-fortified formula, and infants in the control group were given formula without iron (regular formula). The mothers of all the infants were asked to report whether their babies had symptoms of colic. They reported colic in 56.8% of infants who received iron-fortified formula and in 40.8% of infants who received regular formula. In this case, ARI = 0.568 − 0.408 = 0.16, and NNH = 1/0.16 = 6.25. This calculation suggests that one of every six or seven infants given iron-fortified formula would develop colic because of the formula, while another two or three infants would develop colic even without iron in the formula.

Although NNT and NNH are helpful for describing the effects of treatment, several points about their use should be emphasized. First, a complete analysis of NNT and NNH should provide confidence intervals for the estimates.[10] (For an introduction to confidence intervals, see Chapter 9) Second, the length of time that treatment is needed to obtain a unit of benefit should also be incorporated (see previous discussion of incidence density). Third, the net benefit from an intervention should be reduced in some way to account for any harm done. This analysis becomes complicated if it is performed with maximum precision, because the investigator needs to calculate the proportion of treated patients who derive benefit only, the proportion who derive harm only, and the proportion who derive both benefit and harm.[11]

5. APPLICATION OF RISK MEASURES TO COUNSELING OF PATIENTS

5.1 CASE RESOLUTION

When counseling patients about potential benefits and harms of medical interventions, we urge students to be careful. The three cancer screening program options presented in the case introduction at the beginning of the chapter are describing the results from a single randomized clinical trial, but they show the impact of expressing the same results in different ways.[12] When we say that a program reduces death rate by 34% compared with no screening program this is the relative risk reduction. The relative risk reduction sounds more impressive and is often used in the lay press, in health pamphlets, and by companies touting the benefits of their medicines and technology. These relative numbers only tell part of the story. When we describe the results of the second program, as producing an absolute reduction in deaths from cancer of 0.06%, this is the absolute risk difference. Absolute numbers are essential but may be hard to find in the literature. The absolute risk looks small, so this method of describing results is often used for describing side effects. In fact, we urge students to look for mismatched framing—where the benefits are presented in relative terms, while the harms or side effects are presented in absolute terms. Unfortunately patients and public health providers are often making decisions based on lopsided information because of this mismatched framing of the data. Finally, when we state that the program prevents 1 death for every 1588 patients screened over 10 years as provided in program option 3, this is the number needed to screen (or NNT). While the three programs all sound quite different, they are just different ways to describe the results of a single clinical trial.

5.2 CONTINUE OUR EXAMPLE OF SMOKING

Suppose a patient is resistant to the idea of quitting smoking but is open to counseling about the topic. Or, suppose a physician has been asked to give a short talk summarizing the effect of smoking on death rates caused by lung cancer. In each of these situations, by using the measures of risk discussed here and summarized in Table 6.2, the physician could present the following estimates of the impact of smoking (although taken from studies in men, the data apply reasonably well to women as well):

- In the United States, smokers are about 22 times as likely as nonsmokers to die of lung cancer.
- About 95 of every 100 lung cancer deaths in people who smoke can be attributed to their smoking.
- About 158,000 deaths annually result from respiratory tract cancer, and because about 88% can be attributed to smoking, smoking is responsible for about 139,000 deaths per year from respiratory tract cancer in the United States.

Assuming that the risk of fatal lung cancer among smokers is 191/100,000 per year, this equals 0.00191 per year (absolute risk increase). If we consider fatal lung cancer as a *harm* and use the NNH approach, 1 divided by 0.00191 yields 523.6, or approximately 524. In round numbers, therefore, we would expect 1 in every 525 adult smokers to die of lung cancer each year.

6. SUMMARY

The practice of clinical medicine includes balancing the benefit versus risk of interventions such as medications, surgery, and vaccinations. Epidemiologic research provides the underlying data on risk versus benefit. Epidemiologic research is usually designed to demonstrate one or more primary contrasts in risk, rate, or odds of disease or exposure. The most straightforward of these measures are the risk difference (attributable risk) and the rate difference, which show in absolute terms how much the risk of one group, usually the group exposed to a risk or preventive factor, differs from that of another group. This contrast can also be expressed as a ratio of risks, rates, or odds; the greater this ratio, the greater the difference resulting from the exposure. The impact of a risk factor on the total burden of any given disease can be measured in terms of an attributable risk percentage for the exposed group or for the population in general. If it is known by how much and in whom a preventive program can reduce the risk ratio, we can then calculate the total benefit of the program, including its cost effectiveness. Measures such as the relative risk reduction (RRR), number needed to treat (NNT), and number needed to harm (NNH) are used to determine the effect of interventions.

REFERENCES

1. Centers for Disease Control. Chronic disease reports: deaths from lung cancer—United States, 1986. *MMWR*. 1989;38:501-505.
2. Doll R, Hill AB. Lung cancer and other causes of death in relation to smoking; a second report on the mortality of British doctors. *Br Med J*. 1956;2:1071-1081.
3. Haynes RB, Sackett DL, Guyatt GH, Tugwell P. *Clinical Epidemiology*: How to Do Clinical Practice Research. 3rd ed. Philadelphia, PA: Lippincott Williams & Wilkins; 2006.
4. Laupacis A, Sackett DL, Roberts RS. An assessment of clinically useful measures of the consequences of treatment. *N Engl J Med*. 1988;318:1728-1733.
5. Baker D. Anticoagulation for atrial fibrillation. White Institute for Health Services Research. *Health Fail Quality Improv Newsl*. September 15, 1997;4.
6. Kumana CR, Cheung BM, Lauder IJ. Gauging the impact of statins using number needed to treat. *JAMA*. 1999;282:1899-1901.
7. Woolf SH. The need for perspective in evidence-based medicine. *JAMA*. 1999;282:2358-2365.
8. Katz DL. *Clinical Epidemiology and Evidence-Based Medicine*. Thousand Oaks, CA: Sage; 2001.
9. Syracuse Consortium for Pediatric Clinical Studies. Iron-fortified formulas and gastrointestinal symptoms in infants: a controlled study. *Pediatrics*. 1980;66:168-170.
10. Altman DG. Confidence intervals for the number needed to treat. *BMJ*. 1998;317:1309-1312.
11. Mancini GB, Schulzer M. Reporting risks and benefits of therapy by use of the concepts of unqualified success and unmitigated failure: applications to highly cited trials in cardiovascular medicine. *Circulation*. 1999;99:377-383.
12. Geyman JP, Wolf FM. Evidence-based medicine. In: Norris TE, Fuller SS, Goldberg HI, Tarczy-Hornoch P, eds. *Informatics in Primary Care. Health Informatics*. New York, NY: Springer; 2002.

SELECT READINGS

Gigerenzer G. Calculated Risks: How to Know When Numbers Deceive You. New York, NY: Simon & Schuster; 2003.
Health News Review. Available at: https://www.healthnewsreview.org/.

REVIEW QUESTIONS

1. A team of researchers hypothesize that watching violent, noneducational cartoons might lead to epilepsy in childhood. Children with and without epilepsy are compared on the basis of hours spent watching violent, noneducational cartoons. Which of the following statements *best* characterizes the assessment of data in such a study?
   A. Absolute and relative measures of risk can be derived.
   B. The difference in level of exposure to a putative risk factor is the basis for comparison.
   C. The risk ratio can be calculated directly.
   D. The temporal association between exposure and outcome can be established with certainty.
   E. The use of healthy controls ensures external validity.

2. The researchers in question 1 do not find statistically significant evidence that cartoons produce epilepsy in childhood. However, determined to show that violent, noneducational cartoons cause harm, they hypothesize that perhaps viewing this type of programming leads to attention deficits. They assemble two groups of children: those who watch violent, noneducational cartoons frequently and those who watch only other types of television programming. Which of the following is a characteristic of such a study?
   A. Additional risk factors cannot be assessed as the study progresses.
   B. Internal validity is independent of confounders.
   C. The two study groups are assembled on the basis of their outcome status.
   D. The most appropriate measure for comparing outcomes in this study would be an odds ratio.
   E. The temporal association between exposure and outcome is uncertain.

3. The risk of acquiring an infection is 300 per 1000 among the unvaccinated and 5 per 1000 among the vaccinated population. Approximately 80% of the population is exposed to the pathogen every year. Which of the following would be true?
   A. The absolute risk reduction is 295.
   B. The relative risk reduction is 5900%.
   C. The population attributable risk percent is 27.
   D. The number needed to treat is 6.2.
   E. The number needed to harm is 38.

4. A study is conducted to determine the effects of prescription stimulant use on an individual's willingness to bungee jump. A total of 500 individuals are assembled on the basis of bungee-jumping status: 250 are jumpers and 250 are not jumpers. Of the 250 jumpers, 150 report prescription stimulant use. Of the 250 nonjumpers, 50 report prescription stimulant use. Most of the nonjumpers take anxiolytics. Which of the following statements is *true*?
   A. Jumpers and nonjumpers should be matched for prescription stimulant use.
   B. The absolute and relative risks of bungee jumping with the use of prescription stimulants can be determined from this study.
   C. This is a cohort study.
   D. This study can be used to calculate an odds ratio.
   E. Unanticipated outcomes can be assessed in this study.

5. Considering the information given in question 4, what is the absolute difference in the risk of jumping between those using prescription stimulants and those not using these drugs?
   A. 0.4
   B. 0.67
   C. 67
   D. 100
   E. It cannot be calculated because this is a case control study

6. Considering the information given in question 4, the odds ratio calculated from this study would give the odds of:
   A. Jumping among stimulant users to jumping among nonstimulant users
   B. Jumping among stimulant users to nonjumping among nonstimulant users
   C. Nonjumping among stimulant users to nonstimulant use among jumpers
   D. Stimulant use among jumpers to stimulant use among nonjumpers
   E. Stimulant use among nonjumpers to nonstimulant use among jumpers

7. Concerning the information given in question 4, the odds ratio in this study is:
   A. 0.2
   B. 0.6
   C. 2
   D. 5
   E. 6

8. Concerning the information given in question 4, the results of this study indicate that:
   A. Bungee jumping and stimulant use are associated.
   B. Bungee jumping and stimulant use are causally related.
   C. Bungee jumping influences one's need for prescription stimulants.
   D. The use of prescription stimulants influences a person's tendency to bungee jump.
   E. There is no association between anxiolytic use and bungee jumping.

9. You decide to investigate the stimulant use–bungee jumping association further. Your new study again involves a total of 500 individuals, with 250 in each group. This time, however, you assemble the groups on the basis of their past history of stimulant use, and you prospectively determine the incidence rate of bungee jumping. You exclude subjects with a prior history of jumping. Over a 5-year period, 135 of the exposed group and 38 of the unexposed group engage in jumping. The relative risk of bungee jumping among the group exposed to stimulant use is:
   A. 2.1
   B. 3.6
   C. 4.8
   D. 6
   E. Impossible to determine based on the study design

10. Now considering the information provided in question 9, among bungee jumpers, what percentage of the total risk for jumping is caused by stimulant use?
   A. 0%
   B. 3.6%
   C. 10%
   D. 36%
   E. 72%

11. Assume that the risk of death in patients with untreated pneumonia is 15%, whereas the risk of death in patients with antibiotic-treated pneumonia is 2%. Assume also that the risk of anaphylaxis with antibiotic treatment is 1%, whereas the risk without treatment is essentially 0%. What is the number needed to treat (NNT) in this scenario?
   A. 1.0
   B. 7.7
   C. 13
   D. 39.4
   E. 100

12. Concerning the information given in question 11, what is the number needed to harm (NNH) in this scenario?
   A. 1.0
   B. 7.7
   C. 13
   D. 39.4
   E. 100

13. Concerning the information given in question 11, what would be the net result of intervention in this scenario?
    A. 1.0 patient saved for each patient harmed
    B. 7.7 patients harmed for each patient saved
    C. 13 patients saved for each patient harmed
    D. 39.4 patients harmed for each patient saved
    E. 100 patients saved for each patient harmed

14. You randomly assign clinical practices to charting with a new electronic medical record (intervention) or charting using paper records (control), and you test whether physicians are satisfied or not (outcome) after 3 months. Of 100 subjects assigned to each condition, you find evidence of satisfaction in 12 in the EMR group and 92 in the paper group. An appropriate measure of association in this study is the:
    A. Incidence density
    B. Power
    C. Likelihood ratio
    D. Odds ratio
    E. Risk ratio

15. Concerning the information given in question 14, the value of the measure identified is:
    A. 0.08
    B. 0.13
    C. 1.3
    D. 8.1
    E. 13.1

ANSWERS AND EXPLANATIONS

1. **B.** This is a case control study. The cases are children who have epilepsy, and the controls are (or should be) children who do not have epilepsy but whose characteristics are otherwise similar to those of the cases. The difference in the level of exposure to a putative risk factor (violent, noneducational cartoons) is the basis for comparison. The use of healthy controls does not ensure that the results will pertain to a general population, so external validity is uncertain (E). In a case control study, the risk ratio cannot be calculated directly, but must be estimated from the odds ratio (C). The temporal relationship between exposure and outcome usually is not known with certainty in this type of study (D); exposure and disease already have occurred at the time of enrollment. Only relative measures of risk can be calculated based on a case control study (A). A cohort study is required to obtain absolute risk.

2. **A.** This is a cohort study. The two groups are assembled on the basis of exposure status (i.e., risk factor status), not outcome status (C), and are then followed and compared on the basis of disease status. Only the risk factors, or exposures, identified at study entry can be assessed as the study progresses. The development of attention deficits in this case are the "disease" or outcome of interest. The temporal association between exposure and outcome should be established to prevent

bias (E); in a cohort study, subjects are generally free of the outcome (disease) at the time of enrollment. The inclusion of subjects who developed attention deficits before the defined exposure would bias the study, so these subjects should be excluded. In all epidemiologic studies, a thorough attempt must be made to control confounders because confounding compromises internal validity (B). The most appropriate means of comparing the two groups in this study is the risk ratio, or relative risk of attention deficits (D). The control group should have been otherwise similar to those who watch violent, noneducational cartoons except that they did not watch this programming.

3. **B.** To determine relative risk reduction, we can first calculate an absolute risk reduction (ARR). $ARR = Risk_{(exposed)} - Risk_{(unexposed)}$. Those exposed to the vaccine have a risk of 5/1000, or 0.005. Those unexposed to the vaccine have a risk of 300/1000, or 0.3. The ARR is thus $0.005 - 0.3 = -0.295$ (not A). Dividing ARR by $Risk_{(exposed)}$ yields the relative risk reduction (RRR), or $-0.295/0.005 = 59 = 5900\%$. In other words, vaccinated people are 59 times less likely to acquire the infection than unvaccinated people. The number needed to treat (NNT) is simply 1/ARR, or 1/–0.295, or –3.4 (not D). In other words, only four people would have to be vaccinated for one to benefit. The number needed to harm (E) cannot be calculated from the information given, since no adverse events of the vaccine are reported. Likewise, the population attributable risk percent (PAR%) cannot be calculated (C). One of two formulas can be used to determine PAR%. The first is as follows:

   This is equivalent to:

   $$PAR\% = \frac{Risk_{(total)} - Risk_{(unexposed)}}{Risk_{(total)}} \times 100$$

   $$PAR\% = \frac{(Pe)(RR-1)}{1+(Pe)(RR-1)} \times 100$$

   where Pe is the proportion of the population exposed, and RR is the relative risk. In the case described in the question, it is impossible to calculate the PAR% because we have not been told the proportion of the population exposed (i.e., vaccinated) for the first formula, and we do not know the Pe for the second formula. To determine the $Risk_{(total)}$ for the first formula, we need to know the proportion of the population vaccinated (in whom the risk of infection is 5 per 1000) and the proportion unvaccinated (in whom the risk is 300 per 1000). With exposure to a preventive measure, such as a vaccine in this case, risk is reduced among the exposed. The risk of the outcome is less among the exposed than among the unexposed, so the PAR would be negative.

4. **D.** The study described is a case control study (not cohort, C). The cases are individuals who have a history of bungee jumping, and the controls are (or should

be) individuals who have no history of bungee jumping but whose characteristics are otherwise similar to those of the cases. The cases and controls should not be matched for prescription stimulant use (A) because this is the exposure of interest. Overmatching is the result when cases and controls are matched on the basis of some characteristic or behavior that is highly correlated with the exposure of interest. Overmatching precludes the detection of a difference in exposure, even if one truly exists. The odds ratio is calculated from a case control study and is used to estimate relative risk. Absolute risk cannot be determined from a case control study (B). In this type of study, the outcome defines the group at study entry; although unanticipated risk factors can be assessed, only the outcome variables chosen as the basis for subject selection can be evaluated (E).

5. **E.** Absolute risk cannot be determined from a case control study because the groups do not represent the population from which they were drawn. All numerical choices (A–D) are incorrect for this reason. Only the odds ratio can be calculated from a case control study.

6. **D.** The odds ratio in a case control study is the odds of the exposure in cases relative to controls. The exposure in this study is prescription stimulant use. Cases are those who bungee jump, whereas controls are those who do not. The odds of using prescription stimulants among cases relative to controls is the outcome of interest. The odds of jumping among stimulant users to jumping among nonstimulant users (A) could also be an odds ratio of interest, but it would come from a different case control study, with a different design, to answer a different question. Specifically, such a study would assemble cases (stimulant users) and controls (nonstimulant users) and look for the exposure (whether they bungee jump or not). The other answers (B, C, and E) are nonsense distracters.

7. **E.** The formula for the odds ratio (OR) is $(a/c)/(b/d)$. This is algebraically equivalent to ad/bc, where a represents cases with the exposure, b represents controls with the exposure, c represents cases without the exposure, and d represents controls without the exposure. Displaying the data from the study in a 2 × 2 table is helpful.

Prescription Stimulant Use	Bungee Jumping	
	Positive	**Negative**
Positive	150 (*a*)	50 (*b*)
Negative	100 (*c*)	200 (*d*)

Cells c and d had to be calculated from the information in the question so that the total in each

column would be 250 (the question tells us there are 250 jumpers and 250 nonjumpers). For this study:

$$OR = (150/100)/(50/200)$$
$$= (150 \times 200)/(50 \times 100)$$
$$= 30,000/5,000 = 6$$

By convention, the OR is expressed with the exposure rate among cases in the numerator. If the investigators were interested in reporting the odds of prescription stimulant use in nonjumpers relative to jumpers, the OR could be expressed as 1/6, or 0.17. Other answer choices (A–D) are nonsense distracters.

8. **A.** The odds of using prescription stimulants are six times as great in cases as they are in controls in this study. There is an apparent association between stimulant use and tendency to jump. There may in fact be no true causal relationship (B) if the findings are (1) caused by chance, (2) biased (e.g., if cases are interviewed more thoroughly or differently than controls with regard to psychotropic use), or (3) confounded by an unmeasured variable (e.g., alcohol consumption). Moreover, even if the relationship were causal, the found association would not tell us anything about the direction; in other words, we cannot determine whether bungee jumping predisposes to stimulant use (C), or vice versa (D), because exposure and outcome are measured simultaneously in a case control study, and the temporal sequence is uncertain. As for anxiolytics, these drugs may or may not be associated with bungee jumping (E). This study did not assess anxiolytic exposure, and the question gives no information about anxiolytic use among jumpers.

9. **B.** This is a cohort study, and the relative risk (or risk ratio) can absolutely be determined (not E). The formula for relative risk (RR) is:

$$RR = \left[a/(a+b) \right]/\left[c/(c+d) \right]$$

where a, b, c, and d are as defined in the explanation of question 7 and in Table 6.1. The 2 × 2 table for this study is as follows:

Prescription Stimulant Use	Bungee Jumping	
	Positive	**Negative**
Positive	135 (*a*)	115 (*b*)
Negative	38 (*c*)	212 (*d*)

Cells b and d had to be calculated from the information in the question so that the total in each row would be 250 (the question tells us there are 250 jumpers and 250 nonjumpers). The risk ratio, or relative risk, is:

$$RR = \left[135/(135+115) \right]/\left[38/(38+212) \right]$$
$$= (135/250)/(38/250)$$
$$= 0.54/0.152 = 3.55 = 3.6$$

Other numerical answer choices (A, C, and D) are nonsense distracters.

10. **E.** The percentage of total risk caused by an exposure among those with the exposure is the attributable risk percent in the exposed, or AR%$_{(exposed)}$. This can be calculated using the risk ratio (RR), which in this case is 3.6:

$$AR\%_{(exposed)} = \frac{RR-1}{RR} \times 100$$
$$= \frac{3.6-1}{3.6} \times 100 = 72.2\%$$

The AR% in this case indicates that among those who use stimulants, almost three-fourths of the total risk for bungee jumping is attributable to the medication, assuming the found association is real and not an artifact of chance, bias, or confounding. Note that these data are fictitious.

11. **B.** The NNT is calculated as 1 divided by the absolute risk reduction (ARR) associated with an intervention. In this scenario the intervention (antibiotic treatment) reduces the risk of death from 15% to 2%, so ARR is 13%, or 0.13. Dividing 0.13 into 1 yields 7.7. This implies that 1 life is saved, on average, for every 7.7 patients treated with antibiotics. The 1.0 (A) represents the percent absolute risk increase of anaphylaxis with antibiotics. The 100 (E) is the number needed to harm (see explanation to answer 12). The 13 (C) is the percent ARR of death with antibiotics. The 39.4 (D) is a nonsense distracter.

12. **E.** When an intervention increases (rather than decreases) the risk of a particular adverse outcome, the number of patients treated, on average, before one patient has the adverse outcome is the NNH. To calculate the NNH, the absolute risk increase (ARI) associated with the intervention is divided into 1. In this scenario there is a 1% risk of anaphylaxis (the adverse outcome) when antibiotic treatment (the intervention) is used, and a 0% risk of anaphylaxis when antibiotic treatment is not used. Antibiotic treatment increases the risk of anaphylaxis by an absolute 1% (0.01). The NNH is 1/0.01, or 100. On average, 100 patients would need to be treated before 1 patient, on average, is harmed by the intervention. Incorrect answer choices (A–D) are explained under answer 11.

13. **C.** If the NNT were greater than the NNH, the intervention would harm more patients than help. Ignoring the issue that the type and degree of harm and help may differ, if the NNH were greater than the NNT, the intervention in question would help more patients than it harmed. In this scenario the NNH (100) is greater than the NNT (7.7); the procedure provides net benefit because fewer patients need to be treated before one is helped than need to be treated before one is harmed. The number of patients benefiting for each one harmed is calculated as follows:

$$NNH/NNT = 100/7.7 = 13$$

This represents 13 lives saved for every case of anaphylaxis induced by the antibiotic treatment. This same conclusion could have been reached by using the ARR and ARI figures. In this case, dividing the ARR (13%) by the ARI (1%) yields 13 as the number helped for each one harmed. When the ARR is greater than the ARI, there is net benefit, with more than one patient helped for each one harmed. By the same reasoning, when the ARI exceeds the ARR, there is net harm, with more than one patient harmed for each one helped. (The actual numbers in this case are fictitious and used for illustration purposes only.) Answers A, B, D, and E are nonsense distracters having numerical values corresponding to the metrics explained in answer 11.

14. **E.** The study described is a cohort study, in which subjects are assembled on the basis of exposure status (charting method) and followed for outcome (physician satisfaction). The risk ratio is the outcome measure of a cohort study with a dichotomous outcome. The odds ratio (D) is used in case control studies rather than cohort studies and is in essence the "risk of having the risk factor." The likelihood ratio (C) is used to evaluate the utility of a diagnostic test. Incidence density (A) is an outcome measure of events per subject per unit of time (e.g., per 100 person-years) and is particularly useful when events may recur in individual participants. Power (B) is used to assess the capacity of a study to detect an outcome difference when there truly is one, given a particular sample size; power is used to avoid beta error (type II or false-negative error).

15. **B.** To calculate the risk ratio (relative risk), the risk of the outcome in the exposed is divided by the risk of the outcome in the unexposed. In this study the outcome is physician satisfaction; the exposure is electronic medical record (EMR) charting; the risk of the outcome in the exposed is 12/100, or 0.12; and the risk of the outcome in the unexposed is 92/100, or 0.92. Dividing 0.12 by 0.92 yields 0.13. This implies that the "risk" of physician satisfaction in those exposed to the EMR was 0.13 times the risk of that outcome in the control group. Note that an "exposure" can increase or decrease the "risk." In this case the "risk" of satisfaction decreases with EMR implementation, and this may be easier to interpret by considering the inverse ratio: risk of unexposed to risk of exposed, or 0.92/0.12 = 7.7; in other words, the risk of satisfaction is 7.7 times greater among physicians using paper charts than among physicians using an EMR, 3 months after EMR implementation. Note also that the outcome in question need not be an adverse outcome, despite the connotation of the term "risk." Answers A, C, D, and E are nonsense distracters.

Understanding the Quality of Medical Data

"Errors are not in the art but in the artificers."

Isaac Newton

CASE INTRODUCTION

A 46-year-old female patient had a skin biopsy for an irregular-appearing lesion. The initial pathology report was "suspicious for invasive melanoma." When the biopsy material was sent for a second opinion, the new interpretation was "mildly dysplastic nevus" (e.g., benign). The patient, a physician and co-author of this textbook (JGE), decided to send her skin biopsy material to a third pathologist—identifying one who had written textbooks on melanoma with decades of clinical experience. This third biopsy interpretation came back in the middle of the diagnostic spectrum: an "atypical Spitz lesion" that can mimic melanoma but is benign (i.e., not invasive melanoma). In summary, the same skin biopsy specimen was sent to three different pathologists and received three vastly different interpretations.

1. GOALS OF DATA COLLECTION AND ANALYSIS

The practice of medicine requires the constant collection, evaluation, analysis, and use of quantitative and qualitative data. The data are used for diagnosis, prognosis, and choosing and evaluating treatments. Similarly, data are used by public health professionals to evaluate programs and decide on priorities going forward. The accuracy of data is obviously important. To the extent that data are inaccurate, we say there is "error" in the data. It may be disquieting to talk about errors in medicine, but errors in data occur and are difficult to eliminate.

The term *error* is used in more than one way. It can be used to mean mistakes in the diagnosis and treatment of patients or to mean more egregious mistakes with clear negligence, such as removing the wrong body part. This meaning of *error* was emphasized in *To Err Is Human: Building a Safer Health System*, a report issued by the US Institute of Medicine.[1] The report caused a considerable stir nationally.[2]

Medical histories, physical examinations, laboratory values, and imaging reports are never perfect because of the limitations of the human process. In clinical medicine and research, it is important to minimize errors in data so that these data can be used to guide, rather than mislead, the individuals who provide the care. The emphasis in this chapter is on ways to measure and improve the quality of medical data.

1.1 PROMOTING ACCURACY AND PRECISION

Two distinct but related goals of data collection are accuracy and precision. **Accuracy** refers to the ability of a measurement to be correct on the average. If a measure is not accurate, it is biased because it deviates, on average, from the true value in one direction or the other, rather than equally in both directions. **Precision,** sometimes known as **reproducibility** or **reliability,** is the ability of a measurement to give the same result or a similar result with repeated measurements of the same factor. **Random error** is nondifferential error because it does not distort data consistently in any one direction. Random error alone, if large, results in lack of precision, but not bias, because distortions from truth may occur comparably in both directions (see discussion of bias in Chapter 4).

To ask whether accuracy or precision is more important in data collection would be like asking which wing of an airplane is more important. As shown in Figs. 7.1 and 7.2, unless both qualities are present, the data would be generally useless. Accuracy is shown in the fact that the mean (average) is the true (correct) value, whereas precision (reliability) is evident in the fact that all values are close to the true value (see Fig. 7.1A). Fig. 7.1B shows a measure that is accurate but not precise, meaning that it gives the correct answer only on the average. Such a measure might be useful for some types of research, but even so, it would not be reassuring to the investigator. For an individual patient, there is no utility in some factor being correct on the average if it is wrong for that patient. To guide diagnosis and treatment, each observation must be correct. Fig. 7.1C shows data that are precise but biased, rather than being accurate, and are misleading. Fig. 7.1D shows data that are neither accurate nor precise and are useless or even dangerous. Fig. 7.2 uses a target and bullet holes to show the same concepts.

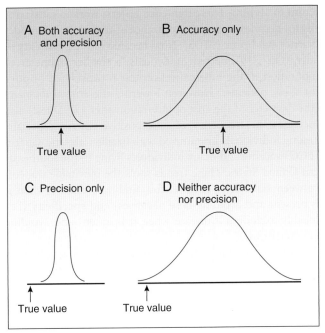

Fig. 7.1 Possible Combinations of Accuracy and Precision in Describing a Continuous Variable. The *x*-axis is a range of values, with the *arrow* indicating the true value. The four curves are the probability distributions of observed values.

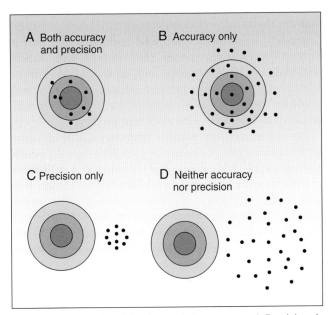

Fig. 7.2 Possible Combinations of Accuracy and Precision in Describing a Continuous Variable. The four targets are used with bullet holes to show the four concepts illustrated in Fig. 7.1 with curves.

1.2 REDUCING ERRORS

As discussed in Chapter 4, there are several types of errors to avoid in the collection of data; this section focuses on errors associated with measurement. A **measurement bias** is a **differential error**—that is, a nonrandom, systematic, or consistent error in which the values tend to be inaccurate in a particular direction. Measurement bias results from measuring the heights of patients with their shoes on or from measuring patient blood pressures with a blood pressure cuff that reads too high or too low. Statistical analysis cannot correct for bias, unless the amount of bias in each individual measurement is known. In the example of the patients' height measurements, bias could be corrected only if the height of each patient's shoe heel were known and subtracted from that patient's reported height.

Although measuring patients in their bare feet could eliminate bias, it would not eliminate **random errors**, or **nondifferential errors.** When data have only random errors, some observations are too high and some are too low. It is even possible for random errors to produce biased results.[3] If there are enough observations, however, data with only random errors usually produce a correct estimate of the average value (see Chapter 9).

1.3 REDUCING VARIABILITY

If the same clinician takes successive measurements of the blood pressure or height of the same person, or if the same clinician examines the same x-ray film or pathology slide several times without knowing that it is the same, there usually are some differences in the measurements or interpretations obtained. This is known as *intraobserver* (*within* observer) **variability.** If two different clinicians measure the same person's blood pressure or examine the same pathology slide independently, there usually are some differences. This is called *interobserver* (*between* observers) **variability.** One goal of data collection is to reduce the amount of intraobserver and interobserver variability. Although much of medicine is still an art, there is also a science in collecting data and studying its quality.

2. STUDYING THE ACCURACY AND USEFULNESS OF MEDICAL TESTS

One way to judge the usefulness of a screening or diagnostic test for a particular disease is to evaluate how often its results are correct in two groups of individuals: (1) a group in whom the disease is known to be *present* and in whom the test results should be positive, and (2) a group in whom the disease is known to be *absent* and in whom the test results should be negative. This form of research is not as easy as it initially might appear because several factors influence whether the results for an individual subject would be accurate and whether the test in general would be useful in diagnosing or screening for a particular disease. These factors include the stage of the disease and the spectrum of disease in the study population. The population in whom the diagnostic or screening test is evaluated should have characteristics similar to the characteristics of the populations in whom the test would be used. For example, data derived from evaluating tests in men or young people may not be as useful in women or old people.[4]

2.1 FALSE-POSITIVE AND FALSE-NEGATIVE RESULTS

In science, if something is said to be true when it is actually false, this is variously called a **type I error,** a **false-positive error,** or an **alpha error.** If something is said to be false when it is actually true, this is called a **type II error,** a **false-negative error,** or a **beta error.** If a benign skin lesion is called invasive melanoma (cancer), that is an example of a false-positive result. If a cancerous skin lesion is called benign, that is a false-negative result.

The **stage of disease** often influences the test results. Tests for infectious diseases, such as some blood tests for human immunodeficiency virus (HIV) and the tuberculin skin test for tuberculosis, are likely to be accurate only after immunity has developed, which might be weeks after the initial infection. Very early in the course of almost any infection, a patient may have no immunologic evidence of infection, and tests done during this time may yield false-negative results.

False-negative results may also occur late in infections such as tuberculosis, when the disease is severe and the immune system is overwhelmed and unable to produce a positive skin test result. This inadequate immune system response is called **anergy** (from Greek, meaning "not working") and can develop with any illness or stress severe enough to cause depression of the immune system.[5] Advanced age also can be a cause of anergy.

The **spectrum of disease** in the study population is important when evaluating a test's potential usefulness in the real world. False-negative and false-positive results can be more of a problem than anticipated. In the case of the tuberculin skin test, false-positive results were formerly found in persons from the southeastern United States. Exposure to atypical mycobacteria in the soil was common in this region, and because there was some cross-reactivity between the atypical mycobacteria and the mycobacteria tested in the tuberculin skin test, equivocal and even false-positive test results were common among this population until standards were tightened. To accomplish this, the use of an antigen called "old tuberculin" was replaced by the use of a *purified protein derivative* (PPD) of mycobacteria at a standardized strength of 5 tuberculin units. The diameter of skin induration needed for a positive test result was increased from 5 mm to 10 mm. These tightened criteria worked satisfactorily for decades, until the appearance of acquired immunodeficiency syndrome (AIDS). Now, because of the possibility of anergy in HIV-infected individuals, a smaller diameter of induration in the tuberculin skin test is considered positive for these patients.[6] However, lowering the *critical diameter* (the diameter of the area of induration after a PPD test) also increases the frequency of false-positive results, especially among individuals immunized with bacille Calmette-Guérin (BCG) vaccine and many individuals living in the southeastern United States. These trends show the inevitable tradeoff between **sensitivity** (i.e., reliably finding a disease when it is present and avoiding false negatives) and **specificity** (i.e., reliably excluding a disease when it is absent and avoiding false positives).

We want the smoke detectors in our homes to go off every time there is a fire (i.e., we want them to be sensitive), but not to be constantly going off when there is no fire (i.e., we want them to be specific).

False-positive and false-negative results are not limited to tests of infectious diseases, as illustrated in the use of serum calcium values to rule out parathyroid disease, particularly hyperparathyroidism, in new patients seen at an endocrinology clinic. Hyperparathyroidism is a disease of calcium metabolism. In an affected patient the serum level of calcium is often elevated, but usually varies from time to time. When the calcium level is not elevated in a patient with hyperparathyroidism, the result would be considered "falsely negative." Conversely, when the calcium level is elevated in a patient without hyperparathyroidism (but instead with cancer, sarcoidosis, multiple myeloma, milk-alkali syndrome, or another condition that can increase calcium level), the result would be considered "falsely positive" for hyperparathyroidism, even though it revealed a different problem.

Fig. 7.3 shows two possible frequency distributions of serum calcium values, one in a population of healthy people without parathyroid disease and the other in a population of patients with hyperparathyroidism. If the calcium level were sufficiently low (e.g., below point A), the patient would be unlikely to have hyperparathyroidism. If the calcium level were sufficiently high (e.g., above point B), the patient would be likely to have an abnormality of calcium metabolism, possibly hyperparathyroidism. If the calcium level were in the intermediate range (between points A and B in Fig. 7.3) in a single calcium test, although the patient probably would not have a disease of calcium metabolism, this possibility could not be ruled out, and if such disease were suspected, serial calcium values and other tests would be obtained.

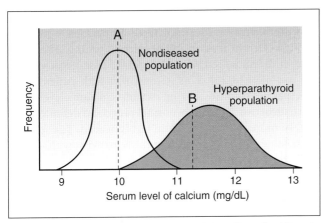

Fig. 7.3 Overlap in Values of Randomly Taken Tests in a Population Mostly of Healthy People *(curve on left)* but with some diseased people *(curve on right)*. A person with a calcium level below point A would be unlikely to have hyperparathyroidism. A person with a calcium level above point B would be likely to have an abnormality of calcium metabolism, possibly hyperparathyroidism. A person with a calcium level between points A and B may or may not have an abnormality of calcium metabolism. (*Note:* The normal range of calcium depends on the method used in a specific laboratory. In some laboratories, the range is 8.5–10.5 mg/dL. In others, as in this illustration, it is 9–11 mg/dL.)

Laboratories publish a range of "normal" values for substances that they measure, such as calcium. A calcium value beyond the normal range for that laboratory requires further diagnostic tests. For many laboratories, a serum calcium of 11 mg/dL is above the upper limit of normal. If the **cutoff point** for the upper limit of normal is set too low, considerable time and money would be wasted following up on false-positive results; if it is set too high, however, persons with the disease might be missed. As discussed subsequently, determining the sensitivity, specificity, and predictive values of a test at different cutoff points would help investigators choose the best cutoff point for that test. It would be convenient if there were no overlaps between the test results in diseased and nondiseased persons. If this were true, the only source of error would be in the performance of the tests. In reality, the distribution of test values in diseased persons often overlaps with the distribution of values in nondiseased persons.

It is easier to visualize the idea of a false-positive error where there is a clear distinction between the diagnosis of disease versus nondisease, as in the evaluation of a spot on a mammogram.[7,8] Even this situation, however, is not always simple. The area in question on a mammogram either does or does not represent breast cancer; a diagnosis of cancer is made only after breast tissue is obtained and reviewed by the pathologist. There may be a true abnormality on the mammogram (e.g., calcifications) without the presence of cancer. If only calcifications without cancer were present, a radiologist's reading of a positive (abnormal) exam would be falsely positive for cancer (the primary concern), but it would be correct about the presence of an abnormality (the calcifications). In contrast, a radiologist's reading of this mammogram as "normal" would be a true negative for cancer, but a false negative for calcifications. Radiologists and pathologists

frequently indicate uncertainty by reporting the results as "abnormality present—possibly/probably not cancer" and recommending that additional tests be done or that the exam be repeated after a defined number of months. Such readings are analogous to laboratory values in the indeterminate range.

2.2 SENSITIVITY AND SPECIFICITY

Sensitivity and specificity are two important measures of test function. They are ways to report the performance of medical tests when the true disease state is known. To calculate these measures, the data concerning the subjects studied and the test results can be put in a 2×2 table of the type shown in Table 7.1. The cells in this table are labeled *a, b, c,* and *d,* as in Table 6.1, but the measures to be calculated are different.

The first column under True Disease Status in Table 7.1 represents all the diseased participants, consisting of those with **true-positive results** (*a*) and those with **false-negative results** (*c*). The second disease status column represents all the healthy participants, consisting of those with **false-positive results** (*b*) and those with **true-negative results** (*d*). When the total in

TABLE 7.1   Standard 2 × 2 Table Comparing Test Results and True Disease Status of Participants Tested

TEST RESULT	TRUE DISEASE STATUS		Total
	Diseased	Nondiseased	
Positive	*a*	*b*	*a + b*
Negative	*c*	*d*	*c + d*
TOTAL	*a + c*	*b + d*	*a + b + c + d*

Interpretation of the Cells
a = Participants with true-positive test result
b = Participants with false-positive test result
c = Participants with false-negative test result
d = Participants with true-negative test result
a + b = All participants with positive test result
c + d = All participants with negative test result
a + c = All participants with the disease
b + d = All participants without the disease
a + b + c + d = All study participants

Formulas
$a/(a + c)$ = Sensitivity
$d/(b + d)$ = Specificity
$b/(b + d)$ = False-positive error rate (alpha error rate, type I error rate)
$c/(a + c)$ = False-negative error rate (beta error rate, type II error rate)
$a/(a + b)$ = Positive predictive value (PPV)
$d/(c + d)$ = Negative predictive value (NPV)
$[a/(a + c)]/[b/(b + d)] = (a/b)/[(a + c)/(b + d)]$ = Likelihood ratio positive (LR+)
$[c/(a + c)]/[d/(b + d)] = (c/d)/[(a + c)/(b + d)]$ = Likelihood ratio negative (LR−)
$(a + c)/(a + b + c + d)$ = Prevalence

the disease column is divided by the total of all the participants studied, the result represents the **prevalence rate** (proportion) of the disease in the study population.

Sensitivity, which refers to the ability of a test to detect a disease when present, is calculated as $a/(a + c)$. If a test is not sensitive, it fails to detect disease in some of the diseased participants, and these participants appear in cell c. The rate at which this occurs is called the **false-negative error rate** and is calculated as $c/(a + c)$. The correct denominator for the false-negative error rate is all those who are diseased, because only those who are diseased are at risk for falsely being called "nondiseased." The sensitivity and the false-negative error rate add up to 1.0 (100%).

Specificity, which refers to the ability of a test to indicate nondisease when no disease is present, is calculated as $d/(b + d)$. If a test is not specific, it falsely indicates the presence of disease in nondiseased subjects, and these subjects appear in cell b. The rate at which this occurs is called the **false-positive error rate.** Because only nondiseased participants are at risk for falsely being called diseased, this rate is calculated as $b/(b + d)$. The specificity and the false-positive error rate add up to 1.0 (100%).

As an example to illustrate what the letters in Table 7.1 imply, suppose that 80 consecutive persons entering an endocrinology clinic have their serum calcium level checked and have a hyperparathyroidism workup to determine whether they have the disease. Also, assume that the upper cutoff point for "normal" serum calcium is 11 mg/dL, so that levels greater than 11 mg/dL are presumptively "test positive" and levels of 11 mg/dL or less are "test negative." Third, assume that the results are as shown in Table 7.2. The following observations could be made. Of the 80 persons

tested, 20 ultimately were shown to have hyperparathyroidism (prevalence of 25%). Of these 20 persons, 12 had an elevated calcium level in initial calcium testing. The sensitivity of the initial test was 60%, and the false-negative error rate was 40% (8/20). This is consistent with patients with hyperparathyroidism having serum calcium levels that alternate between the high-normal range and definite elevation, so more than one calcium test is needed. The specificity in Table 7.2 was higher than the sensitivity, with normal levels correctly identified in 57 of 60 nondiseased persons, indicating 95% specificity. The false-positive error rate was 5% (3/60).

2.3 PREDICTIVE VALUES

Sensitivity and specificity are helpful but do not directly answer two important clinical questions: If a participant's test result is positive, what is the probability that the person has the disease? If the result is negative, what is the probability that the person does not have the disease? These questions, which are influenced by sensitivity, specificity, and prevalence, can be answered by doing a horizontal analysis, rather than a vertical analysis, as in Table 7.1.

In Table 7.1, the formula $a/(a + b)$ is used to calculate the **positive predictive value** (PPV). In a study population, this measure indicates what proportion of the subjects with positive test results had the disease. Likewise, the formula $d/(c + d)$ is used to calculate the **negative predictive value** (NPV), which indicates what proportion of the subjects with negative test results did not have the disease.

In Table 7.2, the positive predictive value is 80% (12/15), and the negative predictive value is 88% (57/65). Based on these numbers, the clinician could not be fully confident in either a positive or a negative test result. Why are the predictive values so low? The predictive values would have been 100% (completely correct) if there were no false-positive or false-negative errors. Medical tests are almost never perfect. This makes predictive values difficult to interpret because, in the presence of false-positive or false-negative findings, the predictive values are influenced profoundly by the prevalence of the condition being sought.[9] Predictive values can be influenced by the prevalence of the condition being assessed, unlike sensitivity and specificity, which are independent of prevalence.

As shown in Table 7.1, the prevalence is the total number of diseased persons $(a + c)$ divided by the total number of persons studied $(a + b + c + d)$. If there is a 1% prevalence of a condition (and most medical conditions are relatively rare), at most there could be an average of 1 true-positive test result out of each 100 persons examined. If there is a 5% false-positive rate (not unusual for many tests), however, 5% of 99 disease-free persons would have false-positive test results. This would mean almost 5 false-positive results of each 100 tests. In this example, almost 5 of every 6 positive test results could be expected to be falsely positive. It almost seems as though probability is conspiring against the use of screening and diagnostic tests in clinical medicine.

TABLE 7.2 **Serum Level of Calcium and True Disease Status of 80 Participants Tested (Fictitious Data)**			
SERUM LEVEL OF CALCIUM	**TRUE DISEASE STATUS**		
	Diseased	**Nondiseased**	**Total**
Positive	12	3	15
Negative	8	57	65
TOTAL	20	60	80

Calculations Based on Formulas in Table 7.1

12/20 = 60% = Sensitivity
57/60 = 95% = Specificity
3/60 = 5% = False-positive error rate (alpha error rate, type I error rate)
8/20 = 40% = False-negative error rate (beta error rate, type II error rate)
12/15 = 80% = Positive predictive value (PPV)
57/65 = 88% = Negative predictive value (NPV)
(12/20)/(3/60) = 12.0 = Likelihood ratio positive (LR+)
(8/20)/(57/60) = 0.42 = Likelihood ratio negative (LR−)
12.0/0.42 = 28.6 = Ratio of LR+ to LR− = Odds ratio
20/80 = 25% = Prevalence of disease

BOX 7.1 Characteristics of Tests Needed to "Rule Out" and "Rule In" a Diagnosis

When a patient presents with complaints of chest pain, the clinician begins by obtaining a history, performing a physical examination, and developing a list of diagnoses that might explain the chest pain. The possible diagnoses have the logical status of hypotheses, and the clinician must order various tests to screen or **rule out** (discard) the false hypotheses. These tests, which include laboratory analyses and imaging procedures, should be highly sensitive. Tests with a high degree of sensitivity have a low false-negative error rate, so they ensure that not many true cases of the disease are missed. Although the clinician does not want false-positive results, they are tolerable at this stage because they can be dealt with by more tests.

After most of the hypothesized diagnoses have been eliminated, the clinician begins to consider tests to **rule in** (confirm) the true diagnosis. These tests should be highly specific. Tests with a high degree of specificity have a small false-positive error rate, so they ensure that not many patients are misdiagnosed as having a particular disease when in fact they have another disease. The clinician does not want to treat patients for diseases they do not have, whether the treatment is surgical or medical.

The principles of testing can be summarized as follows:

1. A **screening test**, which is used to rule out a diagnosis, should have a high degree of **sensitivity.**
2. A **confirmatory test**, which is used to rule in a diagnosis, should have a high degree of **specificity.**

Some recommend the mnemonic **spin** to remember that "**sp**ecificity is needed to rule **in**," and **snout** to remember that "**sen**sitivity is needed to rule **out**."

Whenever clinicians are testing for rare conditions, whether in routine clinical examinations or in large community screening programs, they must be prepared for most of the positive test results to be falsely positive. They must be prepared to follow up with additional testing in persons who have positive results to determine if the disease is truly present. This does not mean that screening tests should be avoided for conditions that have a low prevalence. It still may be worthwhile to do a screening program, because the persons who need follow-up diagnostic tests may represent a small percentage of the total population. A crucial point to remember is that one test does not make a diagnosis, unless it is a **pathognomonic test,** a test that elicits a reaction synonymous with having the disease (a gold standard). Box 7.1 summarizes principles concerning **screening tests** and **confirmatory tests.**

2.4 LIKELIHOOD RATIOS, ODDS RATIOS, AND CUTOFF POINTS

In contrast to predictive values, likelihood ratios are not influenced by the prevalence of the disease. The **likelihood ratio positive** (LR+) is the ratio of the sensitivity of a test to the false-positive error rate of the test. As shown in Table 7.1,

the equation is as follows: $[a/(a + c)] \div [b/(b + d)]$. Because the LR+ is the ratio of something that clinicians do want in a test (sensitivity) divided by something they do not want (false-positive error rate), the higher the ratio, the better the test is. For a test to be good, the ratio should be much larger than 1. The sensitivity and the false-positive error rate are independent of the prevalence of the disease. Their ratio is also independent of the prevalence.

In a similar manner, the **likelihood ratio negative** (LR−) is the ratio of the false-negative error rate divided by the specificity, or $[c/(a + c)] \div [d/(b + d)]$. In this case, because the LR− is the ratio of something clinicians do not want (false-negative error rate) divided by something they do want (specificity), the smaller the LR− (i.e., the closer it is to 0), the better the test is. If the LR+ of a test is large and the LR− is small, the test is probably good.

The LR+ can be calculated from the hypothetical data in Table 7.2. The sensitivity is 12/20, or 60%. The false-positive error rate (1 − specificity) is 3/60, or 5%. The ratio of these is the LR+, which equals 0.60/0.05, or 12.0. Although this looks good, the sensitivity data indicate that, on average, 40% of the diseased persons would be missed. The LR− here would be 8/20 divided by 57/60, or 0.421, which is much larger than acceptable.

Experts in test analysis sometimes calculate the **ratio of LR+ to LR−** to obtain a measure of separation between the positive and the negative test. In this example, LR+/LR− would be 12.0/0.421, which is equal to 28.5, (many consider values <50 indicate weak tests). If the data are from a 2 × 2 table, the same result could have been obtained more simply by calculating the **odds ratio** (*ad/bc*), which here equals $[(12)(57)]/[(3)(8)]$, or 28.5. For a discussion of the concepts of proportions and odds, see Box 7.2.

The LR+ looks better if a high (more stringent) **cutoff point** is used (e.g., a serum calcium level of 13 mg/dL for hyperparathyroidism), although choosing a high cutoff also lowers the sensitivity. This improvement in the LR+ occurs because, as the cutoff point is raised, true-positive results are eliminated at a slower rate than are false-positive results, so the ratio of true positive to false positive increases. The ratio of LR+ to LR− increases, despite the fact that more of the diseased individuals would be missed. The high LR+ means that when clinicians do find a high calcium level in an individual being tested, they can be reasonably certain that hyperparathyroidism or some other disease of calcium metabolism is present. Similarly, if an extremely low cutoff point is used, when clinicians find an even lower value in a patient, they can be reasonably certain that the disease is absent.

Although these principles can be used to create value ranges that allow clinicians to be reasonably certain about a diagnosis in the highest and lowest groups, the results in the middle group or groups (e.g., between points A and B in Fig. 7.3) often remain problematic. Clinicians may be comfortable treating patients in the highest groups and deferring treatment for those in the lowest groups, but they may now need to pursue additional testing for patients whose values fall in the middle. These issues apply when interpreting medical tests such as a ventilation-perfusion scan, the results

BOX 7.2   Concepts of Proportions and Odds

Most people are familiar with proportions (percentages), which take the form $a/(a + b)$. Some may be less familiar, however, with the idea of odds, which is simply a/b. In a mathematical sense, a proportion is less pure because the term a is in the numerator and the denominator of a proportion, which is not true of odds. Odds is the probability that something will occur divided by the probability that it will not occur (or the number of times it occurs divided by the number of times it does not occur). Odds can only describe a variable that is dichotomous (i.e., has only two possible outcomes, such as success and failure).

The odds of a particular outcome (outcome X) can be converted to the probability of that outcome, and vice versa, using the following formula:

$$\text{Probability of outcome } X = \frac{\text{Odds of outcome } X}{1 + \text{Odds of outcome } X}$$

Suppose that the proportion of successful at-bats of a baseball player on a certain night equals 1/3 (a batting average of 0.333). That means there was one success (X) and two failures (Y). The odds of success (number of successes to number of failures) is 1:2, or 0.5. To convert back to a proportion from the odds, put the odds of 0.5 into the previous equation, giving $0.5/(1 + 0.5) = 0.5/1.5 = 0.333$.

If the player goes 1 for 4 another night, the proportion of success is 1/4 (a batting average of 0.250), and the odds of success is 1:3, or 0.333. The formula converts the odds (0.333) back into a proportion: $0.333/(1 + 0.333) = 0.333/1.333 = 0.250$.

---

of which are reported as normal, low probability, indeterminate, or high probability.[10]

Three or more ranges can be used to categorize the values of any test whose results occur along a continuum. In Table 7.3 the results of a serum test formerly used to identify myocardial damage are divided into four ranges.[11] In this classic study, 360 patients who had symptoms suggesting myocardial infarction (MI) had an initial blood sample drawn to determine the level of creatine kinase (CK), an enzyme released into the blood of patients with MI. After the final diagnoses were made, the initial CK values were compared with these diagnoses, and four groups were created. Four levels are too many to measure the sensitivity and specificity in a 2 × 2 table (as in Tables 7.1 and 7.2), but likelihood ratios still can be calculated. The methods of identifying myocardial damage have changed since the time of this report, so these values cannot be applied directly to patient care at present. Troponins are currently used more often than CK, but the data used illustrate the likelihood ratio principle well.

Likelihood ratios can be applied to multiple levels of a test because of a unique characteristic of odds: the result is the same regardless of whether the analysis in a table is done vertically or horizontally. The LR+ is the ratio of two probabilities: the ratio of sensitivity to (1 − specificity). This also can be expressed as $[a/(a + c) \div b/(b + d)]$. When rearranged algebraically, this equation can be rewritten as follows:

$$LR+ = (a/b)/[(a+c)/(b+d)]$$

which is the odds of disease among persons in whom the test yielded positive results, divided by the odds of disease in the entire population. The LR+ indicates how much the odds of disease were *increased* if the test result was *positive*.

Similarly, the LR− is the ratio of two probabilities: the ratio of (1 − sensitivity) to specificity. Alternatively, this can be expressed as $[c/(a + c)] \div [d/(b + d)]$, and the formula can be rearranged algebraically as follows:

$$LR- = (c/d)/[(a+c)/(b+d)]$$

which is the odds of missed disease among persons in whom the test yielded negative results, divided by the odds of disease in the entire population. The LR− shows how much the odds of disease were *decreased* if the test result was *negative*.

Does this new way of calculating the likelihood ratio really work? Compare Table 7.2, in which the LR+ can be calculated as follows and yields exactly the same result as previously obtained:

$$LR+ = (12/3)/(12+8)/(3+57)$$
$$= (12/3)/(20/60)$$
$$= 4/0.333 = 12.0$$

Likewise, the LR− can be calculated as follows and yields the same result as before:

$$LR- = (8/57)/(12+8)/(3+57)$$
$$= (8/57)/(20/60)$$
$$= 0.140/0.333 = 0.42$$

The likelihood ratio (without specifying positive or negative) can be described as the odds of disease given a specified test value divided by the odds of disease in the study population. This general definition of LR can be used for numerous test ranges, as shown for the four ranges of CK results in Table 7.3. If the CK value was 280 IU/L or more, the LR was large (54.8), making it highly probable that the patient had an MI. If the CK was 39 IU/L or less, the LR was small (0.013), meaning that MI was probably absent. The LRs for the two middle ranges of CK values do not elicit as much confidence in the test, however, so additional tests would be needed to make a diagnosis in patients whose CK values were between 40 and 279 IU/L.

In Tables 7.2 and 7.3 the **posttest odds** of disease (a/b) equal the **pretest odds** multiplied by the LRs. In Table 7.2 the pretest odds of disease were 20/60, or 0.333, because this is all that was known about the distribution of disease in the study population before the test was given. The LR+, as calculated previously, turned out to be 12.0. When 0.333 is multiplied by 12.0, the result is 4. This is the same as the posttest odds, which was found to be 12/3, or 4. (See also Bayes theorem in Chapter 13.)

TABLE 7.3 Calculation of Likelihood Ratios for Myocardial Infarction (MI) in Analyzing Performance of a Serum Test With Multiple Cutoff Points (Multiple and Calculable Ranges of Results)

| | DIAGNOSIS OF MI | | |
Serum CK Value[a]	MI Present	MI Absent	Likelihood Ratio
≥280 IU/L	97	1	(97/1)/(230/130) = 54.8
80-279 IU/L	118	15	(118/15)/(230/130) = 4.45
40-79 IU/L	13	26	(13/26)/(230/130) = 0.28
0-39 IU/L	2	88	(2/88)/(230/130) = 0.013
TOTALS	230	130	

[a]The methods of determining serum creatine kinase (CK) values have changed since the time of this report, so these values cannot be applied directly to patient care at present. Troponins are currently used more often than CK, but the data used illustrate the likelihood ratio principle well. Data from Smith AF. Diagnostic Value Of Serum-Creatine-Kinase In A Coronary-Care Unit. *The Lancet.* 1967;290 (7508):178–182. doi:10.1016/s0140-6736(67)90005-0.

2.5 RECEIVER OPERATING CHARACTERISTIC CURVES

In clinical tests used to measure continuous variables such as serum calcium, blood glucose, or blood pressure, the choice of the best cutoff point is often difficult. As discussed earlier, there are few false-positive results and many false-negative results if the cutoff point is very high, and the reverse occurs if the cutoff point is very low. Because calcium, glucose, blood pressure, and other values can fluctuate in any individual, whether healthy or diseased, there is some overlap of values in the "normal" population and values in the diseased population (see Fig. 7.3).

To decide on a good cutoff point, investigators could construct a **receiver operating characteristic** (ROC) **curve**. Beginning with new or previously published data that showed the test results and the true status for *every person tested in a study*, the investigators could calculate the sensitivity and false-positive error rate for several possible cutoff points and plot the points on a square graph. Increasingly seen in the medical literature, ROC curves originated in World War II in evaluating the performance of radar receiver operators: A "true positive" was a correct early warning of enemy planes crossing the English Channel; a "false positive" occurred when a radar operator sent out an alarm but no enemy planes appeared; a "false-negative" occurred when enemy planes appeared without previous warning from the radar operators.

An example of an ROC curve for blood pressure screening is shown in Fig. 7.4 (fictitious data). The *y*-axis shows the **sensitivity** of a test, and the *x*-axis shows the **false-positive error rate** (1 − specificity). Because the LR+ of a test is defined as the sensitivity divided by the false-positive error rate, *the ROC curve can be considered a graph of the LR+*.

If a group of investigators wanted to determine the best cutoff for a blood pressure screening program, they might begin by taking a single initial blood pressure measurement in

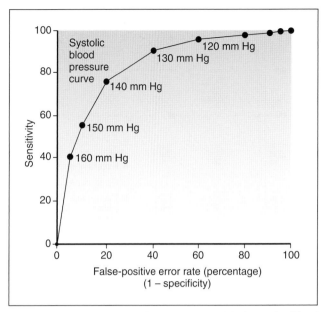

Fig. 7.4 Receiver Operating Characteristic (ROC) Curve for Blood Pressure. ROC curve from a study to determine the best cutoff point for a blood pressure screening program (fictitious data). Numbers beside the points on the curve are the cutoffs of systolic blood pressure that gave the corresponding sensitivity and false-positive error rate.

a large population and then performing a complete workup for persistent hypertension in all of the individuals. Each person would have data on a single screening blood pressure value and an ultimate diagnosis concerning the presence or absence of hypertension. Based on this information, an ROC curve could be constructed. If the cutoff for identifying individuals with suspected high blood pressure were set at 0 mm Hg (an extreme example to illustrate the procedure), *all living* study participants would be included in the group suspected to have hypertension. This means that all of the persons with hypertension would be detected, and the sensitivity would be 100%. However, all of the normal persons also would screen positive for hypertension, so the false-positive error rate would be 100%, and the point would be placed in the upper right (100%-100%) corner of the graph. By similar reasoning, if an extremely high blood pressure, such as 500 mm Hg, was taken as the cutoff to define hypertension, nobody would be detected with hypertension, so sensitivity would be 0%. There would be no false-positive results either, however, so the false-positive error rate also would be 0%. This point would be placed in the lower left (0%-0%) corner of the graph.

Next, the investigators would analyze the data for the lowest reasonable cutoff point—for example, a systolic blood pressure of 120 mm Hg—and plot the corresponding sensitivity and false-positive error rate on the graph. Then they could use 130 mm Hg as the cutoff, determine the new sensitivity and false-positive error rate, and plot the data point on the graph. This would be repeated for 140 mm Hg and for higher values. It is unlikely that the cutoff point for the diagnosis of hypertension would be a systolic blood pressure of less than 120 mm Hg or greater than 150 mm Hg. When all are in place, the points can be connected to resemble Fig. 7.4.

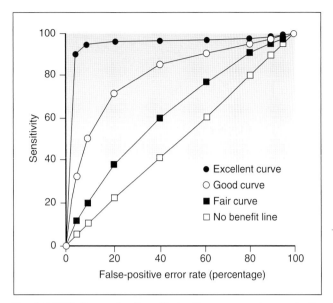

Fig. 7.5 **ROC Curves for Four Tests.** The uppermost curve is the best of the four.

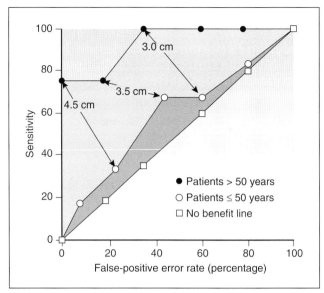

Fig. 7.6 **ROC Curves for a Test to Determine Malignancy Status of Follicular Thyroid Tumor Based on Its Diameter.** *(Upper curve)* Results in patients 50 years or older; *(middle curve)* results in patients younger than 50; *(bottom curve)* line of no benefit from the test. *Numbers beside the points on the curves* are the tumor diameters that gave the corresponding sensitivity and false-positive error rate. (Data courtesy Dr. Barbara Kinder, formerly Department of Surgery, Yale University School of Medicine, New Haven, CT.)

Ordinarily, the best cutoff point would be the point closest to the upper left corner, the corner representing a sensitivity of 100% and a false-positive error rate of 0%.

The ideal ROC curve for a test would rise almost vertically from the lower left corner and move horizontally almost along the upper line, as shown in the uppermost ROC curve in Fig. 7.5, the *excellent curve.* If the sensitivity always equaled the false-positive error rate, the result would be a diagonal straight line from the lower left to the upper right corner, the *no benefit line.* The ROC curve for most clinical tests is somewhere between these two extremes, similar to either the *good curve* or the *fair curve.*

The ROC curve in Fig. 7.6 shows the sensitivity and false-positive error rates found in a study of patients with follicular thyroid tumors.[12] The investigator sought to use the diameter of the tumors as measured at surgery to determine the probability of malignancy. Initially, when the ROC curve was plotted using the tumor diameters of patients of all ages, the curve was disappointing (not shown in Fig. 7.6). When the patients were divided into two age groups (patients <50 and patients ≥50 years old), the diameter of the tumors was found to be strongly predictive of cancer in the older group, but not in the younger group. It is unusual for the curve to hug the axes as it does for the older group, but this was caused by the relatively small number of patients involved (96 patients). In Fig. 7.6 the curve for the older age group can be compared with that for the younger age group. At a tumor diameter of 4.5 cm, the sensitivity in older patients was approximately 75%, in contrast to about 35% in the younger patients, and the corresponding false-positive error rates were 0% and 25%. At a tumor diameter of 3.5 cm, the sensitivities were not greatly different from each other, about 75% in the older patients and 65% in the younger patients, but the corresponding false-positive error rates were very different, about 15% and 45%. At a tumor diameter of 3 cm, the corresponding sensitivities for the older and the younger patients were 100% and 65%, and the false-positive error rates were 35% and 60%, respectively.

Analysis of ROC curves is becoming more sophisticated and popular in fields such as radiology. One method of comparing different tests is to determine the area under the ROC curve for each test and to use a statistical test of significance to decide if the area under one curve differs significantly from the area under the other curve. The greater the area under the curve, the better the test is.[13] In Fig. 7.6 the diagonal line from the lower left to the upper right represents the area of *no benefit,* where the sensitivity and false-positive error rate are the same; the area under this line is 50%. The area under the curve for younger patients is close to 60%, whereas the area under the curve for older patients is near 90%. These data suggest that for older patients, the size of this type of thyroid tumor can help the surgeon decide whether to remove the tumor before receiving a pathology assessment. For younger patients, the tumor diameter does not help in this decision.

3. MEASURING AGREEMENT

An important question in clinical medicine and in research is the extent to which different observations of the same phenomenon differ. If there is high intraobserver and interobserver agreement, as defined at the beginning of this chapter, the data in a study are considered highly reliable and elicit more confidence than if they lack either type of agreement. Reliability is not proof of validity, however. Two observers can report the same interpretation (i.e., show reliability), but both observers could be wrong.

It is not unusual to find disagreement between observers when evaluating the same patient or the same medical data. Similarly, a clinician looking again at the same data (e.g., heart or knee examination, interpretation of x-ray film or pathology slide) may disagree with his or her own previous reading. A study of variability in radiologists' interpretations found that different readers frequently disagreed about the interpretation of a specific mammogram. In two independent readings of the same mammogram, radiologists disagreed with their own previous readings almost as frequently.[8]

3.1 OVERALL PERCENT AGREEMENT

If a test uses a dichotomous variable (i.e., two categories of results, such as positive and negative), the results can be placed in a standard 2×2 table so that observer agreement can be calculated (Table 7.4). Cells a and d represent agreement, whereas cells b and c represent disagreement.

A common way to measure agreement is to calculate the **overall percent agreement.** If 90% of the observations are in cells a and d, the overall percent agreement would be 90%. Nevertheless, merely reporting the overall percent agreement is considered inadequate for numerous reasons. First, the overall percent agreement does not indicate the prevalence of the finding in the participants studied. Second, it does not show how the disagreements occurred. Were the positive and negative results distributed evenly between the two observers,

or did one observer consistently find more positive results than the other? Third, considerable agreement would be expected by chance alone, and the overall percent agreement does not define the extent to which the agreement improves on chance. The prevalence of positive findings and the direction of disagreement between two observers can be reported easily from tables such as Table 7.4. Measuring the extent to which agreement exceeds that expected by chance requires a measurement statistic called the **kappa.**

3.2 KAPPA TEST RATIO

Two clinicians have examined the same 100 patients during the same hour and record either the presence of a heart murmur or the absence of a heart murmur in each patient. For 7 patients, the first clinician reports the absence of a murmur and the second clinician reports the presence of a murmur, and for 3 patients the second clinician reports the absence and the first clinician reports the presence of a murmur. For 30 patients the clinicians agree on the presence of a heart murmur, and for 60 patients the clinicians agree on the absence of a murmur. These results could be arranged in a 2×2 table (Table 7.5). In addition to calculating the overall percent agreement (90%), the kappa test could be performed to determine the extent to which the agreement between the two clinicians improved on chance agreement alone. Even if the two clinicians only guessed about the presence or absence of a murmur, they sometimes would agree by chance.

As shown in Tables 7.4 and 7.5, the **observed agreement** (A_o) is the sum of the actual number of observations in cells a and d. The **maximum possible agreement** is the total number of observations (N). The **agreement expected by chance**

TABLE 7.4 Standard 2 × 2 Table Comparing Test Results Reported by Two Observers

	OBSERVER NO. 1		
OBSERVER NO. 2	Positive	Negative	Total
Positive	a	b	$a + b$
Negative	c	d	$c + d$
TOTAL	$a + c$	$b + d$	$a + b + c + d$

Interpretation of the Cells
a = Positive/positive observer agreement
b = Negative/positive observer disagreement
c = Positive/negative observer disagreement
d = Negative/negative observer agreement

Formulas
$a + d$ = Observed agreement (A_o)
$a + b + c + d$ = Maximum possible agreement (N)
$(a + d)/(a + b + c + d)$ = Overall percent agreement
$[(a + b)(a + c)]/(a + b + c + d)$ = Cell a agreement expected by chance
$[(c + d)(b + d)]/(a + b + c + d)$ = Cell d agreement expected by chance
Cell a agreement expected by chance + Cell d agreement expected by chance = Total agreement expected by chance (A_c)
$(A_o - A_c)/(N - A_c)$ = kappa

TABLE 7.5 Clinical Agreement Between Two Clinicians on Presence or Absence of Cardiac Murmur on Physical Examination of 100 Patients (Fictitious Data)

	CLINICIAN NO. 1		
CLINICIAN NO. 2	Murmur Present	Murmur Absent	Total
Murmur present	30	7	37
Murmur absent	3	60	63
TOTAL	33	67	100

Calculations Based on Formulas in Table 7.4
$30 + 60 = 90$ = Observed agreement (A_o)
$30 + 7 + 3 + 60 = 100$ = Maximum possible agreement (N)
$(30 + 60)/(30 + 7 + 3 + 60) = 90/100 = 90\%$ = Overall percent agreement
$[(30 + 7)(30 + 3)]/100 = [(37)(33)]/100 = 12.2$ = Cell a agreement expected by chance
$[(3 + 60)(7 + 60)]/100 = [(63)(67)]/100 = 42.2$ = Cell d agreement expected by chance
$12.2 + 42.2 = 54.4$ = Total agreement expected by chance (A_c)
$(90 - 54.4)/(100 - 54.4) = 35.6/45.6 = 0.78 = 78\%$ = kappa

(A_c) is the sum of the expected number of observations in cells *a* and *d*. The method used to calculate the expected agreement for the kappa test is the same method used for the chi-square test (see Chapter 10). For a given cell, such as cell *a*, the cell's row total is multiplied by the cell's column total, and the product is divided by the grand total. For cell *a*, the agreement expected by chance is calculated as $[(a + b)(a + c)] \div (a + b + c + d)$.

Kappa is a ratio. The numerator is the observed improvement over chance agreement ($A_o - A_c$), and the denominator is the maximum possible improvement over chance agreement ($N - A_c$). The kappa ratio is a proportion that can take on values from −1 (indicating perfect disagreement) through 0 (representing the agreement expected by chance) to +1 (indicating perfect agreement). Frequently, the results of the kappa test are expressed as a percentage. The following arbitrary divisions for interpreting the results are often used: Less than 20% is negligible improvement over chance, 20% to 40% is minimal, 40% to 60% is fair, 60% to 80% is good, and greater than 80% is excellent.[14] In the example of cardiac murmurs, the kappa test yielded a result of 0.78, or 78%, indicating that the clinician ratings were a "good" improvement on the chance expectation.

The reliability of most tests in clinical medicine that require human judgment seems to fall in the fair or good range. Although the kappa test described here provides valuable data on observer agreement for diagnoses recorded as "present" or "absent," some studies involve three or more outcome categories (e.g., negative, suspicious, or probable). For such data, a **weighted kappa test** must be used. The weighted test is similar in principle to the unweighted test described here, but it is more complex.[15] The weighted test gives partial credit for agreement that is close but not perfect.

In the evaluation of the accuracy and usefulness of a medical laboratory assay, imaging procedure, or any other clinical test, comparing the findings of one observer with the findings of another observer is not as useful as comparing the findings of an observer with the true disease status in the patients being tested. The **true disease status,** which is used to determine the sensitivity and specificity of tests, is considered to be the gold standard, and its use is preferable whenever such data are available. Gold standards seldom exist in clinical medicine, however, and even a small error in the gold standard can create the appearance of considerable error in a test.[16] Studies of the accuracy and usefulness of new medical tests are urgently needed, in addition to studies for many of the older diagnostic tests.

and the gold standard to define accuracy in clinical care and research. She has now expanded her research into pathology and has documented extensive variability in the diagnosis of breast and skin biopsies (Fig. 7.7).[17,18]

One factor leading to the variability among physicians is the lack of carefully gathered and analyzed data using principles described within this text. Another challenge we face in medicine is our expanding labeling of patients as having "atypical" or "abnormal" medical test results, often without a clear benefit to the patients. While many patients and physicians hope and believe that medical data are perfect and can clearly differentiate disease from nondisease, gray areas often exist in the practice of medicine. As William Osler once said, "Medicine is a science of uncertainty and an art of probability."

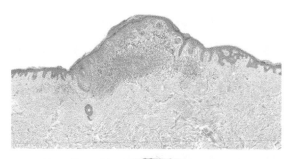

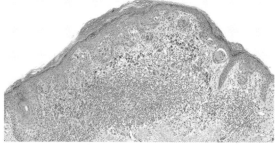

Fig. 7.7 Images of a skin biopsy that was independently interpreted by 36 practicing US pathologists who provided the following diagnoses: 7 pathologists described this biopsy as normal/benign, 10 called this slightly atypical, 8 gave a diagnosis of severely dysplastic nevus, 6 called this melanoma *in situ*, and 5 called this invasive melanoma (*top image* 5× magnification, *bottom image* 10× magnification). Elmore JG, et al in BMJ 2017.

4. SUMMARY

Three important goals of data collection and analysis are the promotion of accuracy and precision (see Figs. 7.1 and 7.2), the reduction of differential and nondifferential errors (nonrandom and random errors), and the reduction in interobserver and intraobserver variability (variability between findings of two observers or between findings of one observer on two occasions). Various statistical methods are available to study the accuracy and usefulness of screening tests and diagnostic (confirmatory) tests in clinical medicine. In general, tests with a high degree of sensitivity and a corresponding low false-negative error rate are helpful for screening patients (for ruling out), whereas tests with a high degree of specificity and a corresponding low false-positive error rate are useful for confirming (ruling in) the diagnosis in patients suspected to have a particular disease. Tables 7.1, 7.2, and 7.3 provide definitions of and formulas for calculating sensitivity, specificity, error rates, predictive values, and likelihood ratios. Tables 7.4 and 7.5 define measures of intraobserver and interobserver agreement and provide formulas for calculating the overall percent agreement and the kappa test ratio.

REFERENCES

1. Kohn LT, Corrigan JM, Donaldson MS, eds. *To Err is Human: Building a Safer Health System. Report of the Institute of Medicine.* Washington, DC: National Academies Press; 2000.
2. Brennan TA. The Institute of Medicine report on medical errors: could it do harm? *N Engl J Med.* 2000;342:1123-1125.
3. Dosemeci M, Wacholder S, Lubin JH. Does nondifferential misclassification of exposure always bias a true effect toward the null value? *Am J Epidemiol.* 1990;132:746-748.
4. Ransohoff DF, Feinstein AR. Problems of spectrum and bias in evaluating the efficacy of diagnostic tests. *N Engl J Med.* 1978;299:926-930.
5. Abbas AK, Lichtman AH, Pober JS. *Cellular and Molecular Immunology.* Philadelphia, PA: Saunders; 1991.
6. Rose DN, Schechter CB, Adler JJ. Interpretation of the tuberculin skin test. *J Gen Intern Med.* 1995;10:635-642.
7. Elmore JG, Barton MB, Moceri VM, Polk S, Arena PJ, Fletcher SW. Ten-year risk of false positive screening mammograms and clinical breast examinations. *N Engl J Med.* 1998;338:1089-1096.
8. Elmore JG, Wells CK, Lee CH, Howard DH, Feinstein AR. Variability in radiologists' interpretations of mammograms. *N Engl J Med.* 1994;331:1493-1499.
9. Jekel JF, Greenberg RA, Drake BM. Influence of the prevalence of infection on tuberculin skin testing programs. *Public Health Rep.* 1969;84:883-886.
10. Stein PD. Diagnosis of pulmonary embolism. *Curr Opin Pulm Med.* 1996;2:295-299.
11. Smith AF. Diagnostic value of serum-creatine-kinase in coronary-care unit. *Lancet.* 1967;2:178-182.
12. Kinder B. Personal communication, 1994.
13. Pepe MS. *The Statistical Evaluation of Medical Tests for Classification and Prediction.* Oxford, UK: Oxford University Press; 2003.
14. Sackett DL, Tugwell P, Haynes RB, Guyatt GH. *Clinical Epidemiology: A Basic Science for Clinical Medicine.* 2nd ed. Boston, MA: Little, Brown; 1991.
15. Cicchetti DV, Sharma Y, Cotlier E. Assessment of observer variability in the classification of human cataracts. *Yale J Biol Med.* 1982;55:81-88.
16. Greenberg RA, Jekel JF. Some problems in the determination of the false positive and false negative rates of tuberculin tests. *Am Rev Respir Dis.* 1969;100:645-650.
17. Elmore JG, Barnhill RL, Elder DE, et al. Pathologists' diagnosis of invasive melanoma and melanocytic proliferations: observer accuracy and reproducibility study. *BMJ.* 2017;357:j2813.
18. Elmore JG, Longton GM, Carney PA, et al. Diagnostic concordance among pathologists interpreting breast biopsy specimens. *JAMA.* 2015;313(11):1122-1132.

SELECT READING

Ransohoff DF, Feinstein AR. Problems of spectrum and bias in evaluating the efficacy of diagnostic tests. *N Engl J Med.* 1978;299:926-930. [Use of diagnostic tests to rule in or rule out a disease.]

REVIEW QUESTIONS

1. This is calculated as $c/(a + c)$.
   A. Accuracy
   B. Alpha error
   C. Beta error
   D. Bias
   E. Cutoff point
   F. False-negative error rate
   G. False-positive error rate
   H. Positive predictive value
   I. Precision
   J. Random error
   K. Sensitivity
   L. Specificity

2. This is the ability of a test to detect a disease when it is present.
   A. Accuracy
   B. Alpha error
   C. Beta error
   D. Bias
   E. Cutoff point
   F. False-negative error rate
   G. False-positive error rate
   H. Positive predictive value
   I. Precision
   J. Random error
   K. Sensitivity
   L. Specificity

3. This is a type I error.
   A. Accuracy
   B. Alpha error
   C. Beta error
   D. Bias
   E. Cutoff point
   F. False-negative error rate
   G. False-positive error rate
   H. Positive predictive value
   I. Precision
   J. Random error
   K. Sensitivity
   L. Specificity

4. This defines normal and abnormal test results.
   A. Accuracy
   B. Alpha error
   C. Beta error
   D. Bias
   E. Cutoff point
   F. False-negative error rate
   G. False-positive error rate
   H. Positive predictive value
   I. Precision
   J. Random error
   K. Sensitivity
   L. Specificity

5. This is the tendency of a measure to be correct on average.
   A. Accuracy
   B. Alpha error
   C. Beta error
   D. Bias
   E. Cutoff point
   F. False-negative error rate
   G. False-positive error rate
   H. Positive predictive value
   I. Precision
   J. Random error
   K. Sensitivity
   L. Specificity

6. This is calculated as $a/(a + c)$.
   A. Accuracy
   B. Alpha error
   C. Beta error
   D. Bias
   E. Cutoff point
   F. False-negative error rate
   G. False-positive error rate
   H. Positive predictive value
   I. Precision
   J. Random error
   K. Sensitivity
   L. Specificity

7. This is the ability of a test to exclude a disease when it is absent.
   A. Accuracy
   B. Alpha error
   C. Beta error
   D. Bias
   E. Cutoff point
   F. False-negative error rate
   G. False-positive error rate
   H. Positive predictive value
   I. Precision
   J. Random error
   K. Sensitivity
   L. Specificity

8. This is a nondifferential error.
   A. Accuracy
   B. Alpha error
   C. Beta error
   D. Bias
   E. Cutoff point
   F. False-negative error rate
   G. False-positive error rate
   H. Positive predictive value
   I. Precision
   J. Random error
   K. Sensitivity
   L. Specificity

9. The closer this is to the upper left corner of an ROC curve, the better it is.
   A. Accuracy
   B. Alpha error
   C. Beta error
   D. Bias
   E. Cutoff point
   F. False-negative error rate
   G. False-positive error rate
   H. Positive predictive value
   I. Precision
   J. Random error
   K. Sensitivity
   L. Specificity

10. This is differential error.
    A. Accuracy
    B. Alpha error
    C. Beta error
    D. Bias
    E. Cutoff point
    F. False-negative error rate
    G. False-positive error rate
    H. Positive predictive value
    I. Precision
    J. Random error
    K. Sensitivity
    L. Specificity

11. As the sensitivity increases, which of the following generally occurs?
    A. The cutoff point decreases
    B. The false-negative error rate increases
    C. The false-positive error rate increases
    D. The specificity increases
    E. The statistical power decreases

12. Two radiologists interpret 100 mammograms. They agree that the results are normal in 70 mammograms and abnormal in 12 mammograms. In the remaining 18 cases, the first radiologist thinks that results are normal in 6 mammograms and abnormal in 12 mammograms, whereas the second radiologist thinks just the opposite. The value of an appropriate measurement of their agreement that takes into consideration chance agreement is:
    A. 6%
    B. 16%
    C. 26%
    D. 46%
    E. 86%

13. The clinicians in a primary care clinic do not know the prevalence of *Chlamydia trachomatis* infection in their community. In screening patients for this infection, they plan to use a test that performed with a sensitivity of 75% and a specificity of 75% in clinical trials. When the clinicians use the test to screen patients for *C. trachomatis* in

their own community, which of the following could they use to help them interpret a positive test result?

A. Kappa
B. Phi
C. LR+
D. Odds ratio
E. RR

14. What is the value for the measure specified in question 13?
   A. 2.6
   B. 3
   C. 5
   D. 8.4
   E. 16

ANSWERS AND EXPLANATIONS

1. **F.** The false-negative error rate is equal to $c/(a + c)$. In a 2 × 2 table, cell c represents the number of participants who have a false-negative test result (participants in whom the disease of interest is present, but the test result is negative). Cell a represents the number of participants who have a true-positive test result. The sum of cells a and c represents all participants who have the disease; this is the denominator and population from which false-negative results are derived. The false-negative error rate is the ratio of participants who have false-negative results to all participants who have the disease, including both those detected and those missed by the diagnostic test.

2. **K.** Sensitivity is defined as the ability of a test to detect true cases of a disease when disease is present. Sensitivity is calculated as the number of true cases of the disease detected by the test (cell a in a 2 × 2 table) divided by all true cases (cell a + cell c).

3. **B.** A false-positive error is also known as a type I error or alpha error. These interchangeable designations refer to situations in which the data indicate that a particular finding (test result or study hypothesis) is true when actually it is not true. Typically, results attributable to chance or random error account for alpha error, although alpha error may result from bias as well. The value of alpha used in hypothesis testing specifies the level at which statistical significance is defined and specifies the cutoff for p values. Under most circumstances, the conventional level of alpha employed is 0.05 (see Chapter 9). The more stringent the value assigned to alpha (i.e., the smaller alpha is), the less likely that a false-positive result would occur. The clinical situation often dictates basic criteria for setting the value of alpha. A false-positive error may be more tolerable in a study involving new therapies that are desperately sought for severely ill patients than in a study involving a preventive intervention to be applied to a healthy population.

4. **E.** In clinical medicine, there are relatively few pathognomonic findings (findings considered definitive of a particular disease and expressed in dichotomous terms as the presence or absence of the disease). Most tests produce results that do not indicate the presence or absence of disease with absolute certainty. The cutoff point indicates the value beyond which a test result is considered abnormal, leading to a diagnosis or suggesting the need for further testing. The cutoff point chosen is influenced by the situational priorities. An initial screening test should be highly sensitive, so the cutoff point for the upper limit of normal values should be set low. A follow-up test should be highly specific, so the cutoff point for the upper limit of normal values should be set high.

5. **A.** Accuracy is the ability to obtain a test result or study result that is close to the true value. Accuracy is to be distinguished from precision, which is the ability to obtain consistent or reproducible results. An accurate result may not be precise. Repeated blood pressure measurements in a group of patients might lead to a correct value of the mean for the group, even if poor technique caused wide variation in individual measurements. A precise result may be inaccurate. The same mean weight might be obtained for a group of participants on consecutive days, but if each measure were obtained with the participants clothed, all the results would be erroneously high. Accuracy and precision are desirable traits in research and diagnostic studies.

6. **K.** Sensitivity is defined as the ability of a test to detect true cases of a disease when disease is present. Sensitivity is calculated as the number of true cases of the disease detected by the test (cell a in a 2 × 2 table) divided by all true cases (cell a + cell c).

7. **L.** Specificity is the capacity of a test to show positive results only in participants who have the disease in question. Alternatively stated, specificity is the ability of a test to exclude a disease when it is absent. A test that is highly specific is a good "rule-in" test, because it reliably indicates the presence of the disease when the result is positive. Specificity is calculated as the number of participants with true-negative test results (cell d in a 2 × 2 table) divided by the total number of participants who do not have the disease (cell b + cell d).

8. **J.** Random error is nondifferential error because it does not distort data consistently in any one direction. Random error may produce some measurements that are too high and others that are too low. The mean may or may not be distorted by random error. Random error affects precision. Bias is differential error because it produces measurements that are consistently too high or too low. Bias affects accuracy.

9. **E.** A cutoff point is used to distinguish normal from abnormal test results. If an upper-limit cutoff point is set too high, the normal range includes many participants with disease. If the upper-limit cutoff point is set too low, many normal participants are said to have

"abnormal" test results. The optimal cutoff point, where all cases of disease are detected with no false-positive results, is represented by the upper left corner of the ROC curve. Such a point virtually never exists and is at best approximated. The closer the cutoff point is to the upper left corner of an ROC curve, the greater the sensitivity, and the lower the false-positive error rate, for a given test.

10. **D.** Bias is differential error because it distorts data in a particular direction (e.g., weighing participants after a meal, taking blood pressure readings after caffeine ingestion or exercise, performing psychometric testing after alcohol ingestion). In contrast to bias, random error is nondifferential error because random error is equally likely to produce spuriously high or spuriously low results.

11. **C.** Sensitivity is the capacity of a test to identify the presence of disease in diseased individuals. The more sensitive a test is, the more likely it is to yield positive results (whether disease is actually present) and the less likely it is to yield negative results. This explains why an increase in sensitivity typically is accompanied by an increase in the false-positive error rate. An increase in sensitivity is also typically accompanied by a decrease in the false-negative error rate (B), which is why a negative result in a highly sensitive test is more likely to be a true negative. As a test's sensitivity increases, its specificity often decreases (D). Specificity is the capacity of a test to identify the absence of disease in nondiseased individuals. The more specific a test, the more readily it yields negative results (whether the disease is actually absent). The cutoff point (A) influences sensitivity and specificity and is generally chosen to strike the "optimal" balance between the two, with optimal dependent on the context and following no general trend. Mathematically, statistical power = 1 − beta. Beta is false-negative error, and (as previously noted) an increase in sensitively tends to lower false-negative error. With a smaller beta, statistical power (E) would increase.

12. **D.** To assess the measure of agreement, kappa, the investigator should begin by setting up a 2×2 table and placing the number of "abnormal" (positive) results and "normal" (negative) results in cells a, b, c, and d:

RADIOLOGIST NO. 2	RADIOLOGIST NO. 1	
	Positive	Negative
Positive	12 (*a*)	6 (*b*)
Negative	12 (*c*)	70 (*d*)

The equation for kappa is as follows:

$$kappa = (A_o - A_c / N - A_c)$$

where N is the sample size; A_o is the observed agreement; and A_c is the total agreement attributable to chance, which is equal to the sum of cell a agreement expected by chance plus cell d agreement expected by chance. N is given as 100. A_o is calculated as $a + d$, so here it is $12 + 70 = 82$. The agreement expected by chance is calculated as follows:

$$\text{for cell } a = [(a+b)(a+c)]/(a+b+c+d)$$
$$= [(12+6)(12+12)]/(12+6+12+70)$$
$$= (18)(24)/100 = 432/100 = 4.32$$
$$\text{for cell } d = [(c+d)(b+d)]/(a+b+c+d)$$
$$= [(12+70)(6+70)]/(12+6+12+70)$$
$$= (82)(76)/100 = 6232/100 = 62.32$$

Based on the previous numbers, the A_c and kappa can be calculated as follows:

$$A_c = 4.32 + 62.32 = 66.64$$
$$kappa = (82-66.64)/(100-66.64)$$
$$= 15.36/33.36 = 0.46 = 46\%$$

13. **C.** The likelihood ratio for a positive test result (LR+) is calculated as the test's sensitivity divided by its false-positive error rate (1 − specificity). The LR+ can be used to estimate the reliability of a positive test result when the prevalence of disease is unknown. It is useful in this context because the components of the LR+ are contained within the columns of a 2×2 table and are independent of disease prevalence. The odds ratio (D) is used to evaluate the outcome of a case control study. The risk ratio, or RR (E), is used to evaluate the outcome of a cohort study. Kappa measures agreement between observers (A), and phi measures the strength of association of a chi-square value (B).

14. **B.** The likelihood ratio for a positive test result (LR+) is a ratio of the sensitivity of the test to the false-positive error rate. The sensitivity is 0.75. The false-positive error rate = (1 − specificity) = (1 − 0.75) = 0.25. Thus the LR+ is 0.75/0.25, or 3.

Biostatistics

8

Describing Variation and Distribution of Data

CHAPTER OUTLINE

"Variability is the law of life, as no two faces are the same, so no two bodies are alike, and no two individuals react alike and behave alike under the abnormal conditions which we know as disease."

William Osler

Statistical methods help clinicians and investigators understand and explain variation in medical data. Variation is evident in almost every human characteristic including blood pressure and other physiologic measurements, disease, environment, and diet, among other aspects of life. A measure of a single characteristic that can vary is called a **variable**.

Statistics can be viewed as a set of tools for working with data and can enable investigators to do the following:

- Describe the patterns of variation in single variables, as discussed in this chapter
- Determine when observed differences are likely to be real differences (Chapter 9)
- Determine the patterns and strength of association between variables (Chapters 10 and 11)
- Apply statistics to the design and interpretation of studies (Chapters 12 and 13)

1. VARIATION

Although variation in clinical medicine may be caused by biologic differences or the presence or absence of disease,

it also may result from differences in the techniques and conditions of measurement, errors in measurement, and random variation. Some types of variation can distort data systematically in one direction, such as measuring and weighing patients while wearing shoes. This form of distortion is called **systematic error** and can introduce bias. Bias in turn may obscure or distort the *truth* being sought in a given study. Other types of variation are random, such as slight, inevitable inaccuracies in obtaining any measure, such as blood pressure. Because **random error** makes some readings too high and others too low, it is not systematic and does not introduce bias. However, by increasing variation in the data, random error increases the noise amidst which the *signal* of association, or cause and effect, must be discerned. The "louder" the noise, the more difficult it is to detect a signal and the more likely to miss an actual signal.

Biologic differences can result from many factors, such as differences in genes, nutrition, environmental exposures, age, sex, and race. For example, tall parents usually have tall children, but other factors also affect height. Malnutrition slows growth in children, and starvation may stop growth altogether, while adequate nutrition allows the full genetic growth potential to be achieved. Polluted water may cause intestinal infections in children, which can retard growth, partly because these infections exacerbate malnutrition.

Variation is seen not only in the **presence or absence of disease**, but also in the **stages or extent of disease**. For example, cancer of the cervix may be in situ, localized, invasive, or metastatic. Also some patients may have multiple diseases (comorbidity), as in the case of insulin-dependent diabetes mellitus that may be accompanied by coronary artery disease and renal disease.

Different conditions of measurement often account for the variations observed in medical data and include factors such as time of day, ambient temperature or noise, and the presence of fatigue or anxiety in the patient. Blood pressure is higher with anxiety or following exercise and lower after sleep. These differences in blood pressure are not errors of measurement, but of the variability of conditions under which the data are obtained. Standardizing conditions is important to avoid variation attributable to them and the introduction of bias.

Different techniques of measurement can produce different results. A blood pressure measurement derived from the use of an intraarterial catheter may differ from a measurement derived from the use of an arm cuff. This may result from differences in the measurement site (e.g., central or distal arterial site), thickness of the arm (which influences readings from the blood pressure cuff), rigidity of the artery (reflecting degree of atherosclerosis), and interobserver differences in the interpretation of blood pressure sounds.

Some variation is caused by **measurement error**. Two different blood pressure cuffs of the same size may give different measurements in the same patient because of defective performance by one of the cuffs. Different laboratory instruments or methods may produce different readings from the same sample. Different x-ray machines may produce images of varying quality. When two clinicians examine the same patient or the same specimen, they may report different results (see Chapter 7). One radiologist may read a mammogram as abnormal and recommend further tests, such as a biopsy, whereas another radiologist may read the same mammogram as normal and not recommend further workup.[1] One clinician may detect a problem, such as a retinal hemorrhage or a heart murmur, and another may fail to detect it. Two clinicians may detect a heart murmur in the same patient but disagree on its characteristics. If two clinicians are asked to characterize a dark skin lesion, one may call it a "nevus," whereas the other may say it is "suspicious for malignant melanoma." A pathologic specimen would be used to resolve the difference, but that, too, is subject to interpretation, and two pathologists might differ.[2]

Variation is a ubiquitous phenomenon in clinical medicine and research. Statistics can help investigators interpret data despite biologic variation; however, many statistical procedures assume that the data are measured without error, systematic or otherwise. While methods are available for dealing with incorrectly measured data, they make additional assumptions about the mechanisms underlying the measurement error. In general, results of research are less biased and subject to error when data are measured as accurately and precisely as possible during the data collection process.

2. STATISTICS AND VARIABLES

2.1 QUANTITATIVE AND QUALITATIVE DATA

The first question to answer before analyzing data is whether the data *describe* a quantitative or a qualitative characteristic. **A quantitative characteristic**, such as a systolic blood pressure measurement or serum sodium level, is characterized using a defined, continuous measurement scale. **A qualitative characteristic**, such as coloration of the skin, is described by its features, generally in words rather than numbers. Normal skin can vary in color from pinkish white through tan to dark brown or black. Medical problems can cause changes in skin color, with *white* denoting pallor, as in anemia; *red* suggesting inflammation, as in a rash or sunburn; *blue* denoting cyanosis, as in cardiac or lung failure; *bluish purple* occurring when blood has been released subcutaneously, as in a bruise; and *yellow* suggesting the presence of jaundice, as in common bile duct obstruction or liver disease.

Examples of disease manifestations that have quantitative and qualitative characteristics are heart murmurs and bowel sounds. Not only does the loudness of a heart murmur vary from patient to patient (and can be described on a 5-point scale), but also the sound may vary from blowing to harsh or rasping in quality. The timing of the murmur in the cardiac cycle also is important.

Variables describe information on characteristics that vary. The qualitative information on colors just described could form a qualitative variable called "skin color." The quantitative information on blood pressure could be contained in variables called *systolic* and *diastolic* blood pressure.

2.2 TYPES OF VARIABLES

Variables can be classified as nominal variables, dichotomous (binary) variables, ordinal (ranked) variables, continuous (dimensional) variables, ratio variables, and risks and proportions (Table 8.1).

2.2.a. Nominal Variables

Nominal variables are naming or categoric variables that are not based on measurement scales or rank order. Examples are blood groups (O, A, B, and AB), occupations, food groups, and skin color. If skin color is the variable being examined, a different number can be assigned to each color (e.g., 1 is bluish purple, 2 is red, 3 is white, 4 is blue, 5 is yellow) before the information is entered into a computer data system. Any number could be assigned to any color, and that would make no difference to the statistical analysis. This is because the number is merely a numerical name for a color, and the size of the number has no inherent meaning. For example, the number given to a particular color has nothing to do with the quality, value, or importance of the color.

TABLE 8.1 Examples of the Different Types of Data

Information Content	Variable Type	Examples
Higher	Ratio	Temperature (Kelvin); blood pressure*
	Continuous (dimensional)	Temperature (Fahrenheit)*
	Ordinal (ranked)	Edema = 3+ out of 5; perceived quality of care = good/fair/poor
	Binary (dichotomous)	Gender = male/female; heart murmur = present/absent
Lower	Nominal	Blood type; skin color = cyanotic/jaundiced/normal

Note: Some variables with more detail may be collapsed into variables with less. For example, hypertension could be described as "165/95 mm Hg" (continuous data), "absent/mild/moderate/severe" (ordinal data), or "present/absent" (binary data). However, one cannot move in the other direction. Understanding the type of variables being analyzed is crucial for deciding which statistical test to use (see Table 10.1).

*For most types of data analysis, the distinction between continuous data and ratio data is unimportant. Risks and proportions sometimes are analyzed using the statistical methods for continuous variables, and sometimes observed counts are analyzed in tables, using nonparametric methods (see Chapter 10).

2.2.b. Dichotomous (Binary) Variables

If all skin colors were included in only one nominal variable, the variable would not distinguish between *normal* and *abnormal* skin color, which is usually the most important aspect of skin color for clinical and research purposes. As discussed, abnormal skin color (e.g., pallor, jaundice, cyanosis) may be a sign of numerous health problems (e.g., anemia, liver disease, cardiac failure). Investigators might choose to create a variable with only two levels: normal skin color (coded as a 1) and abnormal skin color (coded as a 2). This new variable, which has only two levels, is said to be *dichotomous* (Greek, "cut into two").

Many dichotomous variables, such as well/sick, living/dead, and normal/abnormal, have an implied direction that is favorable. Knowing the direction of the more favorable variable would be important for interpreting the data, but not for the statistical analysis. Other dichotomous variables, such as female/male and treatment/placebo, have no inherent qualitative direction.

In many cases, dichotomous variables inadequately describe the information needed. For example, when analyzing outcomes of cancer therapy, it is important to know not only whether the patient survives or dies (a dichotomous variable), but also *how long* the patient survives (time forms a *continuous* variable). A survival analysis or life table analysis that provides estimates related to these outcomes, as described in Chapter 10, may be more clinically relevant. Also, it is important to know the *quality of patients' lives* while they

are receiving therapy, which could be measured with an *ordinal* variable, discussed next. Similarly, for a study of heart murmurs, various types of data may be needed, such as *dichotomous* data concerning a murmur's timing (e.g., systolic or diastolic), *nominal* data on its location (e.g., aortic valve area) and character (e.g., rough), and *ordinal* data on its loudness (e.g., grade III). Dichotomous, nominal, and often ordinal variables are referred to as **discrete variables** because the numbers of possible values they can take are countable.

2.2.c. Ordinal (Ranked) Variables

Many types of medical data can be characterized in terms of three or more qualitative values that have a clearly implied direction from better to worse. An example might be "satisfaction with care" that could take on the values of "very satisfied," "fairly satisfied," or "not satisfied." These data are not measured on a meaningful quantitative measurement scale, but form ordinal (i.e., ordered or ranked) variables.

There are many clinical examples of ordinal variables. The amount of swelling in a patient's legs is estimated by a clinician and is usually reported as "none" or 1+, 2+, 3+, or 4+ pitting edema (puffiness). A patient may have a systolic murmur ranging from 1+ to 6+. Pain may be reported as being absent, mild, moderate, or severe; or described by patients on a scale from 0 to 10, with 0 being no pain and 10 the worst imaginable pain. However, the utility of these scales to quantify subjective assessments, such as pain intensity, is unclear.

Although ordinal variables are not defined by a quantitative measurement scale, the ordering of variables provides additional meaning to them. It is possible to see the relationship between two ordinal categories and know whether one category is better or worse than another. As described in Chapter 10, ordinal variables often require special techniques of analysis.

2.2.d. Continuous (Dimensional) Variables

Many types of medically important data are measured on continuous (dimensional) measurement scales. Patients' heights, weights, systolic and diastolic blood pressures, and serum glucose levels all are examples of data measured on continuous scales. Continuous data show not only the position of the different observations relative to each other, but also the extent to which one observation differs from another. For measures that can be expressed in different ways, such as blood pressure, continuous data often enable investigators to make more detailed inferences than ordinal or nominal data.

2.2.e. Ratio Variables

If a continuous scale has a true 0 point, the variables derived from it can be called ratio variables. The Kelvin temperature scale is a ratio scale because 0 degrees on this scale is absolute 0. The centigrade temperature scale is a continuous scale, but not a ratio scale because 0 degrees on this scale does not mean the absence of heat. For some purposes, it may be useful to know that 200 units of something is twice as large as 100 units, information provided only by a ratio scale. For most statistical analyses, however, including significance testing, the distinction between continuous and ratio variables is not important.

2.2.f. Risks and Proportions as Variables

As discussed in Chapter 2, a risk is the conditional probability of an event (e.g., death or disease) in a defined population in a defined period. Risks and proportions, which are two important types of measurement in medicine, share some characteristics of a discrete variable and some characteristics of a continuous variable. It makes no conceptual sense to say that a "fraction" of a death occurred or that a "fraction" of a person experienced an event. It does make sense, however, to say that a discrete event (e.g., death) or a discrete characteristic (e.g., presence of a murmur) occurred in a fraction of a population. Risks and proportions are variables created by the ratio of counts in the numerator to counts in the denominator. Risks and proportions can be analyzed using the statistical methods for continuous variables (see Chapter 9); and observed counts can be analyzed in tables using statistical methods for analyzing discrete data (see Chapter 10).

2.3 COUNTS AND UNITS OF OBSERVATION

The unit of observation is the person or thing from which the data originated. Common examples of units of observation in medical research are persons, animals, and cells. Units of observation may be arranged in a frequency table, with one characteristic on the x-axis, another characteristic on the y-axis, and the appropriate counts in the cells of the table. Table 8.2, which provides an example of this type of 2 × 2 table, shows that among 71 young adults studied, 63% of women and 57% of men previously had their cholesterol levels checked. Using these data and the chi-square test described in Chapter 10, one can determine whether the difference in the percentage of women and men with cholesterol checks was likely a result of chance variation (in this case the answer is yes).

2.4 COMBINING DATA

A continuous variable may be converted to an ordinal variable by grouping units with similar values together. Three or more groups must be formed when converting a continuous variable to an ordinal variable. For example, the individual

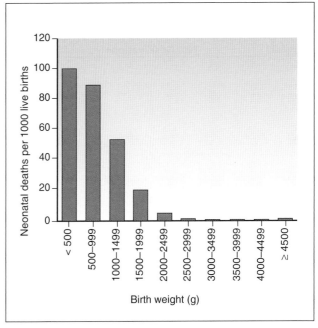

Fig. 8.1 Histogram Showing Neonatal Mortality Rate by Birth Weight Group, All Races, United States, 1980. (Data from Buehler JW, Kleinman JC, Hogue CJ, et al: Birth weight-specific infant mortality, United States, 1960 and 1980. *Public Health Rep* 102: 151–161, 1987.)

birth weights of infants (a continuous variable) can be converted to ranges of birth weights (an ordinal variable), as shown in Fig. 8.1.[3] When the data are presented as categories or ranges (e.g., <500, 500–999, 1000–1499 g), information is lost because the individual weights of infants are no longer apparent. An infant weighing 501 g is in the same category as an infant weighing 999 g, but the infant weighing 999 g is in a different category from an infant weighing 1000 g, just 1 g more. The result of forming several groups is that it creates an ordinal variable that progresses from the lightest to the heaviest birth weight (or vice versa). The advantage to combining data is that percentages can be created, and the relationship of birth weight to mortality is easier to show.

If a continuous variable, such as birth weight, is divided into only two groups, a *dichotomous* variable is created. Dividing infant birth weight into two groups can create a dichotomous variable of infants weighing less than 2500 g (low birth weight) and infants weighing 2500 g or more (normal birth weight). While this may be useful when addressing specific clinical questions, in general, more information is lost when fewer groups are formed from a continuous variable.

3. FREQUENCY DISTRIBUTIONS

3.1 FREQUENCY DISTRIBUTIONS OF CONTINUOUS VARIABLES

A frequency distribution can be shown by creating a table that lists the values of the variable according to the frequency with which the value occurs. A plot or histogram of the **frequency distribution** shows the values of the variable along

TABLE 8.2 **Standard 2 × 2 Table Showing Gender of 71 Participants and Whether Serum Total Cholesterol Was Checked**			
	CHOLESTEROL LEVEL (NO. OF PARTICIPANTS)		
GENDER	**Checked**	**Not Checked**	**Total**
Female	17 (63%)	10 (37%)	27 (100%)
Male	25 (57%)	19 (43%)	44 (100%)
TOTAL	42 (59%)	29 (41%)	71 (100%)

Data from unpublished findings in a sample of 71 young adults in Connecticut.

TABLE 8.3 Serum Levels of Total Cholesterol Reported in 71 Participants*

Cholesterol Value (mg/dL)	No. Observations	Cholesterol Value (mg/dL)	No. Observations	Cholesterol Value (mg/dL)	No. Observations
124	1	164	3	196	2
128	1	165	1	197	2
132	1	166	1	206	1
133	1	169	1	208	1
136	1	171	4	209	1
138	1	175	1	213	1
139	1	177	2	217	1
146	1	178	2	220	1
147	1	179	1	221	1
149	1	180	4	222	1
151	1	181	1	226	1
153	2	184	2	227	1
158	3	186	1	228	1
160	1	188	2	241	1
161	1	191	3	264	1
162	1	192	2	—	—
163	2	194	2	—	—

*In this data set, the mean is 179.1 mg/dL, and the standard deviation is 28.2 mg/dL.
Data from unpublished findings in a sample of 71 young adults in Connecticut.

one axis and the frequency of the value along the other axis. Data are usually easier to interpret from a histogram than from a list of values. Table 8.3 and Fig. 8.2 show the distribution of the levels of total cholesterol among 71 young adults.

3.1.a. Range of a Variable

A frequency distribution can be described, although imperfectly, using only the lowest and highest numbers in the data

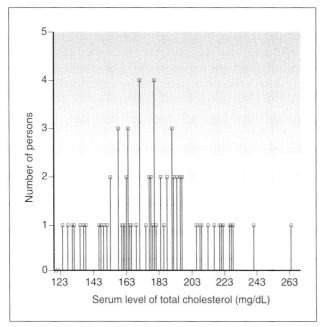

Fig. 8.2 Histogram Showing Frequency Distribution of Serum Levels of Total Cholesterol. As reported in a sample of 71 participants; data shown here are same data listed in Table 8.3; see also Figs. 8.4 and 8.5. (Data from unpublished findings in a sample of 71 young adults in Connecticut.)

set. For example, the cholesterol levels in Table 8.3 vary from a low value of 124 mg/dL to a high value of 264 mg/dL. The distance between the lowest and highest observations is called the **range** of the variable.

3.1.b. Real and Theoretical Frequency Distributions

Real frequency distributions are those obtained from actual data or a sample, and theoretical frequency distributions are calculated using assumptions about the population from which the sample was obtained. Most measurements of continuous data in medicine and biology tend to approximate a particular theoretical distribution known as the **normal distribution**. It is also called the **Gaussian distribution** (after Johann Karl Gauss, who was one of the first to describe it).

The normal (Gaussian) distribution looks something like a bell seen from the side (Fig. 8.3). Real samples of data, however, are seldom if ever perfectly smooth and bell shaped. The plot of the frequency distribution of total cholesterol values among the 71 young adults shows peaks and valleys when the data are presented in the manner shown in Fig. 8.2. This should not cause concern, however, if partitioning the same data into reasonably narrow ranges results in a bell-shaped frequency distribution. When the cholesterol levels from Table 8.3 and Fig. 8.2 are partitioned into seven groups with narrow ranges (of 20-mg/dL width), the resulting frequency distribution appears almost perfectly normal (Gaussian) (Fig. 8.4). If the sample size had been much larger than 71, the distribution of raw data might have looked more Gaussian (see Fig. 8.2).

In textbooks, smooth, bell-shaped curves are often used to represent the **expected or theoretical distribution of the observations** (the height of the curve on the y-axis) for the

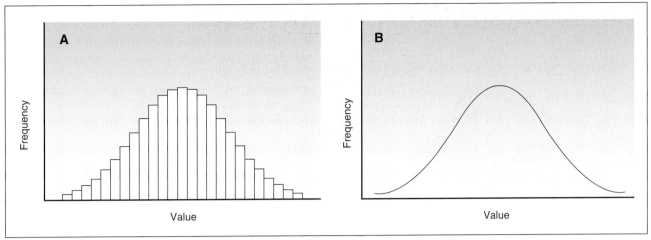

Fig. 8.3 Normal (Gaussian) Distribution, With Value Shown on *x*-axis and Frequency on *y*-axis. (A) Probability distribution of data, plotted as a histogram with narrow ranges of values on the *x*-axis. (B) A simplified version of the normal (Gaussian) distribution.

different possible values on a measurement scale (on the *x*-axis) (see Fig. 8.3). A perfectly smooth, bell-shaped Gaussian distribution actually indicates that the *y*-axis is usually describing the frequency with which the corresponding values in the *x*-axis are *expected* to be found. With an intuitive feeling for the meaning of Fig. 8.3, it is easier to understand the medical literature, statistical textbooks, and problems presented on examinations.

Although the term "normal" distribution is used in this book and frequently in the literature, there is no implication that data not conforming strictly to this distribution are somehow

"abnormal." Even if the underlying distribution is not normal, many of the statistical tests we discuss in this text can be approximated by using the normal distribution if the sample size is large enough (see central limit theorem in Chapter 9).

3.1.c. Histograms, Frequency Polygons, and Line Graphs

Figures in the medical literature show data in several ways, including histograms, frequency polygons, and line graphs. As shown earlier, a **histogram** is a bar graph in which the number of units of observation (e.g., persons) is shown on the *y*-axis, the measurement values (e.g., cholesterol levels) are shown on the *x*-axis, and the frequency distribution is illustrated by a series of vertical bars. In a histogram, the area of each bar represents the relative proportion of all observations that fall in the range represented by that bar. Fig. 8.2 is a histogram in which each bar represents a single numerical value for the cholesterol level. An extremely large number of observations would be needed to obtain a smooth curve for such single values. A smoother distribution is obtained by combining data into narrow ranges on the *x*-axis (see Fig. 8.4).

A **frequency polygon** is a shorthand way of presenting a histogram by putting a dot at the center of the top of each bar and connecting these dots with a line to create a graph. Fig. 8.5 shows a frequency polygon that was constructed from the histogram shown in Fig. 8.4. Although histograms are generally recommended for presenting frequency distributions, the shape of the distribution is seen more easily in a frequency polygon than in a histogram. Frequency polygons are typically appropriate when the underlying variable is assumed to be continuous.

Several types of **line graphs** can be used to depict relationships between incidence rates on the *y*-axis and time on the *x*-axis. An **epidemic time curve** is a histogram in which the *x*-axis is time and the *y*-axis is the number of *incident* cases in each time interval (see Fig. 3.11). An **arithmetic line graph** places both the *x*-axis and *y*-axis on an arithmetic scale, such as illustrated by a graph of the incidence rates of reported salmonellosis in the United States during several decades

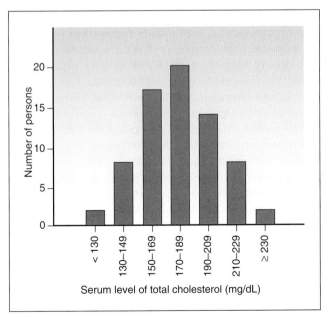

Fig. 8.4 Histogram Showing Frequency Distribution of Serum Levels of Total Cholesterol. As reported in a sample from the 71 participants in Table 8.3, grouped in ranges of 20 mg/dL. The individual values for the 71 participants are reported in Table 8.3 and shown in Fig. 8.2. The mean is 179.1 mg/dL and the median is 178 mg/dL. The original data are needed to calculate these estimates and determine the range. The histogram shows how these data form a normal (Gaussian) distribution, although the *N* is relatively small.

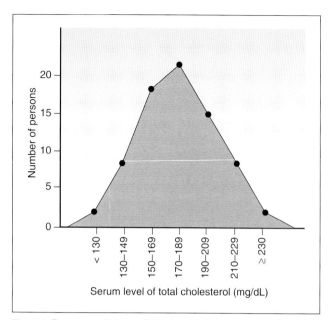

Fig. 8.5 Frequency Polygon Showing the Frequency Distribution of Serum Levels of Total Cholesterol. As reported in a sample from the 71 participants in Table 8.3, grouped in ranges of 20 mg/dL. Data for this polygon are the same as the data for the histogram in Fig. 8.4. Individual values for the 71 participants are reported in Table 8.3 and Fig. 8.2.

(Fig. 3.1). A **semilogarithmic line graph** uses an arithmetic scale for the *x*-axis and a logarithmic scale for the *y*-axis to amplify the lower end of the scale. Although semilogarithmic line graphs make the absolute magnitude of changes appear less striking, they have advantages. These include enabling the detail of changes in very low rates of disease to be seen, which can be difficult on an arithmetic scale. They also can depict proportionately similar changes as parallel lines. For example, if a decline in deaths is proportionately similar to the decline in reported cases of disease, the case fatality ratio (~10%) would remain fairly constant over time. Semilogarithmic line graphs also allow for a wide range of values to be plotted in a single, readable graph. Although unusual, data on both the *x*-axis and the *y*-axis might be displayed on logarithmic scales; such a plot would be a **fully logarithmic line graph**.

3.1.d.   Parameters of a Frequency Distribution

Frequency distributions from continuous data are defined by two types of descriptors known as parameters: measures of central tendency and measures of dispersion. The measures of central tendency locate observations on a measurement scale and are similar to a street address for the variable. The measures of dispersion suggest how widely the observations are spread out, as with indicating the property lines for a given address. In the case of a normal (Gaussian) distribution, the bell-shaped curve can be fully described using only the mean (a measure of central tendency) and the standard deviation (a measure of dispersion).

Measures of central tendency. The first step in examining a distribution is to look for the central tendency of the observations. Most types of medical data tend to clump in such a way that the *density* of observed values is greatest near the center of the distribution. In the case of the observed cholesterol values listed in Table 8.3 and depicted graphically in Fig. 8.2, there appears to be some tendency for the values to cluster near the center of the distribution. However, this tendency is more clearly visualized when the values from Table 8.3 and Fig. 8.2 are grouped in ranges of 20 mg/dL, as shown in Fig. 8.4. The next step is to examine the distribution in greater detail and determine the mode, median, and mean that describe the three measures of central tendency.

Mode. The most commonly observed value (i.e., the value that occurs most frequently) in a data set is called the mode. The mode is of some clinical interest, but seldom of statistical utility. A frequency distribution typically has a mode at more than one value. For example, in Fig. 8.2, the most commonly observed cholesterol levels (each with four observations) are 171 mg/dL and 180 mg/dL. In this case, although the frequency distribution in the sample is bimodal, it is likely that the distribution in the population has only one mode. In other cases, the population distribution may be truly bimodal, usually because the population contains two subgroups, each of which has a different distribution that peaks at a different point. For example, distributions of height could show different modes for men and women. More than one mode also can be produced artificially by what is known as *digit preference*, when observers tend to favor certain numbers over others. For example, persons who measure blood pressure values tend to favor even numbers, particularly numbers ending in zero (e.g., 120 mm Hg).

Median. The median of a sample is the middle observation when data have been arranged in order from the lowest value to the highest value. The median value in Table 8.3 is 178 mg/dL. When there is an even number of observations, the median is considered to lie halfway between the two middle observations. For example, in Table 8.4, which shows the high-density lipoprotein (HDL) cholesterol values for 26 adults, the two middle observations are the 13th and 14th observations. The corresponding values for these are 57 and 58 mg/dL, so the median is 57.5 mg/dL.

The median HDL value is also called the 50th percentile observation because 50% of the observations lie at that value or below. Percentiles frequently are used in educational testing and in medicine to describe normal growth standards for children. They also are used to describe the LD_{50} for experimental animals, defined as the dose of an agent (e.g., a drug) that is lethal for 50% of the animals exposed to it. Because the median is not sensitive to extreme values, it is often a more useful summary of the typical study participant when the data are skewed, for example in survival analysis, health care utilization, and economics. However, the median is seldom used to make complicated inferences from medical data, because it does not lend itself to the development of advanced statistics.

Mean. The mean of a sample is the average value, or the sum (Σ) of all the observed values (x_i) divided by the total number of observations (N):

$$\text{Mean} = \bar{x} = \frac{\sum (x_i)}{N}$$

TABLE 8.4 Raw Data and Results of Calculations in Study of Serum Levels of High-Density Lipoprotein (HDL) Cholesterol in 26 Participants

Parameter	Raw Data or Results of Calculation
No. observations, or N	26
Initial HDL cholesterol values (mg/dL) of participants	31, 41, 44, 46, 47, 47, 48, 48, 49, 52, 53, 54, 57, 58, 58, 60, 60, 62, 63, 64, 67, 69, 70, 77, 81, and 90
Highest value (mg/dL)	90
Lowest value (mg/dL)	31
Mode (mg/dL)	47, 48, 58, and 60
Median (mg/dL)	(57 + 58)/2 = 57.5
Sum of the values, or sum of x_i (mg/dL)	1496
Mean, or $\bar{x}$ (mg/dL)	1496/26 = 57.5
Range (mg/dL)	90 − 31 = 59
Interquartile range (mg/dL)	64 − 48 = 16
Sum of $(x_i - \bar{x})^2$, or TSS	4298.46 mg/dL squared*
Variance, or s^2	171.94 mg/dL†
Standard deviation, or s	$\sqrt{171.94}$ = 13.1 mg/dL

*For a discussion and example of how statisticians measure the total sum of the squares (TSS), see Box 8.3.
†Here, the following formula is used:

$$\text{Variance} = s^2 = \frac{\sum(x_i^2) - \frac{(\sum x_i)^2}{N}}{N-1} = \frac{90,376 - \frac{2,238,016}{26}}{25}$$

$$= \frac{90,376 - 86,077.54}{25} = \frac{4298.46}{25} = 171.94$$

where the subscript letter i means "the value of x for individual i, where i ranges from 1 to N." The mean ($\bar{x}$) has practical and theoretical advantages as a measure of central tendency. It is simple to calculate, and the sum of the deviations of observations from the mean (expressed in terms of negative and positive numbers) equals zero, which provides a simple check of the calculations. The mean also has mathematical properties that enable the development of advanced statistics (Box 8.1). Most descriptive analyses of continuous variables and advanced statistical analyses use the mean as the measure of central tendency. Table 8.4 gives an example of the calculation of the mean.

Measures of dispersion. After the central tendency of a frequency distribution is determined, the next step is to determine how spread out (dispersed) the numbers are. This can be done by calculating measures based on percentiles or measures based on the mean.

Measures of Dispersion Based on Percentiles.
A percentile of a distribution is a point at which a certain percentage of the

BOX 8.1 Properties of the Mean

1. The mean of a random sample is an unbiased estimator of the mean of the population from which it came.
2. The mean is the mathematical expectation. As such, it is different from the mode, which is the value observed most often.
3. For a set of data, the sum of the squared deviations of the observations from the mean is smaller than the sum of the squared deviations from any other number.
4. For a set of data, the sum of the squared deviations from the mean is fixed for a given set of observations. (This property is not unique to the mean, but it is a necessary property of any good measure of central tendency.)

observations lie below the indicated point when all the observations are ranked in descending order. The median, discussed previously, is the 50th percentile because 50% of the observations are below it. The 75th percentile is the point at or below which 75% of the observations lie, whereas the 25th percentile is the point at or below which 25% of the observations lie.

In Table 8.4 the overall range of HDL cholesterol values is 59 mg/dL, reflecting the distance between the highest value (90 mg/dL) and the lowest value (31 mg/dL) in the data set. After data are ranked from highest to lowest, they can be divided into quarters (*quartiles*) according to their rank. In the same table, the 75th and 25th percentiles are 64 mg/dL and 48 mg/dL, and the distance between them is 16 mg/dL. This distance is called the *interquartile range*, sometimes abbreviated Q3-Q1. Because of the tendency of data to cluster around a measure of central tendency, the interquartile range is usually considerably smaller than half the size of the overall range of values, as in Table 8.4. (For more on these measures, see later discussion of quantiles.)

The advantage of using percentiles is that they can be applied to any set of continuous data, even if the data do not form any known distribution. Because few tests of statistical significance have been developed for use with medians and other percentiles, the use of percentiles in medicine is mostly limited to description. In this descriptive role, percentiles are often useful in clinical and education research.

Measures of Dispersion Based on the Mean. Mean deviation, variance, and standard deviation are three measures of dispersion based on the mean.

Mean Absolute Deviation. Mean absolute deviation is seldom used, but helps define the concept of dispersion. Because the mean has many advantages, it might seem logical to measure dispersion by taking the average deviation from the mean. That proves to be useless, however, because the sum of the deviations from the mean is zero. This inconvenience can be solved easily by computing the mean absolute deviation, which is the average of the absolute value of the deviations from the mean, as shown in this formula:

$$\text{Mean deviation} = \frac{\sum(|x_i - \bar{x}|)}{N}$$

Because the mean absolute deviation does not have mathematical properties on which to base many statistical tests, the formula has not come into popular use. Instead the variance has become the fundamental measure of dispersion in statistics that are based on the normal distribution.

Variance. The variance for a set of observed data is the sum of the squared deviations from the mean, divided by the number of observations minus 1:

$$\text{Variance} = s^2 = \frac{\sum(x_i - \bar{x})^2}{N-1}$$

The symbol for a variance calculated from observed data (a sample variance) is s^2. In the previous formula, squaring solves the problem that the deviations from the mean add up to zero. Dividing by $N-1$ (called **degrees of freedom**; see Box 10.2), instead of dividing by N, is necessary for the sample variance to be an unbiased estimator of the population variance. A simple explanation for this denominator is that when the mean is known, and all observations except the last one have been established, the value of the final observation becomes fixed and is not free to vary.

BOX 8.2   Properties of the Variance

1. For an observed set of data, when the denominator of the equation for variance is expressed as the number of observations minus 1 (i.e., $N-1$), the variance of a random sample is an unbiased estimator of the variance of the population from which it was taken.
2. The variance of the sum of two independently sampled variables is equal to the sum of the variances.
3. The variance of the difference between two independently sampled variables is equal to the sum of their individual variances as well. (The importance of this should become clear when the t-test is considered in Chapter 9.)

The *numerator of the variance* (i.e., sum of squared deviations of observations from the mean) is an extremely important measure in statistics. It is usually called either the **sum of squares** (SS) or the **total sum of squares** (TSS). The TSS measures the total amount of variation in a set of observations. Box 8.2 lists the mathematical properties of variance that permit the development of statistical tests, and Box 8.3

BOX 8.3   How Do Statisticians Measure Variation?

In statistics, variation is measured as the sum of the squared deviations of the individual observations from an expected value, such as the mean. The mean is the mathematical expectation (expected value) of a continuous frequency distribution. The quantity of variation in a given set of observations is the numerator of the variance, which is known as the sum of the squares (SS). The sum of the squares of a dependent variable sometimes is called the total sum of the squares (TSS), which is the total amount of variation that needs to be explained.

For illustrative purposes, assume the data set consists of these six numbers: 1, 2, 4, 7, 10, and 12. Assume that x_i denotes the individual observations, $\bar{x}$ is the mean, N is the number of observations, s^2 is the variance, and s is the standard deviation.

Part 1 Tabular Representation of the Data

	x_i	$(x_i - \bar{x})^2$	$\bar{x}_i$
	1	-5	25
	2	-4	16
	4	-2	4
	7	$+1$	1
	10	$+4$	16
	12	$+6$	36
Sum, or Σ	36	0	98

Part 2 Graphic Representation of Data Shown in Third Column of Previous Table, $(x_i-\bar{x})^2$, for Each of the Six Observations

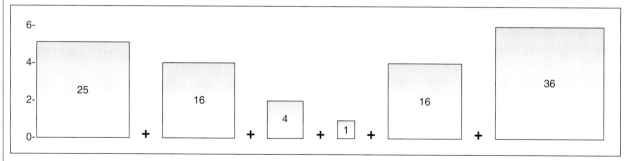

Part 3 Calculation of Numbers That Describe a Distribution (i.e., the Parameters)

$\sum(x_i) = 36$ $\sum(x_i - \bar{x})^2 = \text{TSS} = 98$

$N = 6$ $s^2 = \text{TSS}/(N-1) = 98/5 = 19.6$

$\bar{x} = 6$ $s = \sqrt{19.6} = 4.43$

explains how statisticians measure variation. Understanding the concept of variation makes statistics easier to comprehend.

For simplicity of calculation, another (but algebraically equivalent) formula is used to calculate the variance. It is the sum of the squared values for each observation minus a correction factor (to correct for the fact that the deviations from zero, rather than the deviations from the mean, are being squared), all divided by $N - 1$:

$$\text{Variance} = s^2 = \frac{\sum(x_i^2) - \left[\frac{(\sum x_i)^2}{N}\right]}{N-1}$$

Table 8.4 illustrates the calculation of variance using this second formula.

Standard Deviation. The variance tends to be a large and unwieldy number, and since it is calculated using the sum of squared deviations from the mean, it is measured on a different scale than the original data. The **standard deviation**, which is the square root of the variance, usually is used to describe the amount of spread in the frequency distribution. Conceptually, the standard deviation is an average of the deviations from the mean. The symbol for the standard deviation of an observed data set is *s*, and the formula is as follows:

$$\text{Standard deviation} = s = \sqrt{\frac{\sum(x_i - \bar{x})^2}{N-1}}$$

In an observed data set, the term $\bar{x} \pm s$ represents 1 standard deviation above and below the mean, and the term $\bar{x} \pm 2s$ represents 2 standard deviations above and below the mean. One standard deviation falls well within the range of observed numbers in most data sets and has a known relationship to the normal (Gaussian) distribution. This relationship often is useful in drawing inferences in statistics.

For a continuous distribution, as shown in Fig. 8.6, the area under the curve from A to B is the probability of randomly drawing a point that lies within the interval from A to B. For a normal (Gaussian) distribution in particular, the area under the curve between 1 standard deviation above and below the mean is 68% of the total area. Two standard deviations above and below the mean include 95.4% of the area (i.e., 95.4% of the observations) in a normal distribution. Exactly 95% of the observations from a normal frequency distribution lie between 1.96 standard deviations below the mean and 1.96 standard deviations above the mean. The formula $\bar{x} \pm 1.96$ for standard deviations is often used in clinical studies to show the extent of variation in clinical data.

3.1.e. Problems in Analyzing a Frequency Distribution

In a normal (Gaussian) distribution, the following holds true: mean = median = mode. In an observed data set, however, there may be skewness, kurtosis, and extreme values, in which case the measures of central tendency may not follow this pattern.

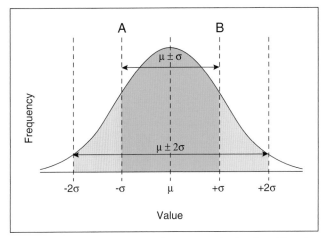

Fig. 8.6 Theoretical Normal (Gaussian) Distribution Showing where 1 and 2 Standard Deviations Above and Below the Mean Would Fall. Lowercase Greek letter mu (μ) stands for the mean in the theoretical distribution, and Greek sigma (σ) stands for the standard deviation in the theoretical population. (The italic Roman letters *x* and *s* apply to an observed sample from the population.) The area under the curve represents all the observations in the distribution. One standard deviation above and below the mean, *shown in dark blue* and represented by the distance from point *A* to point *B*, encompasses 68% of the area under the curve, and 68% of the observations in a normal distribution fall within this range. Two standard deviations above and below the mean, represented by the areas *shown in dark and light blue*, include 95.4% of the area under the curve and 95.4% of the observations in a normal distribution.

Skewness and kurtosis. A horizontal stretching of a frequency distribution to one side or the other, so that one tail of observations is longer and has more observations than the other tail, is called **skewness**. When a histogram or frequency polygon has a longer tail on the left side of the diagram, as in Figs. 8.7 and 8.8A, the distribution is said to be "skewed to the left." If a distribution is skewed, the mean is found farther in the direction of the long tail than the median because the mean is more heavily influenced by extreme values.

A quick way to obtain an approximate idea of whether a frequency distribution is skewed is to compare the mean and the median. If these two measures are close to each other, the distribution is probably not skewed. In the data from Table 8.3, the mean equals 179.1 mg/dL, and the median equals 178 mg/dL. These two values are very close, and as Fig. 8.4 shows, the distribution also does not appear to be skewed.

Kurtosis is characterized by a vertical stretching or flattening of the frequency distribution. As shown in Fig. 8.8, a kurtotic distribution could appear more peaked or more flattened than the normal bell-shaped distribution.

Significant skewness or kurtosis can be detected by statistical tests. Many statistical tests assume that the data are normally distributed, and the tests may not be valid when used to compare distributions with extreme deviations from normal. The statistical tests discussed in this book are relatively robust, meaning that as long as the data are not overly skewed or kurtotic, the results can be considered valid. Even if significant deviations from normality are suspected, the

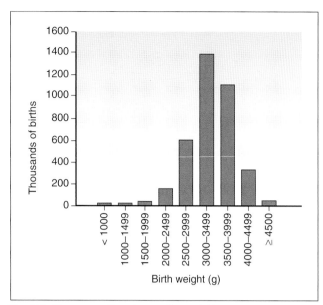

Fig. 8.7 Histogram Showing a Skewed Frequency Distribution.
Values are for thousands of births by birth weight group, United States, 1987. Note the long "tail" on the left. (Data from National Center for Health Statistics: *Trends in low birth weight: United States, 1975-85.* Series 21, No 48, Washington, DC, 1989, Government Printing Office.)

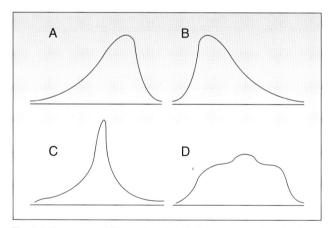

Fig. 8.8 Examples of Skewed and Kurtotic Frequency Distributions.
Distribution *A* is skewed to the left; distribution *B* is skewed to the right; they have the long tail to the left (A) and to the right (B) of the peak. Distribution *C* is kurtotic, with abnormal peaking; distribution *D* is kurtotic, with abnormal flattening compared with the normal distribution.

tests will perform well with large enough sample sizes. Kurtosis is seldom discussed as a problem in the statistical or medical literature, although skewness is observed frequently, and adjustments for skewness are made when needed.

Extreme values (outliers). One of the most perplexing problems for the analysis of data is how to treat a value that is abnormally far above or below the mean. This problem is suggested in the data set of cholesterol values shown in Table 8.3 and Fig. 8.2. The standard deviation of the distribution in the data set is 28.2 mg/dL, so that if the distribution were normal, 95% of the cholesterol values would be expected to be between 123.8 and 234.4 mg/dL (i.e., the

mean $\pm$ 1.96 standard deviations = 179.1 mg/dL $\pm$ the product of 1.96 $\times$ 28.2). Ninety-nine percent of the values would be expected to be found within the range of the mean $\pm$ 2.58 standard deviations, which in this case would be between 106.3 and 251.9 mg/dL.

When the data are observed visually in Fig. 8.2, everything looks normal below the mean; the lowest value is 124 mg/dL, which is within the 95% limits. The upper value is 264 mg/dL, however, which is beyond the 99% limits of expectation and looks suspiciously far from the other values. Because many people have these high total cholesterol values, and because the observation is almost within the 99% limits, there is probably no reason to believe that the value is erroneous (although there might be a reason to be clinically concerned with such a high cholesterol value in a young person). Plausibility is a gauge to be used when considering the reliability of outlying data. Before analyzing the data set, the investigator should check the original source of data, to ensure this value is what the laboratory reported.

3.1.f. Methods of Depicting a Frequency Distribution

In the medical literature, histograms and line graphs are used to illustrate frequency distributions, as defined earlier with frequency polygons. Other methods of visually displaying data include stem and leaf diagrams, quantiles, and boxplots, that can be printed out when using computer programs such as the Statistical Analysis System (SAS) (https://www.sas.com/en_us/software/stat.html) or Statistical Package for the Social Sciences (SPSS) (http://www.spss.com/). Fig. 8.9 plots the HDL cholesterol values for 26 young adults provided in Table 8.4.

Stem and leaf diagrams. As shown in Fig. 8.9, the stem and leaf diagram has three components. The **stem**, which is the vertical column of numbers on the left, represents the value of the left-hand digit (in this case, the 10s digit). The **leaf** is the set of numbers immediately to the right of the stem and is separated from the stem by a space (as here) or by a vertical line. Each of the numbers in the leaf represents the single number digit in one of the 26 observations in the data set of HDL cholesterol values. The stem and leaf value shown on the top line of the diagram represents 90 mg/dL. The # **symbol** to the right of the leaf tells how many observations were seen in the range indicated (in this case, 1 observation of 90 mg/dL). Observations that can be made quickly from viewing the stem and leaf diagram include the following:

1. The highest value in the data set is 90 mg/dL.
2. The lowest value is 31 mg/dL.
3. There are eight observations in the range of the 40s, consisting of 41, 44, 46, 47, 47, 48, 48, and 49.
4. When the diagram is viewed with the left side turned to the bottom, the distribution looks fairly normal, although it has a long tail to the left (i.e., it is skewed to the left).

```
Stem Leaf                          #              Boxplot
   9 0                             1                 0
   8 1                             1
   7 07                            2                 |
   6 0023479                       7              +-----+
   5 234788                        6              *--+--*
   4 14677889                      8              +-----+
   3 1                             1
     ----+----+----+----+                           |
Multiply Stem.Leaf by 10**+ 1
```

Quantiles (Percentiles)

100% Max	90	99%	90
75% Q3	64	95%	81
50% Med	57.5	90%	77
25% Q1	48	10%	44
0% Min	31	5%	41
		1%	31
Range	59		
Q3 - Q1	16		
Mode	47		

Fig. 8.9 Stem and Leaf Diagram, Boxplot, and Quantiles (Percentiles). For the data shown in Table 8.4, as printed by the Statistical Analysis System (SAS). See the text for a detailed description of how to interpret these data.

Quantiles. Below the stem and leaf diagram in Fig. 8.9 is a display of the quantiles (percentiles). The data include the *maximum* (100% of the values were at this level or below) and *minimum* (0% of the values were below this level); the 99%, 95%, 90%, 10%, 5%, and 1% values; the *range*; the *mode*; and the *interquartile range* (from the 75th percentile to the 25th percentile, abbreviated Q3-Q1).

Boxplots. The modified boxplot is shown to the right of the stem and leaf diagram in Fig. 8.9 and provides an even briefer way of summarizing the data.

In the boxplot, the rectangle formed by four plus signs (+) and the horizontal dashes (—) depicts the interquartile range. The two asterisks (*) connected by dashes depict the median. The mean, shown by the smaller plus sign (+), is very close to the median. Outside the rectangle there are two vertical lines, called the "whiskers" of the boxplot. The whiskers extend as far as the data, but no more than 1.5 times the interquartile range above the 75th percentile and 1.5 times the interquartile range below the 25th percentile. They show the range where most of the values would be expected, given the median and interquartile range of the distribution. Values beyond the whiskers but within 3 interquartile ranges of the box are shown as a 0, and values more extreme than this are shown with an asterisk. In Fig. 8.9, all the observed data values except the value of 90 mg/dL might reasonably have been expected. This value may be an outlier observation, however, as indicated by the 0 near the top, just above the top of the upper whisker.

It takes only a quick look at the boxplot to see how wide the distribution is, whether it is skewed, where the interquartile range falls, how close the median is to the mean, and how many (if any) observations might reasonably be considered outliers.

3.1.g. Use of Unit-Free (Normalized) Data

Data from a normal (Gaussian) distribution can be described completely by the mean and the standard deviation. The same set of data, however, would provide different values for the mean and standard deviation depending on the choice of **units of measurement**. For example, the same person's height may be expressed as 66 inches or 167.6 cm, and an infant's birth weight may be recorded as 2500 g or 5.5 lb. Because the units of measurement differ, so do the numbers, although the true height and weight are the same. To eliminate the effects produced by the choice of units, the data can be put into a unit-free form by a procedure called normalization. The result is that each item of data is measured as the number of standard deviations above or below the mean for that set of data.

The first step in normalizing data is to calculate the mean and standard deviation. The second step is to set the mean equal to zero by subtracting the mean from each observation in whatever units have been used. The third step is to measure each observation in terms of the number of standard deviations it is above or below the mean. The normalized values obtained by this process are called *z values*, which are sometimes used in clinical medicine (e.g., bone density measurements to test for osteoporosis). The formula for creating individual *z* values (z_i) is as follows:

$$z_i = \frac{x_i - \bar{x}}{s}$$

Where x_i represents individual observations, $\bar{x}$ represents the mean of the observations, and s is the standard deviation. Suppose that the goal is to standardize blood pressure values for a group of patients whose systolic blood pressures were observed to have a mean of 120 mm Hg and a standard deviation of 10 mm Hg. If two of the values to be standardized were 140 mm Hg and 115 mm Hg, the calculations would be as follows:

$$\frac{140-120}{10}=+2.0 \quad \frac{115-120}{10}=-0.5$$

A distribution of z values always has a mean of 0 and a standard deviation of 1. These z values may be called by various names, often **standard normal deviates**.

Clinically, z values are useful for determining how extreme an observed test result is. For example, in Table 8.3 the highest total cholesterol value observed among 71 persons was 264 mg/dL, 23 points higher than the next highest value. Is this cholesterol value suspect? When the previous formula is used, the z value is $(264 - 179.1)/28.2 = +3.0$. This means that it is 3 standard deviations above the mean. Usually, about 1% of observed values are 2.58 standard deviations or more away from the mean. Because this is the only one of the 71 observed values this high, and such values are often seen clinically, there is no reason to suppose

it is an error. Plausibility is important when evaluating outliers. For example, a height of 10 feet for a person would be suspect because it falls outside of human experience.

3.2 FREQUENCY DISTRIBUTIONS OF DICHOTOMOUS DATA AND PROPORTIONS

Dichotomous data can be seen in terms of flipping a coin. When a fair coin is flipped, on average it is expected to land with the heads side up for half the flips and with the tails side up for half the flips. In this case, the probability of heads is equal to 0.5, and the probability of tails is equal to 0.5. The sum of all the probabilities for all the possible outcomes must equal 1.0. Suppose we carry out an experiment where we flip a fair coin 10 times. If we repeat the experiment many times, it would be very rare for the result to be 10 heads or 10 tails. It would less rarely be a combination of 9 heads plus 1 tail, and most frequently would be a combination of 5 heads and 5 tails.

The probabilities of obtaining various combinations of heads and tails from flipping a coin can be calculated by **expanding the binomial formula** $(a + b)^n$, as shown in Box 8.4. In this formula, a is the probability of heads, b is the probability of tails, and n is the number of coin tosses in a trial. If n is large and the experiment is repeated many times (e.g., hundreds of tosses of the coin), and if the coin is

---

BOX 8.4 How to Determine Probabilities by Expanding the Binomial

The basic binomial formula is $(a + b)^n$. The probabilities of getting various combinations of heads and tails from flipping an unbiased coin can be calculated by expanding this formula. Although the example of heads/tails is used here, the formula and concepts described can also be applied to the probabilities of life/death associated with particular diagnoses, success/failure in treatment, and other clinically relevant dichotomous data.

When the binomial formula is applied to flipping a coin in an unbiased manner, a is the probability of obtaining heads, b is the probability of obtaining tails, and n is the number of trials (coin tosses). The process of calculating the probabilities is called expanding the binomial, and the distribution of probabilities for each combination is the binomial distribution.

With one flip of the coin, there is a 0.5 (50%) chance of heads and a 0.5 (50%) chance of tails, with the sum of 1.0.

Two flips of the coin could produce the following outcomes: two heads, one head and one tail (in either the head/tail or tail/head order), or two tails. What are the probabilities of these possible outcomes? The answer is given by the previous formula, with $n = 2$. It is $(a + b)$ times itself:

$$(a+b)^2 = a^2 + 2ab + b^2$$
$$= (0.5)(0.5) + 2(0.5)(0.5) + (0.5)(0.5)$$
$$= 0.25 + 0.50 + 0.25$$

In other words, with two flips of a coin, the probabilities of the various possible outcomes are as follows:

Two heads = 0.25
One head and one tail (in either order) = 0.25 + 0.25 = 0.50
Two tails = 0.25
The sum of the probabilities = 1.0

Three flips of a coin could produce the following outcomes: three heads, two heads and one tail, two tails and one head, or three tails. The probabilities, calculated by using the formula $(a + b)^3$, are as follows:

Three heads = a^3 = $(0.5)^3$ = 0.125
Two heads and one tail = $3(a^2)(b)$ = $(3)(0.25)(0.5)$ = 0.375
One head and two tails = $3(a)(b^2)$ = $(3)(0.5)(0.25)$ = 0.375
Three tails = b^3 = $(0.5)^3$ = 0.125
The sum of the probabilities = 1.0

If a biased coin (e.g., $a = 0.4$ and $b = 0.6$) were tossed three times, the probabilities would be as follows:

Three heads = a^3 = $(0.4)^3$ = 0.064
Two heads and one tail = $3(a^2)(b)$ = $(3)(0.16)(0.6)$ = 0.288
One head and two tails = $3(a)(b^2)$ = $(3)(0.4)(0.36)$ = 0.432
Three tails = b^3 = $(0.6)^3$ = 0.216
The sum of the probabilities = 1.0

The coefficients for expanding $(a + b)^n$ can be found easily using a Pascal triangle, in which each coefficient is the sum of the two above.

$n =$	Coefficients	Examples
1	1 1	$1a + 1b$
2	1 2 1	$1a^2 + 2ab + 1b^2$
3	1 3 3 1	$1a^3 + 3(a^2)(b) + 3(a)(b^2) + 1b^3$
4	1 4 6 4 1	$1a^4 + 4(a^3)(b) + 6(a^2)(b^2) + 4(a)(b^3) + 1b^4$

If the probabilities from tossing an unbiased coin are plotted as histograms, as the number of coin tosses becomes greater, the probabilities look more and more like a normal (Gaussian) distribution.

thrown in an unbiased manner, the distribution of the binomial toss would look much like a normal (Gaussian) distribution. In fact, binomial probabilities can usually be approximated reasonably well using a normal distribution where the mean is equal to $n \times a$ and the standard deviation is equal to $n \times a \times b$.

3.3 FREQUENCY DISTRIBUTIONS OF OTHER TYPES OF DATA

Data from nominal (categoric) and ordinal (ranked) variables are not properly analyzed using tests based on the normal (Gaussian) distribution. These types of data are typically analyzed using **nonparametric tests**, which are statistical methods that make few or no assumptions about the underlying distribution of the data. For example, the analysis of counts in frequency tables, known as the *chi-square distribution*, is particularly important in medicine (e.g., Table 8.2) (see Chapter 10). The chi-square analysis is a nonparametric test because it does not assume that the data follow any particular distribution.

Ordinal data are sometimes analyzed in the medical literature as though they were continuous data, and means and standard deviations are reported. This is usually satisfactory for describing ordinal data, but it is generally not appropriate for significance testing. The preferred tests are discussed in Chapter 10 and include the Wilcoxon and Mann-Whitney U tests. These tests do not require that the data follow any particular distribution, only that the data be ordinal.

The **Poisson distribution** is used to describe uncommon events occurring in time or space or both, and has the property that the mean equals the variance.[4] It is especially useful in evaluating the clustering of rare events, such as suspected clusters of cancer cases.[5] Further discussion of the Poisson distribution is beyond the scope of this text.

4. SUMMARY

Although variation in clinical medicine may be caused by biologic differences or the presence or absence of disease, it may also result from differences in measurement techniques and conditions, errors in measurement, and random variation. Statistics is used to describe and understand variation, but it cannot correct for measurement errors or bias. However, the analysis can adjust for random error in the sense that it can estimate how much of the total variation is caused by random error and how much by a particular factor under investigation.

Fundamental to any analysis of data is an understanding of the types of variables or data being analyzed. Data types include nominal, dichotomous, ordinal, continuous, and ratio data as well as risks, rates, and proportions. Continuous (measurement) data usually show a frequency distribution that can be described in terms of two parameters: a measure of central tendency (of which median and mean are the most important) and a measure of dispersion based on the mean (of which variance and standard deviation are the most

important). The most common distribution is called the normal (Gaussian) bell-shaped distribution; the mean and the median coincide, and 95% of the observations are within 1.96 standard deviations above and below the mean. Occasionally the frequency distribution appears pulled to one side or the other (skewed distribution), in which case the mean is farther in the direction of the long tail than is the median.

Data may be made unit free (may be *normalized*) by creating z values. This is accomplished by subtracting the mean from each value and dividing the result by the standard deviation. This expresses the value of each observation as the number of standard deviations the value is above or below the mean. The probability distribution for aggregates of dichotomous data may be described by the binomial distribution. If the number of trials is large, the binomial distribution can be reasonably approximated by the normal distribution. For studying counts of rare events, the Poisson distribution is most helpful. When we cannot make assumptions about the underlying distribution of the data, nonparametric statistics can be used to study differences and associations among variables.

REFERENCES

1. Elmore JG, Wells CK, Lee CH, Howard DH, Feinstein AR. Variability in radiologists' interpretations of mammograms. *N Engl J Med.* 1994;331:1493-1499.
2. Elmore JG, Barnhill RL, Elder DE, et al. Pathologists' diagnosis of invasive melanoma and melanocytic proliferations: observer accuracy and reproducibility study. *BMJ.* 2017;357:j2813.
3. Buehler JW, Kleinman JC, Hogue CJ, Strauss LT, Smith JC. Birth weight-specific infant mortality, United States, 1960 and 1980. *Public Health Rep.* 1987;102:151-161.
4. Gerstman BB. *Epidemiology Kept Simple.* New York, NY: Wiley-Liss; 1998.
5. Reynolds P, Smith DF, Satariano E, Nelson DO, Goldman LR, Neutra RR. The four county study of childhood cancer: clusters in context. *Stat Med.* 1996;15:683-697.

SELECT READING

Dawson B, Trapp RG. *Basic & Clinical Biostatistics.* 4th ed. New York, NY: Lange Medical Books/McGraw-Hill; 2004.

REVIEW QUESTIONS

1. In drafting *Goldilocks and the Three Bears*, before settling on the ordinal scale of "too hot, too cold, just right," story authors first considered describing the porridge in terms of (a) degrees Kelvin (based on absolute zero), (b) degrees Fahrenheit (with arbitrary zero point), and even (c) "sweet, bitter, or savory." Respectively, these three unused candidate scales are:
   A. Ratio, continuous, nominal
   B. Nominal, ratio, ordinal
   C. Dichotomous, continuous, nominal

D. Continuous, nominal, binary
E. Ratio, continuous, ordinal

2. When a patient is asked to evaluate his chest pain on a scale of 0 (no pain) to 10 (the worst pain), he reports to the evaluating clinician that his pain is an 8. After the administration of sublingual nitroglycerin and high-flow oxygen, the patient reports that the pain is now a 4 on the same scale. After the administration of morphine sulfate, given as an intravenous push, the pain is 0. This pain scale is a:
   A. Continuous scale
   B. Dichotomous scale
   C. Nominal scale
   D. Qualitative scale
   E. Ratio scale

3. Ten volunteers are weighed in a consistent manner before and after consuming an experimental diet for 6 weeks. This diet consists of apple strudel, tomatillo salsa, and gummy bears. (Don't try this at home!) The weights are shown in the accompanying table.

Volunteer	Weight Before Diet (kg)	Weight After Diet (kg)
1	81	79
2	79	87
3	92	90
4	112	110
5	76	74
6	126	124
7	80	78
8	75	73
9	68	76
10	78	76

The mean weight before the intervention is:
   A. $(81 + 79 + 92 + 112 + 76 + 126 + 80 + 75 + 68 + 78)/10$
   B. $(81 + 79 + 92 + 112 + 76 + 126 + 80 + 75 + 68 + 78)/(10 - 1)$
   C. $(81 + 79 + 92 + 112 + 76 + 126 + 80 + 75 + 68 + 78)^2/10$
   D. $(81 + 79 + 92 + 112 + 76 + 126 + 80 + 75 + 68 + 78)/10^2$
   E. Not possible to calculate from the given data

4. Regarding question 3, the median weight after the intervention is:
   A. $(76 + 79)/2$
   B. $(78 + 79)/2$
   C. $(79 + 87 + 90 + 110 + 74 + 124 + 78 + 73 + 76 + 76)/2$
   D. $(74 + 124)/2$
   E. $(73 + 124)/2$

5. Regarding question 3, the mode of the weights before the intervention is:
   A. Greater than the mode of weights after the intervention
   B. Less than the mode of weights after the intervention
   C. The same as the mode of weights after the intervention
   D. Undefined
   E. Technically equal to every value of weight before the intervention

6. Regarding question 3, assuming a mean weight of m, the variance of the weights before the intervention is:
   A. $(81 + 79 + 92 + 112 + 76 + 126 + 87 + 75 + 68 + 78) - m^2/10$
   B. $[(81 + 79 + 92 + 112 + 76 + 126 + 87 + 75 + 68 + 78) - m]^2/(10 - 1)$
   C. $[(81 - m) + (79 - m) + (92 - m) + (112 - m) + (76 - m) + (126 - m) + (87 - m) + (75 - m) + (68 - m) + (78 - m)]^2/(10 - 1)$
   D. $[(81 - m) + (79 - m) + (92 - m) + (112 - m) + (76 - m) + (126 - m) + (87 - m) + (75 - m) + (68 - m) + (78 - m)]^2/(10 - m)$
   E. $[(81 - m)^2 + (79 - m)^2 + (92 - m)^2 + (112 - m)^2 + (76 - m)^2 + (126 - m)^2 + (87 - m)^2 + (75 - m)^2 + (68 - m)^2 + (78 - m)^2]^2/(10 - 1)$

7. Regarding question 3, to determine whether this diet is effective in promoting weight loss, you intend to perform a statistical test of significance on the differences in weights before and after the intervention. Unfortunately you do not know how to do this until you read Chapter 10. What you do know now is that to use a parametric test of significance:
   A. The data in both data sets must be normally distributed (Gaussian)
   B. The data must not be skewed
   C. The distribution of weight in the underlying population must be normal (Gaussian)
   D. The means for the two data sets must be equal
   E. The variances for the two data sets must be equal

8. Regarding question 3, for distribution A in Fig. 8.8 (see text):
   A. The distribution is normal (Gaussian)
   B. Mean > median > mode
   C. Mean < median < mode
   D. Mean = median = mode
   E. Outliers pull the mean to the right

ANSWERS AND EXPLANATIONS

1. **A.** Scales based on true or absolute zero, such as the Kelvin temperature scale, are ratio. On a ratio scale, 360 degrees (hot porridge) would be twice as hot as 180 degrees (subfreezing porridge). The same would not be true on a scale such as Fahrenheit with an

arbitrary zero point; 200°F (hot porridge) would not be twice as hot as 100°F (lukewarm porridge). The Fahrenheit scale is not ratio, but only continuous. Data in named categories without implied order, such as "sweet, bitter, or savory," are nominal (i.e., categoric). For these reasons, answer A is correct and B, C, D, and E are incorrect. None of the candidate scales demonstrates binary (i.e., dichotomous) variables (C or D). Dichotomous (or binary) is just a special case of nominal (or categoric) when there are only two possible categories (e.g., yes/no, true/false, positive/negative, yummy/yucky).

2. **E.** The scale described is a ratio scale (i.e., for a continuous variable with a true 0 point). The pain scale has a true 0, indicating the absence of pain. A score of 8 on the scale implies that the pain is twice as severe as pain having a score of 4. Of course, the exact meaning of "twice as much pain" may be uncertain, and the concept of "pain" itself is quite subjective. Thus as opposed to other ratio scales (e.g., blood pressure), which have greater comparability between individuals, on a pain scale one person's 4 may be another's 7. For the clinician attempting to alleviate a patient's pain, this potential difference is of little importance. The pain scale provides essential information about whether the pain for a given individual is increasing or decreasing and by relatively how much. Although the pain scale is indeed continuous (A), it is a special and more specific case of continuous (i.e., ratio). Dichotomous scales (B) are binary (only two options) and are a special case of nominal scales (C). Neither binary nor nominal applies to the 0 to 10 pain scale discussed in this question. Qualitative measures (D) are completely devoid of objective scales by definition.

3. **A.** The mean is the sum of all the observed values in a data set divided by the number of observations (10 in this case). Calculating the mean is thus not impossible (E) and not represented by B, C, or D, which are each undefined measures.

4. **B.** The median is the middle observed value in a data set after the data have been arranged in ascending order. The data provided here can be ordered as 73, 74, 76, 76, 78, 79, 87, 90, 110, and 124. In a set of an even number of observed values, the median is the average of the $N/2$ and $(N/2) + 1$ data points. In this case, $N/2 = 5$ and $(N/2) + 1 = 6$, and the average of the fifth data point (78) and sixth data point (79) is $(78 + 79)/2$, or 78.5. Choices A, C, D, and E are all unhelpful quantities: A is the mean of the first and last data points from the order given; C provides half the total weight of all

persons; D is the mean of the fifth and sixth data points from the order given; and E is the mean of the highest and lowest data points, providing the halfway point between these two extremes (in a normal distribution, this value would be equal to the mean, median, and mode).

5. **E.** The mode is the most frequently occurring value in a set of data and is thus not undefined (D). Before the intervention, there are 10 different values for weight. Each value occurs only once. Thus there is a 10-way tie for the most frequently occurring value in the set, and technically each point can be considered a mode (i.e., the data set is decamodal). Since there is no one mode before the intervention, it would be incorrect to speak of a single value as being greater than (A), less than (B), or equal to (C) the mode of weights after the intervention

6. **E.** The variance is the square of the standard deviation. The numerator for variance is $\Sigma(x_i - \bar{x})^2$. In other words, after the mean is subtracted from the first observation and the difference is squared, the process is repeated for each observation in the set, and the values obtained are all added together. The numerator is then divided by the degrees of freedom ($N - 1$). In this case of observed weights before the intervention, N is 10. Choice D uses the wrong degrees of freedom; as does A, which in addition to B and C, uses the wrong calculation for the numerator.

7. **C.** All so-called parametric tests of significance rely on assumptions about the parameters that define a frequency distribution (e.g., mean and standard deviation). To employ parametric methods of statistical analysis, the data being analyzed need not be normally distributed (A) and may be skewed (B). Neither the means (D) nor the variances (E) of two data sets under comparison need to be equal. However, the means of repeated samples from the underlying population from whom the samples are drawn should be normally distributed. To employ a parametric test of significance, one should assume that the distribution of weight in the general population is normal, but even this assumption usually can be relaxed because of the central limit theorem (see Chapter 10).

8. **C.** The distribution in Fig. 8.8 is left skewed. Outliers in the data pull what might otherwise be a normal distribution (A) to the left (not right, E). Whereas for normally distributed data, the mean = median = mode (D); for left-skewed data, the mean < median < mode, not the other way around as would be the case for a right-skewed distribution (B).

Testing Hypotheses

"Extraordinary claims require extraordinary proof."

Carl Sagan

With the nature of variation, types of data and variables, and characteristics of data distribution reviewed in Chapter 8 as background, we now explore how to make inferences from data and test hypotheses using statistical methods.

1. STATISTICAL INFERENCE

Inference means the drawing of conclusions from data. *Statistical inference* can be defined as the drawing of conclusions from quantitative or qualitative information using the methods of statistics to describe and arrange the data and to test suitable hypotheses.

1.1 DIFFERENCES BETWEEN DEDUCTIVE AND INDUCTIVE REASONING

Because data do not provide its own interpretations, it must be interpreted through **inductive reasoning** (from Latin, meaning "to lead into"). This approach to reasoning is less familiar to most people than **deductive reasoning** (Latin, "to lead out from"), which is learned from mathematics, particularly from geometry.

Deductive reasoning proceeds *from the general* (i.e., from assumptions, propositions, or formulas considered true) *to the specific* (i.e., to specific members belonging to the general category). Consider the following two propositions:
- All Americans believe in democracy
- This person is an American

If both propositions are true, then the following deduction must be true:
- This person believes in democracy

Deductive reasoning is of special use in science after hypotheses are formed. Using deductive reasoning, an investigator can say, "*If* the following hypothesis is true, *then* the following prediction or predictions also should be true." If a prediction can be tested empirically, the hypothesis may be rejected or not rejected on the basis of the findings. If the data are inconsistent with the predictions from the hypothesis, the hypothesis must be rejected or modified. Even if the data are consistent with the hypothesis, however, they cannot prove that the hypothesis is true, as shown in Chapter 4 (see Fig. 4.2).

Clinicians often proceed from formulas accepted as true and from observed data to determine the values that variables must have in a certain clinical situation. For example, if the amount of a medication that can be safely given per kilogram of body weight is known, it is simple to calculate how much of that medication can be given to a patient weighing 50 kg. This is deductive reasoning because it proceeds from the general (a formula) to the specific (the patient).

Inductive reasoning, in contrast, seeks to find valid generalizations and general principles from data. Statistics, the quantitative aid to inductive reasoning, proceeds *from the specific* (i.e., from data) *to the general* (i.e., to formulas or conclusions about the data). By sampling a population and determining the age and the blood pressure of the persons in the sample (the specific data), an investigator, using statistical methods, can determine the general relationship between age and blood pressure (e.g., blood pressure increases with age).

1.2 DIFFERENCES BETWEEN MATHEMATICS AND STATISTICS

The differences between mathematics and statistics can be illustrated by showing that they approach the same basic equation in two different ways:

$$y = mx + b$$

This equation is the formula for a straight line in analytic geometry. It is also the formula for simple regression analysis in statistics, although the letters used and their order customarily are different.

In the mathematical formula the b is a constant and stands for the *y-intercept* (i.e., value of y when the variable x equals 0). The value m also is a constant and stands for the *slope* (amount of change in y for a unit increase in the value of x). The important point is that in mathematics, one of the variables (x or y) is unknown and needs to be calculated, whereas the formula and the constants are known. In statistics the reverse is true. The variables x and y are known for all persons in the sample, and the investigator may want to determine the linear relationship between them. This is done by *estimating* the slope and the intercept, which can be done using the form of statistical analysis called *linear regression* (see Chapter 10).

As a general rule, what is known in statistics is unknown in mathematics, and vice versa. In statistics the investigator starts from specific observations (data) to induce (estimate) the general relationships between variables.

2. TESTING HYPOTHESES

Hypotheses are predictions about what the examination of appropriately collected data will show. This discussion introduces the basic concepts underlying common tests of statistical significance such as t-tests. These tests determine the probability that an observed difference between means, for example, represents a true, statistically significant difference (i.e., a difference probably not caused by chance). They do this by determining whether the observed difference is convincingly different from what was expected from the *model*. In basic statistics the model is usually a *null hypothesis* that there will be no difference between the means.

The discussion in this section focuses on the justification for and interpretation of the **_p value_**, which is the probability that under a given statistical model, some summary of the data (called a test statistic) would be at least as large as one observed by chance. The p value is obtained by calculating the test statistic using the observed data and comparing it to its null distribution, which is the distribution of the test statistic under the null hypothesis. The use of p values in medical research is designed to minimize the likelihood of making a false-positive conclusion. False-negative conclusions are discussed more fully in Chapter 12 in the section on sample size.

2.1 FALSE-POSITIVE AND FALSE-NEGATIVE ERRORS

Science is based on the following set of principles:
- Previous experience serves as the basis for developing hypotheses
- Hypotheses serve as the basis for developing predictions
- Predictions must be subjected to experimental or observational testing
- If the predictions are consistent with the data, they are retained, but if they are inconsistent with the data, they are rejected or modified

When deciding whether data are consistent or inconsistent with the hypotheses, investigators are subject to two types of error. An investigator could assert that the data support a hypothesis, when in fact the hypothesis is false; this would be a **false-positive error**, also called an **alpha error** or a **type I error**. Conversely, they could assert that the data do not support the hypothesis, when in fact the hypothesis is true; this would be a **false-negative error**, also called a **beta error** or a **type II error**.

Based on the knowledge that scientists become attached to their own hypotheses, and the conviction that the proof in science (as in courts of law) must be "beyond a reasonable doubt," investigators historically have been particularly careful to avoid false-positive error. This is probably best for theoretical science in general. It also makes sense for hypothesis testing related specifically to medical practice, where the greatest imperative is "first, do no harm" (Latin *primum non nocere*). Although it often fails in practice to avoid harm, medicine is dedicated to this principle, and the high standards for the avoidance of type I error reflect this. However, medicine is subject to the harms of error in either direction. False-negative error in a diagnostic test may mean missing a disease until it is too late to institute therapy, and a false-negative error in the study of a medical intervention may mean overlooking an effective treatment. Therefore researchers need to strike a balance between the risks of making a type I or type II error.

Box 9.1 shows the usual sequence of statistical testing of hypotheses. Analyzing data using these five basic steps is discussed next.

2.1.a. Develop Null Hypothesis and Alternative Hypothesis

The first step consists of stating the null hypothesis and the alternative hypothesis. The **null hypothesis** usually states that there is no association between variables in a data set. For example, the null hypothesis for the data presented in Table 8.2 is that there is no true difference between the percentage of men and the percentage of women who had previously had their serum cholesterol levels checked.

It may seem backward to begin the process by asserting that something is *not* true, but it is much easier to disprove an assertion than to prove something is true. If the data are not consistent with the null hypothesis, it should be rejected in favor of the alternative hypothesis. Because the null hypothesis stated there was no difference between means, and that was rejected, the **alternative hypothesis** states that there *must* be a true difference between the groups being compared. However, if the data are consistent with a hypothesis, this still does not prove the hypothesis, because other hypotheses may fit the data equally well or better.

Consider a hypothetical clinical trial of a drug designed to reduce high blood pressure among patients with essential hypertension (hypertension occurring without a known cause, such as hyperthyroidism or renal artery stenosis). One group of patients would receive the experimental drug and the other group (the control group) would receive a placebo. The null hypothesis might be that, after the intervention, the average change in blood pressure in the treatment group will not differ from the average change in blood pressure in the control group. If a test of significance (e.g., t-test on average change in systolic blood pressure) forces rejection of the null hypothesis, the alternative hypothesis—that there was a true difference in the average change in blood pressure between the two groups—would be accepted. As discussed later, there is a statistical distinction between hypothesizing that a drug will or will not *change* blood pressure, versus hypothesizing whether a drug will or will not *lower* blood pressure. The former does not specify a directional inclination *a priori* (before the fact) and suggests a "two-tailed" hypothesis test. The latter suggests a directional inclination and thus a "one-tailed" test.

2.1.b. Establish Alpha Level

Second, before doing any calculations to test the null hypothesis, the investigator must establish a criterion called the **alpha level**, which is the highest risk of making a false-positive error that the investigator is willing to accept. By custom, the level of alpha is usually set at alpha = 0.05. This says that the

investigator is willing to run a 5% risk (but no more) of being in error when rejecting the null hypothesis and asserting that the treatment and control groups truly differ. In choosing an arbitrary alpha level, the investigator inserts value judgment into the process. Because that is done before the data are collected, however, it avoids the post hoc (after the fact) bias of adjusting the alpha level to make the data show statistical significance after the investigator has looked at the data.

2.1.c. Perform Test of Statistical Significance

When the alpha level is established, the next step is to obtain the **p value** for the data. To do this, the investigator must perform a suitable statistical test of significance on appropriately collected data, such as data obtained from a randomized controlled trial (RCT). This chapter and Chapter 10 focus on some suitable tests. The *p* value obtained by a statistical test (e.g., t-test, described later) gives the probability of obtaining a result as or more extreme than the observed result by chance rather than as a result of a true effect, assuming that the null hypothesis is true. When the probability of an outcome being caused by chance is sufficiently remote, the null hypothesis is rejected. The *p* value states specifically just how remote that probability is.

Usually if the observed *p* value in a study is 0.05 or less, it is considered sufficient evidence that a real difference exists between groups. Although setting alpha at 0.05 or less is arbitrary, this level has become so customary that it is usually necessary to justify choosing a different alpha.. Similarly, two-tailed tests of hypothesis, which require a more extreme result to reject the null hypothesis than do one-tailed tests, are the norm. Consequently, a one-tailed test should be well justified, such as when the directional effect of a given intervention is known with confidence (e.g., it can be neutral or beneficial, but is certain not to be harmful) (see later discussion).

2.1.d. Compare *p* Value Obtained with Alpha

After the *p* value is obtained, it is compared with the alpha level previously chosen.

2.1.e. Reject or Fail to Reject Null Hypothesis

If the *p* value is found to be greater than the alpha level, the investigator fails to reject the null hypothesis. Failing to reject the null hypothesis is not the same as accepting the null hypothesis as true. Rather, it is similar to a jury's finding that the evidence did not prove guilt (or in the example here, did not prove the difference) beyond a reasonable doubt. In the United States a court trial is not designed to prove innocence. The defendant's innocence is assumed and must be disproved beyond a reasonable doubt. Similarly, in statistics, a lack of difference is assumed and it is up to the statistical analysis to show that the null hypothesis is unlikely to be true. The rationale for using this approach in medical research is similar to the rationale in the courts. Although the courts are able to convict the guilty, the goal of exonerating the innocent is an even higher priority. In medicine, confirming the benefit of a new treatment is important, but avoiding the use of ineffective therapies is an even higher priority (first, do no harm).

If the *p* value is found to be less than or equal to the alpha level, the next step is to reject the null hypothesis in favor of the **alternative hypothesis**, that is, the hypothesis that there is in fact a real difference or association. Although it may seem awkward, this process is now standard in medical science and has yielded considerable scientific benefits.

2.2 VARIATION IN INDIVIDUAL OBSERVATIONS AND IN MULTIPLE SAMPLES

Tests of significance are particularly useful in comparing differences between two means or proportions of a variable (e.g., a decrease in blood pressure). The two comparison groups often include a treatment group and a control group. In the example of the experimental drug to reduce blood pressure in hypertensive patients, the investigators would measure the blood pressures of the study participants under experimental conditions before and after the new drug or placebo is given. They would determine the average change in the treatment group and the average change in the control group and use statistical tests to determine whether the difference is large enough to be unlikely to have occurred by chance alone.

Why not just inspect the means to see if they are different? This is inadequate because it is unknown whether the observed difference is unusual or whether a difference that large might be found frequently if the experiment is repeated. Although investigators examine findings in particular patients, their real interest is in determining whether the findings of the study could be generalized to other, similar hypertensive patients. To generalize beyond the participants in the single study, the investigators must know the extent to which the differences discovered in the study are reliable. The estimate of reliability is given by the **standard error**, which is not the same as the standard deviation discussed in Chapter 8.

2.2.a. Standard Deviation and Standard Error

Chapter 8 focused on individual observations and the extent to which they differed from the mean. One assertion was that a normal (Gaussian) distribution could be completely described by its mean and standard deviation. Fig. 8.6 showed that, for a truly normal distribution, 68% of observations fall within the range described as the mean $\pm$ 1 standard deviation, 95.4% fall within the range of the mean $\pm$ 2 standard deviations, and 95% fall within the range of the mean $\pm$ 1.96 standard deviations. This information is useful in describing individual observations (raw data), but it is not directly useful when comparing means or proportions.

Because most research is done on samples rather than on complete populations, investigators need to have some idea of how close the mean of the study sample is to the real-world mean (i.e., mean in underlying population from whom the sample came). For 100 samples (such as in multicenter trials), the means of each sample would differ from the others, but they would cluster around the true mean of the total study sample. Sample means can be plotted like individual observations and have their own distributions. Owing to the central limit theorem (CLT, discussed later), the distribution of the sample means will also follow a normal (Gaussian) distribution with its own mean and standard deviation in large enough samples. The standard deviation of the sampling distribution of the means is called the standard error of the mean (SEM), because it helps estimate the probable error of the sample mean's estimate of the true population mean.

The SEM is a parameter that enables the investigator to do two things that are essential to the function of statistics. One is to estimate the probable amount of error around a quantitative assertion (called confidence limits). The other is to perform tests of statistical significance.

The data shown in Table 9.1 can be used to explore the concept of the SEM. The table lists the systolic and diastolic blood pressures of 26 young adults. To determine the range of expected variation in the estimate of the mean blood pressure obtained from the 26 young adults, the investigator would need an unbiased estimate of the variation in the underlying population. How can this be done with only one small sample?

The formula for calculating the SEM is as follows:

$$\text{Standard error of the mean} = \text{SEM} = \frac{\text{SD}}{\sqrt{N}}$$

TABLE 9.1 Systolic and Diastolic Blood Pressure Values of 26 Young Adults

| | BLOOD PRESSURE (mm Hg) | | |
Participant	Systolic	Diastolic	Gender
1	108	62	F
2	134	74	M
3	100	64	F
4	108	68	F
5	112	72	M
6	112	64	F
7	112	68	F
8	122	70	M
9	116	70	M
10	116	70	M
11	120	72	M
12	108	70	F
13	108	70	F
14	96	64	F
15	114	74	M
16	108	68	M
17	128	86	M
18	114	68	M
19	112	64	M
20	124	70	F
21	90	60	F
22	102	64	F
23	106	70	M
24	124	74	M
25	130	72	M
26	116	70	F

Data from unpublished findings in a sample of 26 young adults in Connecticut.

The larger the sample size (*N*), the smaller the standard error, and the better the estimate of the population mean. Ideally when the true standard deviation in the population is known, this formula gives an unbiased estimate of the population standard error. When estimating the standard deviation using the square root of the sample variance (see Chapter 8), the estimate of the SEM will be biased. However, this is not usually a problem because bias decreases with increasing sample size.

In the medical literature, means are often reported either as the mean ± 1 SD or as the mean ± 1 SE. Reported data must be examined carefully to determine whether the SD or the SE is shown. Either is acceptable in theory because an SD can be converted to an SE, and vice versa, if the sample size is known. Many journals have a policy, however, stating whether the SD or SE must be reported. In either case, the sample size should always be shown.

2.2.b. Confidence Intervals

A confidence interval provides the same service as a *p* value, indicating statistical significance. However, it is typically more useful than simply reporting a *p* value because it shows what range of values, with 95% confidence, is likely to contain the value representing the "true" effect of the intervention. When a confidence interval is narrow, it defines the true effect within a small range of possible values; when the interval is wide, even if significant, it suggests the true effect lies within a wide range of possible values.

While the SD shows the variability of individual observations, the SE shows the variability of means. The mean ± 1.96 SD estimates the range in which 95% of individual observations would be expected to fall, whereas the mean ± 1.96 SE estimates the interval in which 95% of the means of repeated samples of the same size would be expected to fall. The lower and upper boundaries of this interval are called the 95% confidence interval, which represents a range of values that a researcher can be 95% confident contains the mean. Note that this is not the same as saying that there is a 95% probability that the confidence interval contains the true value, because once the interval is generated, it either does or does not contain the true value and is therefore not random. Other confidence intervals, such as the 99% confidence interval, also can be determined easily. Box 9.2 shows the calculation of the SE and the 95% confidence interval for the systolic blood pressure data in Table 9.1.

Confidence intervals can be used as a test to determine whether a mean or proportion differs significantly from a **fixed value**. A common situation is testing to see whether a risk ratio or an odds ratio differs significantly from the ratio of 1.0 (which means no difference). If a 95% confidence interval for such a ratio contains the value 1.0, this means that 1.0 is a plausible value for the ratio and the estimated ratio is not significantly different from 1.0 at an alpha of 0.05. For example, if a risk ratio has a point estimate of 1.7 and a 95% confidence interval of 0.92 to 2.70, it would not be statistically significantly different from 1.0 at an alpha of 0.05 because the confidence interval includes 1.0. If the same estimated risk ratio had a 95% confidence interval between 1.02 and 2.60, however, it would be statistically significantly different from a risk ratio of 1.0 at an alpha of 0.05 because 1.0 does not fall within the 95% confidence interval shown. Because it is common practice to set alpha to 0.05, it is

---

> **BOX 9.2   Calculation of Standard Error and 95% Confidence Interval for Systolic Blood Pressure Values of 26 Adults**
>
> **Part 1 Beginning Data (see Table 9.1)**
> Number of observations, or N = 26
> Mean, or $\bar{x}$ = 113.1 mm Hg
> Standard deviation, or SD = 10.3 mm Hg
>
> **Part 2 Calculation of Standard Error (SE)**
>
> $$SE = SD/\sqrt{N} = 10.3/\sqrt{26} = 10.3 / 51 = 2.02 \text{ mm Hg}$$
>
> **Part 3 Calculation of 95% Confidence Interval (95% CI)**
>
> $$\begin{aligned}
> 95\% \text{ CI} &= \text{mean} \pm 1.96 \text{ SE} \\
> &= 113.1 \pm (1.96)(2.02) \\
> &= 113.1 \pm 3.96 \\
> &= \text{between } 113.1 - 3.96 \text{ mm Hg and } 113.1 \\
> &\quad + 3.96 \text{ mm Hg} \\
> &= 109.1 \text{ mm Hg, } 117.1 \text{ mm Hg}
> \end{aligned}$$

usually permissible to omit the alpha level when reporting the results of a statistical analysis unless a different alpha is chosen.

3. TESTS OF STATISTICAL SIGNIFICANCE

The tests described in this section allow investigators to compare two parameters, such as means or proportions, and to determine whether the difference between them is statistically significant. Typically when we are interested in carrying out tests of differences between means, we use a **t-test** (commonly referred to as a two-sample t-test or paired t-test depending on whether the data are independent, as discussed later), where we use the t distribution to decide whether our critical ratio is large enough to reject the null hypothesis. When we are interested in carrying out a test of differences between **proportions**, we use a **z-test**, which uses the standard normal distribution (a normal distribution with a mean of 0 and a SD of 1) to decide whether the observed difference is large enough to reject the null hypothesis. All these tests make comparisons possible by calculating the appropriate form of a ratio, called a **critical ratio**.

3.1 CRITICAL RATIOS

Critical ratios are the means by which many tests of statistical significance enable clinicians to obtain a *p* value that is used to decide on the null hypothesis. A critical ratio is the ratio of an estimate of a parameter (e.g., a difference between means from two sets of data) divided by the **standard error** (SE) of the estimate (e.g., the standard error of the difference between the means). The general formula for tests of significance is as follows:

$$\text{Critical ratio} = \frac{\text{Parameter}}{\text{SE of that parameter}}$$

When applied to the t-test, the formula becomes:

$$\text{Critical ratio} = t = \frac{\text{Difference between two means}}{\text{SE of the difference between the two means}}$$

When applied to a z-test, the formula becomes:

$$\text{Critical ratio} = z = \frac{\text{Difference between two proportions}}{\text{SE of the difference between two proportions}}$$

The value of the critical ratio (e.g., t or z) is found in the appropriate table (of t or z values) to determine the corresponding p value. (Note that statistical software packages [e.g., SAS, STATA, SPSS] generate the p value for many statistical tests automatically.) For any critical ratio, the larger the ratio, the less likely it is that the difference between means or proportions is due to random variation (i.e., the more likely the difference can be considered statistically significant and real). Unless the total sample size is small (e.g., <10), the finding of a critical ratio of greater than about 2 for t-tests and z-tests usually indicates that the difference is statistically significant. This enables the investigator to reject the null hypothesis. The statistical tables adjust the critical ratios for the sample size by means of the degrees of freedom (see discussion later in the chapter).

The reason that a critical ratio works is complex and can best be explained using an example. Assume that an investigator conducted 1000 different clinical trials of the same *ineffective* antihypertensive drug, and each trial had the same large sample size. In each trial, assume that the investigator obtained an average value for the change in blood pressure in the experimental group ($\bar{x}_E$) and an average value for the change in blood pressure in the control group ($\bar{x}_C$). For each trial, there would be two means, and the difference between the means could be expressed as $\bar{x}_E - \bar{x}_C$. In this study the null hypothesis would be that any difference between means is not a real difference.

If the null hypothesis were true (i.e., no true difference), chance variation would still cause $\bar{x}_E$ to be greater than $\bar{x}_C$ about half the time, despite the drug's lack of effect. The reverse would be true, also by chance, about half the time. On average, however, the differences between the two means would be near zero, reflecting the drug's lack of effect.

If the values representing the difference between the two means in each of the 1000 clinical trials were plotted on a graph, the distribution curve would appear normal (Gaussian), with an average difference of 0, as in Fig. 9.1A. Chance variation would cause 95% of the values to fall within the large central zone, which covers the area of 0 ± 1.96 SE and is lightly

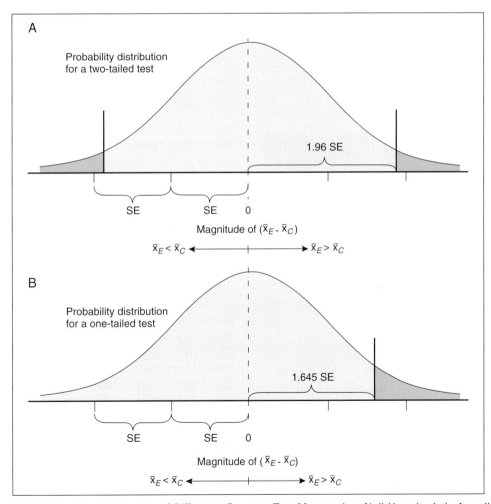

Fig. 9.1 Probability Distribution of Difference Between Two Means when Null Hypothesis is Actually True (i.e., when there is no Real Difference between the Two Means). *(Dark area)* Zone for rejecting the null hypothesis. *(Light area)* Zone for failing to reject the null hypothesis. (A) When a two-tailed test is used, there is a rejection zone on each side of the distribution. (B) When a one-tailed test is used, there is a rejection zone on only one side. *SE,* Standard error; $\bar{x}_E$, mean for experimental group; $\bar{x}_C$, mean for control group.

colored. This is the zone for *failing to reject* the null hypothesis. Outside this zone is the zone for *rejecting* the null hypothesis, which consists of two dark-colored areas (Fig. 9.1A).

By setting alpha at 0.05, the investigator is willing to take a 5% risk (i.e., a 1-in-20 risk) of a false-positive assertion, but is not willing to take a higher risk. This implies that if alpha is set at 0.05, and if 20 data sets of two research samples that are *not* truly different are compared, one "statistically significant" difference would be expected by chance alone. If only one clinical trial was performed, and if the ratio of the difference between the means of the two groups was outside the area of 0 ± 1.96 SE of the difference, either the study was a rare example (i.e., <5% chance) of a false-positive difference or there was a true difference between the groups. Some false-positive results are to be expected in the medical literature. They are inevitable, which is why follow-up studies are performed to confirm the findings.

3.2 DEGREES OF FREEDOM

The term *degrees of freedom* refers to the number of observations that are free to vary. Box 9.3 presents the idea behind this important statistical concept. Generally speaking, the degrees of freedom for a t-test are equal to the total sample size minus 1 degree of freedom for each mean that is calculated. In a two-sample t-test, 2 degrees of freedom are lost because two means are calculated (one mean for each group whose means are to be compared). The general formula

---

BOX 9.3 **Idea Behind the Degrees of Freedom**

The term *degrees of freedom* refers to the number of observations (N) that are free to vary. A degree of freedom is lost every time a mean is calculated. Why should this be?

Before putting on a pair of gloves, a person has the freedom to decide whether to begin with the left or right glove. When the person puts on the first glove, however, he or she loses the freedom to decide which glove to put on last. If centipedes put on shoes, they would have a choice to make for the first 99 shoes, but not for the 100th shoe. Right at the end, the freedom to choose (vary) is restricted.

In statistics, if there are two observed values, only one estimate of the variation between them is possible. Something has to serve as the basis against which other observations are compared. The mean is the most solid estimate of the expected value of a variable, so it is assumed to be fixed. This implies that the numerator of the mean (the sum of individual observations, or the sum of x_i), which is based on N observations, is also fixed. When $N - 1$ observations (each of which was, presumably, free to vary) have been added up, the last observation is not free to vary because the total values of the N observations must add up to the sum of x_i. For this reason, 1 degree of freedom is lost each time a mean is calculated. When estimating the variance of a sample, the proper variance is the sum of squares divided by the degrees of freedom $(N - 1)$.

---

for the degrees of freedom for a two-sample t-test is $N_1 + N_2 - 2$, where N_1 is the sample size in the first group and N_2 is the sample size in the second group.

3.3 USE OF t-TESTS

One of the more common uses of t-tests is to compare the means of a continuous variable in two research samples, such as a treatment group and a control group. This is done by determining whether the difference between the two observed means exceeds the difference that would be expected by chance from the two random samples.

3.3.a. Sample Populations and Sizes

If the two research samples come from two different groups (e.g., a group of men and a group of women), a two-sample t-test is used. If the two samples come from the same group (e.g., pretreatment and posttreatment values for the same study participants), the paired t-test is used. The main difference between the two-sample t-test and the paired t-test is in the degrees of freedom.

The two-sample t-test and the paired t-test depend on certain assumptions, including the assumption that the data being studied are normally distributed in the larger population from which the sample came. Very seldom, however, are observed data perfectly normally distributed. This does not invalidate the t-test because there is a convenient theorem that rescues the t-test (and much of statistics as well). The **central limit theorem** can be derived theoretically or observed by experimentation. According to the theorem, for reasonably large samples (e.g., ≥30 observations of blood pressure in each sample), the sampling distribution of the means is approximately *normal* (Gaussian), even if the data in individual samples have skewness, kurtosis, or unevenness. Thus in large enough samples the answers we get from t-tests and z-tests will be approximately the same.

3.3.b. Two-Sample t-Test

A t-test can be one tailed or two tailed. The calculations are the same, but the interpretation of the resulting *t* differs.

Calculation of the value of t. In both two-sample and paired t-tests, the test statistic *t* is calculated by taking the observed difference between the means of the two groups (the numerator) and dividing this difference by the standard error of the difference between the means of the two groups (the denominator). Before *t* can be calculated, the **standard error of the difference between the means** (SED) must be determined. The basic formula for this is the square root of the sum of the respective population variances, each divided by its own sample size.

For a theoretical distribution, the correct equation for the SED would be as follows:

$$\text{SED of } \mu_E - \mu_C = \sqrt{\frac{\sigma_E^2}{N_E} + \frac{\sigma_C^2}{N_C}}$$

BOX 9.4 Formula for Standard Error of Difference between Means

The standard error equals the standard deviation (σ) divided by the square root of the sample size (N). Alternatively, this can be expressed as the square root of the variance (σ^2) divided by N:

$$\text{Standard error} = \text{SE} = \frac{\sigma}{\sqrt{N}} = \sqrt{\frac{\sigma^2}{N}}$$

As mentioned in this chapter (see Box 9.2), the variance of a difference is equal to the sum of the variances if the two groups are independent. The variance of the difference between the mean of an experimental group (μ_E) and the mean of a control group (μ_C) could be expressed as follows: $\sigma_E^2 + \sigma_C^2$.

As shown in the previous equation, a standard error can be written as the square root of the variance divided by the sample size, allowing the equation to be expressed as:

$$\text{Standard error of } \mu_E - \mu_C = \sqrt{\frac{\sigma_E^2}{N_E} + \frac{\sigma_C^2}{N_C}}$$

where the Greek letter μ is the population mean, E is the experimental population, C is the control population, σ^2 is the variance of the population, and N is the number of observations in the population. The rationale behind this formula is discussed in Box 9.4.

The theoretical formula requires that the population variances be known, which usually is not true with experimental data. Nevertheless, if the sample sizes are large enough (e.g., if the total of the two samples is ≥ 30), the previous formula can be used with the sample variances substituted for the population variances because of the central limit theorem. When dealing with samples, instead of using Greek letters in the formulas, the italic Roman symbol $\bar{x}$ is used to indicate the mean of the sample, and the italic Roman symbol s^2 is used to indicate the variance:

$$\text{Estimate of the SED of } \bar{x}_E - \bar{x}_C = \sqrt{\frac{s_E^2}{N_E} + \frac{s_C^2}{N_C}}$$

Because the t-test typically is used to test a null hypothesis of *no difference between two means*, the assumption generally is made that there is also no difference between the variances, so **a pooled estimate of the SED** (SED_P) may be used instead. In this case, if the combined sample size is large enough (e.g., ≥ 30 in the combined sample), the previous formula for the estimate of the standard error of the difference becomes:

$$\text{SED}_P \text{ of } \bar{x}_E - \bar{x}_C = \sqrt{s_P^2 \left(\frac{1}{N_E} + \frac{1}{N_C}\right)}$$
$$= \sqrt{s_P^2 \left[(1/N_E) + (1/N_C)\right]}$$

The s_P^2, called the **pooled estimate of the variance**, is a weighted average of s_E^2 and s_C^2. The s_P^2 is calculated as the sum of the two sums of squares divided by the combined degrees of freedom:

$$s_P^2 = \frac{\sum(x_1 - \bar{x}_E)^2 + \sum(x_C - \bar{x}_C)^2}{N_E + N_C - 2}$$

Note that if the variances are not known ahead of time, they need to be estimated separately. Thus it can be useful to have the sample sizes in the two groups be comparable to check the assumption that the variances are actually equal. If it turns out that the variance of one sample is much greater than the variance of the other, more complex formulas are needed.[1] Putting all of this together, when using a t-test to test the null hypothesis of no difference in group means, the t statistic and its degrees of freedom are defined as:

$$t = \frac{\bar{x}_E + \bar{x}_C - 0}{\sqrt{s_P^2 \left[(1/N_E) + (1/N_C)\right]}}$$
$$df = N_E + N_C - 2$$

The 0 in the numerator of the equation for t was added for correctness because the t-test determines if the difference between the means is significantly different from zero. Because the 0 does not affect the calculations in any way, however, it is usually omitted from t-test formulas.

The same formula, recast in terms to apply to any two independent samples (e.g., samples of men and women), is as follows:

$$t = \frac{\bar{x}_1 - \bar{x}_2 - 0}{\sqrt{s_P^2 \left[(1/N_1) + (1/N_2)\right]}}$$
$$df = N_1 + N_2 - 2$$

in which $\bar{x}_1$ is the mean of the first sample, $\bar{x}_2$ is the mean of the second sample, s_P^2 is the pooled estimate of the variance, N_1 is the size of the first sample, N_2 is the size of the second sample, and df is the degrees of freedom. The 0 in the numerator indicates that the null hypothesis states the difference between the means would not be significantly different from zero.[*] The df is needed to enable the investigator to refer to the correct line in the table of the values of t and their relationship to the p value.

Box 9.5 shows the use of a t-test to compare the mean systolic blood pressures of the 14 men and 12 women whose data were given in Table 9.1. Box 9.6 presents a different and more visual way of understanding the t-test.

---

[*]The value stated in the null hypothesis could be different from zero. In that case, the test would determine whether the observed difference between means is greater than the number in the null hypothesis, which might be a minimum goal. Because the 0 (or other number) does not contribute to the variance, it does not alter the denominator. Because the hypothesis still asserts there is "no difference" in the numerator, it is still a null hypothesis.

BOX 9.5   Calculation of Results from Two-Sample t-Test Comparing Systolic Blood Pressure of 14 Male Participants with 12 Female Participants

Part 1 Beginning Data (see Table 9.1)
Number of observations, or $N = 14$ for males, or M; 12 for females, or F
Mean, or $\bar{x} = 118.3$ mm Hg for males; 107.0 mm Hg for females
Variance, or $s^2 = 70.1$ mm Hg for males; 82.5 mm Hg for females
Sum of $\left(\bar{x}_i - \bar{x}\right)^2$, or TSS = 911.3 mm Hg for males; 907.5 mm Hg for females
Alpha value for the t-test = 0.05

Part 2 Calculation of t Value Based on Pooled Variance (s_P^2) and Pooled Standard Error of the Difference (SED_P)

$$s_P^2 = \frac{TSS_M + TSS_F}{N_M + N_F - 2} = \frac{911.3 + 907.5}{14 + 12 - 2} = \frac{1818.8}{24} = 75.78 \text{ mm Hg}$$

$$SED_p = \sqrt{S_P^2[(1/N_M) + (1/N_F)]}$$

$$= \sqrt{75.78[(1/14) + (1/12)]}$$

$$= \sqrt{75.78(0.1548)} = \sqrt{11.73} = 3.42 \text{ mm Hg}$$

$$t = \frac{\bar{x}_M - \bar{x}_F - 0}{\sqrt{S_P^2[(1/N_M) + (1/N_F)]}} = \frac{\bar{x}_M - \bar{x}_F - 0}{SED_p}$$

$$= \frac{11.83 + 107.0 - 0}{3.42} = \frac{11.30}{3.42} = 3.30$$

Part 3 Alternative Calculation of t Value Based on SED Equation Using Observed Variances for Males and Females, Rather Than Based on SED_P Equation Using Pooled Variance

$$SED = \sqrt{\frac{S_M^2}{N_M} + \frac{S_F^2}{N_M}} = \sqrt{\frac{70.1}{14} + \frac{82.5}{12}}$$

$$= \sqrt{5.01 + 6.88} = \sqrt{11.89} = 3.45 \text{ mm}$$

$$t = \frac{\bar{x}_M - \bar{x}_F - 0}{SED}$$

$$= \frac{118.3 + 107.0 - 0}{3.45} = \frac{11.30}{3.45} = 3.28$$

Compared with the equation in Part 2, the equation in Part 3 usually is easier to remember and to calculate, and it adjusts for differences in the variances and the sample sizes. The result here ($t = 3.28$) is almost identical to that earlier ($t = 3.30$), even though the sample size is small. However, note that if we decide to use this formula, we cannot use the degrees of freedom calculation in Part 4 and instead have to use a more complicated formula known as the Welch-Satterthwaite equation.

Part 4 Calculation of Degrees of Freedom (df) for t-Test and Interpretation of t Value

$$df = N_M + N_F - 2 = 14 + 12 - 2 = 24$$

For a t value of 3.30, with 24 degrees of freedom, p value is less than 0.01, as indicated in the table of the values of t. This means that the male participants have a significantly different (higher) systolic blood pressure than the female participants in this data set.

The t-test is designed to help investigators distinguish *explained variation* from *unexplained variation* (random error or chance). These concepts are similar to the concepts of *signal* and background *noise* in radio broadcast engineering. Listeners who are searching for a particular station on their radio dial find background noise on almost every radio frequency. When they reach the station they want to hear, they may not notice the background noise because the signal is much stronger than the noise. Because the radio can amplify a weak signal greatly, the critical factor is the ratio of the strength of the signal to the strength of the background noise. The greater the ratio, the clearer the station's sound. The closer the ratio is to 1.0 (i.e., the point at which the magnitude of the noise equals that of the signal), the less satisfactory is the sound the listener hears.

In medical studies the particular factor being investigated is similar to the radio signal, and random error is similar to

BOX 9.6 Does the Eye Naturally Perform ± t-Tests?

The paired diagrams in this box show three patterns of overlap between two frequency distributions (e.g., a treatment group and a control group). These distributions can be thought of as the frequency distributions of systolic blood pressure values among hypertensive patients after randomization and treatment either with an experimental drug or with a placebo. The treatment group's distribution is shown in gray, the control group's distribution is shown in blue, and the area of overlap is shown with gray and blue hatch marks. The means are indicated by the vertical dotted lines. The three different pairs show variation in the spread of systolic blood pressure values.

Examine the three diagrams. Then try to guess whether each pair was sampled from the same universe (i.e., was not significantly different) or was sampled from two different universes (i.e., was significantly different).

Most observers believe that the distributions in pair A look as though they were sampled from different universes. When asked why they think so, they usually state that there is little overlap between the two frequency distributions. Most observers are not convinced that the distributions in either pair B or pair C were sampled from different universes. They say that there is considerable overlap in each of these pairs, and this makes them doubt that there is a real difference. Their visual impressions are indeed correct.

It is not the absolute distance between the two means that leads most observers to say "different" for pair A and "not different" for pair B, because the distance between the means was drawn to be exactly the same in pairs A and B. It is also not the absolute amount of dispersion that causes them to say "different" for pair A and "not different" for pair C, because the dispersions were drawn to be the same in pairs A and C. The essential point, which the eye notices, is the ratio of the distance between the means to the variation around the means. The greater the distance between the means for a given amount of dispersion, the less likely it is that the samples were from the same universe. This ratio is exactly what the t-test calculates:

$$t = \frac{\text{Distance between the means}}{\text{Variation around the means}}$$

where the variation around the means is expressed as the standard error of the difference between the means. The eye naturally does a t-test, although it does not quantify the relationship as precisely as does the t-test.

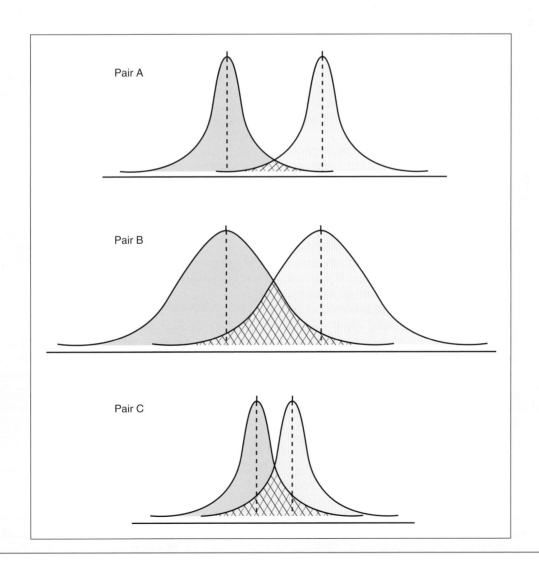

background noise. Statistical analysis helps distinguish one from the other by comparing their strength. If the variation caused by the intervention is considerably larger than the variation caused by random factors (i.e., in the t-test the ratio is >1.96), the effect of the intervention becomes detectable above the statistical *noise* of random factors.

Interpretation of the results. If the value of *t* is large, the *p* value is small because it is unlikely that a large t ratio would be obtained by chance alone. If the *p* value is 0.05 or less, it is customary to reject the hypothesis that there is no difference. Such findings are called "statistically significant." Conceptually the *p* value is the probability of being in error if the null hypothesis of no difference between the means is rejected.

One-tailed and two-tailed ± t-tests. The conceptual diagram in Fig. 9.1 shows the theory behind the acceptance and rejection regions for the one-tailed and two-tailed types of t-test. These tests are also sometimes called a *one-sided test* or a *two-sided test*.

In the two-tailed test the alpha (e.g., of 0.05) is equally divided at the ends of the two tails of the distribution (see Fig. 9.1A). The two-tailed test is generally recommended, because most of the time the difference could go in either direction and the tests of hypothesis should account for both possibilities. For example, it is important to know if a new treatment is significantly better than a standard or placebo treatment, but it is also important to know if a new treatment is significantly worse. In this situation the two-tailed test provides an accepted criterion for when a difference shows the new treatment to be better or worse.

Sometimes only a one-tailed test is appropriate. Suppose that a new therapy is known to cost much more than the currently used treatment. It would not be used if it were worse than the current therapy, but it also would not be used if it were merely as good as the current therapy. It would be used only if it were significantly better than the current therapy. Under these circumstances, some investigators consider it acceptable to use a one-tailed test because they are concerned only with whether the new treatment is better; if it is not better, it will not be recommended. In this situation the 5% rejection region for the null hypothesis is all at one tail of the distribution (see Fig. 9.1B) instead of being evenly divided between extremes of the two tails.

In the one-tailed test the null hypothesis nonrejection region extends only to 1.645 standard errors above the "no difference" point of 0. In the two-tailed test, it extends to 1.96 SE above and below the "no difference" point. This makes the one-tailed test more robust, that is, more able to detect a significant difference, if it is in the expected direction. Many investigators dislike one-tailed tests because they believe that if an intervention is significantly worse than the standard therapy, that fact should be documented scientifically. Most reviewers and editors require that the use of a one-tailed significance test be justified. The two-tailed test is more *conservative*, making it more difficult to reject the null hypothesis when the outcome is in the expected direction.

> ## BOX 9.7 Implications of Choosing a One-Tailed or Two-Tailed Test of Significance
>
> For students who are confused by the implications of choosing a one-tailed or two-tailed test, a football analogy may be helpful. The coach of a football team wants to assess the skill of potential quarterbacks. He is unwilling to allow mere completion of a pass to serve as evidence of throwing accuracy because he knows that a pass could be completed by chance, even if the football did not go where the quarterback intended. Because the coach is an amateur statistician, he further infers that if the quarterback were to throw randomly, the ball would often land near the center of the field and would less often land way off toward one sideline or the other. The distribution of random throws on the 100-foot-wide field might even be Gaussian (thinks the coach).
>
> The coach asks quarterback applicants to throw to a receiver along the sideline. The coach announces that each applicant has a choice: (1) He may pick one side ahead of time and complete a pass to that side within 5 feet of the sideline; or (2) he may throw to either side, but then must complete the pass within 2.5 feet of the sideline. The coach's null hypothesis is simply that the quarterback would not be able to complete a pass within the specified zone. In either case, a complete pass outside the specified zone would be attributed to chance because it is not what was intended.
>
> The coach does not give applicants the option of throwing to either side and completing the pass within 5 feet of the sideline. If the coach were to allow applicants to elect this option, the coach would reject his null hypothesis on the basis of chance 10% of the time, and he is unwilling to take so great a risk of selecting a lucky but unskillful quarterback.
>
> The quarterback has more room to work with if he prefers to throw to one side (one-tailed test) and can count on throwing in only that direction. If he is unsure in which direction he may wish to throw, he can get credit for a completed pass in either direction (two-tailed test), but has only a narrow zone for which to aim.

The implications of choosing a one-tailed or two-tailed test are explored further in Box 9.7.

3.3.c. t Distribution

The t distribution was described by Gosset, who used the pseudonym "Student" when he wrote the description. The normal (Gaussian) distribution is also called the z distribution. The t distribution looks similar to the z distribution except that its tails are wider and its peak is slightly less high, depending on the sample size. The t distribution is needed in smaller samples due to the additional uncertainty that arises from having to estimate the standard deviations of the populations. The larger the sample size, the smaller the errors, and the more the t distribution looks like the normal (Gaussian) distribution.

3.3.d. Paired t-Test

In many medical studies, individuals are followed over time to see if there is a change in the value of a continuous variable. Typically this occurs in a before-and-after experiment, such as one testing to see if there is a decrease in average blood pressure after treatment or a reduction in weight after the use of a special diet. In this type of comparison, an individual patient serves as their own control. The appropriate statistical test for this type of data is the paired t-test. For paired data, a paired t-test is more powerful for detecting differences than a two-sample t-test, because it considers the correlation between the observations. Variation that is detected in the paired t-test is presumably attributable to the intervention or to changes over time in the same person.

Calculation of the value of t. To calculate a paired t-test, a new variable must be created. This variable, called *d*, is the difference between the values before and after the intervention for each individual studied. The paired t-test is a test of the null hypothesis that, on average, the difference is equal to zero, which is what would be expected if there were no changes over time. Using the symbol $\bar{d}$ to indicate the mean observed difference between the before and after values, the formula for the paired t-test is as follows:

$$t_{paired} = t_p = \frac{\bar{d}_l - 0}{\text{Standard error of } \bar{d}}$$
$$= \frac{\bar{d} - 0}{\sqrt{\frac{s_d^2}{N}}}$$
$$df = N - 1$$

The numerator contains a 0 because the null hypothesis says that the observed difference will not differ from zero; however, the 0 does not enter into the calculation and can be omitted. Because the 0 in this formula is a constant, it has no variance, and the only error in estimating the mean difference is its own standard error.

The formulas for the two-sample t-test and the paired t-test are similar: the ratio of a difference to the variation around that difference (the standard error). In the two-sample t-test, each of the two distributions to be compared contributes to the variation of the difference, and the two variances must be added. In the paired t-test, there is only one frequency distribution, that of the before-after difference in each person. In the paired t-test, because only one mean is calculated ($\bar{d}$), only 1 degree of freedom is lost; the formula for the degrees of freedom is $N - 1$.

Interpretation of the results. The values of *t* and their relationship to *p* are shown in a statistical table in the Appendix (see Table C). If the value of *t* is large for the given degrees of freedom, the *p* value will be small because it is unlikely that a large t ratio would be obtained by chance alone. If the *p* value is 0.05 or less, it is customary to assume that there is a real difference (i.e., that the null hypothesis of no difference can be rejected).

3.4 USE OF z-TESTS

A z-test is used to compare differences in proportions and the critical ratio follows a standard normal (Gaussian) distribution.

This differs from a t-test, which is often used to compare differences in means and the test statistic follows a t distribution. In medicine, examples of proportions that are frequently studied are sensitivity, specificity, positive predictive value, risks, and percentages of people with symptoms, illness, or recovery. Frequently the goal of research is to see if the proportion of patients surviving in a treated group differs from that in an untreated group. This can be evaluated using a z-test for proportions.

Calculation of the Value of z

As discussed earlier (see Critical Ratios earlier in the chapter), z is calculated by taking the observed difference between the two proportions (the numerator) and dividing it by the standard error of the difference between the two proportions (the denominator). For purposes of illustration, assume that research is being conducted to see whether the proportion of patients surviving in a treated group is greater than that in an untreated group. For each group, if *p* is the proportion of successes (survivals), then $1 - p$ is the proportion of failures (nonsurvivals). If *N* represents the size of the group on whom the proportion is based, the parameters of the proportion could be calculated as follows:

$$\text{Variance (proportion)} = \frac{p(1 - \curlywedge p)}{N}$$
$$\text{Standard error (proportion)} = SE_p = \sqrt{\frac{p(1 - p)}{N}}$$
$$\text{95\% Confidence interval} = 95\% \ CI = p \pm 1.96 \ SE_p$$

If there is a 0.60 (60%) survival rate after a given treatment, the calculations of SE_p and the 95% confidence interval (CI) of the proportion, based on a sample of 100 study subjects, would be as follows:

$$SE_p = \sqrt{(0.6)(0.4)/100}$$
$$= \sqrt{0.24/100}$$
$$= 0.049$$
$$95\% \ CI = 0.6 \pm (1.96)(0.049)$$
$$= 0.6 \pm 0.096$$
$$= \text{between } 0.6 - 0.096 \text{ and } 0.6 + 0.096$$
$$= 0.504, 0.696$$

The result of the CI calculation means that we can say with 95% confidence that the true proportion is in the interval (50.4%, 69.6%).

Now that there is a way to obtain the standard error of a proportion, the standard error of the difference between proportions also can be obtained, and the equation for the z-test can be expressed as follows:

$$z = \frac{p_1 - p_2 - 0}{\sqrt{\bar{p}(1 - \bar{p})[(1/N_1) + (1/N_2)]}}$$

in which p_1 is the proportion of the first sample, p_2 is the proportion of the second sample, N_1 is the size of the first sample, N_2 is the size of the second sample, and $\bar{p}$ is the mean proportion of successes in all observations combined. The 0 in the numerator indicates that the null hypothesis states that the difference between the proportions will not be significantly different from zero.

Interpretation of the Results

The previous formula for z is similar to the formula for t in the two-sample t-test, as described earlier (see the pooled variance formula). Because the variance and the standard error of the proportion are based on a theoretical distribution (normal approximation to the binomial distribution), however, the z distribution is used instead of the t distribution in determining whether the difference is statistically significant. When the z ratio is large, as when the t ratio is large, the difference is more likely to be real.

The computations for the z-test appear different from the computations for the chi-square test (see Chapter 10), but when the same data are set up as a 2×2 table the results are identical. Most people find it easier to do a chi-square test than to do a z-test for proportions, but both tests accomplish the same goal.

3.5 USE OF OTHER TESTS

Chapter 10 discusses other statistical significance tests used in the analysis of two variables (bivariate analysis). Chapter 11 discusses tests used in the analysis of multiple independent variables (multivariable analysis).

4. SPECIAL CONSIDERATIONS

4.1 VARIATION BETWEEN GROUPS VERSUS VARIATION WITHIN GROUPS

If the differences between two groups are found to be statistically significant, it is appropriate to ask why the groups are different and how much of the total variation is explained by the variable defining the two groups, such as treatment versus control. A straightforward comparison of the heights of men and women can be used to illustrate the considerations involved in answering the following question: Why are men taller than women? Although biologists might respond that genetic, hormonal, and perhaps nutritional factors explain the differences in height, a biostatistician would take a different approach. After first pointing out that individual men are not always taller than individual women, but that the average height of men is greater than that of women, the biostatistician would seek to determine the amount of the total variation in height that is explained by the gender difference and whether the difference is more than would be expected by chance.

For purposes of this discussion, suppose that the heights of 200 randomly selected university students were measured,

that 100 of these students were men and 100 were women, and that the unit of measure was centimeters. As discussed in Chapter 8, the **total variation** would be equal to the sum of the squared deviations, which is usually called the **total sum of squares** (TSS) but is sometimes referred to simply as the **sum of squares** (SS). In the total group of 200 students, suppose that the total SS (the sum of the squared deviations from the average height for all 200 students) was found to be 10,000 cm². This number is the total amount of variation that needs to be explained in the data set. The biostatistician would begin by seeking to determine how much of this variation was caused by gender and how much was caused by other factors.

Fig. 9.2 shows a hypothetical frequency distribution of the heights of a sample of women *(black marks)* and a sample of men *(blue marks),* indicating the density of observations at the different heights. An approximate normal curve is drawn over each of the two distributions, and the overall mean *(grand* mean) is indicated by the vertical dotted line, along with the mean height for women (a *gender mean)* and the mean height for men (a *gender mean).*

Measuring the TSS (the total unexplained variation) from the grand mean yielded a result of 10,000 cm². Measuring the SS for men from the mean for men and the SS for women from the mean for women would yield a smaller amount of unexplained variation, about 6000 cm². This leaves 60% of the variation still to be explained. The other 40% of the variation is explained, however, by the variable gender. From a statistical perspective, *explaining variation* implies reducing the unexplained SS. If more explanatory variables (e.g., age, height of father, height of mother, nutritional status) are analyzed, the unexplained SS may be reduced still further, and even more of the variation can be said to be explained.

The following question is even more specific: Why is the shortest woman shorter than the tallest man? Statistically there are two parts to the explanation:

- She is a member of the class (group) of individuals (women) who have a shorter mean height than do men
- She is the shortest of her group of women, and the man selected is the tallest of the group of men, so they are at the opposite extremes of height within their respective groups

The greater the distance between the means for men and women, the greater the proportion of the variation likely to be explained by **variation between groups**. The larger the standard deviation of heights of women and men, the greater the proportion of the variation likely to be explained by **variation within groups**. The within-groups variation might be reduced still further, however, if other independent variables were added.

Suppose that all women were of equal height, all men were of equal height, and men were taller than women (Fig. 9.3A). What percentage of the variation in height would be explained by gender and what percentage would be unexplained? The answer is that all the variation would be caused by gender (between-groups variation); and because there

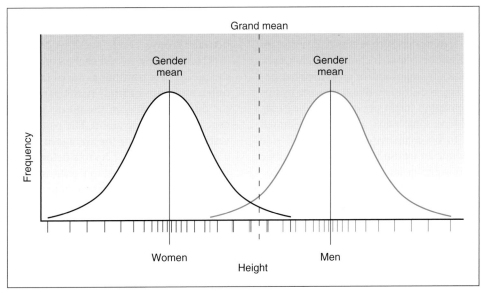

Fig. 9.2 Hypothetical Frequency Distribution of Heights. From a sample of women (*black marks* along *x*-axis) and a sample of men (*blue marks* along *x*-axis), indicating the density of observations at the different heights. An approximate normal curve is drawn over each of the two distributions, and the overall mean (grand mean) is indicated by the *vertical dashed line*, along with the mean height for women (a gender mean) and the mean height for men (a gender mean).

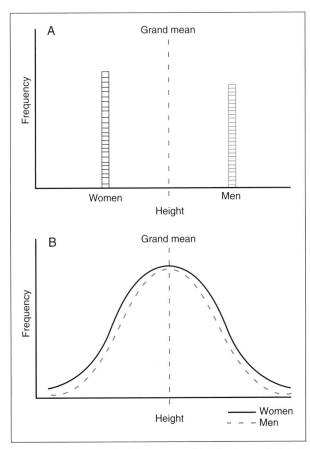

Fig. 9.3 Two Hypothetical Frequency Distributions of Heights. From a sample of women (*black lines*) and a sample of men (*blue lines*). (A) How the distribution would appear if all women were of equal height, all men were of equal height, and men were taller than women. (B) How the distribution would appear if women varied in height, men varied in height, but the mean heights of men and women were the same.

is no within-groups variation, no variation would be left unexplained.

Alternatively, suppose that women varied in height, that men varied in height, and that the mean heights of the men and women were the same (see Fig. 9.3B). Now what percentage of the variation in height would be explained by gender and what percentage would be unexplained? The answer: None of the variation would be caused by gender; all of it would be left unexplained.

This simple example shows that statistics ultimately attempts to divide the total variation into a part that is explained by the independent variables (called the model) and a part that is still unexplained. This activity is called analyzing variation or analyzing the TSS. A specific method for doing this under certain circumstances and testing hypotheses at the same time is called **analysis of variance** (ANOVA) (see Chapter 11).

4.2 CLINICAL IMPORTANCE AND EXTERNAL VALIDITY VERSUS STATISTICAL SIGNIFICANCE

A frequent error made by investigators has been to find a statistically significant difference, reject the null hypothesis, and recommend the finding as being useful for determining disease etiology, making a clinical diagnosis, or treating disease, without considering whether the finding is clinically important or whether it has external validity. Testing for statistical significance is important, because it helps investigators reject assertions that are not true. Even if a finding is **statistically significant**, however, it may not be **clinically significant** or **scientifically important**. For example, with a very large sample size it is possible to show that an average decrease of 2 mm Hg in blood pressure with a certain medication is statistically significant. Such a small decrease in blood pressure would not be of much clinical use, however, and would not be clinically important in an individual patient. However, an average reduction in blood pressure by this amount in a large population might prevent some heart attacks and strokes and have some value, although the limited benefits would need to be compared with costs and side effects. Sometimes a clinician treating a patient and a public health practitioner considering an intervention with wide population impact interpret research findings differently.

In addition, before the findings of a study can be put to general clinical use, the issue of whether the study has **external validity**, or generalizability, must be addressed. In a clinical trial of a new drug, one must ask whether the **sample** of patients in the study is representative of the **universe** of patients for whom the new drug eventually might be used. Studies can lack external validity because the **spectrum of disease** in the sample of patients is different from the spectrum of disease in the universe of patients. Types, stages, and severity of disease can vary. The spectrum must be defined clearly in terms of the criteria for including or excluding patients, and these criteria must be reported with the findings. If patients with a severe form of the disease were excluded from the study, this **exclusion criterion** must be reported because the results of the study would not be generalizable to patients with severe disease. (See the discussion of the Physicians' Health Study in Chapter 4; the results from a study of healthy, compliant physicians might not be generalizable to all adults.)

The study also can lack external validity because the **spectrum of individual characteristics** in the sample of patients was different from the spectrum of individual characteristics in the universe of patients. The sample could differ from most patients on the basis of age, gender, income or educational level, or ethnic background, among other characteristics.

5. SUMMARY

Statistics is an aid to inductive reasoning, which is an effort to find generalizable relationships and differences in observed data. It is the reverse process from mathematics, which is the attempt to apply known formulas to specific data to predict an outcome. Statistics helps investigators reach reasonable conclusions and estimations from observed data and provide approximate limits to the probability of being in error when making conclusions and estimations from the data. Significance testing starts with the statement of a null hypothesis, such as that there is no true difference between the mean of a measure from an experimental group and the mean from a control group. The next step is to calculate a test statistic (usually a critical ratio) and its associated p value to estimate the probability of being wrong if the null hypothesis is rejected. If the re-

sults of the significance test allow the investigator to reject the null hypothesis, then there is evidence of a difference between groups.

The two-sample t-test enables the investigator to compare the means of a continuous variable (e.g., weight) from two different groups of study participants to determine whether the difference between the means is greater than would be expected by chance alone. The paired t-test enables the investigator to evaluate the average in a continuous variable in a group of study participants before and after an intervention is given. In contrast to t-tests, which compare the difference between means, z-tests compare the difference between proportions.

REFERENCES

1. Moore DS, McCabe GP. *Introduction to the Practice of Statistics*. 7th ed. New York, NY: Freeman; 2010.

SELECT READINGS

Dawson B, Trapp RG. *Basic & Clinical Biostatistics*. 4th ed. New York, NY: Lange Medical Books/McGraw-Hill; 2004.

Silver N. *The Signal and the Noise: Why So Many Predictions Fail— but Some Don't*. New York, NY: Penguin Press; 2012.

REVIEW QUESTIONS

1. In your work at a local hospital, the first three medical interns you meet report feeling much better since they started taking a commonly prescribed antidepressant. You reluctantly draw the conclusion that internship is associated with depression. Drawing this conclusion is an example of:
   A. Hypothesis testing
   B. Inductive reasoning
   C. Deductive reasoning
   D. Interpolation
   E. Extrapolation

2. When 100 students were asked to read this chapter, the mean amount of time it took for each student to vaguely comprehend the text was 3.2 hours, with a 95% confidence interval of 1.4 to 5.0 hours. The 95% confidence interval in this case represents:
   A. The sample mean of 3.2 ± 1 standard deviation
   B. The population mean of 3.2 ± the standard error
   C. The maximum and minimum possible values for the true population mean
   D. The range of values for which we can be 95% confident contains the sample mean
   E. The range of values for which we can be 95% confident contains the population mean

3. The basic goal of hypothesis testing in clinical medicine is:
   A. To confirm the alternative hypothesis
   B. To determine if there is a meaningful difference in outcome between groups
   C. To establish a p value
   D. To establish an alpha value
   E. To establish a beta value

4. Alpha, in statistical terms, represents:
   A. False-negative error
   B. Sample size
   C. Selection bias
   D. Type I error
   E. 1 – beta

5. Statistical significance is achieved when:
   A. Alpha is greater than or equal to p
   B. Beta is greater than or equal to alpha
   C. p is greater than or equal to alpha
   D. p is greater than or equal to beta
   E. The result is two tailed

6. For a test of the latest athlete's foot treatment, alpha is set at 0.01 and beta is set at 0.30. In a two-tailed test, the new treatment is superior to the standard of care at $p = 0.04$, producing feet that are 1 point less malodorous on a 100-point olfactory assault scale in 5% of patients. This result:
   A. Shows a statistically significant difference between therapies
   B. Shows a clinically meaningful difference between therapies
   C. Would be less significant if the test were one tailed
   D. Favors continued use of the standard of care in clinical practice
   E. Would allow investigators to reject the null hypothesis

7. Six volunteers have gone on a high–oat bran cholesterol-lowering diet for 3 months. Pretrial and posttrial cholesterol values are as follows:

	CHOLESTEROL LEVEL (mg/dL)	
Subject	Pretrial	Posttrial
1	180	182
2	225	220
3	243	241
4	150	140
5	212	222
6	218	216

What is the standard error for these data?
   A. $33.8\sqrt{7}$
   B. $33.8\sqrt{6}$
   C. $33.8\sqrt{5}$
   D. $\sqrt{33.8}/6$
   E. $\sqrt{33.8}/5$

8. In the trial described in question 7, the appropriate test of statistical significance is:
   A. The critical ratio
   B. The odds ratio
   C. The two-sample t-test
   D. The paired t-test
   E. The z-test

9. In the trial described in question 7, by mere inspection of the data, what can you conclude about the difference in pretrial and posttrial cholesterol values?
   A. Even if clinically significant, the difference cannot be statistically significant
   B. Even if statistically significant, the difference is probably not clinically significant
   C. If clinically significant, the difference must be statistically significant
   D. If statistically significant, the difference must be clinically significant
   E. The difference cannot be clinically or statistically significant

10. In the trial described in question 7, the difference between pretrial and posttrial cholesterol values ultimately is not statistically significant. Before concluding that oat bran does not reduce cholesterol levels, you would want to consider:
    A. Type II error
    B. The alpha level
    C. The critical ratio
    D. The p value
    E. Type I error

ANSWERS AND EXPLANATIONS

1. **B.** A logical progression from the specific to the general, inductive reasoning is a process in which one draws conclusions about general associations based on specific data. In this example, based on the specific experience of three medical interns (obviously a small and limited sample), you draw a general association between internship and depression. In contrast, deductive reasoning (C) involves making specific predictions based on general rules or hypotheses. For example, if it was established as a general rule that medical interns tend to be miserable and depressed, you might predict there would be a good chance that any specific intern you met would be taking (or needing) an antidepressant. Hypothesis testing (A) involves running an experiment to test predictions. For instance, holding the general rule that medical interns tend to be miserable and depressed, we might predict that antidepressants would benefit such interns, and we could randomize a sample of interns to antidepressant or placebo to test this hypothesis. Interpolation (D) is the process of

predicting new data points within a given data range. For example, in a plot of depression severity versus daily work hours, if we know how depressed interns are who work 10 hours per day, and how depressed interns are who work 14 hours per day, we can interpolate how depressed an intern who works 12 hours per day might be. Extrapolation (E) is the prediction of new data points outside of known range. In the example, we would have to extrapolate how depressed an intern who works 16 hours per day would be since this data point would be outside the known range of depression severity when working 10–14 hours per day.

2. **E.** The 95% confidence interval is the range of values around which we can be reasonably certain the population mean should be. Specifically, an investigator can be 95% confident that the true population mean lies within this range. The sample mean (D) serves as the midpoint of the 95% confidence interval. The sample mean can be determined with complete confidence (it is calculated directly from known sample values); thus there is a 100% chance that the 95% confidence interval contains the sample mean, and a 0% chance that the value falls outside this range. The sample mean ± 1 standard deviation (A) is a convention for reporting values in the medical literature. The sample mean ± 1 standard error is also sometimes seen in medical literature, but not the population mean ± standard error (B), because usually the population mean is not known. To determine the maximum and minimum possible values for a population mean (C), you would need to have a 100% confidence interval (i.e., the sample mean ± infinity standard errors). In other words, all possible values would have to be known.

3. **B.** The fundamental goals of hypothesis testing in clinical medicine are to determine whether differences between groups exist, are large enough to be statistically significant (i.e., not likely the result of random variation), and substantial enough to be clinically meaningful (i.e., matter in terms of clinical practice). The p value (C) allows you to determine if a result is statistically significant. However, this value does not tell you whether observed differences between groups are clinically important (vs. being too small to affect patient care). Only consideration of trial findings in the context of other clinical knowledge can answer the question, "Is the difference large enough to mean something in practice?" Also, a p value is only interpretable in the context of a predetermined alpha value. Both the alpha value (D) and beta value (E) should be established before hypothesis testing begins and are therefore not themselves goals of conducting hypothesis tests. Alpha and beta are preconditions influencing the stringency of statistical significance

and investigators' ability to detect a difference between groups. Both alpha and beta influence the likelihood of rejecting the null hypothesis. Conventionally, trials in clinical medicine are set up to reject the null hypothesis rather than confirm the alternative hypothesis (A).

4. **D.** The value of alpha represents the probability of committing type I error (i.e., false-positive error; or probability of believing an association exists when in fact it does not). By convention, alpha is set at 0.05, indicating that a statistically significant result is one with no more than a 5% chance of false-positive error occurring (i.e., error caused by chance or random variation). The smaller the value of alpha, the less likely one is to make a type I error. False-negative error (A)—type II error or the probability of believing an association does not exist when one in fact does—is represented by beta. The quantity 1 – beta (E) is power (a.k.a. sensitivity), the likelihood of finding an association when one actually exists. Alpha influences sample size (B) but does not represent sample size directly. Alpha is entirely unrelated to selection bias (C). *Note:* In addition to representing type I or false-positive error, the Greek letter alpha (α) is also often used in statistics to represent the intercept in regression equations, where it has an entirely different meaning (see Chapter 11).

5. **A.** The value of p is the probability that an observed outcome difference is caused by random variation, or chance, alone. Alpha is the maximum risk that one is willing to take on the observed outcome difference being caused by chance. One rejects the null hypothesis ("no difference") whenever p is less than or equal to the preselected value of alpha. By convention, alpha is usually set at 0.05 so p of 0.05 or less indicates statistical significance in most cases. Answer choice C reverses the relationship between p and alpha. Statistical significance has little to do with beta (B and D); beta is important only in setting how much false-negative error one is willing to accept. By convention, beta is set at 0.2, meaning one is willing to accept a 20% chance of not finding a difference when a difference actually exists. Beta influences power (i.e., sensitivity) and affects the sample size needed to detect the statistically significant difference set by alpha. Whether a test is one tailed or two tailed (E) affects the p at which a result is "statistically significant," but the number of tails (i.e., whether the hypothesis is one tailed and directional or two tailed and nondirectional) does not itself equate to statistical significance.

6. **D.** The p value in this case is not less than the predetermined alpha of 0.01. Thus the result shows no statistically significant difference between therapies (A) and would therefore not allow investigators to reject the null hypothesis of no difference between therapies (E).

The new treatment does not appear to be different from usual therapy in a statistically significant way; thus the results of the study favor continued use of the standard of care. The difference between therapies would have been more significant by a one-tailed test (C), although even if p were then less than alpha, the clinical difference seems trivial. Even for feet that are malodorous, a 1-point difference on a 100-point scale for only 5% of the treated patients would not be clinically meaningful (B).

7. **B.** The standard error (SE) is the standard deviation (SD) divided by the square root of the sample size, or SE $= SD/\sqrt{3N}$. In this case, SD is 33.8 and the sample size is 6. Thus answer choices A, C, D, and E are incorrect. The SE is smaller than the SD. This is to be expected conceptually and mathematically. Conceptually, SD is a measure of dispersion (variation) among individual observations, and SE is a measure of variation among means derived from repeated trials. One would expect that mean outcomes would vary less than their constituent observations. Mathematically, SE is SD divided by the square root of the sample size. The larger the sample size, the smaller the SE and the greater the difference between the SD and SE.

8. **D.** A t-test is appropriate whenever two means are being compared and the population data from which the observations are derived are normally distributed. When the data represent pretrial and posttrial results for a single group of subjects (i.e., when participants serve as their own controls), the paired t-test is appropriate. Conversely, when the two means are from distinct groups, a two-sample t-test (C) is appropriate. The paired t-test is more appropriate in detecting a statistically significant difference than the two-sample t-test when the data are paired because the variation has been reduced to that from one group rather than two groups. A critical ratio (A) is not a specific test of statistical significance, but a metric common across many tests of statistical significance: a ratio of some parameter over the standard error for that parameter allowing for the calculation of a p value. In the case of t-tests (paired or two-sample tests), the parameter in question is the difference between two means. The odds ratio (B) relates to the odds of observing a critical ratio as large or larger than one observed (see Chapter 6). The odds ratio would be appropriate if, for example, one were looking at participants with low versus high cholesterol values and comparing who had eaten oat bran and who had not. The z-test (E) is appropriate when considering differences in proportions rather than means (e.g., proportion of high-cholesterol participants having eaten oat bran vs. proportion of low-cholesterol participants having eaten oat bran).

9. **B.** Statistical significance and clinical significance are not synonymous. A clinically important intervention might fail to show statistical benefit over another intervention in a trial if the sample size is too small to detect the difference. Conversely, a statistically significant difference in outcomes may result when the sample size is very large, but the magnitude of difference may have little or no clinical importance. In the cholesterol-lowering diet described, inspection of the pretrial and posttrial data suggests that the data are unlikely to result in statistical significance, but one cannot be certain of this without formal hypothesis testing (and formal testing confirms there is no effect). Regardless, the data do not show a clinically significant effect, because greater changes in cholesterol would be needed to affect clinical outcomes (e.g., heart attacks) or even intermediate outcomes (e.g., reductions in cholesterol toward target levels). In contrast to statistical significance, which is purely numerical, clinical significance is the product of judgment. Statistical and clinical significance are separate, nondependent considerations and thus answer choices C and D are incorrect. Answers A and E are incorrect because the difference could conceivably be statistically significant, but there is no way to tell by mere inspection alone.

10. **A.** A negative result in a trial may indicate that the null hypothesis is true (that there is in fact no difference) or it may be caused by type II error (false-negative error). Beta error generally receives less attention in medicine than alpha error. Consequently, the likelihood of a false-negative outcome is often unknown. A negative result can occur if the sample size is too small, if an inadequate dosage is administered (e.g., of oat bran in this case), or if the difference one is trying to detect is too large (e.g., one greater than needed for clinical significance). (See Chapter 12 for further discussion of type II error and the related concept of power.) Changing the alpha level (B)—specifically, increasing it—would make it more likely that an observed difference achieves statistical significance. For example, if the difference between pretrial and posttrial values had $p = 0.25$, this would not be significant at alpha $= 0.05$. However, it would be significant had one reset alpha, for example, to 0.3. The problem with such a strategy is that one always sets alpha before doing a trial. To reset alpha later would be difficult to justify and in most cases unethical. Moreover, setting alpha at 0.3 means one would be willing to accept a 30% chance of finding a difference when a difference does not actually exist (i.e., 30% risk of type I error) (E). Beta is also set before the trial and cannot be changed after the trial. However, if one truly believes oat bran lowers cholesterol despite a result showing no difference,

one should consider beta and use this consideration to redesign a trial with a new, lower beta (i.e., lower chance of false-negative error, higher sensitivity, and higher power). For example, one might run the trial again enrolling a larger number of volunteers or giving a larger dose of oat bran to see if this improves the situation. The critical ratio (C) is set by the statistical test chosen and is unmodifiable. In this case the critical ratio is the difference in pretrial and posttrial means over the standard errors of the pretrial and posttrial means. The p value (D) derives from running the statistical test and informs one how likely a difference as large could have been found by chance alone.

Analyzing Relationships Between Two Variables

CHAPTER OUTLINE

"Numbers have an important story to tell. They rely on you to give them a clear and convincing voice."

Stephen Few

Several statistical tests can be used to analyze the relationships between two or more variables. This chapter focuses on **bivariate analysis**, which is the analysis of the relationship between two variables. Bivariate analysis typically assigns one variable as an independent (possibly causal) variable and one as a dependent (outcome) variable, although bivariate analysis does not require variation in one variable to be a consequence of the other variable. Chapter 11 focuses on **multivariable analysis**, or the analysis of the relationship of more than one independent variable to a single dependent variable. The term *multivariate* technically refers to analysis of multiple dependent variables, such as in longitudinal analyses, although it is often inappropriately used interchangeably with the term *multivariable*.

Statistical tests are chosen for a specific data analysis based on the types of clinical data to be analyzed and the research design. The statistical test must be appropriate for the scientific metrics used (e.g., comparisons of means or rates). In general, the analytic approach begins with a prespecified analysis plan. Before analysis, data for individual variables are studied by determining distributions and outliers and searching for errors. Then bivariate analysis can be performed to test hypotheses and determine relationships. Only after these procedures have been done, and if there is more than one independent variable to consider, is multivariable analysis appropriate.

1. CHOOSING AN APPROPRIATE STATISTICAL TEST

Statistical testing is not required when the results of interest are purely descriptive, such as percentages, sensitivity, or specificity. Statistical testing is necessary when the investigator wants to formally evaluate whether there are meaningful differences in a characteristic between groups or over time, for example. Observed differences may be the result of random chance or may represent meaningful associations; statistical testing is intended to make this distinction.

TABLE 10.1   **Choice of Appropriate Statistical Significance Test in Bivariate Analysis (Analysis of One Independent Variable and One Dependent Variable)**

VARIABLES TO BE TESTED			
First Variable	**Second Variable**	**Appropriate Tests of Significance**	**Examples**
Continuous (C)	Continuous (C)	Pearson correlation coefficient (*r*); linear regression	Age (C) and measured systolic blood pressure (C)
	Ordinal (O)	ANOVA (F-test) or Spearman correlation coefficient (*rho*)	Age (C) and levels of satisfaction (O)*
	Dichotomous unpaired (DU)	Two-sample t-test	Systolic blood pressure (C) and stroke (yes/no) (DU)
	Dichotomous paired (DP)	Paired t-test	Difference in systolic blood pressure (C) before vs. after treatment (DP)
	Nominal (N)	ANOVA (F-test)	Hemoglobin level (C) and blood type (N)
Ordinal (O)	Ordinal (O)	Spearman correlation coefficient (*rho*); Kendall correlation coefficient (*tau*)	Correlation of care (O) and severity of illness (O)
	Dichotomous unpaired (DU)	Mann-Whitney U-test	Satisfaction (O) and cancer (yes/no) (DU)
	Dichotomous paired (DP)	Wilcoxon matched-pairs signed-ranks test	Difference in satisfaction (O) before vs. after a program (DP)
	Nominal (N)	Kruskal-Wallis test	Satisfaction (O) and ethnicity (N)
Dichotomous (D)	Dichotomous unpaired (DU)	Chi-square test; Fisher exact probability test	Success/failure (D) in treated/untreated groups
	Dichotomous paired (DP)	McNemar chi-square test	Change in success/failure (D) before vs. after treatment (DP)
	Nominal (N)	Chi-square test	Success/failure (D) and blood type (N)
Nominal (N)	Nominal (N)	Chi-square test	Ethnicity (N) and blood type (N)

*The following is an example of satisfaction described by an ordinal scale: "very satisfied," "somewhat satisfied," "neither satisfied nor dissatisfied," "somewhat dissatisfied," and "very dissatisfied."

Table 10.1 shows various tests of statistical significance that are available for bivariate (two-variable) analysis. The **types of variables** and the research design provide a general guide for determining which test or tests are appropriate. There are many kinds of variables, some of the most commonly used include *continuous* (e.g., levels of glucose in blood samples), *ordinal* (e.g., rankings of very satisfied, satisfied, and unsatisfied), *nominal* (e.g., race), and *dichotomous* (e.g., alive vs. dead). The term *nominal* can be used to refer to both polytomous and dichotomous data since dichotomous data is a subtype of polytomous data in which there are just two groups.

The type of research design is important when choosing a statistical test. Many of the statistical procedures outlined in this text, such as the two-sample t-test or z-test, assume that the sampling is done in such a way that all observations are independent. If, however, the research design involves, for example, *before-and-after comparisons* in the same study participants, or involves comparisons of matched pairs of study participants, a paired design may be needed for appropriately evaluating statistical significance (e.g., a *paired* t-test for a continuous outcome, McNemar's test for a dichotomous outcome). It is often important to consider which variables in the study are considered outcomes (dependent variables) and which are considered exposures (independent variables), or whether the relationship does not require this differentiation.

2. INFERENCES (PARAMETRIC ANALYSIS) FROM CONTINUOUS DATA

The distribution of a continuous variable is often characterized by a measure of location (e.g., the mean and a measure of its variation, such as the standard deviation). These quantities are referred to as **parameters**. Assumptions about the distributional form of data serve as the basis of statistical procedures on estimates of the parameters. These methods of analysis are referred to as *parametric*, in contrast to *nonparametric* methods, for which distributional assumptions about the outcome are not required. This section describes parametric analysis of continuous data.

Studies may involve evaluating the association between one variable that is continuous (e.g., systolic blood pressure) and another variable that is categorical (e.g., treatment groups). As shown in Table 10.1, a t-test may be appropriate for analyzing associations between a continuous and a dichotomous variable, while a one-way analysis of variance (ANOVA) is appropriate for analyzing the relationship between a continuous variable and a variable that has more than two groups. Chapter 9 discusses the use of two-sample and paired t-tests in detail and introduces the concept of ANOVA (see Variation Between Groups Versus Variation Within Groups).

The best way to evaluate the relationship between two continuous variables, such as the association between systolic and diastolic blood pressures, is to plot the data on a joint distribution graph for visual inspection (see next section) and then perform correlation analysis and simple linear regression analysis.

2.1 JOINT DISTRIBUTION GRAPH

The raw data concerning the systolic and diastolic blood pressures of 26 young adults were introduced in Chapter 9 and listed in Table 9.1. These same data can be plotted on a joint distribution graph, as shown in Fig. 10.1. The data lie generally along a straight line, from the lower left to the upper right on the graph, and all the observations except one are fairly close to the line.

As indicated in Fig. 10.2, the Pearson linear correlation between two variables, labeled x and y, can range from non-existent ($r = 0$) to strong ($r = +/- 1$). If the correlation is positive, this means that an increase in x is associated with an increase in y. Conversely, a negative correlation means that the value of y decreases as the value of x increases. Based on Fig. 10.1, there appears to be a real relationship between diastolic and systolic blood pressure and this relationship is positive and almost perfectly linear. The graph does not provide quantitative information about how strong the association is (although it looks strong to the eye), and the graph does not reveal the probability that such a relationship could have occurred by chance. To answer these questions more precisely, it is necessary to use the techniques of correlation analysis or simple linear regression.

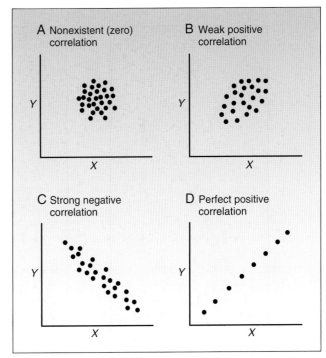

Fig. 10.2 Four possible patterns in joint distribution graphs. As seen in examples (A) to (D), the correlation between two continuous variables, labeled **X** and **Y**, can range from nonexistent to perfect. If the value of y increases as x increases, the correlation is positive. If y decreases as x increases, the correlation is negative.

2.2 PEARSON CORRELATION COEFFICIENT

Even without plotting the observations for two continuous variables on a graph, the strength of their linear relationship can be determined by calculating the **Pearson product-moment correlation coefficient**. This coefficient is given the symbol r, referred to as the **Pearson r**, which varies from -1 to $+1$. An estimate of $r = -1$ indicates the two variables have a perfect negative or inverse linear relationship, $r = +1$ indicates that they have a perfect positive or direct linear relationship, and 0 indicates that the two variables are not linearly associated. The r value is rarely found to be -1 or $+1$, but frequently there is an imperfect correlation between the two variables, resulting in r values between 0 and 1 or between 0 and -1. Because the Pearson correlation coefficient is strongly influenced by extreme values, it is important to plot the data to determine if the resulting r is heavily influenced by any outliers (Fig. 10.3).

The formula for the correlation coefficient r is shown here. The numerator is an estimate of the sample covariance. The **covariance** is a measure of the magnitude and direction of how x and y tend to jointly vary. When marked on a graph, this usually gives a rectangular area, in contrast to the sum of squares, which are squares of the deviations from the mean. The denominator of r is the standard deviations of the x and y variables:

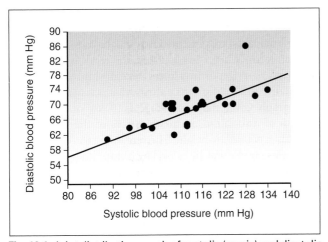

Fig. 10.1 Joint distribution graph of systolic (x-axis) and diastolic (y-axis) blood pressure values of 26 young adult participants. The raw data for these participants are listed in Table 9.1. The correlation between the two variables is strong and positive.

$$r = \frac{\sum (x_i - \bar{x})(y_i - \bar{y})}{\sqrt{\sum (x_i - \bar{x})^2 \sum (y_i - \bar{y})^2}}$$

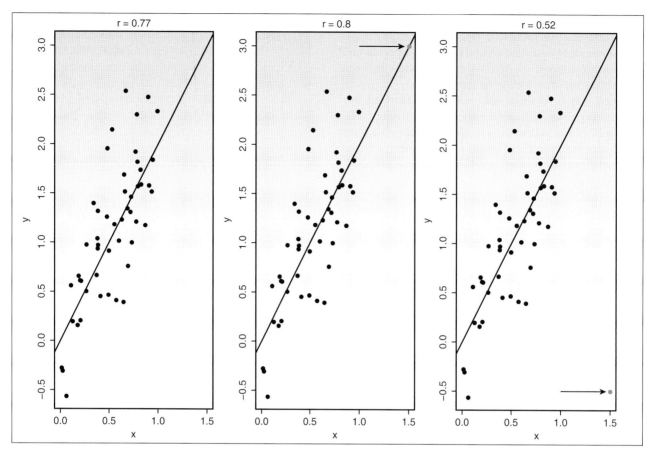

Fig. 10.3 Outliers in Linear Models. In the figures above, the solid line illustrates the true relationship between x and y for the black points. In the left figure, the estimated Pearson correlation is 0.77. In the middle figure a blue point has been added to the plot (see arrow pointing to the new blue point). Even though the blue point is far outside the range of the black points, it lies directly on the line and therefore has little effect on the estimated Pearson correlation coefficient. In the figure on the right, the blue point has been moved far off of the line (see arrow pointing to this blue point). This point is an outlier that changes the correlation between x and y from 0.77 to 0.52. (image courtesy of Martiniano J. Flores, PhD.)

Using statistical computer programs, investigators can determine whether the value of r is greater than would be expected by chance alone (i.e., whether the two variables are statistically associated). Most statistical programs provide the p value along with the correlation coefficient, but the p value of the correlation coefficient can be calculated easily. Its associated t statistic can be calculated from the following formula, and the p value can be determined from a table of t[1]:

$$t = r\frac{\sqrt{n-2}}{\sqrt{1-r^2}} \qquad df = N-2$$

As with every test of significance, for a given nonzero association, the larger the sample size, the more likely it is to be statistically significant. A weak correlation in a large sample might be statistically significant, even if it is not etiologically or clinically important (see later and Box 10.5). The converse may also be true; a result that is statistically weak still may be of public health and clinical importance if it pertains to a large portion of the population.

There is no statistical method for estimating clinical importance, but with continuous variables, a valuable concept is the **strength of the association**, measured by the square of the correlation coefficient, or R^2 ("R-squared"). R^2 is the proportion of variation in y (usually the outcome) explained by x (the exposure). It is an important parameter in model assessment.

For purposes of showing the calculation of r and R^2, a small set of data is introduced in Box 10.1. The data, consisting of the observed heights (variable x) and weights (variable y) of eight participants, are presented first in tabular form and then in graph form. When r is calculated, the result is 0.96, which indicates a strong positive linear relationship and provides quantitative information to confirm what is visually apparent in the graph. Given that r is 0.96, R^2 is $(0.96)^2$ or 0.92. A 0.92 strength of association means that 92% of the variation in weight is *explained* by height. The remaining 8% of the variation in this sample may be caused by factors other than height.

2.3 LINEAR REGRESSION ANALYSIS

Linear regression is related to correlation analysis, but it produces two parameters that can be useful for interpreting the relationships between variables: the slope and the intercept. **Linear regression** assumes a model where the variation of one variable (y) is considered to be a consequence of the other (predictor) variable (x). In simple correlation analysis, the two variables are treated more equally (symmetrically) since the correlation between x and y is the same as the correlation between y and x. More specifically, regression quantifies how the mean difference in the outcome y changes with a one-unit difference in x.

The formula for a straight line, in general, is $y = a + bx$ (see Chapter 9). The variable y corresponds to the ordinate of an observation (y-axis); x is the abscissa (x-axis); a is the regression constant (value of y when value of x is 0); and b is the slope (change in value of y for a unit change in value of x). Simple linear regression is used to estimate the slope of the line (b) and the y-intercept (a). In the example using heights and weights, the slope is used to summarize the expected increase in weight for a 1-cm increase in height. The intercept tells us the expected value of y for a person with an

average x value of zero, and thus it is most useful when the value of x is clinically meaningful.

When the usual statistical notation is used for a regression of y on x, the formulas for the slope (b) and y-intercept (a) are estimated as follows:

$$b = \frac{\sum(x_i - \bar{x})(y_i - \bar{y})}{\sum(x_i - \bar{x})^2}$$
$$a = \bar{y} - b\bar{x}$$

Box 10.1 shows the calculation of the slope (b) for the observed heights and weights of eight participants. The graph in Box 10.1 shows the linear relationship between the height and weight data, with the regression line inserted. In these

---

BOX 10.1   Analysis of Relationship Between Height and Weight (Two Continuous Variables) in Eight Study Participants

Part 1 Tabular and Graphic Representation of the Data

Participant	Variable x (Height, cm)	Variable y (Weight, kg)
1	182.9	78.5
2	172.7	60.8
3	175.3	68.0
4	172.7	65.8
5	160.0	52.2
6	165.1	54.4
7	172.7	60.3
8	162.6	52.2

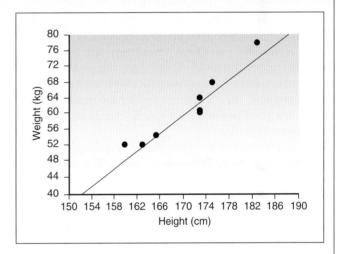

Part 2 Data Calculations

$\sum(x_i) = 1364 \, cm$

$\sum(y_i) = 492.2 \, kg$

$N = 8$

$\bar{x} = 1364 / 8 = 170.50 \, cm$

$\bar{y} = 492.2 / 8 = 61.53 \, kg$

$\sum(x_i - \bar{x})(y_i - \bar{y}) = 456.88$

$\sum(x_i - \bar{x})^2 = 393.1$

$\sum(y_i - \bar{y})^2 = 575.1$

Note: Characteristics of the distribution can be calculated from the raw data, including the number of observations, the sum of their values, the mean, the variance, the standard deviation, and tests of normality.

Part 3 Calculation of Pearson Correlation Coefficient (r) and Strength of Association of Variables (R^2)

$$r = \frac{\sum(x_i - \bar{x})(y_i - \bar{y})}{\sqrt{\sum(x_i - \bar{x})^2 \sum(y_i - \bar{y})^2}}$$

$$= \frac{456.88}{\sqrt{(393.1)(575.1)}} = \frac{456.88}{\sqrt{226,071.8}} = \frac{456.88}{475.47} = 0.96$$

$$r^2 = (0.96)^2 = 0.92 = 92\%$$

Interpretation: The two variables are highly correlated. The association between the two variables is strong and positive with 92% of variation in weight (y) explained by variation in height (x).

Continued

BOX 10.1   Analysis of Relationship Between Height and Weight (Two Continuous Variables) in Eight Study Participants—cont'd

Part 4 Calculation of the Slope (*b*) for a Regression of Weight (*y*) on Height (*x*)

$$b = \frac{\sum(x_i - \bar{x})(y_i - \bar{y})}{\sum(x_i - \bar{x})^2} = \frac{456.88}{393.1} = 1.16$$

Interpretation: There is a 1.16-kg increase in weight (*y*) for each 1-cm increase in height (*x*). The *y*-intercept, which indicates the value of *x* when *y* is 0, is not meaningful in the case of these two variables and it is not calculated here. Variables can often be centered so that the intercept is meaningful. For example, using (height – mean height) sets a *y*-intercept that could indicate the expected weight for someone with average height in the sample.

Data from unpublished findings in a sample of eight young adults in Connecticut.

eight participants, the slope is 1.16, meaning that there is an average difference of 1.16 kg of weight for every 1-cm difference in height.

Linear regression analysis enables investigators to predict the value of *y* from the values that *x* takes. The formula for linear regression is a form of statistical modeling, where the adequacy of the model is determined by how closely the value of *y* can be predicted from the other variable. For example, how much the systolic blood pressure increases, on the average, for each added year of age. Linear regression is useful in answering routine questions in clinical practice, such as, "How much exercise do I need to do to raise my HDL 10 points, or lose 10 pounds?" Such questions involve the magnitude of change in a given factor, *y*, for a specific change in behavior, or exposure, *x*.

Just as it is possible to set confidence intervals around parameters such as means and proportions (see Chapter 9), it is possible to set confidence intervals around the parameters of the regression, the slope, and the intercept using computations based on linear regression formulas. Most statistical computer programs perform these computations, and moderately advanced statistics books provide the formulas.[2] Multiple linear regression and other methods involved in the analysis of more than two variables are discussed in Chapter 11.

3. INFERENCES (NONPARAMETRIC ANALYSIS) FROM ORDINAL DATA

Medical data are often ordinal, meaning the observations can be ranked from the lowest value to the highest value, but they are not measured on an exact scale. In some cases, investigators assume that ordinal data meet the criteria for continuous (measurement) data and analyze these variables as though they had been obtained from a measurement scale. To study patients' satisfaction with the care in a hospital, investigators might assume that the conceptual distance between "very satisfied" (e.g., coded as a 3) and "fairly satisfied" (coded as a 2) is equal to the difference between "fairly satisfied" (coded as a 2) and "unsatisfied" (coded as a 1). If the investigators are willing to make these assumptions, the data might be analyzed using the parametric statistical methods discussed here, such

as t-tests, analysis of variance, and analysis of the Pearson correlation coefficient.

If investigators are not willing to assume that an ordinal variable can be analyzed as though it were continuous, bivariate statistical tests for ordinal data can be used[1,3] (see Table 10.1 and later description). Tests specific for ordinal data are **nonparametric**. Hand calculation of tests for ordinal data is extremely tedious and prone to errors, thus the use of a computer for these calculations is customary.

3.1 MANN-WHITNEY U-TEST

The test for ordinal data that is similar to the two-sample t-test is the **Mann-Whitney U-test** (often referred to as the Wilcoxon rank-sum test). *U*, similar to *t*, designates a probability distribution. In the Mann-Whitney test, all the observations in a study of two samples (e.g., experimental and control groups) are ranked numerically from the smallest to the largest without regard to whether the observations came from the experimental group or from the control group. Next, the observations from the experimental group are identified, the values of the ranks in this sample are summed, and the average rank and the variance of those ranks are determined. The process is repeated for the observations from the control group.

The Mann-Whitney test defines the null hypothesis as a 50:50 chance that a randomly selected observation from one population (*x*) would be larger than an observation from the other population (*y*). If the null hypothesis is true, the average ranks of the two samples should be similar. If the average rank of one sample is considerably greater than that of the other sample, the null hypothesis probably can be rejected, but a test of significance is needed to be sure.

3.2 WILCOXON MATCHED-PAIRS SIGNED-RANKS TEST

The rank-order test that is comparable to the paired t-test is the **Wilcoxon matched-pairs signed-ranks test**. In this test, all the observations in a study of two samples are ranked numerically from the largest to the smallest, without regard to whether the observations came from the first sample (e.g., pretreatment sample) or from the second sample (e.g., post-treatment sample). After pairs of data are identified (e.g., pretreatment and posttreatment observations are linked), the pretreatment-posttreatment difference in rank is identified for each pair. For example, if for a given pair the pretreatment observation scored 7 ranks higher than the posttreatment observation, the difference would be noted as −7. If in another pair the pretreatment observation scored 5 ranks lower than the posttreatment observation, the difference would be noted as +5. Each pair would be scored in this way. The rank-order test defines the null hypothesis as the "median pairwise mean" is equal to zero, in the absence of additional assumptions for the underlying characteristic (e.g., symmetry). If the null hypothesis is true, the sum of the positive and negative scores should be close to zero. If the average difference is considerably different from zero, the null hypothesis can be rejected.

3.3 KRUSKAL-WALLIS TEST

If the investigators of a study involving continuous data want to compare the means of three or more groups simultaneously, the appropriate test is a one-way analysis of variance (a one-way ANOVA), usually called an F-test. The comparable test for ordinal data is called the Kruskal-Wallis test or the **Kruskal-Wallis one-way ANOVA**. As in the Mann-Whitney U-test, for the Kruskal-Wallis test, all the data are ranked numerically and the rank values are summed in each of the groups to be compared. The Kruskal-Wallis test seeks to determine if the average ranks from three or more groups differ from one another more than would be expected by chance alone. It is another example of a critical ratio (see Chapter 9), in which the magnitude of the difference is in the numerator and a measure of the random variability is in the denominator. If the ratio is sufficiently large, the null hypothesis is rejected.

3.4 SPEARMAN AND KENDALL CORRELATION COEFFICIENTS

When relating two *continuous* variables to each other, investigators often use regression analysis when the variation of one of the two variables is considered to be a consequence of the other variable; or correlation analysis, when either there is no prespecified need to evaluate one of the variables being dependent upon the other, or if the two variables are being treated symmetrically. For *ordinal* data, the **Spearman rank correlation coefficient** (*rho*) and **Kendall rank correlation coefficient** (*tau*) are used to assess associations between variables. Unlike the Pearson correlation coefficient *r* which measures the strength of linear associations among variables, *rho* measures the strength of any strictly increasing or decreasing relationship between variables, even if the relationship is nonlinear. The tests for *rho* and *tau* usually give similar results, but *rho* is more often used in the medical literature, perhaps because of its conceptual similarity to the Pearson *r*. The *tau* may give better results with small sample sizes.

3.5 SIGN TEST AND THE MOOD MEDIAN TEST

Sometimes an experimental intervention produces positive results on many different measurements, but few if any of the individual outcome variables show a difference that is statistically significant. When clinically appropriate, the **sign test** can be used to compare the results in the experimental group with those in the control group. If the null hypothesis is true (i.e., there is no real difference between the groups), by chance, the experimental group should perform better on about half the measurements, and the control group should perform better on the other half.

For paired data (i.e., each person is his or her own control), the sign test can determine whether there is a significant change in the response in the experimental group. The only data needed for the sign test are the records of whether, on average, the experimental participants or the control participants scored "better" on each outcome variable (by what amount is not important). If the average score for a given variable is better in the experimental group, the result is recorded as a plus sign (+); if the average score for that variable is better in the control group, the result is recorded as a minus sign (−); and if the average score in the two groups is exactly the same, no result is recorded and the variable is omitted from the analysis. Because under the null hypothesis the expected proportion of plus signs is 0.5 and of minus signs is 0.5, the test compares the observed proportion of successes with the expected value of 0.5.

The **Mood median test** compares two independent samples to determine whether they have the same median. Like the sign test, the null hypothesis states there is no difference between the two groups. In the Mood median test, each observation is compared to the overall median when the two groups are pooled together. If an observation is above the pooled median, it is recorded as a plus sign (+), and if not, it is recorded as a minus (−) sign. A 2 × 2 table indicating the numbers of pluses and minuses within each group is constructed and a chi-square test is performed (see upcoming discussion) to determine whether the proportions of pluses in each group are the same. The null hypothesis is rejected if the medians of the two groups are not the same.

4. INFERENCES (NONPARAMETRIC ANALYSIS) FROM DICHOTOMOUS AND NOMINAL DATA

As indicated in Table 10.1, the chi-square test, Fisher exact probability test, and McNemar chi-square test can be used in the analysis of dichotomous data, although they are based on different statistical theory. Usually the data are first arranged in a 2 × 2 table in order to test the null hypothesis that the variables are independent.

4.1 2 × 2 CONTINGENCY TABLE

Data arranged as in Box 10.2 form what is known as a *contingency table*, because it is used to determine whether the distribution of one variable is conditionally dependent (contingent) on the other variable. More specifically, Box 10.2 provides an example of a 2 × 2 contingency table, meaning that it has two cells in each direction. Generally, 2 × 2 tables are constructed with the outcome or dependent variable in the columns and the exposure in the rows. In this case, the table shows the data for a study of 91 patients who had a myocardial infarction.[4] One variable is treatment (propranolol vs. a placebo) and the other is outcome (survival for at least 28 days vs. death within 28 days).

A cell is a specific location in a contingency table. In this case, each cell shows the observed number, the expected number, and the percentage of study participants in each treatment group who lived or died. In Box 10.2 the top left cell indicates that 38 patients who were treated with propranolol survived the first 28 days of observation, that they represented 84% of all patients who were treated with propranolol, and that 33.13 patients treated with propranolol were expected to survive the first 28 days of observation, based on the null hypothesis. The methods for calculating the percentages and expected counts are discussed subsequently.

The other three cells indicate the same type of data (observed number, expected number, and percentage) for patients who died after propranolol treatment, patients who survived after placebo treatment, and patients who died after placebo treatment. The bottom row shows the column totals, and the right-hand column shows the row totals.

If there are more than two cells in each direction of a contingency table, the table is called an $R \times C$ table, where R stands for the number of rows and C stands for the number of columns. Although the principles of the chi-square test are valid for $R \times C$ tables, the subsequent discussion focuses on 2 × 2 tables for the sake of simplicity.

4.2 CHI-SQUARE TEST OF INDEPENDENCE

Along with t-tests, another statistical test commonly reported in the medical literature is the **chi-square test** of the independence of two variables in a contingency table.[5] The chi-square test is another example of a common approach to statistical analysis known as **statistical modeling**, which seeks to develop a statistical expression (the model) that predicts the behavior of a dependent variable on the basis of knowledge of one or more independent variables. The process of comparing the **observed counts** with the **expected counts**—that is, of comparing O with E—is called a **goodness-of-fit test**, because the goal is to see how well the observed counts in a contingency table fit the counts expected on the basis of the model. Usually the model in such a table is the null hypothesis that the two variables are independent of each other. If the chi-square value is small, the null hypothesis provides a good fit and it is not rejected. If the chi-square value is large,

however, the data do not fit the hypothesis well and the null hypothesis is rejected.

Box 10.2 illustrates the steps and considerations involved in constructing a 2 × 2 contingency table and in calculating the chi-square value. For the data presented in Box 10.2, the null hypothesis is that treating the myocardial infarction patients with propranolol is not associated with the percentage of patients who survived for at least 28 days. Treatment is the independent variable and the outcome of survival is the dependent variable. The alternative hypothesis is that the outcome (survival or death) is associated with treatment.

4.2.a. Calculation of Percentages

Each of the four cells of Box 10.2 shows an observed count and a percentage. The percentage in the first cell of the contingency table is calculated by dividing the number of propranolol-treated patients who survived (38) by the total number of propranolol-treated patients (45), which equals 84%. This percentage is calculated as the frequency distribution of the dependent variable (survival) within the propranolol-treated group.

If treatment was influenced by survival, rather than vice versa, the percentage would be calculated by dividing the number of propranolol-treated patients who survived (38) by the total number of survivors (67), but this arrangement does not make sense. The way the percentages are calculated affects the way people think about and interpret the data, but it does not influence the way the chi-square test is calculated. The appropriate way to calculate the percentages in a contingency table is to calculate the frequency distribution of the dependent variable within each category of the independent variable.

4.2.b. Calculation of Expected Counts

In Box 10.2, the propranolol-treated group consists of 45 patients, the placebo-treated group consists of 46 patients, and the total for the study is 91 patients. The observed counts indicate how many of each group actually survived, whereas the expected counts indicate how many of each group would be expected to survive if the method of treatment made no difference (i.e., if survival were independent of treatment). The formula for calculating the expected count in one cell of the table (here the top left cell) is as follows:

$$E_{1,1} = \frac{Row_1 \; total}{Study \; total} \times Column_1 \; total$$

where $E_{1,1}$ is defined as the expected value of the cell in row_1, $column_1$. The same is done for each cell in the table.

In Box 10.2, if survival were independent of the treatment group, 45 of 91 (or 49.45%) of the observations in each column would be expected to be in the top row, because that is the overall proportion of patients who received propranolol. It follows that 0.4945×67 (or 33.13) observations (the total in $column_1$) would be expected in the left upper cell, whereas 0.4945×24 (or 11.87) observations (the total in $column_2$) would be expected in the right upper cell. The *expected* counts may include fractions, and the sum of the expected

BOX 10.2 Chi-Square Analysis of Relationship Between Treatment and Outcome (Two Nonparametric Variables, Unpaired) in 91 Participants

Part 1 Beginning Data, Presented in a 2 × 2 Contingency Table, Where O Denotes Observed Counts and E Denotes Expected Counts

| | OUTCOME | | | | Total | |
| | Survival for at Least 28 Days | | Death before 28 days | | | |
TREATMENT	No.	(%)	No.	(%)	No.	(%)
Propranolol (O)	38	(84)	7	(16)	45	(100)
Propranolol (E)	33.13		11.87		45	
Placebo (O)	29	(63)	17	(37)	46	(100)
Placebo (E)	33.87		12.13		46	
Total	67	(74)	24	(26)	91	(100)

Part 2 Calculation of the Chi-Square (χ^2) Statistic

$$\chi^2 = \sum \left[\frac{(O-E)^2}{E} \right]$$

$$= \frac{(38-33.13)^2}{33.13} + \frac{(7-11.87)^2}{11.87} + \frac{(29-33.87)^2}{33.87} + \frac{(17-12.13)^2}{12.13}$$

$$= \frac{(4.87)^2}{33.13} + \frac{(-4.87)^2}{11.87} + \frac{(-4.87)^2}{33.87} + \frac{(4.87)^2}{12.13}$$

$$= \frac{23.72}{33.13} + \frac{23.72}{11.87} + \frac{23.72}{33.87} + \frac{23.72}{12.13}$$

$$= 0.72 + 2.00 + 0.70 + 1.96 = 5.38$$

Part 3 Calculation of Degrees of Freedom (df) for Contingency Table, Based on Number of Rows (R) and Columns (C)

$$df = (R-1)(C-1) = (2-1)(2-1) = 1$$

Part 4 Determination of the p Value

Value from the chi-square table for 5.38 on 1 df: $0.01 < p < 0.025$ (statistically significant)

Exact p from a computer program: 0.0205 (statistically significant)

Interpretation: The results noted in this 2 × 2 table are statistically significant. That is, it is highly probable (only 1 chance in about 50 of being wrong) that the investigator can reject the null hypothesis of independence and accept the alternative hypothesis that propranolol affects the outcome of myocardial infarction (the effect observed to be in a positive direction).

Data from Snow PJ: Effect of propranolol in myocardial infarction. *Lancet* 2:551–553, 1965.

counts in a given row should equal the sum of the observed counts in that row (33.13 + 11.87 = 45). By the same logic, 50.55% of observations would be expected to be in the bottom row, with 33.87 in the left lower cell and 12.13 in the right lower cell, so that the row total equals the sum of the observed counts (33.87 + 12.13 = 46). Finally, as shown in Box 10.2, the column totals for expected counts should add up to the column totals for observed counts.

The *expected* counts in *each cell* of a 2 × 2 contingency table should equal 5 or more, or the assumptions and approximations inherent in the chi-square test are not valid. For a study involving a larger contingency table (an $R \times C$ table), the investigator can allow up to 20% of the expected cell counts to be less than 5. If these conditions are not met, the Fisher exact probability test (see later in the chapter) should be used instead of the chi-square test.

4.2.c. Calculation of the Chi-Square Statistic

When the observed (O) and expected (E) counts are known, the chi-square (χ^2) statistic can be calculated. One of two methods can be used, depending on the size of the counts.

Method for large numbers. In Box 10.2, the investigators begin by calculating the chi-square statistic for each cell in the table, using the following formula:

$$\frac{(O-E)^2}{E}$$

The numerator is the square of the deviation of the observed count in a given cell from the count that would be expected in that cell if the null hypothesis were true. This is similar to the numerator of the variance, which is expressed as $\sum(x_i - \bar{x})^2$, where x_i is the *observed* value and $\bar{x}$ (the mean) is the *expected* value (see Chapter 8). The denominator for variance is the degrees of freedom ($N - 1$), however, the denominator for chi-square is the expected number (E).

To obtain the total chi-square statistic for a 2×2 table, the investigators add up the chi-square statistics for the four cells:

$$\chi^2 = \sum\left[\frac{(O-E)^2}{E}\right]$$

The basic statistical method for measuring the total amount of variation in a data set, the total sum of squares (TSS), is rewritten for the chi-square test as the sum of $(O - E)^2$.

Box 10.2 shows how chi-square is calculated for the study of 91 patients with myocardial infarction. Before the result ($\chi^2 = 5.38$) can be interpreted, the degrees of freedom must be determined.

4.2.d. Determination of Degrees of Freedom

As discussed in Chapter 9 and Box 9.3, the term *degrees of freedom* refers to the number of observations that can be considered to be free to vary. A statistician needs some solid (nonvarying) place to begin. According to the null hypothesis, the best estimate of the expected counts in the cells of a contingency table is given by the row and column totals, so they are considered to be fixed (in the same way as is the mean when calculating a variance). An observed count can be entered freely into one of the cells of a 2×2 table (e.g., top left cell), but when that count is entered, none of the other three cells are free to vary. This means that a 2×2 table has only 1 degree of freedom.

Another look at Box 10.2 helps explain why there is only 1 degree of freedom in a table with two rows and two columns. If 38 is entered freely in the top left cell, the only possible number that can go in the cell immediately to the right of it is 7, because the two numbers in the top row must equal the *fixed* row total of 45. Similarly, the only possible number that can go in the cell directly below is 29, because the column must add up to 67. Finally, the only possible number for the remaining cell is 17, because the row total must equal 46 and the column total must equal 24. This is illustrated in Fig. 10.4, where the cells that are free to vary are shown in white, the cells that are not free to vary are shown in light blue, and the fixed row and column totals are shown in dark blue. The top table in the figure corresponds to the table in Box 10.2.

The same principle applies to contingency tables with more than two rows and columns. In $R \times C$ contingency tables, imagine that the right-hand column and the bottom row are never free to vary because they must contain the numbers that make the totals come out right (see the bottom table in Fig. 10.4). The formula for degrees of freedom in a contingency table of any size is as follows:

$$df = (R-1)(C-1)$$

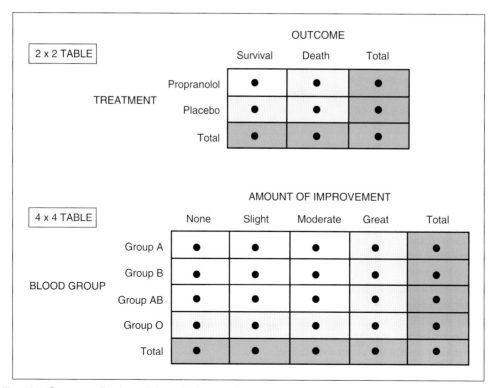

Fig. 10.4 Conceptualization of the calculation of the degrees of freedom *(df)* in a 2×2 contingency table *(top)* and in a 4×4 contingency table *(bottom)*. A *white* cell is free to vary, a *light-blue* cell is not free to vary, and a *dark-blue* cell is a row or column total. The formula is $df = (R - 1)(C - 1)$, where R denotes the number of rows and C denotes the number of columns. For 2×2 table, $df = 1$; for 4×4 table, $df = 9$.

where *df* denotes degrees of freedom, *R* is the number of rows, and *C* is the number of columns.

4.2.e. Interpretation of Results

After the chi-square statistic and the degrees of freedom are known, a standard table of chi-square statistics can be consulted to determine the corresponding *p* value. The *p* value indicates the probability that a chi-square statistic as large or larger would have resulted from chance alone. For data shown in Box 10.2, the chi-square statistic is 5.38 with 1 degree of freedom, and the *p* value listed for that chi-square statistic in the standard table for a two-tailed test is between 0.01 and 0.025 ($0.01 < p < 0.025$). Most computer programs provide the exact *p* value when calculating a chi-square; for the data in Box 10.2, the *p* value is 0.0205. Because the observed *p* is less than alpha (alpha = 0.05), the results are considered statistically significant, the null hypothesis that propranolol made no difference is rejected, and there is evidence for the alternative hypothesis that propranolol is associated with survival.

Hypotheses for chi-square tests are inherently two sided. However, if the investigator wants to test the null hypothesis that the propranolol-treated group has a higher survival rate than the placebo-treated group, a one-sided two-sample test of proportions could be used.

4.3 CHI-SQUARE TEST FOR PAIRED DATA (MCNEMAR TEST)

The chi-square test as just described is useful for comparing the distribution of a categoric variable in two or more groups, but a different test is needed to compare *before-and-after findings* in the *same individuals* or to compare findings in a matched analysis. The appropriate test for this situation for dichotomous variables is the McNemar chi-square test.

4.3.a. McNemar Test of Before-and-After Comparisons

The discussion of t-tests in Chapter 9 noted that when doing a before-and-after study, a research participant serves as his or her own control. Here it is appropriate to use the paired t-test, instead of the two-sample t-test. In the case of a matched 2 × 2 table, it is appropriate to use the **McNemar test**, which is a type of paired chi-square test of data with 1 degree of freedom.[1]

Suppose that an investigator wants to see how attitudes about visiting Paris changed among audience members after attending a particular Broadway show. The researcher enrolls 200 willing audience members who complete questionnaires indicating their interest in visiting Paris both before and after the show, and their responses are recorded as either positive or negative (i.e., dichotomous responses). The data could be set up in a 2 × 2 table with the preshow opinion on the left axis and the postshow opinion at the top, as shown in

Box 10.3. Each of the four cells represents one of the following four possible combinations:

- Cell *a* = Positive opinion before and after (no change)
- Cell *b* = Change from positive to negative opinion
- Cell *c* = Change from negative to positive opinion
- Cell *d* = Negative opinion before and after (no change)

According to the hypothetical data from 200 audience members who participated in the study, the overall percentage reporting a favorable opinion of visiting Paris decreased from 86% (172 of 200) before the show to 79% (158 of 200) after the show, presumably reflecting a response to the show content. The null hypothesis to be tested is that the show produced no true change in audience opinion, and the following formula would be used:

$$\text{McNemar} \chi^2 = \frac{\left(|b-c|-1\right)^2}{b+c}$$

The formula uses only cells *b* and *c* in the 2 × 2 table, because cells *a* and *d* do not correspond to changes of opinion and do not contribute to the standard error. Note also that the formula tests data with 1 degree of freedom. The subtraction of 1 in the numerator is called a correction for continuity.

The McNemar chi-square statistic for the data shown in Box 10.3 is 5.63. This result is statistically significant ($p < 0.025$), so that the null hypothesis is rejected. Care must be taken when interpreting these data, however, because the test of significance only states the following: "Among audience members *who changed their opinions*, the proportion of people who changed from positive to negative is different from the proportion of people who changed from negative to positive." Any adequate interpretation of the data also would need to indicate the following:

1. Of the audience members, 75% had a positive opinion throughout the study.
2. The percentage of the audience who changed their opinion is relatively small (15%).

4.3.b. McNemar Test of Matched Data

In medical research, the McNemar chi-square test is used frequently in case control studies, where the cases and controls are *matched* on the basis of characteristics such as age, gender, and residence, then *compared* for the presence or absence of a specific risk factor. Under these circumstances, the data can be set up in a 2 × 2 table similar to that shown in Box 10.4.

To illustrate the use of the McNemar test in matched data, the observations made in an actual case control study are discussed here and reported in the second part of Box 10.4.[6] In this study the investigator examines the association between mycosis fungoides (a type of lymphoma that begins in the skin and eventually spreads to internal organs) and a history of employment in an industrial environment with exposure to cutting oils. After matching 54 participants who had the disease (the cases) with 54 participants who did not have the disease (the controls), the investigator recorded whether the study participants had a history of this type of industrial employment.

BOX 10.3   McNemar Chi-Square Analysis of Relationship Between Data Before and Data After an Event (Two Dichotomous Variables, Paired) in a Study of 200 Participants

Part 1 Standard 2 × 2 Table Format on Which Equations Are Based

| | FINDINGS AFTER EVENT | | |
FINDINGS BEFORE EVENT	Positive	Negative	Total
Positive	a	b	$a + b$
Negative	c	d	$c + d$
Total	$a + c$	$b + d$	$a + b + c + d$

Part 2 Data for Study of Opinions of Audience Members Toward Travel to Paris Before and After Seeing a Particular Broadway Show

| | POSTSHOW OPINION | | |
PRESHOW OPINION	Positive	Negative	Total
Positive	150	22	172
Negative	8	20	28
Total	158	42	200

Part 3 Calculation of the McNemar Chi-Square (χ^2) Statistic

$$\text{McNemar}\,\chi^2 = \frac{\left(|b - c| - 1\right)^2}{b + c}$$

$$= \frac{\left(|22 - 8| - 1\right)^2}{22 + 8} = \frac{(13)^2}{30} = \frac{169}{30} = 5.63$$

Part 4 Calculation of Degrees of Freedom (*df*) for Contingency Table, Based on Number of Rows (*R*) and Columns (*C*)

$$df = (R - 1)(C - 1) = (2 - 1)(2 - 1) = 1$$

Part 5 Determination of the *p* Value

Value from the chi-square table for 5.63 with 1 *df*: $p < 0.025$ (statistically significant)

Interpretation: Among audience members who changed their opinions, the proportion of people who changed from positive to negative is different from the proportion of people who changed from negative to positive.

When the McNemar chi-square formula is used to test the null hypothesis that prior occupation is not associated with the development of mycosis fungoides (see Box 10.4), the chi-square statistic is 5.06. Because the result is statistically significant ($p = 0.021$), the null hypothesis is rejected, and results provide evidence for the alternative hypothesis that mycosis fungoides is associated with industrial exposure.

A matched odds ratio also can be calculated (see Chapter 6). When the data are set up as in Box 10.4, the ratio is calculated simply as b/c. Here the ratio is 13/3, or 4.33, indicating that the *odds* of acquiring mycosis fungoides is more than four times as great in participants with a history of industrial exposure than those without such a history.

4.4 FISHER EXACT PROBABILITY TEST

When one or more of the expected counts in a 2 × 2 table is small (i.e., <2), the chi-square test cannot be used. It is possible, however, to calculate the exact probability of finding the observed numbers by using the **Fisher exact probability test**. The formula is as follows:

$$\text{Fisher}\,p = \frac{(a + b)!\,(c + d)!\,(a + c)!\,(b + d)!}{N!\,a!\,b!\,c!\,d!}$$

where p is probability; a, b, c, and d denote values in the top left, top right, bottom left, and bottom right cells in a 2 × 2 table; N is the total number of observations; and ! is the symbol for factorial. For example, the factorial of $4 = 4! = 4 \times 3 \times 2 \times 1$.

The Fisher exact probability test would be extremely tedious to calculate manually, because unless one of the four cells contains a 0, the sum of more than one calculation is needed. Most commercially available statistical packages now calculate the Fisher probability automatically when an appropriate situation arises in a 2 × 2 table.

BOX 10.4 McNemar Chi-Square Analysis of Relationship Between Data from Cases and Data from Controls (Two Dichotomous Variables, Paired) in Case-Control Study of 54 Participants

Part 1 Standard 2 × 2 Table Format on Which Equations Are Based

	CONTROLS		
CASES	Risk Factor Present	Risk Factor Absent	Total
Risk Factor Present	a	b	$a + b$
Risk Factor Absent	c	d	$c + d$
Total	$a + c$	$b + d$	$a + b + c + d$

Part 2 Data for Case Control Study of Relationship Between Mycosis Fungoides (Disease) and History of Exposure to Industrial Environment Containing Cutting Oils (Risk Factor)

	CONTROLS		
CASES	History of Industrial Exposure	No History of Industrial Exposure	Total
History of Industrial Exposure	16	13	29
No History of Industrial Exposure	3	22	25
Total	19	35	54

Part 3 Calculation of the McNemar Chi-Square (χ^2) Statistic

$$\text{McNemar}\,\chi^2 = \frac{\left(|b-c|-1\right)^2}{b+c}$$

$$= \frac{\left(|13-3|-1\right)^2}{13+3} = \frac{(9)^2}{16} = \frac{81}{16} = 5.06$$

Part 4 Calculation of Degrees of Freedom (df) for Contingency Table, Based on Number of Rows (R) and Columns (C)

$$df = (R-1)(C-1) = (2-1)(2-1) = 1$$

Part 5 Determination of the p Value
Value from the chi-square table for 5.06 on 1 df: $p = 0.021$ (statistically significant)

Interpretation: The data presented in this 2 × 2 table are statistically significant. The cases (participants with mycosis fungoides) were more likely than expected by chance alone to have been exposed to an industrial environment with cutting oils than were the controls (participants without mycosis fungoides).

Part 6 Calculation of the Odds Ratio (OR)

$$OR = b/c = 13/3 = 4.33$$

Interpretation: When a case and a matched control differed in their history of exposure to cutting oils, the odds that the case was exposed was 4.33 times as great as the odds that the control was exposed.

Data from Cohen SR: *Mycosis fungoides: clinicopathologic relationships, survival, and therapy in 54 patients, with observation on occupation as a new prognostic factor (master's thesis)*, New Haven, CT, 1977, Yale University School of Medicine.

4.5 STANDARD ERRORS FOR DATA IN 2 × 2 TABLES

Standard errors for proportions, risk ratios, and odds ratios are sometimes calculated for data in 2 × 2 tables, although for use of larger $R \times C$ tables, a referent group must be chosen for each comparison.

4.5.a. Standard Error for a Proportion

In a 2 × 2 table, the proportion of success (defined, for example, as survival) can be determined for each of the two levels (categories) of the independent variable, and the standard error can be calculated for each of these proportions. This is valuable when an objective of the study is to estimate the true proportions of success when using a new treatment.

In Box 10.2, the proportion of 28-day survivors in the propranolol-treated group is 0.84 (shown as 84% in the percentage column), and the proportion of 28-day survivors in the placebo-treated group is 0.63. Knowing this information allows the investigator to calculate the standard error and the 95% confidence interval for each result (i.e., proportion of 28-day survivors) by the methods described earlier (see z-tests in Chapter 9). In Box 10.2, when the calculations are performed for the proportions surviving, the 95% confidence interval for survival in the propranolol-treated group is expressed as (0.73, 0.95). This means that if this study were repeated many times, 95% of all confidence intervals would contain the true proportion of survival in the population of propranolol-treated patients. The confidence interval for the placebo-treated group is expressed as (0.49, 0.77).

4.5.b. Standard Error for a Risk Ratio

If a 2 × 2 table is used to compare the proportion of disease in two different exposure groups or is used to compare the proportion of success in two different treatment groups, the relative risk or relative success can be expressed as a risk ratio. Standard errors can be set around the risk ratio. If the 95% confidence limits exclude the value of 1.0, there is a statistically significant difference between the risks at an alpha level of 5%.

In Box 10.2, because the proportion of 28-day survivors in the propranolol-treated group is 0.84 and the proportion of 28-day survivors in the placebo-treated group is 0.63, the risk ratio is 0.84/0.63, or 1.34. This ratio indicates that for the patients with myocardial infarction studied, the 28-day survival probability with propranolol is 34% better than that with placebo.

There are several approaches to computing the standard error of a risk ratio. Because all the methods are complicated, they are not shown here, but are provided in every major statistical computer package. When the risk ratio in Box 10.2 is analyzed by the Taylor series approach used in the EPI-INFO computer package, for example, the 95% confidence interval around the risk ratio of 1.34 is reported as (1.04, 1.73).[7] Thus, the true risk ratio has a 95% probability of being between 1.04 and 1.73. This result confirms the chi-square test finding of statistical significance, because the 95% confidence interval does not include a risk ratio of 1.0 (which means no true difference between the groups).

4.5.c. Standard Error for an Odds Ratio

If a 2 × 2 table provides data from a case control study, the odds ratio can be calculated. Although Box 10.2 is best analyzed by a risk ratio, because the study method is a randomized controlled trial rather than a case control study, the odds ratio also can be examined. Here the odds of surviving in the propranolol-treated group are 38/7, or 5.43; and the odds of surviving in the placebo-treated group are 29/17, or 1.71. The odds ratio is 5.43/1.71, or 3.18, which is much larger than the risk ratio. As emphasized in Chapter 6, the odds ratio is a good estimate of the risk ratio only if the risk being studied by a case control study is rare. Because the risk event (mortality)

in Box 10.2 is not rare, the odds ratio is not a good estimate of the risk ratio.

Calculating the standard error for an odds ratio is also complicated and is not discussed here. When the odds ratio in Box 10.2 is analyzed by the Cornfield approach used in the EPIINFO 5.01 computer package, the 95% confidence interval around the odds ratio of 3.18 is reported as (1.06, 9.85).[7] The lower-limit estimate of 1.06 with the odds ratio is close to the lower-limit estimate of 1.04 with the risk ratio, and it confirms statistical significance. The upper-limit estimate for the odds ratio is much larger than that for the risk ratio, however, because the odds ratio itself is much larger than the risk ratio.

4.6 STRENGTH OF ASSOCIATION AND CLINICAL UTILITY OF DATA IN 2 × 2 TABLES

Earlier in this chapter the strength of the linear association between two continuous variables was measured as R^2. For the data shown in 2 × 2 tables, an alternative method is used to estimate the strength of association. A fictitious scenario and set of data are used here to illustrate how to determine strength of association and why it is important to examine associations for strength and statistical significance.

Assume that a master's degree student conducted a study to determine if there is a true difference between the results of a certain blood test in men compared with women. After obtaining the data shown in the first part of Box 10.5, the student calculated the chi-square statistic and found that the difference is not statistically significant ($\chi^2 = 0.32$; $p = 0.572$). The student's advisor pointed out that even if the difference had been statistically significant, the data would not have been clinically useful because of the small gender difference in the proportion of participants with positive findings in the blood test (52% of men vs. 48% of women).

The student decided to obtain a PhD and continued to study the same topic. Believing that small numbers were the problem with the master's thesis, this time the student decided to obtain blood test findings in a sample of 20,000 participants, half from each gender. As shown in the second part of Box 10.5, the difference in proportions is the same as before (52% of men vs. 48% of women), so the results are still clinically unimportant (i.e., trivial). Now, however, the student obtains a statistical association that is highly statistically significant ($\chi^2 = 32.0$; $p < 0.0001$).

Findings can have statistical significance, especially if the study involves a large number of participants, and at the same time have little or no clinical value. This example illustrates an interesting point. Because the sample size in the PhD study is 100 times as large as that in the master's study, the chi-square statistic for the data in the PhD study (given identical proportions) also is 100 times as large. As a next step, it would be helpful to measure the strength of the association in Box 10.5 to show whether the magnitude of the association is not important, even though it is statistically significant.

In 2 × 2 tables, the strength of association is measured using the *phi* (Φ) coefficient, which basically adjusts the

BOX 10.5   Analysis of Strength of Association (phi) Between Blood Test Results and Gender (Two Nonparametric Variables, Unpaired) in Initial Study of 200 Participants and Subsequent Study of 20,000 Participants (Fictitious Data)

Part 1 Data and Calculation of *phi* Coefficient for Initial Study (Master's Thesis)

	GENDER				Total	
BLOOD TEST RESULT	**Male**		**Female**			
	No.	**(%)**	**No.**	**(%)**	**No.**	**(%)**
Positive	52	(52)	48	(48)	100	(50)
Negative	48	(48)	52	(52)	100	(50)
Total	100	(100)	100	(100)	200	(100)

Chi-square (χ^2) statistic: 0.32
Degrees of freedom (*df*): 1
p value: 0.572 (not statistically significant)

$$phi = \sqrt{\frac{\chi^2}{N}} = \sqrt{\frac{0.32}{200}} = \sqrt{0.0016} = 0.04$$

Interpretation: The association between gender and the blood test result is neither statistically significant nor clinically important.

Part 2 Data and Calculation of *phi* Coefficient for Subsequent Study (PhD Dissertation)

	GENDER				Total	
BLOOD TEST RESULT	**Male**		**Female**			
	No.	**(%)**	**No.**	**(%)**	**No.**	**(%)**
Positive	5,200	(52)	4,800	(48)	10,000	(50)
Negative	4,800	(48)	5,200	(52)	10,000	(50)
Total	10,000	(100)	10,000	(100)	20,000	(100)

Chi-square (χ^2) statistic: 32.0
Degrees of freedom (*df*): 1
p value: <0.0001 (highly statistically significant)

$$phi = \sqrt{\frac{\chi^2}{N}} = \sqrt{\frac{32}{20,000}} = \sqrt{0.0016} = 0.04$$

Interpretation: The association between gender and the blood test result is statistically significant. It is clinically unimportant (i.e., it was trivial), however, because the *phi* value is 0.04 and the proportion of chi-square explained by the blood test result is only (0.04)^2, or 0.0016, much less than 1%.

chi-square statistic for the sample size. It can be considered as analogous to the correlation coefficient (*r*) for the data in a 2 × 2 table. The formula is as follows:

$$phi = \sqrt{\frac{\chi^2}{N}}$$

The *phi* value in the first part of Box 10.5 is the same as that in the second part (i.e., 0.04), because the strength of the association is the same, very small. If *phi* is squared (similar to R^2), the proportion of variation in chi-square that is explained by gender in this example is less than 0.2%, which is extremely small. Although *phi* is not accurate in larger ($R \times C$)

tables, a related test, called the **Cramer V**, can be used in these tables.[8]

Every association should be examined for strength of association, clinical utility, and statistical significance. Strength of association can be shown by a risk ratio, a risk difference, an odds ratio, an R^2 value, a *phi* value, or a Cramer *V* value. A statistically significant association implies that the association is real (i.e., not caused by chance alone), but not that it is important. A **strong association** is likely to be important if it is real. Looking for statistical significance *and* strength of association is as important to statistical analysis as having the right *and* left wings on an airplane.

There is a danger of automatically rejecting as unimportant statistically significant associations that show only limited strength of association. As discussed in Chapter 6, the risk ratio (or odds ratio if from a case control study) and the prevalence of the risk factor determine the population attributable risk. For a prevalent disease such as myocardial infarction, a common risk factor that showed a risk ratio of only 1.3 could be responsible for a large number of preventable infarctions. In general, **clinical significance** depends on the magnitude of effect in an individual, and the population prevalence of the factor in question. A small change in blood pressure or low-density lipoprotein (LDL) cholesterol that might be trivial in an individual could translate to many lives saved if a large population is affected.

4.7 SURVIVAL ANALYSIS

In clinical studies of medical or surgical interventions for cancer, success usually is measured in terms of the length of time that some desirable outcome (e.g., survival or remission of disease) is maintained. An analysis of the time-related patterns of survival typically involves using variations of life table techniques that were first developed in the insurance field. Insurance companies needed to know the risk of death in their insured populations so that they knew what rates to charge for the company to make profit.

The mere reporting of the proportion of patients who are alive at the termination of a study's observation period is inadequate, because it does not account for how long the individual patients were observed and it does not consider when they died or how many were lost to follow-up. Techniques that statisticians use to control for these problems include the following:

- Person-time methods
- Survival analysis using the *actuarial life table method* or the *Kaplan-Meier method*

Survival analysis requires that the dependent (outcome) variable be dichotomous (e.g., survival/death, success/failure) and that the time to failure or loss to observation be known.

4.7.a. Person-Time Methods

In a survival study, some participants are lost to follow-up, some survive through the end of the study, and others die during the observation period. To control for the fact that the length of observation varies from participant to participant, the person-time methods, introduced in an earlier discussion of incidence density (see Chapter 2), can be used to calculate the likelihood of death. Briefly, if one person is observed for 3 years and another person is observed for 1 year, the total duration of observation would be equal to 4 person-years. Calculations can be made on the basis of years, months, weeks, or any other unit of time. The results can be reported as the number of events (e.g., deaths or remissions) per person-time of observation.

Person-time methods are useful if the risk of death or some other outcome does not change greatly over the follow-up period. If the risk of death does change with the amount of time elapsed since baseline (e.g., amount of time since diagnosis of a disease or since entry into a study), person-time methods are not helpful. For example, certain cancers tend to kill quickly if they are going to be fatal, so the amount of risk per person-time depends on whether most of the years of observation were soon after diagnosis or much later. As mentioned in Chapter 2, person-time methods are especially useful for studies of phenomena that can occur repeatedly over time, such as otitis media, episodes of angina pectoris, and exacerbations of asthma.

4.7.b. Life Table Analysis

In follow-up studies of a single dichotomous outcome such as death, some participants may be lost to follow-up (unavailable for examination) and some may be censored (when a patient is terminated from a study early because the patient entered late and the study is ending). The most popular solution to this problem is to use life table analysis. The two main methods of life table analysis—the actuarial method and the Kaplan-Meier method—treat losses to follow-up and censorship in slightly different ways. However, both methods make it possible to base the analysis on the findings in all the participants for whom data are available. Both methods require the following information for each patient:
1. Date of entry into the study.
2. Reason for withdrawal: loss to follow-up, or censorship, or occurrence of the outcome (often death).
3. Date of withdrawal: date of death for patients who died, the last time seen alive for patients who were lost to follow-up, and the date withdrawn alive for patients who were censored.

If different treatment groups are being compared, the method also requires knowing in which group each study participant was enrolled.

Life table methods do not eliminate the bias that occurs if the losses to follow-up occur more frequently in one group than in another, particularly if the characteristics of the patients lost from one group differ greatly from those of the patients lost from the other group. For example, in a clinical trial comparing the effects of an experimental antihypertensive drug with the effects of an established antihypertensive drug, the occurrence of side effects in the group treated with the experimental drug might cause many in this group to drop out of the study and no longer maintain contact with the investigators. The life table method is a powerful tool, however, if the losses are few, if the losses represent a similar percentage of the starting numbers in the groups to be compared, and if the characteristics of those who are lost to follow-up are similar. Survival methods are usually considered the method of choice for describing dichotomous outcomes in longitudinal studies such as randomized clinical trials.

In statistics it is always crucial to look at the raw data; and nowhere is this more important than in survival analysis, where examining the pattern of survival differences may be more important for making a clinical decision than examining whether the difference is statistically significant.

For example, a surgical therapy for cancer might result in a greater initial mortality but a higher 5-year survival (i.e., the therapy is a "kill or cure" method), whereas a medical therapy may result in a lower initial mortality, but also a lower 5-year survival. It might be important for patients to know this difference when choosing between these therapies. Patients who preferred to be free of cancer quickly and at all costs might choose the surgical treatment. In contrast, patients who wanted to live for at least a few months to finish writing a book or to see the birth of a first grandchild might choose the medical treatment.

Actuarial method. The **actuarial method**, which was developed to calculate risks and premium rates for life insurance companies and retirement plans, was the basis of the earlier methods used in life table analysis. In medical studies the actuarial method is used to calculate the survival rates of patients during fixed intervals such as years. First, it determines the number of people surviving to the beginning of each interval. Next, it assumes that the individuals who were censored or lost to follow-up during the interval were observed for only half that interval. Finally, the method calculates the mortality rate for that interval by dividing the number of deaths in the interval by the total person-years of observation in that interval for all those who began the interval.

The survival rate for an interval (p_x) is 1.0 minus the mortality rate. The rate of survival of the study group to the end of three of the fixed intervals (p_3) is the product of the survival of each of the three component intervals. For example, assume that the intervals are years; the survival rate to the end of the first interval (p_1) is 0.75 (i.e., 75%); for participants who began the second year, the survival rate to the end of the second interval (p_2) is 0.80; and for participants who began the third year, the survival rate to the end of the third interval (p_3) is 0.85. These three numbers would be multiplied together to arrive at a 3-year survival rate of 0.51, or 51%.

An important example of a study in which the actuarial method was used is the US Veterans Administration study of the long-term effects of coronary artery bypass grafts versus medical treatment of patients with stable angina.[9] Fig. 10.5 shows the 11-year cumulative survival for surgically and medically treated patients who did not have left main coronary artery disease, but were nevertheless at high risk according to angiographic analysis in the study.

The actuarial method also can be used in studies of outcomes other than death or survival. Investigators used this method in a study of subsequent pregnancies among two groups of teenage mothers.[10] The mothers in one group were enrolled in special programs to help them complete their education and delay subsequent pregnancies, whereas the mothers in the other group had access to the services that are usually available. The actuarial method was used to analyze data concerning the number and timing of subsequent pregnancies in each group. When tests of significance were performed, the observed differences between the groups were found to be statistically significant.

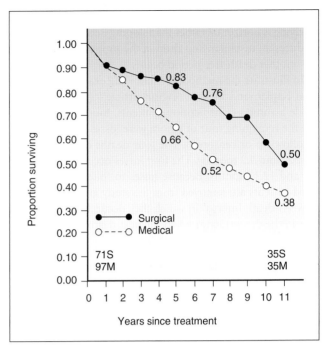

Fig. 10.5 Graph showing results of survival analysis using actuarial method. From a study of long-term effects of coronary artery bypass grafts versus medical treatment of patients with stable angina. Depicted here is the 11-year cumulative survival for surgically and medically treated patients who did not have left main coronary artery disease but were nevertheless at high risk according to angiographic analysis in the study. Numbers of patients at risk at the beginning and end of the study are given at the bottom of the figure, where *S* denotes surgical and *M* denotes medical. (From Veterans Administration Coronary Artery Bypass Surgery Cooperative Study Group: Eleven-year survival in the veterans administration randomized trial of coronary bypass surgery for stable angina. *N Engl J Med* 311:1333–1339, 1984.)

The actuarial method is still used for studies with large numbers of participants. However, the Kaplan-Meier method is more commonly used because of its many advantages, particularly when the sample size is small.

Kaplan-Meier method. The Kaplan-Meier method has become the most commonly used approach to survival analysis in medicine.[11] In the medical literature it is usually referred to as the **Kaplan-Meier life table method**. It also is sometimes referred to as the **product-limit method**, because it takes advantage of the *N*-year survival rate (P_N) being equal to the product of all the survival rates of the individual intervals (e.g., p_1, p_2) leading up to time *N*.

The Kaplan-Meier method is different from the actuarial method in that it calculates a new line of the life table every time a new death occurs. Because deaths occur unevenly over time, the intervals are uneven and numerous. Thus the graph of a Kaplan-Meier life table analysis often resembles uneven stair steps.

In a Kaplan-Meier analysis, the deaths are not viewed as occurring during an interval. Rather, they are seen as instantaneously terminating one interval and beginning a new interval at a lower survival rate. The periods of time between when deaths occur are *death-free intervals*, and the proportion surviving between deaths does not change, although losses to follow-up and censorship are applied during this interval.

During the death-free intervals, the curve of the proportion surviving is horizontal rather than sloping downward. A death produces an instantaneous drop in the proportion surviving, and another death-free period begins.

To illustrate the method, the following example was taken from Kaplan and Meier's original article[11] (Box 10.6). The article assumed eight fictitious patients, four of whom died and the remaining four of whom were losses (i.e., either lost to follow-up or censored). The four deaths occurred at 0.8, 3.1, 5.4, and 9.2 months. The four losses occurred at 1.0, 2.7, 7.0, and 12.1 months. Because losses to follow-up and censored patients are removed from the study group during the between-death interval in which they occur, they do not appear in the denominator when the next death occurs.

In Box 10.6, p_x is the proportion surviving interval x (i.e., from the time of the previous death to just before the next death), and P_x is the proportion surviving from the beginning of the study to the end of that interval. (P_x is obtained by multiplying together the p_x values of all the intervals up to and including the row of interest.) The p_x of the first interval is always 1 because the first death ends the first study interval, and all the patients not lost to follow-up survive until the first death.

To illustrate the use of Kaplan-Meier analysis in practice, Fig. 10.6 shows a Kaplan-Meier life table of the probability of remaining relapse free over time for two groups of patients who had cancer of the bladder.[12] All the patients had organ-confined transitional cell cancer of the bladder with

---

BOX 10.6 Survival Analysis by Kaplan-Meier Method in Eight Study Participants

Part 1 Beginning Data

Timing of deaths in four participants: 0.8, 3.1, 5.4, and 9.2 months
Timing of loss to follow-up or censorship in four participants: 1.0, 2.7, 7.0, and 12.1 months

Part 2 Tabular Representation of Data

No. Months at Time of Subject's Death	No. Living Just Before Subject's Death	No. Living Just After Subject's Death	No. Lost to Follow-up Between This and Next Subject's Death	Fraction Surviving After This Death	p_x	Survival Interval (for p_x)	P_x Surviving to End of Interval
—	—	—	—	—	1.000	0 < 0.8	1.000
0.8	8	7	2	7/8	0.875	0.8 < 3.1	0.875
3.1	5	4	0	4/5	0.800	3.1 < 5.4	0.700
5.4	4	3	1	3/4	0.750	5.4 < 9.2	0.525
9.2	2	1	0	1/2	0.500	9.2 <12.1	0.263
No deaths	1	1	1	1/1	1.000	>12.1	0.263

Note: p_x is the proportion surviving interval x (i.e., from time of previous death to just before next death), and P_x is the proportion surviving from the beginning of the study to the end of that interval.

Part 3 Graphic Representation of Data

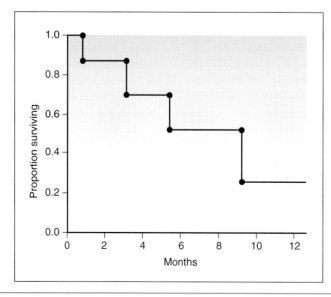

Data from Kaplan EL, Meier P: Nonparametric estimation from incomplete observations. *J Am Stat Assoc* 53:457–481, 1958.

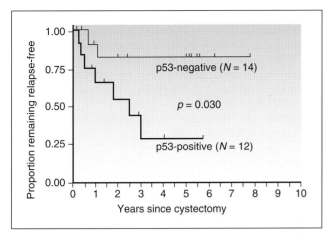

Fig. 10.6 Graph showing life table analysis using Kaplan-Meier method. From a study of the probability of remaining relapse free over time for two groups of patients who had organ-confined transitional cell cancer of the bladder with deep invasion into the muscularis propria (stage 3a disease), but without regional lymph node metastases. One group consisted of 14 patients with negative results in a test for p53 protein in the nuclei of tumor cells, and the other group consisted of 12 patients with positive results in the same test. (From Esrig D, Elmajian D, Groshen S, et al: Accumulation of nuclear p53 and tumor progression in bladder cancer. *N Engl J Med* 331:1259–1264, 1994.)

deep invasion into the muscularis propria (stage 3a disease), but without regional lymph node metastases. One group consisted of 14 patients with negative results in a test for p53 protein in the nuclei of tumor cells, and the other group consisted of 12 patients with positive results in the same test. Despite small numbers, the difference in the survival curves for the p53-positive group and the p53-negative group is visually obvious and found to be statistically significant ($p = 0.030$).

4.7.c. Tests of Significance for Differences in Survival

Two or more life table curves can be tested to see if they are significantly different from each other. Statistical computer packages do this by using complicated tests, such as the Breslow test and the Cox test. However, there are reasonably good simple tests of significance for differences between actuarial survival curves (z-test for proportions) and between Kaplan-Meier curves (e.g., the logrank test).

Significance tests for proportions. See Chapter 9 for a discussion of t-tests and z-tests. The t-test for a difference between actuarial curves depends on the Greenwood formula for the standard error of a proportion and is not described here.[1,13]

Logrank test. Despite its name, the logrank test does not deal with logarithms or with ranked data. The test is often used to compare data in studies involving treatment and control groups and to test the null hypothesis that each group has the same death rate over time.

In the logrank test, each time a death occurs the investigator calculates the probability that the observed death would have occurred in the treatment group and the

probability that it would have occurred in the control group, if the null hypothesis were true. These probabilities are proportional to the number of survivors to that point in time in each group. Suppose the study started with 100 patients in each group, but at a certain point there are 60 left in the treatment group and 40 in the control group. Under the null hypothesis, the probability that the next death would occur in the treatment group is 0.6, and the probability that the next death would occur in the control group is 0.4.

Within each study group, the expected probabilities for each death are summed to form the total expected number of deaths (E) for that group. The actual deaths in each group also are summed to form the observed number of deaths (O). Then the observed deaths are compared with the expected deaths using the following chi-square test on 1 degree of freedom:

$$\text{logrank } \chi^2 = \sum \frac{\left(O_T - E_T\right)^2}{E_T} + \frac{\left(O_C - E_C\right)^2}{E_C}$$

where O_T and E_T are the observed and expected deaths in the treatment group, and where O_C and E_C are the observed and expected deaths in the control group. Only two terms are needed, because the expected counts are not determined from row and column totals in a 2 × 2 table, but instead are obtained by an independent method. There is only 1 degree of freedom here because the total number of deaths is already known; and when the number of deaths in one of the two groups is known, the number of deaths in the other group is fixed and is no longer free to vary.

Proportional hazards models (Cox models). The Kaplan-Meier approach has been made even more powerful by the development of statistical models that enable dichotomous outcomes to be used as dependent variables in multiple logistic regression analyses, despite losses to follow-up and censorship of patients. Although a detailed discussion of these models is beyond the scope of this book, students should be aware that they are called **proportional hazards models** or, in some studies, **Cox models**, and that their application in clinical trials is common.[14-17]

5. SUMMARY

Bivariate analysis studies the relationship between one independent variable and one dependent variable. The relationship between two continuous variables should first be examined graphically. Then the data can be analyzed statistically to determine whether there is a real relationship between the variables, the relationship is linear or nonlinear, the association is positive or negative, and the association is sufficiently strong that it is not likely to have occurred by chance alone. The strength of a linear association between two continuous variables can be determined by calculating the value of R^2, and the impact that variable x has on variable y can be determined by calculating the slope of the regression line.

Correlation and regression analyses indicate whether there is an association between two continuous variables such as weight (y) and height (x). Correlation estimates the strength of the relationship between y and x, and R^2 describes what proportion of the variation in y is explained by the variation in x. Simple linear regression estimates the value of y when the value of x is zero, and it predicts the degree of expected change in y when x changes by one unit of measure.

Different statistical tests are used for ordinal data. The relationship between an ordinal variable and a dichotomous variable can be determined by the Mann-Whitney U-test, while the Wilcoxon matched-pairs signed-ranks test compares paired data (before/after). The Spearman and Kendall correlation coefficients (*rho* and *tau*) measure the correlation between two ordinal variables. The Kruskal-Wallis test compares the means of three or more groups simultaneously.

Analyzing the relationships between nominal variables (including dichotomous variables) usually begins by placing the data for the two variables in a contingency table. Useful summaries of the table include calculating proportions of observations in each cell and then calculating risk ratios or risk differences (in cohort studies) or odds ratios (for case control studies). The null hypothesis of independence between the two variables is usually tested by using the chi-square test for unpaired data. When the expected numbers are small in one or more cells, the Fisher exact probability test must be used in the analysis of dichotomous unpaired data. For paired or matched dichotomous data, the McNemar chi-square test for paired data may be used. For data in 2×2 tables, the *phi* coefficient can be used to test the strength of association.

Survival analysis employs various methods to study dichotomous outcome variables (e.g., death/survival) over time. Although the actuarial method of analysis is sometimes still used, the Kaplan-Meier (product-limit) method has become the most frequently used approach. Life table curves are constructed from the data, and two or more curves can be tested to see if they are significantly different. For actuarial curves, significance tests for proportions can be used. For Kaplan-Meier curves, the logrank test is the most straightforward test of statistical significance. Proportional hazards (Cox) models are used to perform a survival analysis while controlling for many variables.

REFERENCES

1. Dawson B, Trapp RG. *Basic and Clinical Biostatistics.* 4th ed. New York, NY: Lange Medical Books/McGraw-Hill; 2004.
2. Holford TR. *Multivariate Methods in Epidemiology.* New York, NY: Oxford University Press; 2002.
3. Siegel S. *Nonparametric Statistics for the Behavioral Sciences.* New York, NY: McGraw-Hill; 1956.
4. Snow PJ. Effect of propranolol in myocardial infarction. *Lancet.* 1965;2:551-553.
5. Emerson JD, Colditz GA. Use of statistical analysis. *N Engl J Med.* 1983;309:709-713.
6. Cohen SR: *Mycosis Fungoides: Clinicopathologic Relationships, Survival, and Therapy in 54 Patients, with Observation on Occupation as a new Prognostic Factor (Master's Thesis).* New Haven, CT: Yale University School of Medicine; 1977.
7. Dean AG, Arner TG, Sunki GG, et al. *Epi Info™, a Database and Statistics Program for Public Health Professionals.* Atlanta, GA, USA: CDC; 2011.
8. Feinstein AR. *Principles of Medical Statistics.* Boca Raton, FL: Chapman & Hall/CRC; 2002.
9. Veterans Administration Coronary Artery Bypass Surgery Cooperative Study Group. Eleven-year survival in the veterans administration randomized trial of coronary bypass surgery for stable angina. *N Engl J Med.* 1984;311:1333-1339.
10. Currie JB, Jekel JF, Klerman LV. Subsequent pregnancies among teenage mothers enrolled in a special program. *Am J Public Health.* 1972;62:1606-1611.
11. Kaplan EL, Meier P. Nonparametric estimation from incomplete observations. *J Am Stat Assoc.* 1958;53:457-481.
12. Esrig D, Elmajian D, Groshen S, et al. Accumulation of nuclear p53 and tumor progression in bladder cancer. *N Engl J Med.* 1994;331:1259-1264.
13. Cutler SJ, Ederer F. Maximum utilization of the life table method in analyzing survival. *J Chronic Dis.* 1958;8:699-712.
14. Schneider M, Zuckerman IH, Onukwugha E, et al. Chemotherapy treatment and survival in older women with estrogen receptor-negative metastatic breast cancer: a population-based analysis. *J Am Geriatr Soc.* 2011;59:637-646.
15. Thourani VH, Keeling WB, Kilgo PD, et al. The impact of body mass index on morbidity and short- and long-term mortality in cardiac valvular surgery. *J Thorac Cardiovasc Surg.* 2011;142:1052-1061.
16. Appleby PN, Allen NE, Key TJ. Diet, vegetarianism, and cataract risk. *Am J Clin Nutr.* 2011;93:1128-1135.
17. Park JY, Mitrou PN, Keogh RH, et al. Self-reported and measured anthropometric data and risk of colorectal cancer in the EPIC-Norfolk study. *Int J Obes (Lond).* 2012;36:107-118.

SELECT READING

Lee ET. *Statistical Methods for Survival Data Analysis.* Belmont, CA: Lifetime Learning Publications; 1980.

REVIEW QUESTIONS

1. A joint distribution graph can be used to display:
   A. Causality
   B. Correlation
   C. Kurtosis
   D. Power
   E. Specificity

2. A direct correlation is noted between the number of times per year one puts on boxing gloves and the frequency of being punched in the head. The correlation coefficient (r) in this case:
   A. Cannot be determined because the data are dichotomous
   B. May be close to 1
   C. May be greater than 1
   D. Must be less than 0.05
   E. Must be statistically significant

3. In linear regression, the slope represents:
   A. The value of x when y is zero
   B. The value of y when x is zero
   C. The error in the line describing the relationship between x and y
   D. The change in y when x changes by 1 unit
   E. The mathematical value of (y/x) minus the y-intercept

4. A distinction between one-tailed and two-tailed tests of significance is that a one-tailed test:
   A. Does not affect statistical significance but does affect power
   B. Does not affect the performance of the statistical test but does affect the conversion to a p value
   C. Is based on the number of independent variables
   D. Requires that the sample size be doubled
   E. Should be performed during data analysis

5. A study is conducted to determine the efficacy of influenza vaccine. Volunteers agree to participate for 2 years. During the first year, participants are randomly assigned to be injected with either an inert substance (a placebo) or the active vaccine. During the second year, each participant who previously received the placebo is given the active vaccine, and each who previously received the active vaccine is given the placebo. Each participant serves as his or her own control. All incident cases of influenza are recorded, and the occurrence of influenza when vaccinated is compared with the occurrence when unvaccinated. The appropriate test of significance for this study is the:
   A. Kaplan-Meier method
   B. Kruskal-Wallis test
   C. Mann-Whitney U-test
   D. McNemar test
   E. Pearson correlation coefficient

6. Two groups of participants are assembled on the basis of whether they can identify a newt in a pondlife sample. The groups are then asked to rate the probability that industrial emissions cause global warming, using a scale with five choices, ranging from "improbable" to "highly probable." The industrial emissions data in this study are:
   A. Continuous
   B. Pseudocontinuous
   C. Dichotomous
   D. Nominal
   E. Ordinal

7. In regard to the scenario in question 6, to analyze the responses of the two groups statistically, researchers might compare the data on the basis of:
   A. Means
   B. Ranking
   C. Standard deviation
   D. Standard error
   E. Variance

8. In regard to the scenario in question 6, the appropriate statistical method for the analysis would be:
   A. Chi-square analysis
   B. Linear regression analysis
   C. Nonparametric analysis
   D. Fisher exact probability test
   E. Two-sample t-test

9. Given the following data comparing two drugs, A and B, you can conclude:

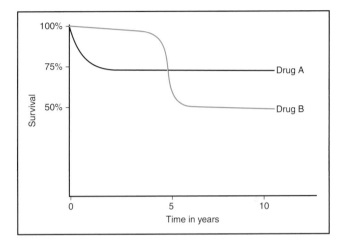

   A. Drug A shows superior survival at 5 years
   B. Drug B shows superior survival at 5 years
   C. A rational patient would choose drug A
   D. A rational patient would choose drug B
   E. Drug A is initially less beneficial than drug B

ANSWERS AND EXPLANATIONS

1. **B.** A joint distribution graph is a plot of the relationship between two continuous variables. The more closely the data points cluster about a line, the greater the linear correlation between the two variables. If two variables are related in a nonlinear manner, the correlation may not be displayed as a line but as a curvilinear distribution of data points (e.g., S-shaped, U-shaped, or J-shaped curve). Methods for calculating the correlation coefficient in such a setting are available, but their description is beyond the scope of this text. Correlation alone does not establish causality (A). For example, someone who owns a car is also likely to own a television set, but ownership of one item does not cause ownership of the other item. Joint distributions do not display kurtosis (C), a measure of how peaked or spread out a probability distribution is; power (D), probability of detecting an association when one exists (also known as sensitivity); or specificity (E), probability of not detecting an association when there actually is no true association.

2. **B.** The Pearson product-moment correlation coefficient, also referred to as the r value, is a measure of the linear

relationship between two continuous variables. Its value range is the same as that for the slope of a line, from −1 (perfect inverse, or negative, correlation), through 0 (no correlation), to +1 (perfect direct, or positive, correlation). A correlation such as the one in the question could produce a correlation coefficient close to 1. However, the correlation coefficient can never be greater than 1 (C), nor can any correlation coefficient ever be less than −1. The correlation coefficient could theoretically be less than 0.05 (D), but such a value is near zero, implying an essentially nonexistent correlation. The correlation does not have to be statistically significant (E). If the sample size is small, the associations (correlation) cannot be measured with much precision, and even a large correlation could have a wide confidence interval and could be nonsignificant. Although the question does not reveal the actual data, the description of the variables gives enough information to show the data are not dichotomous (A), that is, variables are not constrained to only two possible values. Correlation requires that both the variables being compared be continuous (i.e., data can assume any numerical value) or at least pseudocontinuous/interval (i.e., data can assume any integer value). In this case the variables are the number of times putting on gloves expressed as a natural number (i.e., 0, 1, 2, 3) and the frequency of being hit as a fraction or ratio (e.g., 2 of 3 times).

3. **D.** Simple linear regression is a method of describing the association between two variables using a straight line. The slope of the line describes the unit change in y (the dependent variable) for every unit change in x (the independent variable). If the mathematical formula for a line is $y = \alpha + \beta x$ (where β is the slope and α is the y-intercept), then the mathematical formula for the slope is $(y - \alpha)/x$, not $(y/x) - \alpha$ (E). The y-intercept and x-intercept can also be determined from the equation. The y-intercept is the value of y when x is zero (B); the value in this case is $y = \beta(0) + \alpha = \alpha$. (Note: The α here has an entirely different meaning than that used to represent false-positive error.) The x-intercept is the value of x when y is zero (A); the value in this case is $x = (0 - \alpha)\beta = -\alpha/\beta$. Most often, the line used to represent an association between two variables is just an approximation; the actual relationship will almost never be precisely linear. To account for the imprecision, our formula should include an error term (e.g., $y = \alpha + \beta X + \epsilon$), which, no matter how it is symbolized (ϵ in this case), is separate and entirely different from the slope (C). (Note: Slope symbolized as β here has an entirely different meaning than that used to represent false-negative error.)

4. **B.** The choice of a one-tailed or two-tailed test of significance should be made before a study is conducted, not during data analysis (E). The choice of a one-tailed test versus a two-tailed test is based on the hypothesis to be tested, not the number of independent variables (C). If the outcome can differ from the null hypothesis in only one direction (e.g., if you are comparing a placebo with an antihypertensive drug that you are thoroughly convinced would not cause the blood pressure to increase), a one-tailed test of significance is appropriate. If the outcome may differ from the null hypothesis in either direction (e.g., if you are comparing a placebo with a type of drug that may cause the blood pressure to increase or decrease), a two-tailed test of significance is warranted. The stipulation of a one-tailed or a two-tailed test affects the associated p value. When a one-tailed test is chosen, statistical significance (i.e., a p value less than alpha) is more readily achieved, because the extreme 5% of the distribution that differs sufficiently from the null hypothesis to warrant rejection of the null hypothesis (when alpha is set at 0.05) is all to one side. When a two-tailed test of significance is chosen, the rejection region is divided into two areas, with half (or 0.025 of the distribution when alpha is set at 0.05) at either extreme of the curve. Thus choosing a one-tailed test affects both significance level and power (A). A one-tailed test inherently has greater power to detect a statistically significant difference in an expected direction and thus would not require a doubling of sample size (D); if anything, a smaller sample size would be required for a one-tailed test. The implications of choosing a one-tailed test or a two-tailed test are discussed in the chapter.

5. **D.** In the study described, the outcome for each participant is binary (dichotomous)—that is, the disease (influenza) occurs or does not occur. The proportion of participants who acquire the disease in the year they were vaccinated is compared with the proportion of participants who acquire it in the year they were not vaccinated. Chi-square analysis is appropriate for this sort of comparison, and because each participant in the study serves as his or her own control, the McNemar test (chi-square test for paired data) is used. The contingency table for such a test contains paired data and would be set up as follows:

Year Not Vaccinated	Year Vaccinated	
	Diseased	Nondiseased
Diseased	a	b
Nondiseased	c	d

The numbers placed in the various cells would represent the following:
- In cell a, participants who acquired influenza when vaccinated and not vaccinated
- In cell b, participants who acquired influenza only when not vaccinated
- In cell c, participants who acquired influenza only when vaccinated
- In cell d, participants who remained free of influenza whether vaccinated or not

Kaplan-Meier method (A) is a type of survival analysis or life table analysis, considering length of survival time (or perhaps influenza-free time, as in this case). Had data been collected such that a vaccinated group and separate unvaccinated group were followed for their time until contracting influenza, then the Kaplan-Meier method may have been appropriate. The Kruskal-Wallis test (B) is appropriate when rather than two dichotomous variables you have a dichotomous (or nominal/categorical) dependent variable and an ordinal independent variable. If you were comparing who contracted flu among those vaccinated with a low-, medium-, or high-dose vaccine, the Kruskal-Wallis test might be appropriate. The Mann-Whitney U-test (C) could also be appropriate in this case; it is similar to the Kruskal-Wallis test except the dependent variable can only be dichotomous (vs. dichotomous or nominal/categorical). The Pearson correlation coefficient (E) is appropriate for comparing two different (continuous or pseudocontinuous) variables, when the relationship between the variables is approximately linear. If you wanted to compare concentration of flu vaccine to some continuous measure of immunologic response, a Pearson correlation coefficient may be appropriate.

6. **E.** Ordinal data are data that can be ranked from lowest to highest, but on scales that are subjective and that do not necessarily have equal intervals between values, as interval/pseudocontinuous data (B) do, or that can assume any value between intervals, as with continuous data (A). Unlike nominal (D) or dichotomous data (C), which are merely categoric without direction (e.g., red, yellow, blue or yes, no, respectively), the scale in the described study clearly has directionality (with choices ranging from "improbable" to "highly probable").

7. **B.** Researchers often use the nonparametric methods of statistical analysis for ordinal data, such as comparative approaches based on rankings. Ordinal data do not have a mean (A) or a definable variance (E) and cannot be characterized by a standard deviation (C) or standard error (D).

8. **E.** Nonparametric methods of statistical analysis are often used for ordinal data and are based on the ranking of the data. To analyze the probability that industrial emissions cause global warming (ordinal responses provided by the two groups of participants), the Mann-Whitney U-test or Kruskal-Wallis test would be appropriate (see Table 10.1). The chi-square test (A) and its nonparametric counterpart, the Fisher exact probability test (D), are appropriate when dealing with nominal/categoric data (including dichotomous data). Linear regression (B) requires a continuous outcome. If in this case we were looking not at the presence or absence of newts but the number of newts in a pond sample, and we had some measure of global warming as an independent variable, then linear regression might be appropriate provided certain assumptions were met (although Poisson regression, describing uncommon events, would probably be more appropriate in such a case; see Chapter 11). A two-sample t-test (E) could be used if we had a continuous measure of global warming as our dependent variable (e.g., concentration of carbon emissions in the atmosphere) and a dichotomous outcome (e.g., newts vs. no newts).

9. **E.** The figure shows a life table analysis with perplexing results: survival curves that cross. At 5 years, neither drug A (A) nor drug B (B) shows superior survival. Five years is the intersection point where survival is momentarily the same for the two drugs: 75%. With drug A, a number of patients seem to die rapidly, but then survival for remaining patients is stable at about 75%. Drug B shows immediate but short-lived high survival. With drug B, almost all patients live until about year 4, when a large percentage start dying precipitously. Deaths in patients taking drug B do not plateau until about year 6, and then the surviving 50% of patients go on for the next 4 years with no fatal events. From the figure we can conclude that drug A is initially less beneficial than drug B. However, it is unclear overall which drug is better. If a rational patient had to choose one drug or the other, whether he or she would choose drug A (C) or drug B (D) would depend on individual preferences, life considerations, and priorities. It would also depend on knowing what the natural history of survival is for the disease untreated (e.g., if the natural history of the disease is that almost 100% of patients survive to year 8 and 90% survive to year 10 untreated, then neither drug is a good option because both produce premature mortality).

Analyzing Relationships Between Multiple Variables

"An approximate answer to the right problem is worth a good deal more than an exact answer to an approximate problem."

John Tukey

1. OVERVIEW OF MULTIVARIABLE STATISTICS

Statistical models that have one outcome variable, but more than one independent variable are generally called multivariable models (or multivariate models, although many statisticians reserve this term for models with multiple dependent variables).[1] Multivariable models are intuitively attractive to investigators, because they seem more "true to life" than models with only one independent variable. A bivariate (two-variable) analysis, described in Chapter 10, simply indicates whether there is significant movement in Y in tandem with movement in X. Multivariable analysis allows for an assessment of the influence of change in X and change in Y once the effects of other factors (e.g., A, B, and C) are considered.

Multivariable analysis helps us to understand the relative importance of different independent variables for explaining the variation in a dependent (outcome) variable (y) when they act alone and when they work together (interaction). There may be considerable overlap in the ability of different independent variables to explain a dependent variable. For example, in the first two decades of life, age and height predict body weight, but age and height are usually correlated. During the growth years, height and weight increase with age, so age can be considered the underlying explanatory variable and height can be viewed as an *intervening variable* influencing weight. Children grow at different rates, so height would add additional explanatory power to that of age. Children who are tall for their age, on the average, also would be heavier than children of the same age who are short for their age. Each independent variable may share explanatory power with other independent variables and explain some of the variation in y beyond what any other variable explains.

All statistical equations attempt to model reality. However, they may represent only one dimension of reality, such as the effect of one variable (e.g., a nutrient) on another variable (e.g., growth rate of an infant). For a simple model to be of scientific value, the research design must try to equalize all the factors other than the independent and dependent variables being studied. In animal studies, this might be achieved by using genetically identical animals. Except for some observational studies of identical twins, this cannot be done for humans.

For *experimental* research involving humans, the first step is to make the experimental and control groups similar by randomizing the allocation of study participants to study groups. Sometimes randomization is impossible, however, or important factors may not be adequately controlled by this strategy. One way to remove the effects of these unwanted factors is to control for them by using **multivariable statistical analysis.** Common uses include:

1. Equalizing research groups (i.e., make them as comparable as possible) when studying the effects of medical or public health interventions.
2. Building models from *observational studies* that help investigators understand which factors affect the risk of different diseases in populations (assisting clinical and public health efforts to promote health and prevent disease and injury).

3. Creating *clinical indices* that can suggest the risk of disease in well people or a certain diagnosis, complications, or death in ill people.

Multivariable analysis does not enable an investigator to ignore the basic principles of good research design, however, because multivariable analysis also has many limitations. Although the statistical methodology and interpretation of findings from multivariable analysis are difficult for many clinicians, the methods and results are reported routinely in the medical literature.[2,3] To be intelligent consumers of the medical literature, health care professionals should at least understand the use and interpretation of the findings of multivariable analysis as usually presented.

2. ASSUMPTIONS UNDERLYING MULTIVARIABLE METHODS

Several important assumptions underlie most multivariable methods commonly used in medical research. Most methods of regression analysis assume that the average value of the outcome can be represented in terms of a linear function of the covariates (assumption of **linearity**). The effects of independent variables are assumed to be independent (assumption of **independence**), and if not, testing of interaction is warranted. This involves entering a term in a multivariable equation that represents the interaction between two of the independent variables. The assumption of **homoscedasticity** refers to homogeneity of all levels of the independent variables. In other words, it is assumed that variance and error are constant across a range of values for a given variable in the equation. Computer software packages for multivariable analysis provide ways to test these assumptions. For our purposes in this chapter, we accept that the conditions of these assumptions are satisfied.

2.1 CONCEPTUAL UNDERSTANDING OF EQUATIONS FOR MULTIVARIABLE ANALYSIS

One reason many people are put off by statistics is that the equations look like a jumble of meaningless symbols. That is especially true of multivariable techniques, but it is possible to understand the equations conceptually. Suppose a study is designed to predict the prognosis (in terms of survival months) of patients at the time of diagnosis for a certain cancer. Clinicians might surmise that to predict the length of survival for a patient, they would need to know at least four factors: the patient's *age*; anatomic *stage* of the disease at diagnosis; degree of systemic *symptoms* from the cancer, such as weight loss; and presence or absence of other diseases, such as renal failure or diabetes (*comorbidity*). That prediction equation could be written conceptually as follows:

$$\text{Cancer prognosis varies with Age, Stage, Symptoms,}$$
$$\text{and Comorbidity} \tag{11.1}$$

This statement could be made to look more mathematical simply by making a few slight changes:

$$\text{Cancer prognosis} \approx \text{Age} + \text{Stage} + \text{Symptoms} + \text{Comorbidity} \tag{11.2}$$

The four independent variables on the right side of the equation are almost certainly not of exactly equal importance. Equation 11.2 can be improved by giving each independent variable a **coefficient**, which is a **weighting factor** measuring its *relative importance* in predicting prognosis. The equation becomes:

$$\text{Cancer prognosis} \approx (\text{Weight}_1 \times Age) + (\text{Weight}_2 \times Stage) +$$
$$(\text{Weight}_3 \times Symptoms) +$$
$$(\text{Weight}_4 \times Comorbidity) \tag{11.3}$$

Before Equation 11.3 can become useful for estimating survival for an individual patient, two other factors are required: (1) a measure to quantify the *starting point* for the calculation, and (2) a measure of the *error* in the predicted value of *y* for each observation (because statistical prediction is almost never perfect for a single individual). By inserting a *starting point* and an *error term*, the $\approx$ symbol (meaning "varies with") can be replaced by an equal sign. Abbreviating the weights with a *W*, the equation now becomes:

$$\text{Cancer prognosis} = \text{Starting Point} + (W_1 \times Age) + (W_2 \times Stage) +$$
$$(W_3 \times Symptoms) + (W_4 \times Comorbidity) +$$
$$\text{Error Term} \tag{11.4}$$

This equation now can be rewritten in common statistical symbols: y is the dependent (outcome) variable (cancer prognosis) and is customarily placed on the left. Then x_1 (age) through x_4 (comorbidity) are the independent variables, and they are lined up on the right side of the equation; b_i is the statistical symbol for the weight of the *i*th independent variable; a is the starting point, usually called the regression constant; and e is the error term. Purely in statistical symbols, the equation can be expressed as follows:

$$y = a + b_1 x_1 + b_2 x_2 + b_3 x_3 + b_4 x_4 + e \tag{11.5}$$

Although Equation 11.5 looks complex, it really means the same thing as Equations 11.1 through 11.4.

What is this equation really saying? It states that the dependent variable (*y*) can be *predicted* for each person at diagnosis by beginning with a standard *starting point* (*a*), then making an adjustment for the new information supplied by the first variable (age), plus a further adjustment for the information provided by the second variable (anatomic stage), and so on, until an *adjustment* is made for the last independent variable (comorbidity) and for the almost inevitable error in the resulting prediction of the prognosis for any given study participant.

2.2 BEST ESTIMATES

In the example of cancer prognosis, to calculate a general prediction equation (the index we want for this type of patient), the investigator would need to know values for the regression constant (a) and the slopes (b_i) of the independent variables that would provide the best prediction of the value of y. These values would have to be obtained by a research study, preferably on two sets of data, one to provide the estimates of these parameters and a second (validation set) to determine the reliability of these estimates. The investigator would assemble a large group of newly diagnosed patients with the cancer of interest, record the values of the independent variables (x_i) for each patient at diagnosis, and follow the patients for a long time to determine the length of survival (y_i). The goal of the statistical analysis would be to solve for the best estimates of the regression constant (a) and the coefficients (b_i). When the statistical analysis has provided these estimates, the formula can take the values of the independent variables for new patients to predict the prognosis. The statistical research on a sample of patients would provide estimates for a and b, and then the equation could be used clinically.

How does the statistical equation know when it has found the best estimates for the regression constant and the coefficients of the independent variables? A little statistical theory is needed. The investigator would already have the observed y value and all the x values for each patient in the study and would be looking for the best values for the starting point and the coefficients. Because the error term is unknown at the beginning, the statistical analysis uses various values for the coefficients, regression constant, and observed x values to *predict* the value of y, which is called "y-hat" ($\hat{y}$). If the values of all the observed b's and x's are inserted, the following equation can be solved:

$$\hat{y} = a + b_1 x_1 + b_2 x_2 + b_3 x_3 + b_4 x_4 \qquad (11.6)$$

This equation is true because $\hat{y}$ is only an estimate, which can have error. When Equation 11.6 is subtracted from Equation 11.5, the following equation for the error term emerges:

$$(y - \hat{y}) = e \qquad (11.7)$$

This equation states that the error term (e) is the difference between the *observed* value of the outcome variable y for a given patient and the *predicted* value of y for the same patient. How does the computer program know when the best estimates for the values of a and b_i have been obtained? They have been achieved in this equation *when the sum of the squared error terms has been minimized*. That sum is expressed as:

$$\sum (y_i - \hat{y})^2 = \sum (y_O - y_E)^2 = \sum e^2 \qquad (11.8)$$

This idea is not new because, as noted in previous chapters, variation in statistics is measured as the sum of the squares of the observed value (O) minus the expected value (E). In multivariable analysis, the error term e is often called a **residual**.

In straightforward language, the best estimates for the values of a and b_1 through b_i are found when the total quantity of error (measured as the sum of squares of the error term, or most simply e^2) has been *minimized*. The values of a and the several bs that, taken together, give the smallest value for the squared error term are the best estimates that can be obtained from the set of data. Appropriately enough, this approach is called the **least-squares solution**, because the process is stopped when the sum of squares of the error term is the least.

2.3 GENERAL LINEAR MODEL

The multivariable equation shown in Equation 11.6 is usually called the *general linear model*. The model is general because there are many variations regarding the types of variables for y and x_i and the number of x variables that can be used. The model is linear because it is a linear combination of the x_i terms. For the x_i variables, a variety of transformations might be used to improve the model's "fit" (e.g., square of x_i, square root of x_i, or logarithm of x_i). The combination of terms would still be linear, however, if all the coefficients (the b_i terms) were to the first power. The model does not remain linear if any of the coefficients is taken to any power other than 1 (e.g., b^2). Such equations are much more complex and are beyond the scope of this discussion.

Numerous procedures for multivariable analysis are based on the general linear model. These include methods with such imposing designations as analysis of variance (ANOVA), analysis of covariance (ANCOVA), multiple linear regression, multiple logistic regression, the log-linear model, and discriminant function analysis. As discussed subsequently and outlined in Table 11.1, the choice of which procedure to use depends primarily on whether the dependent and independent variables are continuous, dichotomous, nominal, or ordinal. Knowing that the procedures listed in Table 11.1 are all variations of the same theme (the general linear model) helps to make them less confusing. Detailing these methods is beyond the scope of this text but readily available both online and in print.[4]

2.4 USES OF MULTIVARIABLE STATISTICS

Straightforward bivariate findings and relationships are usually presented by a contingency table or a graph (see Chapter 10). Subtle findings and interactions among multiple independent variables are difficult to detect using tables, however, and thus multivariable analysis is usually required. Multivariable analysis can often tease out how variables work *synergistically* (with each other to strengthen an effect) and *antagonistically* (against each other to weaken an effect).

Multivariable techniques enable investigators to determine whether there is an interaction between variables. **Interaction** is present when the value of one independent variable influences the way another independent variable explains y. For example, a large blood pressure survey in

TABLE 11.1 Choice of Appropriate Statistical Significance Test in Multivariable Analysis (Analysis of One Dependent Variable and More than One Independent Variable)

VARIABLES TO BE TESTED		
Dependent Variable	Independent Variables*	Appropriate Tests of Significance
Continuous	All categoric	Analysis of variance (ANOVA)
	Categoric and continuous	Analysis of covariance (ANCOVA)
		Multiple linear regression
Ordinal	All continuous	Multiple linear regression
	Categoric or continuous	Ordinal logistic regression or cumulative logit models (modification to logistic regression for ordinal outcomes)
Dichotomous	All categoric	Logistic regression; log-linear analysis
	Categoric and continuous	Logistic regression†
	All continuous	Logistic regression
Nominal	All categoric	Log-linear analysis
	Categoric and continuous	Multinomial logistic regression (modification to logistic regression for nominal outcomes)
	All continuous	Discriminant function analysis; or group the continuous variables and perform log-linear analysis

*Categoric variables include dichotomous and nominal variables.
†If the outcome is a time-related dichotomous variable (e.g., live/die), proportional hazards (Cox) models are best.

Connecticut found that in African Americans younger than 50, hypertension was more likely to occur in men than in women.[5] In people older than 50, however, that trend was reversed, and hypertension was more likely to occur in women than in men. For these relationships, there is an interaction between age and gender when explaining the prevalence rate of hypertension.

The net effect of the complex calculations of multivariable analysis is to help the investigators determine which of the independent variables are the strongest predictors of y, and which of the independent variables overlap with one another in their ability to predict y, or oppose each other, or interact.

In a clinical setting, such as an emergency department, it is helpful to have a scale or index that predicts whether a patient with chest pain is likely to have a myocardial infarction. Several multivariable techniques might be used to develop such a **prediction model**, complete with coefficients for use in prediction. Logistic regression was used to develop a prognostic index for 4-year mortality in older adults, for example.[6] Using various combinations of symptoms, signs, laboratory values, and electrocardiographic findings, investigators developed estimates for the probability of myocardial infarction and other diseases.[7,8] More recently, multiple logistic regression has become a common technique for developing clinical prediction models (see next section). Although such clinical prediction models usually work well on average, their predictions for an individual patient may be less satisfactory. Clinical prediction models are applied increasingly to chronic disease as well as acute disease.[9]

Multivariable analysis also can be used to develop clinical prediction models for the risk of disease or death among the general population, based on their known risk factors.

Investigators in the Framingham Heart Study used multivariable analysis to develop prediction equations for the 8-year risk of developing cardiovascular disease in people with various combinations of risk factors: smoking, elevated cholesterol levels, hypertension, glucose intolerance, and left ventricular hypertrophy (see Table 5.2 and reference/website listed). These prediction equations, or updated versions, are being used in various health risk assessment programs, as well as by health insurers interested in the costs and likely benefits associated with interventions directed toward the modification of specific chronic disease risk factors.

As stated earlier, an increasingly important role for multivariable analysis in clinical research is to adjust for intergroup differences that arise from observational research. For example, the relation between blood pressure and mortality from coronary heart disease in men across different countries was studied after using multivariable statistical methods to adjust for age, total cholesterol level, and cigarette smoking.[10] One strategy for this purpose is called **propensity matching**. This is typically used in observational cohort studies, where preexisting demographic and clinical differences exist between people who received some type of treatment and people who did not receive the treatment because the allocation to treatment was not randomized. Study participants who received treatment are matched with participants who did not receive treatment who have a similar **propensity score** (based on multivariable analysis). The objective is to make the matched groups who did and did not receive the treatment similar on all relevant variables except the treatment.[10,11] It is hoped that this will accomplish approximately the same goal as randomization and allow meaningful conclusions about the effects of treatment, even from nonrandomized studies.

3. PROCEDURES FOR MULTIVARIABLE ANALYSIS

As shown in Table 11.1, the choice of an appropriate statistical method for multivariable analysis depends on whether the dependent and independent variables are continuous, ordinal, dichotomous, or nominal. In cases in which more than one method could be used, the final choice depends on the investigator's experience, personal preference, and comfort with methods that are appropriate. Because there are many potential pitfalls in the use of multivariable techniques in medical research, these techniques should not be used without experience or expert advice, and as a general rule there should be at least 10 observations for each independent variable in the multivariable equation.[2]

3.1 ANALYSIS OF VARIANCE (ANOVA)

If the dependent variable is continuous and all the independent variables are categoric (i.e., nominal, dichotomous, or ordinal), the correct technique to use is analysis of variance (ANOVA). ANOVA is based on the general linear model and can be used to analyze the results of an experimental study. If the design includes only one independent variable (e.g., treatment group), the technique is a bivariate analysis called **one-way ANOVA** (see Chapter 9), regardless of how many different treatment groups are compared. If it includes more than one independent variable (e.g., treatment group, age group, and gender), the technique is a multivariate analysis called **N-way ANOVA** (the N standing for the number of different independent variables).

3.1.a One-Way ANOVA (F-Test)

One-way ANOVA is a method of bivariate analysis. Suppose a team of investigators wants to study the effects of drugs A and B on blood pressure. They might randomly allocate hypertensive patients into four treatment groups: patients taking drug A alone, patients taking drug B alone, patients taking drugs A and B in combination, and patients taking a placebo. Alternatively, they might choose to compare three different dosage patterns of the same drug against a placebo. The investigators could measure systolic blood pressure (SBP) before and after treatment in each patient and calculate a *difference score* (posttreatment SBP − pretreatment SBP) for each study participant. This difference score would become the dependent (outcome) variable. A mean difference score would be calculated for each of the four treatment groups (three drug groups and one placebo group) so that these mean scores could be compared by using ANOVA.

The investigators would want to determine whether the differences (presumably declines) in SBP found in one or more of the drug groups are large enough to be clinically important. A decrease in mean SBP from 150 to 148 mm Hg would be too small to be clinically useful. If the results are not clinically useful, there would be little point in doing a test of significance. If one or more of the groups showed a clinically important decrease in SBP compared with the placebo, however, the investigators would want to determine whether the difference was likely to have occurred by chance alone. To do this, an appropriate statistical test of significance is needed.

A two-sample t-test could be used to compare each pair of groups, but this would require six different t-tests: each of the three drug groups (A, B, and AB) versus the placebo group; drug A versus drug B; drug A versus drug combination AB; and drug B versus drug combination AB. Testing these six hypotheses raises the problem of multiple comparisons (see Chapter 12, section 3 Controlling for the Testing of Multiple Hypotheses). Even if the investigators decided that the primary comparison should be each drug or the drug combination with the placebo, this still would leave three hypotheses to test instead of just one. If two or three treatment groups performed significantly better than the placebo group, it would be necessary to determine if one of the treatment groups was significantly superior to the others.

The best approach when analyzing such a study would be first to perform an F-test (i.e., one-way ANOVA). The F-test is a type of *super t-test* that allows the investigator to compare more than two means simultaneously. In the antihypertensive drug study, the *null hypothesis* for the F-test is that the mean change in blood pressure $(\overline{d})$ will be the *same* for all four groups $(\overline{d}_A = \overline{d}_B = \overline{d}_{AB} = \overline{d}_P)$. This would indicate that all samples were taken from the same underlying population (called a *universe*), and that any observed differences between the means are caused by chance variation.

When creating the F-test, Fisher reasoned that there were two different ways to estimate the variance. One estimate is called **between-groups** variance and is based on the variation between (or among) the means. The other is called **within-groups** variance and is based on the variation within the groups (i.e., variation around the group means). Assuming the null hypothesis that all the study groups were sampled from the same population (i.e., the treatments made no difference), these two estimates of variance should be similar. The ratio of the between-groups variance to the within-groups variance is called *F* (in honor of Fisher). It is another form of *critical ratio* that enables a decision to be made either to reject or not to reject the null hypothesis. The F-test has the same general form as other critical ratios: the ratio of a measure of the effect (the differences between means) divided by a measure of the variability of the estimates. There is a nice relationship between hypothesis testing using ANOVA and hypothesis testing using a two-sample t-test. When comparing the means between two groups, the *p* value using an ANOVA to calculate the critical ratio *F* will be the exact same *p* value as using the t statistic from a two-sample t-test. In fact, in this case, it can be shown that $F = t^2$.

In ANOVA the two measures of variance are called the **between-groups mean square** and the **within-groups mean square**. (Mean square is simply the ANOVA name for variance, which is defined as a sum of squares [SS] divided by the appropriate number of degrees of freedom [*df*]). The ratio of the two measures of variance can be expressed as follows:

$$F \text{ ratio} = \frac{\text{Between-groups variance}}{\text{Within groups variance}}$$
$$= \frac{\text{Between-groups mean square}}{\text{Within groups mean square}}$$

If the F ratio is close to 1.0, the two estimates of variance are similar and the null hypothesis—that all the means came from the same underlying population—is not rejected. This occurs when the treatment has too small an effect to push apart the observed means of the different groups. If the F ratio is much larger than 1.0, however, some force, presumably the treatment, caused the means to differ, so the null hypothesis of no difference is rejected. The assumptions for the F-test are similar to those for the t-test. First, the dependent variable (in this case, blood pressure difference scores) should be normally distributed, although with large samples this assumption can be relaxed because of the central limit theorem. Second, the several samples of the dependent variable should be independent random samples from populations with approximately equal variances. This need for

equal variances is more acute in the F-test than it is in the t-test, where an adjustment is available to correct for a large difference between the two variances. As with the t-test, the F-test requires that an alpha level be specified in advance. After the F statistic has been calculated, its *p* value can be looked up in a table of the F distribution to determine whether the results are statistically significant. With the F-test, this task is more complicated than with the t-test, however, because ANOVA has two different degrees of freedom to deal with: one for the numerator (the model mean square) and one for the denominator (the error mean square), as explained in Box 11.1.

If the results *are* statistically significant, the investigators must take additional steps to determine which of the differences between means are greater than would be expected by chance alone. In the case of the example introduced earlier involving four treatment groups (drug A alone, drug B alone, drugs A and B combined, and placebo), overall statistical significance could be found if any of the following were true:

1. The mean difference of one group differed greatly from that of the other three groups.
2. The means of two groups differed greatly from those of the remaining two groups.

BOX 11.1 **Analysis of Variance (ANOVA) Table**

The goal of ANOVA, stated in the simplest terms, is to explain (i.e., to model) the total variation found in one analysis. Because the total variation is equal to the sum of squares (SS) of the dependent variable, the process of explaining that variation entails partitioning the SS into component parts. The logic behind this process was introduced in Chapter 9 (see the section on variation between groups versus variation within groups). That discussion focused on the example of explaining the difference between the heights of men and women using fictitious data. The heights of 100 female and 100 male university students were measured, the total variation (SS from the grand mean) was found to be 10,000 cm², and 4000 cm² of the variation was attributed to gender. Because that example is uncomplicated and involves round numbers, it is used here to illustrate the format for an ANOVA table.

Source of Variation	Sum of Squares (SS)	Degrees of Freedom (*df*)	Mean Square (MS)	*F* Ratio
Total	10,000	199		
Model (gender)	4,000	1	4000.0	132.0
Error	6,000	198	30.3	

The model in this example has only one independent variable—gender, considered here as a dichotomous variable. In the SS column the figure of 4000 represents the amount of variation explained by gender (i.e., the between-groups SS noted in the ANOVA), and 6000 represents the amount of SS not explained by gender (i.e., the within-groups variation). In the *df* column the total *df* is listed as 199, reflecting there were 200 participants and that 1 *df* was lost in calculating the grand mean for

all observations. The *df* for the model is calculated as the number of categories (groups) minus 1. Gender has only two categories (men and women), so 1 *df* is assigned to it. The *df* for error is calculated as the total *df* minus the number of *df* assigned to the model: 199 − 1 = 198.

The mean square is simply another name for variance and is equal to the SS divided by the appropriate *df*: 4000/1 = 4000.0 for the model mean square, and 6000/198 = 30.3 for the error mean square.

The F ratio is a ratio of variances, or in ANOVA-speak, a ratio of mean squares. Specifically, the F ratio here is calculated by dividing the model mean square by the error mean square: 4000/30.3 = 132.0. To look up the *p* value that corresponds to this F ratio in the table of F distributions, it is necessary to know the *df* for the denominator and the *df* for the numerator. In this case, as described previously, the *df* for the numerator would be 1, and the *df* for the denominator would be 198. Because the F ratio is so large, 132.0, the *p* value would be extremely small ($p < 0.00001$), and the null hypothesis that there is no true (average) difference between the mean heights of men and women would be rejected.

If there was more than one independent variable in the model being analyzed, there would be more entries under the column showing the source of variation: total, model, *interaction*, and error. The model also would contain separate lines for the other independent variable(s), such as height of the participant's mother. The *interaction* term refers to the portion of the variation caused by interactions between the independent variables in the model (here that might be written as *gender × mother-height*). The error SS would be the variation not explained by either of the independent variables or their interaction.

When performed using standard software packages, the full results automatically include the critical ratio and the *p* value, along with other details.

3. The means of the four groups were strung along a line (e.g., if drugs A and B combined showed the best results, drug A second-best results, drug B third-best results, and placebo least impressive results).

4. There are no mean differences that are significantly different from that of the other groups. While less common, it is possible for the overall test to be statistically significant, but none of the individual comparisons reach statistical significance.

Most advanced statistical computer packages include options in the ANOVA program that allow investigators to determine which of the differences are true differences; this involves making adjustments for more than one hypothesis being tested simultaneously.[12] Although a detailed discussion of the various adjustment methods is beyond the scope of this book, it is important for readers to understand the logic behind this form of analysis and to recognize the circumstances under which one-way ANOVA is appropriate. As an example of the use of ANOVA, a clinical trial was performed in which asthma patients were randomized into three treatment groups: one who received 42 μg of salmeterol two times daily, one who received 180 μg of albuterol four times daily, and one who received a placebo.[13] At the beginning and end of the study, the investigators measured the asthma patients' forced expiratory volume in 1 second (FEV_1), and they used F-tests to compare the changes in FEV_1 values seen in the three different treatment groups. Based on the results of one-way ANOVA, they concluded that salmeterol was more effective than albuterol or placebo in increasing the morning peak expiratory flow rate.

3.1.b. *N*-Way ANOVA

The goal of ANOVA is to explain (to model) as much variation in a continuous variable as possible, by using one or more categoric variables to predict the variation. If only one independent variable is tested in a model, it is called an F-test, or a one-way ANOVA. If two or more independent variables are tested, it is called a two-way ANOVA or an *N*-way ANOVA (the *N* specifying how many independent variables are used).

In ANOVA, if one variable for an F-test is gender (see Box 11.1), the total sum of squares (SS) in the dependent variable can be partitioned into a contribution from gender and residual noise. If two independent variables are tested in a model, and those variables are treatment and gender, the total amount of variation is divided into how much variation is caused by each of the following: independent effect of treatment, independent effect of gender, interaction between (i.e., joint effect of) treatment and gender, and error. If more than two independent variables are tested, the analysis becomes increasingly complicated, but the underlying logic remains the same. As long as the research design is "balanced" (i.e., there are equal numbers of observations in each of the study groups), *N*-way ANOVA can be used to analyze the individual and joint effects of categorical independent variables and to partition the total variation into the various component parts. If the design is not balanced, most computer programs provide an alternative method to do an approximate ANOVA; for example, in SAS, the PROC GLM procedure can be used. The details of such analyses are beyond the scope of this book.

As an example, *N*-way ANOVA procedures were used in a study to determine whether supplementing gonadotropin-releasing hormone with parathyroid hormone would reduce the osteoporosis-causing effect of gonadotropin-releasing hormone.[14] The investigators used ANOVA to examine the effects of treatment and other independent variables on the bone loss induced by estrogen deficiency.

3.2 ANALYSIS OF COVARIANCE (ANCOVA)

Analysis of variance and analysis of covariance are methods for evaluating studies in which the dependent variable is continuous (see Table 11.1). If the independent variables are all of the categorical type (nominal, dichotomous, or ordinal), ANOVA is used. If some of the independent variables are categoric and some are continuous, however, **ANCOVA** is appropriate. ANCOVA could be used, for example, in a study to test the effects of antihypertensive drugs on SBP in participants of varying age. The change in SBP after treatment (a continuous variable) is the dependent variable, and the independent variables might be age (a continuous variable) and treatment (a categoric variable). One study used ANCOVA to evaluate the results of a controlled clinical trial of dichloroacetate to treat lactic acidosis in adult patients.[15] ANCOVA adjusted the dependent variable for the pretreatment concentrations of arterial blood lactate in the study participants and tested the difference between the adjusted means of the treatment groups.

3.3 MULTIPLE LINEAR REGRESSION

Multiple linear regression is a commonly used technique that can include both continuous and categoric predictors. It can be used to identify the strength of the relationship between one dependent variable and multiple independent variables, describe the effects of change on dependent variables that independent variables may have, and predict future values of dependent variables when values of the independent variables are prespecified. The formula looks like the general linear model formula shown in Equation 11.6.

Performing an analysis using any type of regression must begin with descriptive statistics of all variables to be included to determine if any outliers or data errors are present. It is essential to examine if there is a relationship between each potential independent variable with the independent variable. For continuous independent variables it is important to assess whether the relationship with the dependent variable is linear and, if not, a nonlinear relationship may be investigated.

It is also important to examine the independent variables for multicollinearity, which occurs when one or more independent variables is highly associated with other independent variables. If multicollinearity is present, the model can produce parameter estimates with a high degree of uncertainty. Thus it is important to remove independent variables that are highly correlated with each other.

An important concern when generating multiple regression models is to avoid overfitting the models, which can occur when including too many variables in the model. The variables included in linear models can be chosen by using content experts or variable selection procedures. Variable selection procedures can include **stepwise methods** (forward selection, backward elimination, or stepwise regression) or criterion-based methods (e.g., Mallows' Cp, Akaike Information Criterion [AIC], or Bayesian Information Criterion [BIC]). The explanatory strength of all the variables entered (i.e., their adjusted or predicted R^2, modifications for the multivariable context to the R^2 discussed in Chapter 10) can also be used to examine the strength of the model. Finally, an assessment of diagnostics (residual plots, QQ-plots, Cook's distance, influential values) is crucial to determine if the results of the model can be interpreted with accuracy.

Multiple linear regression is often used in clinical, economic, and health services research when the dependent variable is continuous, such as the amount of profit (or loss) in dollars for a hospital over a time period.

3.4 OTHER PROCEDURES FOR MULTIVARIABLE ANALYSIS

Multiple logistic regression is an appropriate procedure when the outcome variable in a clinical prediction model is dichotomous (e.g., improved/unimproved or survived/died). Where linear regression models the expected change in y for a one-unit change in one of the predictors, holding all of the others constant, logistic regression models the expected change in the odds for a one-unit increase in the predictor. As in multiple linear regression, issues of overfitting, multicollinearity, and checking of diagnostics are all fundamental to the development of a useful logistic regression model. This procedure was used to test a model that was developed to predict on admission to the hospital whether patients with bacterial meningitis would experience a good outcome (complete recovery) or a poor outcome (residual neurologic sequelae or death).[16]

A commonly used regression model for survival data is the **Cox proportional hazards model**, which is used to test for differences in the instantaneous hazard of death or some other event between groups. It also is used to determine which variables are associated with better survival. For example, Cox models have been used to compare the relapse-free survival of two groups of patients with rectal cancer: patients treated with radiation plus a protracted infusion of fluorouracil and patients given a bolus injection of fluorouracil.[17] The mechanics of such methods are beyond the scope of this text, but knowing when they are warranted is important in interpreting the medical literature.

4. SUMMARY

Multivariable analysis involves statistical methods for determining how well several independent (possibly causal) variables, separately and together, explain the variation in a single, dependent (outcome) variable. In medical research, there are three common uses for multivariable analysis: (1) to improve the testing of an intervention in a clinical trial by controlling for the effects of other variables on the outcome variable; (2) to shed light on the etiology or prognosis of a disease in observational studies by estimating the relative impact of one or more independent variables on the risk of disease or death; and (3) to develop weights for the different variables used in a diagnostic or prognostic scoring system. As shown in Table 11.1, the choice of an appropriate procedure to be used for multivariable analysis depends on whether the dependent and independent variables are continuous, dichotomous, nominal, ordinal, or a combination of these. Because the use of multivariable techniques has many potential problems and limitations in clinical research, these procedures should be used and interpreted with understanding and care.

REFERENCES

1. Kleinbaum DG. *Applied Regression Analysis and Other Multivariable Methods*, 4th ed. Belmont, CA: Brooks/Cole; 2008.
2. Horton NJ, Switzer SS. Statistical methods in the journal. *N Engl J Med*. 2005;353:1977-1979.
3. Arbogast PG, Ray WA. Performance of disease risk scores, propensity scores, and traditional multivariable outcome regression in the presence of multiple confounders. *Am J Epidemiol*. 2011;174:613-620.
4. Holford TR. *Multivariate Methods in Epidemiology*. New York, NY: Oxford University Press; 2002.
5. Freeman Jr DH, D'Atri DA, Hellenbrand K, et al. The prevalence distribution of hypertension: Connecticut adults 1978-1979. *J Chronic Dis*. 1983;36:171-181.
6. Lee SJ, Lindquist K, Segal MR, Covinsky KE. Development and validation of a prognostic index for 4-year mortality in older adults. *JAMA*. 2006;295:801-808.
7. Yoo HH, De Paiva SA, Silveira LV, Queluz TT. Logistic regression analysis of potential prognostic factors for pulmonary thromboembolism. *Chest*. 2003;123:813-821.
8. Ayanian JZ, Landrum MB, Guadagnoli E, Gaccione P. Specialty of ambulatory care physicians and mortality among elderly patients after myocardial infarction. *N Engl J Med*. 2002;347:1678-1686.
9. D'Agostino Jr RB. Propensity score methods for bias reduction in the comparison of a treatment to a non-randomized control group. *Stat Med*. 1998;17:2265-2281.
10. Nakayama M, Osaki S, Shimokawa H. Validation of mortality risk stratification models for cardiovascular disease. *Am J Cardiol*. 2011;108:391-396.
11. van den Hoogen PC, Feskens EJ, Nagelkerke NJ, Menotti A, Nissinen A, Kromhout D. The relation between blood pressure and mortality due to coronary heart disease among men in different parts of the world. *N Engl J Med*. 2000;342:1-8.

12. Dawson B, Trapp RG. *Basic & Clinical Biostatistics*. 4th ed. New York, NY: Lange Medical Books/McGraw-Hill; 2004.

13. Pearlman DS, Chervinsky P, LaForce C, et al. A comparison of salmeterol with albuterol in the treatment of mild-to-moderate asthma. *N Engl J Med*. 1992;327:1420-1425.

14. Finkelstein JS, Klibanski A, Schaefer EH, Hornstein MD, Schiff I, Neer RM. Parathyroid hormone for the prevention of bone loss induced by estrogen deficiency. *N Engl J Med*. 1994;331:1618-1623.

15. Stacpoole PW, Wright EC, Baumgartner TG, et al. A controlled clinical trial of dichloroacetate for treatment of lactic acidosis in adults. *N Engl J Med*. 1992;327:1564-1569.

16. Aronin SI, Peduzzi P, Quagliariello VJ. Community-acquired bacterial meningitis: risk stratification for adverse clinical outcome and effect of antibiotic timing. *Ann Intern Med*. 1998;129:862-869.

17. O'Connell MJ, Martenson JA, Wieand HS, et al. Improving adjuvant therapy for rectal cancer by combining protracted-infusion fluorouracil with radiation therapy after curative surgery. *N Engl J Med*. 1994;331:502-507.

SELECT READING

Feinstein AR. *Multivariable Analysis: An Introduction*. New Haven, CT: Yale University Press; 1996.

REVIEW QUESTIONS

1. A multivariable analysis is needed when:
   A. Multiple groups of participants are being compared
   B. Multiple outcome variables are under investigation
   C. Multiple repetitions of an experiment are planned
   D. Multiple confounders need to be controlled simultaneously
   E. Multiple investigators will be repeating analyses for comparability

2. A multivariable model is best exemplified by which of the following statements?
   A. Height and weight vary together.
   B. Height and weight vary with age.
   C. Height varies with weight and age.
   D. Height varies with gender.
   E. Height varies with gender, and weight varies with age.

3. The basic equation for a multivariable model generally includes a dependent (outcome) variable (y); a starting point or regression constant (a); weights or coefficients (the b terms); and a residual or error term (e). The least-squares solution to a multivariable equation is determined when:
   A. The model is statistically significant
   B. The residual is maximized
   C. The value of a is minimized
   D. The value of e^2 is minimized
   E. The regression constant is 0

4. In a survival study of patients with pancreatic cancer, one group was treated with a chemotherapeutic agent and another group with a placebo. Which of the following procedures would be best for comparing the survival experience of the two groups over time while adjusting for other variables, such as age, gender, and cancer stage?
   A. ANCOVA
   B. Linear regression analysis
   C. Logrank test
   D. McNemar chi-square test
   E. Proportional hazards (Cox) model

5. You are interested in comparing the effects of various agents on the management of pain caused by osteoarthritis. Pain is measured on a continuous pain scale. You design a study in which equal numbers of patients are assigned to three groups defined by treatment (acetaminophen, ibuprofen, or placebo). Other independent variables are gender, age (dichotomous: <50 years or ≥50 years), and severity of arthritis (categoric: mild, moderate, or severe). Which of the following would be the most appropriate statistical method for analyzing your data?
   A. Logistic regression analysis
   B. One-way ANOVA
   C. N-way ANOVA
   D. ANCOVA
   E. Wilcoxon matched-pairs signed-ranks test

6. Concerning question 5, to calculate an F ratio, you must first establish:
   A. The between-groups mean square and the degrees of freedom
   B. The between-groups variance and within-groups variance
   C. The degrees of freedom and the value of p
   D. The least squares and the residual
   E. The standard error and the mean for each group

ANSWERS AND EXPLANATIONS

1. **D.** Multivariable analyses allow investigators to examine associations among multiple independent variables and an outcome variable simultaneously. Often, only one of the independent variables will be of interest to investigators, and others will be potential confounders. However, independent variables may also exert a truly meaningful effect on the outcome or function as effect modifiers (see Chapter 4). Multivariable analyses allow investigators to estimate the association between the independent variable of interest and the outcome, controlling for or adjusting for the potential influence of possible confounding variables in the regression model. Multiple groups of participants (A), multiple investigators (E), or multiple repetitions of the experiment planned (C) have no bearing on whether investigators choose multivariable analytic techniques. If multiple outcomes are under investigation (B), what is needed is multivariate analysis.

2. **C.** Multivariable models may be expressed conceptually and mathematically. A conceptual understanding of multivariable analysis is facilitated by a verbal description of the relationships under study. To conform to the requirements for multivariable analysis, the model must postulate the influence of more than one independent variable on one, and only one, dependent (outcome) variable. In general, such a model, expressed in words, would take the following form: dependent variable y varies with independent variables x_1, x_2, and so on. The only choice provided that fits this pattern is C; the other answer choices are all bivariable associations.

3. **D.** The basic equation for a multivariable model is as follows:

$$y = a + b_1 x_1 + b_2 x_2 + b_3 x_3 + b_4 x_4 + e$$

The outcome variable is y, the regression constant or starting point is a, the b terms represent weights, and e is the residual or error term. The goal of the least-squares approach to multivariable analysis is to find the model that produces the smallest sum of squares of the error term, e. The error term is also called the residual, and the least-squares solution minimizes, versus maximizes (B), this value. The values of a and the b_is that lead to this result, which are not minimized (C), maximized, or set at zero (E), produce the best fit or model. The least-squares model may or may not be statistically significant (A), depending on the strength of association between the independent and dependent variables under investigation.

4. **E.** In a survival study showing the proportion surviving after a fixed number of months, the outcome variable is dichotomous (live/die). Consequently, a standard chi-square can be used to test the hypothesis of independence, or the McNemar chi-square (D) can be used for paired data. A survival study can provide much more information about the participants in each group, however, than simply the proportion of participants who were alive at the end of the study. In a study that may span years, the timing of death is equally important. Intergroup comparison should address the distribution and the number of deaths. The logrank test (C) is designed for making such a comparison, but it cannot adjust for other independent variables. The multivariable method appropriate for survival analysis is the proportional hazards (Cox) model, a method now usually employed in the analysis of clinical trial data. ANCOVA (A) is a multivariable method used with a continuous outcome variable, when the independent variables are a mix of continuous and categoric. Linear regression (B) is either a bivariable method or, in the case of multiple linear regression, a multivariable method; it is also used to analyze a continuous outcome variable, regardless of the type of independent variables.

5. **C.** As shown in Table 11.1, ANOVA is appropriate when the outcome variable is continuous, and multiple independent variables are categoric. The study described meets these criteria. The method is N-way ANOVA, rather than one-way ANOVA (B), because the model includes several different independent variables. ANCOVA (D) would not be appropriate in this case because at least one of the independent variables has to be continuous to employ this method. Logistic regression (A) is for dichotomous, not continuous, outcomes. The Wilcoxon signed-ranks test (E) is a nonparametric test requiring a single dichotomous independent variable and dependent/matched groups; if investigators had been looking at pain on a scale of 10 for a given group of individuals before and after acetaminophen treatment, the Wilcoxon matched-pairs signed-ranks test may have been appropriate.

6. **B.** The F ratio is simply the ratio of between-groups variance to within-groups variance. In ANOVA, variance is often called the mean square, which is different from the least squares or the residual (D) of linear regression. One does not need to know the standard error or the mean for each group (E) to calculate an F ratio. Likewise, degrees of freedom (A and C) are not needed to calculate an F ratio. However, degrees of freedom are needed to determine the p value from an F ratio (e.g., using a table of the F distribution).

Using Statistics to Design Studies:
Sample Size Calculation, Randomization, and Controlling for Multiple Hypotheses

With Martiniano J. Flores

CHAPTER OUTLINE

"Absence of evidence is not evidence of absence."

Carl Sagan

When correctly designed, analyzed, and interpreted, randomized controlled trials (RCTs) are the best method to determine whether a clinical or public health intervention works. Randomization reduces selection bias by distributing important demographic, social, and biologic characteristics between comparison groups by chance. In theory, with randomization, groups are similar enough that any differences in outcomes between intervention and control groups can be attributed to the effect of the intervention. One of the most important uses of statistics in designing studies is to determine the required sample sizes for comparing groups such that if a difference between groups truly exists, the study will likely detect it. Other uses of statistics in RCTs include methods of randomization and controlling for the testing of multiple hypotheses.

1. SAMPLE SIZE

From a statistical standpoint, the determination of sample size is essential to the likelihood of finding statistical significance if a difference between groups truly exists. Sample size calculations are also critical in planning clinical research, because it is usually the most important factor in determining the time and funding necessary to perform the study.

Individuals responsible for evaluating and funding clinical studies look closely at the assumptions used to estimate the number of study participants needed and at the way in which calculations of sample size are performed. Part of their task when reviewing the sample size is to determine whether the proposed research is realistic (e.g., whether adequate participants are included in the intervention and control groups in a RCT, or in the groups of cases and controls in a case control study). In research reported in the literature, inadequate sample size may explain why expected results are not statistically significant.

Statisticians are probably consulted more often to determine a sample size calculation for an investigator planning a study than for any other reason. Sample size calculations can be confusing, even for investigators who perform ordinary statistical analyses without trouble. As a test of intuition regarding sample size, try to answer the following three questions.

How would the sample size calculation be affected if:
1. The outcome has a high amount of variability?
2. The investigator wants the result to be extremely close to the true value (i.e., have narrow confidence limits)?
3. The investigator wants to detect an extremely small difference between comparison groups?

If your intuition suggested that all these requirements would create the need for a larger sample size, you would be correct. If intuition did not suggest the correct answers, review these questions again after reading the following information about how the basic formulas for sample size are derived.

Other factors affecting the number of participants required for a study include whether the:

1. Research design involves *paired data* (e.g., each subject has a pair of observations from two points in time—before treatment and after treatment) or *unpaired data* (e.g., observations are compared between an experimental group and a control group).
2. Investigator chooses the usual alpha level (*p* value of 0.05 or confidence interval of 95%) or chooses a smaller level of alpha.
3. Investigator chooses the usual power (80%) for detecting group differences or chooses a higher level of power.
4. Alpha chosen is one sided or two sided (see upcoming discussion).

1.1 BETA (FALSE-NEGATIVE) ERROR

A beta error occurs when results of a study are negative when they are actually positive. If a difference is examined with a t-test, and it is statistically significant at the prestated level of alpha (e.g., 0.05), there is no need to worry about a false-negative (beta) error. However, what if a reported finding seems to be clinically important, but it is not "statistically significant" in the study? Here the question of a possible false-negative (beta) error becomes important. In many cases, beta error may have occurred because the sample size was too small. When planning a study, investigators need to avoid the likelihoods of both alpha (false-positive) and beta (false-negative) errors, and users of research results should be on the lookout for these problems as well. The relationship between the results of a study and the true status can be seen in a *truth table* (Table 12.1). Notice the similarity of Table 12.1 to the relationship between a test result and the disease status (see Table 7.1).

A seminal article illustrated the need to be concerned about beta error by identifying many RCTs with inadequate sample sizes.[1] In 94% of 71 *negative* RCTs of new therapies published in prominent medical journals, the sample sizes were too small to detect a 25% improvement in outcome with reasonable (90%) assurance. In 75% of the studies, the sample sizes were too small to detect a 50% improvement in outcome with the same level of assurance. Additional research indicates that this problem has persisted over time.[2]

TABLE 12.1 "Truth Table" Showing Relationship Between Study Results and True Status

STUDY RESULT	TRUE STATUS	
	True Difference	No Difference
Statistically significant difference	True-positive result	False-positive result (alpha error)
Not statistically significant	False-negative result (beta error)	True-negative result

A study with a large beta error has a low sensitivity for detecting a true difference because, as discussed in Chapter 7:

$$\text{Sensitivity} + \text{False negative (beta) error} = 1.00$$

When investigators speak of a research study versus a clinical test, however, they often use the term "statistical power" instead of "sensitivity." With this substitution in terms:

$$\text{Statistical power} + \text{Beta error} = 1.00$$

which means statistical power is equal to $(1 - \text{beta error})$. When calculating a sample size, if the investigators accept a 20% possibility of missing a true finding (beta error $= 0.2$), the study has a statistical power of 0.8, or 80%. That means the investigators are 80% confident that they would be able to detect a true mean difference of the size they specify with the sample size they determine. The best way to incorporate beta error into a study is to include it beforehand in the determination of sample size.

1.2 DERIVATION OF BASIC SAMPLE SIZE FORMULA

Statistical power is the probability of rejecting the null hypothesis, given that it is in fact false. Represented as an equation, power is

$$\text{Power} = P\left(\text{Reject null hypothesis given that it is false}\right)$$

In sample size calculations, the basic question is: If the true difference between groups is equal to some value *d*, what is the sample size needed to ensure a power of $(1-\beta)$ for detecting this difference? The basic procedure for deriving the appropriate sample size involves two steps. The first step is to determine the conditions that will reject the null hypothesis. This will result in a formula that contains the sample size *N*. The next step is to solve the equation in terms of *N*. To show how this works in practice, it is easiest to start with a *one-sided paired t-test* (see Chapter 9). The formula for the test statistic in a paired t-test is given by $t = \dfrac{\bar{d} - 0}{\dfrac{\text{SD}}{\sqrt{N}}}$, where $\bar{d}$ is an estimate of *d* and zero is in the numerator because the null hypothesis tests whether the group means are equivalent. The null hypothesis is rejected when $t > t_{1-\alpha,\text{df}}$, which is the rejection region associated with the T table given in the Appendix. However, the properties of the *t* distribution generally make the sample size calculation intractable analytically. Therefore, one can assume a large sample size and approximate the rejection region using the Z table, thereby rejecting if $t > z_{1-\alpha}$. If "Power" is replaced with $(1-\beta)$ in the power formula, and "Reject the null hypothesis given that it is false" is replaced with $t > z_{1-\alpha}$, the equation becomes

$$P\left(\frac{\bar{d}\sqrt{N}}{\text{SD}} > z_{1-\alpha}\right) = 1 - \beta$$

where the t statistic was rearranged to put the sample size on top. Finally, assuming the true difference between the groups is *d*, after some algebra and using the properties of normal distribution, the equation can be rewritten as

$$\frac{d\sqrt{N}}{SD} - z_{1-\alpha} = z_{1-\beta}$$

where $z_{1-\beta}$ can be found using a Z table. Solving for N,

$$N = \frac{\left(z_{1-\alpha} + z_{1-\beta}\right)^2 SD^2}{d^2}$$

Notice in the sample size formula there are four items to choose: (1) the α level, which represents the willingness to make a false-positive error; (2) the β level, which represents the willingness to make a false-negative error; (3) the hypothesized variability (SD) in the population; and (4) the hypothesized true group difference d. All values except the variance must come from clinical and research judgment, although the estimated variance should be based on knowledge of data. If the outcome variable being studied is continuous, such as blood pressure, the estimate of variance can be obtained from the literature or from a small pilot study.

How do each of these quantities affect the required sample size?

1. For the alpha level, to have considerable confidence that a mean difference shown in a study is real, the analysis must produce a small p value for the observed mean difference, which implies that the value for $z_{1-\alpha}$ was large. Because $z_{1-\alpha}$ is in the numerator of the sample size formula, the larger $z_{1-\alpha}$ is, the larger the N (sample size) that is needed. For a two-tailed test, a p value of 0.05 (the α level chosen) would require a $z_{1-\alpha}$ of 1.96. To be even more confident, the investigator might set alpha at 0.01. This would require a $z_{1-\alpha}$ of 2.58. Assuming the standard beta error of 0.2, this means that decreasing the probability of making a false-positive error from 5% to 1% would require the sample size to be increased by about 50%.

2. Similarly, wanting a greater probability of rejecting a false null hypothesis, means wanting a smaller false-negative error. This means the beta is to be smaller (or equivalently, $[1 - \beta]$ is larger). This will increase $z_{1-\beta}$, which leads to an increase in the sample size. The takeaway is that wanting a smaller chance of getting the wrong conclusion, whether false positive or false negative, requires a larger sample size.

3. The larger the variance (SD²), the larger the sample size must be, because the variance is in the numerator of the formula for N. This makes sense intuitively because with a large variance (and large standard error), a larger N is needed to compensate for the greater uncertainty of the estimate.

4. If the investigator wanted to detect with confidence a very small difference between the mean values of two study groups (i.e., a small $\bar{d}$), a very large N would be needed because the difference (squared) is in the denominator. The smaller the denominator is, the larger the ratio is, and the larger the N must be. A precise estimate and a large sample size are needed to detect a small difference.

Whether a small difference is considered clinically important often depends on the topic of research. Studies showing that a new treatment for hypertension reduces the systolic blood pressure by 1 to 2 mm Hg would be considered clinically trivial. Studies showing that a new treatment for pancreatic cancer improves the survival rate by 10% (0.1) would be considered a major advance. Clinical judgment is involved in determining the minimum difference that should be considered clinically important.

1.3 STEPS IN CALCULATION OF SAMPLE SIZE

The first step in calculating a sample size that would detect a true treatment effect is to choose the appropriate formula to use based on the type of study. Two common formulas for calculating sample size for studies using t-tests or testing differences in proportions are discussed in this chapter and listed in Table 12.2, and their use is illustrated in Boxes 12.1, 12.2, 12.3 and 12.4.[3]

The N determined using these formulas is only for the experimental group. If there is a control group, it is common practice to assume that its sample size is the same as the experimental group. For some studies, investigators may find it easier to obtain control participants than cases. In general, the sample size formulas can be simplified by assuming that the number of controls is equal to some fraction of the number of cases. For example, when cases are scarce or costly, it is possible to increase the sample size by matching two or three controls with each case in a case control study or by obtaining two or three control group participants for each experimental participant in a clinical trial. The incremental benefits in statistical power decline, however, as the number of controls per cases increases, so it is seldom cost effective to have more than three controls for each case.

The application of the formulas described here assumes the research objective is to have equal numbers of experimental and control participants. If the number of control subjects is planned to be much greater than the number of cases, the sample size formulas discussed in this chapter would need to be modified.[4]

TABLE 12.2 Formulas for Calculation of Sample Size for Study Designs Common in Medical Research

Type of Study*	Appropriate Formula
Studies using two-sample t-test	$N = \dfrac{\left(z_{1-\alpha} + z_{1-\beta}\right)^2 \times 2 \times SD^2}{d^2}$
Studies using a test of differences in proportions	$N = \dfrac{\left(z_{1-\alpha} + z_{1-\beta}\right)^2 \times 2 \times \bar{p}(1-\bar{p})}{d^2}$

*The appropriate formula is based on the study design and type of outcome data. In these formulas, N = sample size; $z_{1-\alpha}$ = z value for alpha error; $z_{1-\beta}$ = z value for beta error; SD^2 = variance; $\bar{p}$ = mean proportion of success; and d^2 = mean difference to be detected. See Boxes 12.1 to 12.4 for examples of calculations using these formulas.

BOX 12.1 Calculation of Sample Size for a Study Using the Paired t-Test and Assuming 50% Power

Part 1 Data on Which the Calculation is Based

Study Characteristic	Assumptions Made by Investigator
Type of study	Before-and-after study of antihypertensive drug
Data sets	Pretreatment and posttreatment observations in the same participants
Variable	Systolic blood pressure
Losses to follow-up	None
Standard deviation (SD)	15 mm Hg
Variance (SD^2)	225 mm Hg
Data for alpha ($z_{1-\alpha}$)	$p = 0.05$; 95% confidence desired (two-tailed test); $z_{1-\alpha} = 1.96$
Difference to be detected d	≥10 mm Hg difference between pretreatment and posttreatment blood pressure values

Part 2 Calculation of Sample Size (N)

$$N = \frac{z_{1-\alpha}^2 \times s^2}{d^2}$$
$$= \frac{1.96^2 \times 15^2}{10^2}$$
$$= 9 \text{ participants total}$$

Interpretation: Only nine participants are needed for this study because each paired subject serves as his or her own control in a before-and-after study, thereby greatly reducing the variance (i.e., variance between a subject before and after a particular treatment is almost certain to be much less than the variance between one person and another). The relatively low power of the study also reduces the sample size considerably. When the estimated N is a fraction, the N should be rounded up to insure adequate sample size.

BOX 12.2 Calculation of Sample Size for a Study Using Two-Sample t-Test Assuming 50% Power

Part 1 Data on Which the Calculation Is Based

Study Characteristic	Assumptions Made by Investigator
Type of study	Randomized controlled trial of antihypertensive drug
Data sets	Observations in one experimental group and one control group of the same size
Variable	Systolic blood pressure
Losses to follow-up	None
Standard deviation (SD)	15 mm Hg
Variance (SD^2)	225 mm Hg
Data for alpha ($z_{1-\alpha}$)	$p = 0.05$; 95% confidence desired (two-tailed test); $z_{1-\alpha} = 1.96$
Difference to be detected (d)	≥10 mm Hg difference between mean blood pressure values of the experimental group and the control group

Part 2 Calculation of Sample Size (N)

$$N = \frac{z_{1-\alpha}^2 \times 2 \times s^2}{d^2}$$
$$= \frac{1.96^2 \times 2 \times 15^2}{10^2}$$
$$= 18 \text{ participants per group} \times 2 \text{ groups}$$
$$= 36 \text{ participants total}$$

Interpretation: For the type of study depicted in this box, 18 participants are needed in the experimental group and 18 in the control group, for a total N of 36 study participants. The total N needed in this box is four times as large as the total N needed in Box 12.1, although the values for $z_{1-\alpha}$, SD^2, and d^2 are the same in both boxes. One reason for the larger sample size for a randomized controlled trial is that there are two groups, and the N calculated is for the intervention group only. The other reason is there are two variances to consider (i.e., the intervention and control groups contribute to the overall variance), so the estimated variance must be multiplied by 2.

BOX 12.3 Calculation of Sample Size for a Study Using Two-Sample t-Test Assuming 80% Power

Part 1 Data on Which the Calculation Is Based

Study Characteristic	Assumptions Made by Investigator
Type of study	Randomized controlled trial of antihypertensive drug
Data sets	Observations in one experimental group and one control group of the same size
Variable	Systolic blood pressure
Losses to follow-up	None
Standard deviation (s)	15 mm Hg
Variance (s^2)	225 mm Hg
Data for alpha ($z_{1-\alpha}$)	$p = 0.05$; 95% confidence desired (two-tailed test); $z_{1-\alpha} = 1.96$
Data for beta ($z_{1-\beta}$)	20% beta error; 80% power desired (one-tailed test); $z_{1-\beta} = 0.84$
Difference to be detected (d)	$\geq$10 mm Hg difference between mean blood pressure values of the experimental group and control group

Part 2 Calculation of Sample Size (N)

$$
\begin{aligned}
N &= \frac{\left(z_{1-\alpha} + z_{1-\beta}\right)^2 \times 2 \times s^2}{d^2} \\
&= \frac{\left(1.96 + 0.84\right)^2 \times 2 \times 15^2}{10^2} \\
&= 36 \text{ participants per group} \times 2 \text{ groups} \\
&= 72 \text{ participants total}
\end{aligned}
$$

Interpretation: The total number of participants needed is 72. Including $z_{1-\beta}$ (for beta error) in the calculation approximately doubled the sample size here compared with the sample size in Box 12.2. If the investigators had chosen a smaller beta error, the sample size would have increased even more.

BOX 12.4 Initial and Subsequent Calculation of Sample Size for a Study Using a Test of Differences in Proportions Assuming 80% Power

Part 1A Data on Which the Initial Calculation is Based

Study Characteristic	Assumptions Made by Investigator
Type of study	Randomized controlled trial of a drug to reduce 5-year mortality in patients with a particular form of cancer
Data sets	Observations in one experimental group (E) and one control group (C) of the same size
Variable	$Success$ = 5-year survival after treatment (expected to be 0.6 in experimental group and 0.5 in control group)
	$Failure$ = death within 5 years of treatment
Losses to follow-up	None
Variance, expressed as $\bar{p}(1 - \bar{p})$	$\bar{p} = 0.55$; $(1 - \bar{p}) = 0.45$
Data for alpha ($z_{1-\alpha}$)	$p = 0.05$; 95% confidence desired (two-tailed test); $z_{1-\alpha} = 1.96$
Data for beta ($z_{1-\beta}$)	20% beta error; 80% power desired (one-tailed test); $z_{1-\beta} = 0.84$
Difference to be detected (d)	$\geq$0.1 difference between the success (survival) of the experimental group and that of the control group (i.e., 10% difference because $p_E = 0.6$, and $p_C = 0.5$)

Part 1B Initial Calculation of Sample Size (N)

$$
\begin{aligned}
N &= \frac{\left(z_{1-\alpha} + z_{1-\beta}\right)^2 \times 2 \times \bar{p}(1 - \bar{p})}{d^2} \\
&= \frac{\left(1.96 + 0.84\right)^2 \times 2 \times 0.55 \times 0.45}{0.1^2} \\
&= 388 \text{ participants per group} \times 2 \text{ groups} \\
&= 776 \text{ participants total}
\end{aligned}
$$

Interpretation: A total of 776 participants would be needed, 388 in each group.

BOX 12.4 Initial and Subsequent Calculation of Sample Size for a Study Using a Test of Differences in Proportions Assuming 80% Power—cont'd

Part 2A Changes in Data on Which Initial Calculation Was Based (Because First *N* Was Too Large for Study to Be Feasible; See Text)

Study Characteristic	Assumptions Made by Investigator
Difference to be detected (d)	≥ 0.2 difference between the success (survival) of the experimental group and that of the control group (i.e., 20% difference because $p_E = 0.7$, and $p_C = 0.5$)
Variance, expressed as $\bar{p}(1-\bar{p})$	$\bar{p} = 0.60$; $(1-\bar{p}) = 0.40$

Part 2B Subsequent (Revised) Calculation of Sample Size (*N*)

$$N = \frac{\left(z_{1-\alpha} + z_{1-\beta}\right)^2 \times 2 \times \bar{p}\left(1-\bar{p}\right)}{d^2}$$

$$= \frac{\left(1.96 + 0.84\right)^2 \times 2 \times 0.60 \times 0.40}{0.2^2}$$

$$= 94 \text{ participants per group} \times 2 \text{ groups}$$

$$= 188 \text{ participants total}$$

Interpretation: Now a total of 188 participants would be needed, 94 in each group. As a result of changes in the data on which the initial calculation was based, the number of participants needed would be reduced from 776 to 188.

1.4 SAMPLE SIZE FOR STUDIES USING t-TESTS

Box 12.1 shows the formula and calculations for a paired, before-after study of an antihypertensive drug in patients whose blood pressure is checked before starting the drug and then after taking the drug. A paired t-test would be used for this type of paired data. Given the variance, alpha, and difference chosen by the investigator, only nine participants would be needed altogether. This type of study is efficient in terms of the sample size required. However, even most paired studies require considerably more than nine participants. Also note that a very small sample tends to limit the external validity, or *generalizability*, of a trial because a study based on few participants is less likely to resemble the larger population from which they are drawn.

Box 12.2 shows the formula and calculations for a RCT of an antihypertensive drug in a study for which a *two-sample t-test* would be used. This formula differs from the formula in Box 12.1 only in that the variance estimate must be multiplied by 2. Given the same assumptions as in Box 12.1 concerning variance, alpha, and difference, it would be necessary to have a total of 36 study participants for this RCT (18 in experimental group and 18 in control group), which is four times the number of participants required for the paired, before-after study described in Box 12.1.

The larger sample size is needed in a two-sample t-test for two reasons. First, studies using the two-sample t-test have *two sources of variance* instead of one, because the study and control groups each contribute to the variance (thus the number 2 in the numerator). Second, the N obtained is *only for the intervention group*, and another person serves as the control for each experimental participant (so that the total sample size for equal numbers of cases and controls would be 2N). Although there is no complete agreement on the level of

beta error acceptable for most studies, usually a beta error of 20% is used, corresponding to a z value of 0.84. When this beta estimate is used in Box 12.3, with the same $z_{1-\alpha}$, variance, and mean difference as in Box 12.2, the calculations show that 72 study participants are needed for the RCT. In contrast, with a 50% chance of making a beta error, only 36 participants would be needed, as shown in Box 12.2.

While large sample sizes seem desirable, excessive sample sizes can be problematic. When $z_{1-\alpha}$ and $z_{1-\beta}$ are added together before squaring, as shown in the formula in Box 12.3, the sample size may become quite large. Depending on the value of $z_{1-\beta}$ used, this would at least double and could as much as quadruple the estimated value of N, which could increase the cost of a study. In addition, a needlessly large sample size introduces problems interpreting results. If the sample size is larger than necessary, differences smaller than what the investigators considered to be clinically important are now statistically significant. What do they do now with clinically trivial findings that are nevertheless statistically significant? In the research described in Boxes 12.2 and 12.3, investigators sought to detect a difference of 10 mm Hg or more in systolic blood pressure, presumably because they believed that a smaller difference would be clinically unimportant. With a total sample size of 36 (see Box 12.2), a difference smaller than 10 mm Hg would not be statistically significant. With a total sample size of 72 (see Box 12.3), however, a difference of only 8 mm Hg would be statistically significant ($t = 2.26$; p is approximately 0.03 on 70 df). In cases such as this, it is important to focus on the original hypotheses of the research and clinical significance rather than report every statistically significant finding as important.

In general, investigators usually want the actual sample size to be larger than that calculated from the formulas, particularly if significant losses to follow-up are expected or the accuracy of the variance estimate is uncertain. Further, while it is true that alpha and beta are usually set at 0.05 and 0.2, respectively, these are merely conventions and the values chosen for alpha and beta should also be motivated by the scientific question being asked. For example, for new treatments that have relatively minor side effects, but huge potential benefits, investigators may be willing to make more false-positive errors. Conversely, for treatments that have substantially negative adverse effects and are only slightly better than the current gold standard, investigators need to guard against false-positive errors and may not be particularly worried about making a false-negative error.

1.5 SAMPLE SIZE FOR A TEST OF DIFFERENCES IN PROPORTIONS

Often a dependent variable is measured as success/failure and is described as the proportion of outcomes that represent some form of success, such as improvement in health, remission of disease, or reduction in mortality. In this case, the formula for sample size must be expressed in terms of proportions, as shown in Box 12.4.

Box 12.4 provides an example of how to calculate the sample size for a RCT of a drug to reduce the 5-year mortality in patients with a particular form of cancer. Before the calculations can be made, investigators must decide which values they will use for $z_{1-\alpha}$, $z_{1-\beta}$, variance, and the smallest difference to be detected. For alpha and beta, they decide to use a level of 95% confidence (two-tailed test) and 80% power, so that $z_{1-\alpha}$ equals 1.96 and $z_{1-\beta}$ equals 0.84.

Initially, as shown in the first part of Box 12.4, investigators decide they want to detect a 10% improvement in survival (i.e., difference of 0.1 between 5-year mortality of experimental group and that of control group). They also assume that the survival rate will be 50% (0.5) in the control group and 10% better (0.6) in the experimental group. They assume the mean proportion of success $\bar{p}$ for all participants enrolled in the study will be 0.55. Based on these assumptions, the calculations show that they would need 388 participants in the experimental group and 388 in the control group, for a total of 776 participants. If it is difficult to find that many participants or to fund a study this large, what can be done?

Theoretically any of the estimated values in the formula might be altered. The alpha and beta values used in these boxes ($\alpha = 0.05$ two sided; $\beta = 0.20$ one sided) are the ones customarily used, however, and the best estimate of variance should always be used. The best place to rethink the sample size calculation is the requirement for the minimum clinically important difference. Perhaps a 10% improvement is not large enough to be meaningful. What if it were changed to 20% (a difference of 0.2, based on a survival rate of 70% in the experimental group and 50% in the control group)? As shown in the second part of Box 12.4, changing the improvement requirement to 20% changes the variance estimate, so that $\bar{P}$ now equals 0.6. Based on these revised assumptions, calculations show that investigators would need only 94 participants in the experimental group and 94 in the control

group, for a total of 188 participants. A study with this smaller sample size seems much more reasonable to perform and less costly. However, it is very important that we be sure that 20% is a reasonable difference to expect, because if the sample size calculation assumes a difference of 20%, but the true difference is only 10%, then there is a 51% chance of missing the difference. Therefore, if the investigators really believe the difference they chose is clinically important they should try to obtain funding for the large sample required.

When choosing the 10% difference initially, investigators may have intuitively assumed (incorrectly) that it is easier to detect a small difference than a large one. Alternately, they may have had an interest in detecting a small difference, even though it would not be clinically important. In either case, the penalty in sample size may alert investigators to the statistical realities of the situation and force them to think seriously about the smallest difference that would be clinically important.

2. RANDOMIZING STUDY PARTICIPANTS

Randomized clinical trials and field trials require that the allocation of study participants to an intervention or a control status be done by **randomization**. There is a distinction between randomization (i.e., allocating the available participants to one or another study group) and **random sampling** (i.e., selecting a small group for study from a much larger group of potential study participants). Randomization is often used in clinical trials. It is an important technique for achieving internal validity in a study because it reduces the possibility of bias, whereas random sampling helps to ensure external validity because it seeks to ensure a representative sample of participants (see Chapter 4).

2.1 GOALS OF RANDOMIZATION

An experimental design, of which the RCT is the gold standard in clinical research, depends on an **unbiased allocation of study participants** to the experimental and control groups. For most purposes, the best indication of an unbiased allocation is randomization. Contrary to popular opinion, randomization does not guarantee that the two (or more) groups created by random allocation are identical in either size or subject characteristics (although block randomization can guarantee identical group sizes). What randomization does guarantee, if properly done, is that the different groups will be free of selection bias and problems resulting from regression toward the mean.

Selection bias can occur if participants are allowed to choose whether they will be in an intervention or a control group, as occurred in the polio vaccine trials (see Chapter 4). Another form of selection bias, *allocation bias*, can occur if investigators influence the assignment of participants to one group or another. There may be considerable pressure from a patient and family members or other caregivers to alter the randomization process and allow the patient to enroll in the intervention group, especially in studies involving a community intervention, but this pressure must be resisted.[5]

Regression toward the mean, also known as the **statistical regression effect**, is common among patients who were chosen to participate in a study because they had an extreme measurement on some variable (e.g., high number of ear infections during the past year). For many conditions, these patients are likely to have a measurement that is closer to average at a later time (e.g., during the subsequent year) for reasons unrelated to the type or efficacy of the treatment they receive. In a study comparing treatment methods in two groups of patients, both with extreme measurements at the beginning of the study, randomization cannot eliminate the tendency to regress toward the mean. Randomization may *equalize* this tendency between the study groups however, preventing bias in the comparison.

This concept is illustrated by a RCT of surgical treatment (tonsillectomy and adenoidectomy) versus medical treatment (antibiotics) of children with recurrent throat infections conducted in the 1980s when surgery for this condition was common. In this trial, children in both groups had fewer episodes of throat infection in the year after treatment than in the year before treatment (an effect attributed to regression toward the mean), but the surgically treated patients showed more improvement than the medically treated patients (an effect attributed to the intervention).[6]

2.2 METHODS OF RANDOMIZATION

Before-and-after studies sometimes randomize the study participants into two groups, with one group given the experimental intervention first and the other group given the placebo first. Then after a **washout period**, when no intervention is given and physiologic values are expected to return to baseline, the group previously given the experimental intervention crosses over to receiving the placebo, and vice versa. These studies are also referred to as *crossover trials*. By careful analysis it is possible to determine whether being randomized to receive the experimental intervention first or second made any difference in the results.

When a study involving comparison groups is planned, investigators must decide what method of randomization will be used to ensure that each participant has an equal (or at least a known) probability of being assigned to each group. The use of computer-generated random numbers is a common method to keep human preferences from influencing the randomization process. If possible, the study participants should not know the group to which they are assigned. This often can be accomplished by "blinding" the study participants (e.g., using a placebo that looks, tastes, and smells the same as treatment), and blinding the individuals conducting the study, such as those who dispense the treatment, record the findings, and manage the data. If blinding is accomplished for both participants and researchers of the study, it is called a **double-blind** study. Blinding protects against bias in any of the study procedures that might favor one group or another if either the participants or the investigators knows who is receiving the treatment and who is not. Blinding minimizes differences in the ways participants experience the condition or intervention, or how investigators manage study participants or measure outcomes, for example.

The methods described subsequently assume that an equal number of participants is desired in the comparison groups. However, these methods can be modified to provide two or more control participants for each experimental participant.

2.2.a. Simple and Block Randomization

Simple random allocation uses a random-number table or a computerized random-number generator to allocate potential participants to a treatment or control status. If it is important to have equally sized groups, study participants can be randomized two at a time (i.e., block randomization).

2.2.b. Systematic Allocation

In systematic allocation, the first participant is randomly assigned to a group and the next participant is automatically assigned to the alternate group. Subsequent participants are given group assignments on an alternating basis. This method also ensures that the experimental and control groups are of equal size if there is an even number of participants entered in the study. There are advantages to this method beyond simplicity. Usually the variance of the data from a systematic allocation is smaller than that from a simple random allocation, so the statistical power is improved. If there is any form of periodicity in the way participants enter, however, there may be a bias. For example, suppose systematic sampling is used to allocate participants into two groups, and only two participants are admitted each day to the study (e.g., first two new patients who enter the clinic each morning). If each intake day started so that the first patient was assigned to the experimental group and the second was assigned to the control group, all the experimental group participants would be the first patients to arrive at the clinic, perhaps early in the morning. They might be systematically different (e.g., employed, eager, early risers) compared with patients who come later in the day, in which case bias might be introduced into the study. This danger is easy to avoid, however, if the investigator reverses the sequence frequently, sometimes taking the first patient each day into the control group. The convenience and statistical advantages of systematic sampling make it desirable to use whenever possible. The systematic allocation method also can be used for allocating study participants to three, four, or even more groups.

2.2.c. Stratified Allocation

In clinical research, stratified allocation is often called **prognostic stratification**. It is used when investigators want to assign participants to different risk groups depending on baseline variables such as the severity of disease (e.g., stage of cancer) and age. When these risk groups have been created, each stratum can be allocated randomly to the experimental group or the control group. This is usually done to ensure homogeneity of the study groups by severity of disease. If homogeneity was achieved, the analysis can be done for the entire group and as well as within the prognostic groups.

2.3 SPECIAL ISSUES WITH RANDOMIZATION

Randomization does not guarantee that two or more groups will be identical. Suppose an investigator, when checking how similar the experimental and control groups were after randomization, found that the two groups were of different size and that 1 of 20 characteristics being compared showed a statistically significant difference between the groups. Occasional differences being statistically significant does not mean the randomization was biased because some differences are expected by chance. There may be a legitimate concern, however, that some of the observed differences between the randomized groups could confound the analysis. In this case the variables of concern can be controlled for in the analysis.

Although randomization is essential in reducing bias in clinical trials, many other precautions must also be taken to reduce bias, such as ensuring the accuracy of data by blinding participants and observers and standardizing data collection instruments. An additional concern with RCTs is the generalization of study findings. Patients have the right to refuse to participate in a study before or after randomization. This means that most studies include only patients who are willing to participate. Are these patients similar to those who refused to participate, or are they an unusual subset of the entire population being studied? Because these questions are usually unresolved, the results of a clinical trial are most accurately applied to individuals who are similar to the actual participants.

What happens if, after randomization, a participant is not doing well, and the participant or clinician wants to switch from the experimental treatment to another medication? Ethically the participant cannot be forced to continue the study treatment. When the switch occurs, how would the data for this participant be analyzed? The most accepted approach is to analyze the *data as if the patient had remained in the original group*, so that any negative outcomes are assigned to the original treatment. This strategy, called the **intention to treat** approach, is based on the belief that if the participant was doing so poorly as to want to switch, the outcome should be ascribed to the original group. Other investigators prefer to exclude this participant and analyze the data as if the participant had never enrolled in the study. However, this could lead to a smaller and probably biased sample. Still others prefer to reassign the participant to a third group and analyze the data separately from the original groups. In this approach, the original groups change so it is unclear how to interpret results of the remaining groups.

Another problem in randomized trials of treatment effects is deciding what to consider as the starting point for measuring the outcome. If surgical treatment and medical treatment are being compared, should surgical mortality (dying as a result of the surgery) be included as part of the debit side for surgical treatment? Or does measuring the outcome start with the question, "Given survival from the initial surgical procedure, do patients treated surgically or those treated medically do better?"[7] Most investigators recommend beginning the analysis at the time of randomization.

3. CONTROLLING FOR THE TESTING OF MULTIPLE HYPOTHESES

In studies with large amounts of data there is a temptation to use modern computer techniques to see which variables are associated with which other variables and report many associations. This process is sometimes referred to as *data dredging*, and it is often used in medical research. Sometimes, however, this fact is not made clear in the article, thus misleading readers of medical literature, who should be aware of such limitations.

The search for associations can be appropriate as long as the investigator keeps two points in mind. First, the scientific process requires that hypothesis development and hypothesis testing be based on different data sets. One data set is used to develop the hypothesis or model, which is used to make predictions, which are then tested on a new data set. Second, a **correlational study** (e.g., using Pearson correlation coefficient or chi-square test) is useful only for developing hypotheses, not for testing them. Stated in slightly different terms, a correlational study is an initial method to identify associations that might be real. Investigators who keep these points in mind are unlikely to make the mistake of thinking every association found in a data set represents a true association.

One example of the problem of data dredging is a report of an association between coffee consumption and pancreatic cancer. These results were obtained by testing many associations in a large data set without repeating the analysis on another data set to determine whether they were consistent.[8] This approach was severely criticized at the time, and subsequent studies failed to find a true association between coffee consumption and pancreatic cancer.[9]

How does this problem arise? Suppose there are 10 variables in a descriptive study and the investigator wants to associate each one with every other one creating 10×10 possible cells (see Chapter 5 and Fig. 5.6). Ten cells would be each variable times itself, however, which is always a perfect correlation. That leaves 90 possible associations, although half of these would be "$x \times y$" and the other half "$y \times x$." Because the *p* values for bivariate tests are the same regardless of which is considered the independent variable and which is considered the dependent variable, there are only half as many truly independent associations, or 45. If the $p = 0.05$ cutoff point is used for alpha, 5 of 100 independent associations would be expected to occur by chance alone.[10] In the example, it means that slightly more than two *statistically significant* associations would be expected to occur just by chance.

The problem with multiple hypotheses is similar to the problem with multiple associations. In this case, the greater the number of hypotheses that are tested, the more likely it is that at least one of them will be found *statistically significant* by chance alone. One possible way to handle this problem is to lower the *p* value required before rejecting the null hypothesis (e.g., make it <0.05). This was done in a study testing the same medical educational hypothesis at five different hospitals.[11] If the alpha level in the study had been set at 0.05, there would have been almost a 25% probability of finding a statistically significant difference by chance alone in at least one of the five hospitals because each hospital had a 5% ($\alpha = 0.05$) probability of showing a difference from chance alone. To keep the risk of a false-positive finding in the entire study to no more than 0.05, the alpha level chosen for rejecting the null hypothesis was made more stringent by dividing alpha by 5 (number of hospitals) to make it 0.01. This method of adjusting for multiple hypotheses is called the **Bonferroni adjustment to alpha**, and it is quite stringent. Other possible adjustments are less stringent but more complicated statistically and used in different situations. Examples include the Tukey, Scheffe, and Newman-Keuls procedures.[12]

4. SUMMARY

Statisticians are often consulted for help in calculating the sample sizes needed for studies. However, sample sizes can only be estimated when the investigator has determined the information to be used in the calculations. This includes the levels of alpha and beta, the clinically important difference in outcome variables, and expected variance. Randomization and blinding can reduce bias in studies comparing intervention and control groups. Ideally, neither study participants, those providing the intervention, nor those collecting data should know group assignments. The basic methods of random allocation include simple and block random allocation, systematic allocation, and stratified allocation. In the analysis of data, investigators should be alert to the problem of data dredging and understand that testing multiple hypotheses increases the probability of false-positive statistical associations (alpha errors).

REFERENCES

1. Freiman JA, Chalmers TC, Smith Jr H, Kuebler RR. The importance of beta, the type II error and sample size in the design and interpretation of the randomized control trial. Survey of 71 "negative" trials. *N Engl J Med*. 1978;299:690-695.
2. Williams HC, Seed P. Inadequate size of 'negative' clinical trials in dermatology. *Br J Dermatol*. 1993;128:317-326.
3. Chow SC, Wang H, Shao J. *Sample Size Calculations in Clinical Research*. 2nd ed. New York, NY: Chapman & Hall/CRC; 2007.
4. Kelsey JL, Whittemore AS, Evans AS, Thompson WD. *Methods in Observational Epidemiology*. 2nd ed. New York, NY: Oxford University Press; 1996.
5. Lam JA, Hartwell S, Jekel JF. "I prayed real hard, so I know I'll get in": living with randomization. *New Dir Prog Eval*. 1994;63:55-66.
6. Paradise JL, Bluestone CD, Bachman RZ, et al. Efficacy of tonsillectomy for recurrent throat infection in severely affected children. Results of parallel randomized and nonrandomized clinical trials. *N Engl J Med*. 1984;310:674-683.
7. Sackett DL, Gent M. Controversy in counting and attributing events in clinical trials. *N Engl J Med*. 1979;301:1410-1412.
8. MacMahon B, Yen S, Trichopoulos D, Warren K, Nardi G. Coffee and cancer of the pancreas. *N Engl J Med*. 1981;304:630-633.
9. Feinstein AR, Horwitz RI, Spitzer WO, Battista RN. Coffee and pancreatic cancer. The problems of etiologic science and epidemiologic case-control research. *JAMA*. 1981;246:957-961.
10. Jekel JF. Should we stop using the P value in descriptive studies? *Pediatrics*. 1977;60:124-126.
11. Jekel JF, Chauncey KJ, Moore NL, Broadus AE, Gowdy DP. The regional educational impact of a renal stone center. *Yale J Biol Med*. 1983;56:97-108.
12. Dawson B, Trapp RG. *Basic & Clinical Biostatistics*. 4th ed. New York, NY: Lange Medical Books/McGraw-Hill; 2004.

SELECT READING

Dawson B, Trapp RG: *Basic & Clinical Biostatistics*. 4th ed. New York, NY: Lange Medical Books/McGraw-Hill; 2004.

REVIEW QUESTIONS

1. The formula for a paired t-test is as follows:

$$t_a = \frac{\bar{d}}{\dfrac{s_d}{\sqrt{N}}}$$

To determine the needed sample size, this formula is rearranged algebraically to solve for N. In the process, z must be substituted for t because:
   A. t is dependent on degrees of freedom and z is not
   B. z is dependent on degrees of freedom and t is not
   C. t provides too large a sample
   D. t provides too small a sample
   E. z takes beta error into account

2. It is important to consider beta error when:
   A. The difference under consideration is not clinically meaningful
   B. The difference under investigation is statistically significant
   C. The null hypothesis is not rejected
   D. The null hypothesis is rejected
   E. The sample size is excessively large

3. Which one of the following characteristics of a diagnostic test is analogous to the statistical power of a study?
   A. Positive predictive value
   B. Negative predictive value
   C. Sensitivity
   D. Specificity
   E. Utility

4. A study is designed to test the effects of sleep deprivation on academic performance among medical students. Each subject serves as his or her own control. A 10-point difference (10% difference) in test scores is considered meaningful. The standard deviation of test scores in a similar study was 8. Alpha is set at 0.05 (two-tailed test), and beta is set at 0.2. The appropriate sample size is:
   A. $[(0.05)^2 \times 8]/(10)^2$
   B. $[(1.96)^2 \times (8)^2]/(10)^2$
   C. $[(0.05 + 0.2)^2 \times (8)^2]/(10)^2$
   D. $[(1.96 + 0.84)^2 \times (8)^2]/(10)^2$
   E. $[(1.96 + 0.84)^2 \times 2 \times (8)^2]/(10)^2$

5. A different investigator plans a study designed to test the effects of sleep deprivation on academic performance among medical students. Each subject serves as his or her own control. A 10-point difference (10% difference) in test scores is considered meaningful. The standard deviation of test scores in a similar study was 8. Alpha is set at 0.05 (two-tailed test), and beta is set at 0.5. The required sample size for this study is:
A. $[(0.05)^2 \times 8]/(10)^2$
B. $[(1.96)^2 \times (8)^2]/(10)^2$
C. $[(0.05 + 0.2)^2 \times (8)^2]/(10)^2$
D. $[(1.96 + 0.84)^2 \times (8)^2]/(10)^2$
E. $[(1.96 + 0.84)^2 \times 2 \times (8)^2]/(10)^2$

6. A study designed to test the effects of sleep deprivation on academic performance among medical students is conducted by yet another group. The investigators use separate intervention and control groups. A 10-point difference (10% difference) in test scores is considered meaningful. The standard deviation of test scores in a similar study was 8. Alpha is set at 0.05 (two-tailed test), and beta is set at 0.2 (one-tailed test). The values for $z_{1-\alpha}$ and $z_{1-\beta}$, for the variance, and for the minimum difference remain the same. The required sample size for this study is:
A. $[(0.05)^2 \times 8]/(10)^2$
B. $[(1.96)^2 \times (8)^2]/(10)^2$
C. $[(0.05 + 0.2)^2 \times (8)^2]/(10)^2$
D. $[(1.96 + 0.84)^2 \times (8)^2]/(10)^2$
E. $[(1.96 + 0.84)^2 \times 2 \times (8)^2]/(10)^2$

7. A study is designed to test the effects of sleep deprivation on academic performance among medical students. A 10-point difference (10% difference) in test scores is considered meaningful. The standard deviation of test scores in a similar study was 8. Alpha is set at 0.05 (two-tailed test), and beta is set at 0.2. The before-after study in the previous question is revised to detect a difference of only 2 points (2%) in test scores. All other parameters of the original study remain unchanged, except investigators are undecided as to whether to use a single group of participants for test and control conditions or two separate groups of participants. Given this uncertainty, the required sample size would:
A. Be unaffected regardless of whether the study had a single group of participants (serving as their own controls) or two separate groups of participants (test group and control group)
B. Increase regardless of whether the study had a single group of participants (serving as their own controls) or two separate groups of participants (test group and control group)
C. Increase only if the study had a single group of participants serving as their own controls
D. Decrease regardless of whether the study had a single group of participants (serving as their own controls) or two separate groups of participants (test group and control group)

E. Decrease only if the study had a single group of participants serving as their own controls

ANSWERS AND EXPLANATIONS

1. **A.** Both z and t are distributions used to provide unit-free measures of dispersion about a mean value. To know the value of t, degrees of freedom (df) must be known. Unfortunately df depends on N, which is what we are trying solve for, creating a circular problem. A solution to the problem is to substitute z, which is independent of df, not dependent (B). The t distribution is approximated by the z distribution when the sample size is large, but having a large (C) or small (D) sample size does not necessitate substitution with z. Substitution with z confers a slight risk of underestimating the sample size required. Both z and t represent critical ratios to determine the probability of alpha error (false-positive error) if the null hypothesis is rejected. Neither takes beta error (false-negative error) into account (E) when we assume that there is in fact no treatment difference.

2. **C.** Beta error (also called type II error and false-negative error) is the failure to detect a true difference when one exists. Only a negative result (i.e., failure to reject the null hypothesis) is at risk for being a false-negative result. If the null hypothesis is rejected (D) or if the difference under investigation is statistically significant (B), a difference is being detected. Although alpha error (also called type I or false-positive error) may be a possibility in either case, beta error is not a concern. Beta error is the result of inadequate power to detect the difference under investigation and occurs when the sample size is small, not excessively large (E). Either enlarging the sample or reducing the effect size would increase statistical power and help reduce the risk for beta error. However, reducing the effect size (the difference under consideration) might result in a clinically meaningless difference (A). Beta error is a concern when the difference under consideration is clinically meaningful, but not found.

3. **C.** The sensitivity of a diagnostic test, or $a/(a + c)$, is the ability of the test to detect a condition when it is present. Statistical power, or $(1 - \beta)$, is the ability of a study to detect a difference when it exists. The two terms are mathematically equivalent since β, or beta error, equals 1 − sensitivity. Thus power = 1 − (1 − sensitivity) = sensitivity = $a/(a + c)$. Power is essentially unrelated to specificity (D), or positive (A) or negative (B) predictive values. Utility (E) is a term used colloquially to mean "usefulness," and it has other meanings in economics/econometrics, but it is not a term that has statistical meaning.

4. **D.** This is a study for which a paired t-test is appropriate. The corresponding sample size formula, as detailed in Box 12.1, is:

$$N = \frac{z_{1-\alpha}^2 \times s^2}{\bar{d}^2}$$

In this example, however, the value for beta also is specified, so that the formula becomes:

$$N = \frac{\left(z_{1-\alpha} + z_{1-\beta}\right)^2 \times s^2}{\bar{d}^2}$$

The value of $z_{1-\alpha}$ when alpha is 0.05 and the test is two tailed is 1.96. The value of $z_{1-\beta}$ when beta is 20%, or 0.2, is 0.84; $z_{1-\beta}$ is one tailed by convention. The standard deviation (s) is derived from a prior study and is 8. The difference sought is 10 points. Thus $[(1.96 + 0.84)^2 \times (8)^2]/(10)^2$ is the correct sample size formula. The corresponding value calculated from this formula is 6 (5.02 rounded up to smallest number of whole persons). The sample size is so small in this case because of the large difference sought (10% change in test score is substantial), the small standard deviation, and the use of each subject as his or her own control. If each subject had not served as his or her own control and there were two distinct study groups, a larger number of participants would be needed. In such a case, formula E would be correct, representing the sample size calculation for a student t-test. Formula B would be the correct sample size calculation for a paired t-test based on alpha error only. Such a calculation would necessarily result in a sample size smaller than one considering both alpha error and beta error. A and C are nonsense distracters, substituting alpha and beta values for the expected z values at these thresholds.

5. **B.** The sample size calculation here is the same as for question 4, except this time we can remove the beta term because when the power is 50%, the z beta term is equal to zero. Thus in this case the sample size needed is even smaller. In fact the sample size is 3 (rounded up from 2.46). A sample this small may make intuitive sense if you consider how many participants you would need to show that test scores are higher if the test taker is well rested rather than sleep deprived. However, a study with only 50% power is unusual. Incorrect answer choices for this question are in the explanation for question 4.

6. **E.** The formula for this calculation is shown in Box 12.2. The difference between this equation and the equation for the before-and-after study in the previous question is the 2 in the numerator. This equation calculates the sample size for a two-sample t-test (sample needed for each of two separate groups: test and control) rather than a paired t-test (number needed for a single group serving as its own control). The total number of participants in this case is not N (number of participants in each group; such as single group for paired t-test) but $2N$ (number of participants needed in total). In this case the total number of participants needed is 22 (10.04 rounded to 11 and doubled), almost four times the number needed for the analogous paired study. Incorrect answer choices for this question are in the explanation for question 4.

7. **B.** As already demonstrated, if investigators switch from a single study group to two groups, the sample size will necessarily increase considerably (see explanation to question 6). Even if they decide to keep a single study group, however, reducing the difference to be detected necessarily means that the sample size will need to increase substantially. Such increase makes intuitive sense because it is more difficult to detect a smaller difference, so more study participants are required. The sample size will not stay the same (A) or decrease (D and E) in either possible scenario; it will increase in both scenarios, even—and especially—if a single group serving as their own controls is not used (C). In fact, although in the scenario with one study group the sample size needed to detect a 2% difference would be 126 (125.44 rounded up), with two groups the sample size needed for a study with two groups would be 502 (250.88 rounded up and doubled).

13

Using Statistics to Answer Clinical Questions:
Meta-Analysis, Bayes Theorem and Predictive Values of Tests, and Decision Analysis

"It is easy to lie with statistics. It is hard to tell the truth without it."

Andrejs Dunkels

Clinical practice guidelines and standards of care are based on the best available clinical research. This approach to clinical practice is widely referred to as **evidence-based medicine** (EBM). The accessibility of the research literature through internet searches, and methods of clinical epidemiology and biostatistics, provide opportunities to base diagnostic and therapeutic decisions on quantitative information provided by clinical research. EBM requires that clinicians do the following:

- Access the most relevant research data.
- Decide which studies are most trustworthy and applicable to the clinical question under consideration.
- Use appropriate methods available to determine the best diagnostic and therapeutic approaches to each problem.
- Use experience and judgment to apply EBM to individual patients

Many methods described in this text—especially some of the tools discussed in this chapter, such as meta-analysis, Bayes theorem and test performance, and clinical decision analysis—are considered tools for the practice of EBM.

Although there is general agreement about the need to improve clinical decision making and maximize the quality of medical care, opinions differ regarding the extent to which the tools discussed in this chapter are likely to help in actual clinical decision making. While some methods are currently used to guide the care of individual patients, others are more useful in formulating policy and analyzing the effectiveness

and cost effectiveness of medical interventions, such as immunizations and screening programs.[1,2] Even the most highly regarded evidence, such as results of double-blind, placebo-controlled clinical trials, may not be relevant to an individual patient. How well evidence derived from research studies applies to individual circumstances is uncertain and often a matter of clinical judgment.

Regardless of the clinician's approach to using these methods for patient care, they are useful in understanding the quantitative basis for making clinical decisions in the increasingly complex field of medicine.

1. META-ANALYSIS

One of the best ways to reach reliable and clinically applicable conclusions from the medical literature is to base judgments on very large, diverse data sets. *P* values, confidence intervals, and error bars are used to indicate the degree to which a sample population is likely to reflect the real-world experience in the population at large. When the test sample is the population at large, the tools of extrapolated inference are not required.

Although trials involving the entire population are generally not conducted for obvious reasons, large test populations may approximate truth for the population at large better than small populations. A study conducted in a small, select group is much less likely to generalize to other groups than a comparable study in a large, diverse group. Large samples provide the advantages of both statistical power (see Chapter 12) and external validity/generalizability (see Chapter 9), assuming that the population is clearly defined and the sample represents it well. For example, a large trial of breast cancer screening in men would provide little useful information about screening in women, given the marked differences in risk and incidence.

One way to generate data based on large, diverse samples is to conduct a large, multisite intervention trial. This is routinely done with funding from large pharmaceutical companies testing the utility of a proprietary drug, and at times from trials funded by federal agencies. The US National Institutes of Health (NIH) studies such as The Diabetes Prevention Program[3] and the Women's Health Initiative[4] are examples of extremely large, costly, federally funded intervention trials. In both cases, thousands of participants were involved.

Often, however, logistical constraints related to recruitment, time, money, and other resources preclude conducting such large trials. Multiple trials involving small samples are much more common. The aggregation of findings from multiple smaller trials thus becomes an efficient, less costly means of approximating the statistical power and generalizability of much larger trials. The aggregation of findings may be qualitative or quantitative (**meta-analysis**). At times, data aggregation may pertain to a whole domain of medicine rather than a narrowly framed question, for which a method known as evidence mapping is of specific utility.

1.1 SYSTEMATIC REVIEW

A *systematic review* results in the synthesis of multiple studies addressing a similar research question. It requires a comprehensive review of studies that meet prespecified criteria for inclusion, generally pertaining to study population, intervention, comparisons, outcomes, timing, and setting (PICOTS). All relevant studies are identified through searches of electronic databases and other sources; are thoroughly reviewed; and the strengths, weaknesses, risk of bias, and applicability of each are critically appraised using established criteria. There are standard approaches to adjudicating the quality and inclusion of articles for a systematic review. The details of the process are beyond the scope of this text.

According to the Cochrane Collaborative's *Cochrane Handbook for Systematic Review of Interventions*,[5] the salient characteristics of a systematic review include the following:

- A clearly stated set of objectives with predefined eligibility criteria for studies
- Explicit, reproducible methodology
- Systematic search that attempts to identify all studies that would meet the eligibility criteria
- Assessment of the validity of the findings of the included studies, as through the assessment of risk of bias
- Systematic presentation and synthesis of the characteristics and findings of the included studies.

Systematic reviews synthesize results qualitatively when quantitative methods are not appropriate. This occurs when the studies themselves are qualitative,[6] or when trials addressing a given research question differ substantially in measures, methods, or other factors (heterogeneous) and are not amenable to combining data across studies.[7,8] Usually the analysis indicates the number of studies of the outcome in question and provides an impression, although not a statistical measure, of the weight of evidence.

Quantitative synthesis allows for formal statistical analysis and is thus referred to as *meta-analysis* (i.e., "analysis among many"). Whereas a systematic review may or may not include a meta-analysis, a meta-analysis requires a systematic review of the literature to identify studies that serve as data sources.

1.2 QUANTITATIVE META-ANALYSIS

Meta-analysis is a statistical method to aggregate the results of studies to determine the strength of a particular association. **Quantitative meta-analysis** takes one of two forms: either the data are analyzed as reported in the literature or the raw data from multiple studies are obtained and aggregated.[9] A meta-analysis in which raw data are aggregated requires that access to the data be accorded by the investigators responsible for each included trial, because it is not routinely included in publications.

In either type of quantitative meta-analysis, strict criteria are employed for the selection of studies. Despite these criteria, some variability in methods among included studies is inevitable. This is generally measured in a **test of heterogeneity;** details of the test method are available in other sources.[10]

The less variation across the trials included in the meta-analysis, the more meaningful the aggregation of findings tends to be. Typically when only published data are used, trials are displayed on plots that show whether they support an association and, if so, with what degree of statistical significance. This is shown by setting a vertical line at a **relative risk** of 1 (no association), then plotting the 95% confidence intervals for the results of each study included. The generation of these plots, called **forest plots**, requires the conversion of study-specific data into a unit-free, standardized effect size, typically the Cohen D.[11] The Cochrane Collaborative, which provides meta-analytic software called RevMan, uses a comparable measure called Hedges' adjusted g.[5] Fig. 13.1 provides an example of a plot of effect sizes. In addition to results of the statistical analysis, a quantitative meta-analysis provides information on individual trial strengths and weaknesses, comparability of the trials assessed, and distribution of results.

The most rigorous form of meta-analysis is fully quantitative, aggregating individual-level data from multiple trials after ensuring the comparability of subjects and methods among the trials included. Such meta-analyses are relatively rare because they are dependent on the availability of multiple, highly comparable trials. An example is an analysis of angioplasty in acute myocardial infarction, in which the data from 23 separate trials were pooled together and reanalyzed.[12]

Because meta-analyses are typically limited to published data, they often assess the potential influence of publication bias by use of a **funnel plot**.[9,13] In essence, a funnel plot attempts to populate a "funnel" of expected effect sizes around a mean; significant gaps in the funnel, particularly missing studies with null or negative effects, are interpreted to suggest

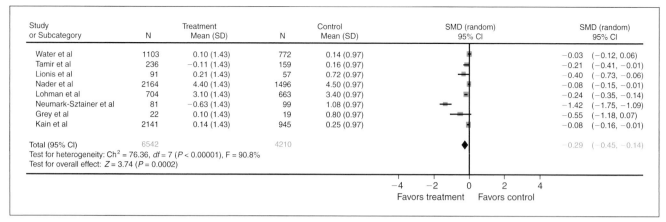

Fig. 13.1 Plot of Standardized Effects Sizes. Each point is the mean effect for a given study, and the lines to either side of it represent the 95% confidence interval (CI). The *vertical line* is the line of unity and represents a null effect; estimates with 95% CI crossing the null line do not support a statistically significant effect; studies with estimates that do not cross the null line do. The *diamond* represents the pooled effects size estimate and its CI. *SMD*, standardized mean difference. This figure is a comparison of nutrition plus physical activity interventions versus control for prevention and treatment of childhood obesity in schools. (Modified from Katz DL, O'Connell M, Njike VY, et al: Strategies for the prevention and control of obesity in the school setting: systematic review and meta-analysis, *Int J Obes Lond* 32:1780–1789, 2008.)

publication bias (a relative reluctance to publish negative findings). Fig. 13.2 shows an example of a funnel plot.

Meta-analysis is predicated on either a **fixed effects** or a **random effects** model. In the fixed effects model the pooled data of the available studies are used to answer the question, "Is there evidence here of an outcome effect?" The data from the selected trials are considered to comprise the entire study sample. In random effects modeling the data from the

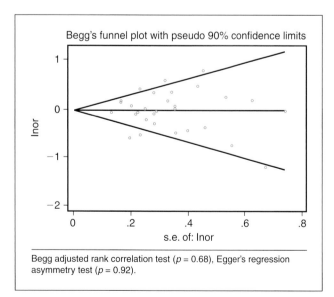

Begg adjusted rank correlation test (*p* = 0.68), Egger's regression asymmetry test (*p* = 0.92).

Fig. 13.2 Funnel Plot Showing Distribution of Trial Results around a Line of Mean Effect. Larger trials generally cluster near the mean effect, and smaller trials to either side of it. If one side of the funnel is relatively vacant of trials compared with the other, publication bias is likely. A symmetric funnel plot argues against an important influence of publication bias, supporting that the results of the meta-analysis are reliable. *lnor,* natural log of the odds ratio; *s.e.,* standard error. (From Botelho F, Lunet N, Barros H: Coffee and gastric cancer: systematic review and meta-analysis, *Cad Saude Publica* 22:889–900, 2006.)

selected trials are presumed to be a representative sample of a larger population of studies. This approach is used to answer the question, "Do the available data indicate that the larger population of data from which they were drawn provides evidence of an outcome effect?"[9]

Although meta-analysis is a useful statistical method, it is subject to important limitations. Aggregated data invariably compound the errors intrinsic to the original sources. Heterogeneity of methods or of study participants may result in the proverbial comparison between apples and oranges. Because of these issues, the results of a meta-analysis of many inadequately designed or executed studies can differ with results of a single large, well-conducted RCT.[14,15]

2. BAYES THEOREM AND PREDICTIVE VALUES OF TESTS

Although it is useful to know the sensitivity and specificity of a test, when a clinician decides to use a certain test on a patient, the following two clinical questions require answers (see Chapter 7):

- If the test results are positive, what is the probability that the patient has the disease?
- If the test results are negative, what is the probability that the patient does not have the disease?

Bayes theorem provides a way to answer these questions, as it is one of the most imposing statistical formulas in medicine. Put in symbols more meaningful in medicine, the formula is as follows:

$$p(D+|T+) = \frac{p(T+|D+)p(D+)}{p(T+)}$$

$$p(D+|T+) = \frac{p(T+|D+)p(D+)}{[p(T+|D+)p(D+)+p(T+|D-)p(D-)]}$$

where p denotes probability, D+ means the patient has the disease in question, D− means the patient does not have the disease, T+ means a certain diagnostic test for the disease is positive, T− means the test is negative, and the vertical line (|) means *conditional on* what immediately follows.

Many clinicians, even those who understand sensitivity, specificity, and predictive values, do not understand Bayes theorem. A close look at the previous equation reveals, however, that Bayes theorem is merely the formula for the **positive predictive value** (PPV), a value discussed in Chapter 7 and illustrated there in a standard 2 × 2 table (see Table 7.1).

The **numerator of Bayes theorem** merely describes **cell *a*** (the true-positive results) in Table 7.1. The probability of being in cell *a* is equal to the prevalence times the sensitivity, where $p(D+)$ is the prevalence (expressed as the probability of being in the diseased column) and $p(T+ | D+)$ is the sensitivity (the probability of being in the top, test-positive row, given the fact of being in the diseased column). The **denominator of Bayes theorem** consists of two terms, the first of which describes **cell *a*** (the true-positive results) and the second of which describes **cell *b*** (the false-positive results) in Table 7.1. In the second term of the denominator, the probability of the false-positive error rate, or $p(T+| D−)$, is multiplied by the prevalence of nondiseased persons, or $p(D−)$. As outlined in Chapter 7, the true-positive results (*a*) divided by the true-positive plus false-positive results (*a* + *b*) gives $a/(a + b)$, which is the positive predictive value.

In genetics, a simpler-appearing formula for Bayes theorem is sometimes used. The numerator is the same, but the denominator is merely $p(T+)$. This makes sense because the denominator in $a/(a + b)$ is equal to all those who have positive test results, whether they are true-positive or false-positive results.

2.1 COMMUNITY SCREENING PROGRAMS

In a population with a low prevalence of a particular disease, most of the positive results in a screening program for the disease would likely be falsely positive (see Chapter 7). Although this fact does not automatically invalidate a screening program, it raises some concerns about cost effectiveness, which can be explored using Bayes theorem.

A program employing the tuberculin tine test to screen children for tuberculosis (TB) is a good example (based on actual experience of Dr. Jekel, original coauthor of this text).[16] This test uses small amounts of tuberculin antigen on the tips of tiny prongs, called tines. The tines pierce the skin on the forearm and leave some antigen behind. The skin is examined 48 hours later, and the presence of an inflammatory reaction in the area where the tines entered is considered a positive result. If the sensitivity and specificity of the test and the prevalence of TB in the community are known, Bayes theorem can be used to predict what proportion of the children with positive test results will have true-positive results (i.e., will actually be infected with *Mycobacterium tuberculosis*).

Box 13.1 shows how the calculations are made. Suppose a test has a sensitivity of 96% ($p[T+|D+] = 0.96$ and $p[T-|D+] = 0.04$) and a specificity of 94% ($p[T-|D-] = 0.94$

BOX 13.1 **Use of Bayes Theorem or 2 × 2 Table to Determine Positive Predictive Value of a Hypothetical Tuberculin Screening Program**

Part 1 Beginning Data

Sensitivity of tuberculin tine test	= 96%	= 0.96
False-negative error rate of test	= 4%	= 0.04
Specificity of test	= 94%	= 0.94
False-positive error rate of test	= 6%	= 0.06
Prevalence of tuberculosis in community	= 1%	= 0.01

Part 2 Use of Bayes Theorem

$$P(D+ | T+) = \frac{P(T+ | D+)P(D+)}{P(T+ | D+)P(D+) + P(T+ | D-)P(D-)}$$

$$= \frac{(\text{Sensitivity})(\text{Prevalence})}{[(\text{Sensitivity})(\text{Prevalence}) + (\text{False Positive Rate})(1 - \text{Prevalence})]}$$

$$= \frac{(0.96)(0.01)}{[(0.96)(0.01) + (0.06)(0.99)]} = \frac{0.0096}{[0.0096 + 0.0594]} = 0.139 = 13.9\%$$

Part 3 Use of 2 × 2 Table, With Numbers Based on Study of 10,000 Persons

TEST RESULT	TRUE DISEASE STATUS (NO.)		Total
	Diseased	Nondiseased	
Positive	96 (96%)	594 (6%)	690 (7%)
Negative	4 (4%)	9,306 (94%)	9,310 (93%)
TOTAL	100 (100%)	9,900 (100%)	10,000 (100%)

Positive predictive value = 96/690 = 0.139 = 13.9%

Data from Jekel JF, Greenberg RA, Drake BM: Influence of the prevalence of infection on tuberculin skin testing programs. *Public Health Reports* 84:883–886, 1969.

and $p[T+|D- = 0.06]$). If the prevalence of TB in the community is 1% ($p[D+] = 0.01$ and $p[D-] = 0.99$), then placing all of these values into Bayes theorem shows that only 13.9% of those with a positive test result would be likely to be infected with TB. Clinicians involved in community health programs can quickly develop a table that lists different levels of test sensitivity, test specificity, and disease prevalence that shows how these levels affect the proportion of positive results that are likely to be true-positive results. Although this calculation is quite straightforward and useful, it is not used often in the early stages of planning screening programs. Before a new test is used, particularly for screening a large population, it is best to apply the test's sensitivity and specificity to the anticipated prevalence of the condition in the population. This helps avoid awkward surprises and is useful in the planning of appropriate follow-up for test-positive individuals. If the primary concern is simply to determine the overall performance of a test, however, likelihood ratios, which are independent of prevalence, are recommended (see Chapter 7).

There is another important point to keep in mind when planning community screening programs. The first time a previously unscreened population is screened, a considerable number of cases of disease may be found, but a repeat screening program soon afterward may find relatively few cases of new disease. This is because the first screening would detect cases that had their onset over *many years* (**prevalent cases**), whereas the second screening primarily would detect cases that had their onset during the interval since the last screening (**incident cases**).

2.2   INDIVIDUAL PATIENT CARE

Suppose a clinician is uncertain about a patient's diagnosis, obtains a test result for a certain disease, and the test is positive. Even if the clinician knows the sensitivity and specificity of the test, to calculate the positive predictive value, whether using Bayes theorem or a 2 × 2 table (e.g., Table 7.1), it is necessary to know the *prevalence of the disease*. In a clinical setting, the prevalence can be considered the *expected prevalence* in the population of which the patient is part. The actual prevalence is usually unknown, but often a reasonable estimate can be made.

For example, a clinician in a general medical clinic sees a male patient who complains of easy fatigability and has a history of kidney stones, but no other signs or symptoms of parathyroid disease on physical examination. The clinician considers the probability of hyperparathyroidism and decides that it is low, perhaps 2% (reflecting that in 100 similar patients, probably only 2 of them would have the disease). This probability is called the **prior probability**, reflecting that it is estimated *before* the performance of laboratory tests and is based on the estimated prevalence of a particular disease among patients with similar signs and symptoms. Although the clinician believes that the probability of hyperparathyroidism is low, he or she orders a serum calcium test to rule out the diagnosis. To the clinician's surprise, the results of the test come back positive, with an elevated level of 12.2 mg/dL. The clinician could order more tests for parathyroid disease,

but even here, some test results might come back positive and some negative.

Under these circumstances, Bayes theorem could be used to help interpret the positive test. A second estimate of disease probability in this patient could be calculated. It is called the **posterior probability**, reflecting that it is made *after* the test results are known. Calculation of the posterior probability is based on the sensitivity and specificity of the test that was performed and on the prior probability of disease before the test was performed, which in this case was 2%. Suppose the serum calcium test had 90% sensitivity and 95% specificity (which implies it had a false-positive error rate of 5%; specificity + false-positive error rate = 100%). When this information is used in the Bayes equation, as shown in Box 13.2, the result is a posterior probability of 27%. This means that the patient is now in a group of patients with a substantial possibility, but still far from certainty, of parathyroid disease. In Box 13.2, the result is the same (i.e., 27%) when a 2 × 2 table is used. This is true because, as discussed, the probability based on the Bayes theorem is identical to the positive predictive value.

In light of the 27% posterior probability, the clinician decides to order a serum parathyroid hormone concentration test with simultaneous measurement of serum calcium, even though this test is expensive. If the parathyroid hormone test had a sensitivity of 95% and a specificity of 98%, and the results turned out to be positive, the Bayes theorem could be used again to calculate the probability of parathyroid disease in this patient. This time, however, the *posterior* probability for the *first* test (27%) would be used as the prior probability for the second test. The result of the calculation, as shown in Box 13.3, is a new probability of 94%. The patient likely has hyperparathyroidism, although lack of true numerical certainty even at this stage is noteworthy.

Why did the posterior probability increase so much the second time? One reason was the *prior probability* was *considerably higher* in the second calculation than in the first (27% vs. 2%), based on the first test yielding positive results in this specific patient. Another reason was the *specificity of the second test was assumed to be high* (98%), which greatly reduced the false-positive error rate and increased the PPV. A highly specific test is useful for "ruling in" disease, which in essence is what has happened here.

2.3   INFLUENCE OF THE SEQUENCE OF TESTING

With an increasing number of diagnostic tests available in clinical medicine, the clinician now needs to consider whether to do many tests simultaneously or to do them sequentially. Tests used to rule out a diagnosis should have a high degree of sensitivity, whereas tests used to rule in a diagnosis should have a high degree of specificity (see Chapter 7 and Box 7.1). The *sequential approach* is best taken as follows:
1. Starting with the most sensitive test.
2. Continuing with increasingly specific tests if the previous test yields positive results.
3. Stopping when a test yields negative results.

BOX 13.2   Use of Bayes Theorem or 2 × 2 Table to Determine Posterior Probability and Positive Predictive Value in Clinical Setting (Hypothetical Data)

Part 1 Beginning Data (Before Performing First Test)

Sensitivity of first test	= 90%	= 0.90
Specificity of first test	= 95%	= 0.95
Prior probability of disease	= 2%	= 0.02

Part 2 Use of Bayes Theorem to Calculate First Posterior Probability

$$P(D+\mid T+) = \frac{P(T+\mid D+)P(D+)}{P(T+\mid D+)P(D+) + P(T+\mid D-)P(D-)}$$

$$= \frac{(0.90)(0.02)}{[(0.90)(0.02)+(0.05)(0.98)]}$$

$$= \frac{0.018}{[0.018+0.049]} = \frac{0.018}{0.067} = 0.269 = 27\%$$

Part 3 Use of a 2 × 2 Table to Calculate First Positive Predictive Value

	TRUE DISEASE STATUS (NO.)		
TEST RESULT	Diseased	Nondiseased	Total
Positive	18 (90%)	49 (5%)	67 (6.7%)
Negative	2 (10%)	931 (95%)	933 (93.3%)
TOTAL	20 (100%)	980 (100%)	1000 (100%)

Positive predictive value = 18/67 = 27%

BOX 13.3   Use of Bayes Theorem or 2 × 2 Table to Determine Second Posterior Probability and Second Positive Predictive Value in Clinical Setting

Part 1 Beginning Data (Before Performing the Second Test)

Sensitivity of second test	= 95%	= 0.95
Specificity of second test	= 98%	= 0.98
Prior probability of disease (see Box 13.2)	= 27%	= 0.27

Part 2 Use of Bayes Theorem to Calculate Posterior Probability

$$P(D+\mid T+) = \frac{P(T+\mid D+)P(D+)}{P(T+\mid D+)P(D+) + P(T+\mid D-)P(D-)}$$

$$= \frac{(0.95)(0.27)}{[(0.95)(0.27)+(0.02)(0.73)]}$$

$$= \frac{0.257}{[0.257+0.0146]} = \frac{0.257}{0.272} = 0.9449 = 94\%$$

Part 3 Use of 2 × 2 Table to Calculate Positive Predictive Value

	TRUE DISEASE STATUS (NO.)		
TEST RESULT	Diseased	Nondiseased	Total
Positive	256 (95%)	15 (2%)	271 (27.1%)
Negative	13 (5%)	716 (98%)	729 (72.9%)
TOTAL	269 (100%)	731 (100%)	1000 (100%)

Positive predictive value = 256/271 = 0.9446* = 94%

*The slight difference in the results for the two approaches is caused by rounding errors. It is not important clinically.

Compared with the simultaneous approach, the sequential approach to testing is more conservative and more economical in the care of outpatients. The sequential approach may increase the length of stay for a hospitalized patient, however, so the cost implications may be unclear.

The sequence of testing may have implications for the overall accuracy. If multiple diagnostic tests are performed at the same time, the natural tendency is to ignore the negative results while seriously considering the positive results. This approach to establishing a diagnosis may not be ideal, however. Even if the tests are performed simultaneously, it is probably best to consider first the results of the most sensitive test. If a negative result is reported for that test, the result is probably a true-negative one (the patient probably does not have the disease). Why? Highly sensitive tests are reliably positive when disease is present and tend to deliver negative results only when disease is truly absent. Simultaneous testing may produce conflicting results, but a careful consideration of each test's result in light of the test's sensitivity and specificity should improve the chances of making the correct diagnosis.

3. DECISION ANALYSIS

A decision-making tool that has come into the medical literature from management science is called **decision analysis**. Its purpose is to improve decision making under conditions of uncertainty. In clinical medicine, decision analysis can be used for an individual patient or for a general class of patients. As a technique, decision analysis is more popular clinically than Bayes theorem; and it is being used with increasing frequency in the literature, particularly to make judgments about a class of patients or clinical problems.

The primary value of decision analysis is to help health care workers understand the following:

- The types of data that must go into a clinical decision.
- The sequence in which decisions need to be made.
- The personal values of the patient that must be considered before major decisions are made.

As a general rule decision analysis is more important as a tool to help clinicians take a disciplined approach to decision making than as a tool for making the actual clinical decisions.

3.1 STEPS IN CREATING A DECISION TREE

The five logical steps to setting up a decision tree are[17]:
a. Identify and set limits to the problem.
b. Diagram the options.
c. Obtain information on each option.
d. Compare the utility values.
e. Perform sensitivity analysis.

3.1.a. Identify the Problem

When identifying a course of clinical action, the clinician must determine the possible alternative clinical decisions, the sequence in which the decisions must be made, and the possible patient outcomes of each decision. The clinical problem illustrated here is whether to remove a gallbladder in a patient with silent gallstones.[18] This clinical decision is useful as a teaching example only, because clinical practice has changed since this decision tree was constructed and surgery for silent gallstones is only indicated for diabetics. Nonetheless, diabetic patients with silent gallstones face a similar decision.

3.1.b. Diagram the Options

Fig. 13.3 provides a simple example of how to diagram the options. The beginning point of a decision tree is the patient's current clinical status. **Decision nodes** (i.e., points where

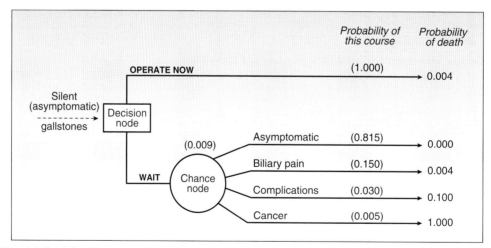

Fig. 13.3 **Decision Tree on Treatment for Silent (Asymptomatic) Gallstones.** The decision node, defined as a point where the clinician has to make a decision, is represented by a *square*. The chance node, defined as a point where the clinician must wait to see the outcome, is represented by a *circle*. If the clinician decides to operate now, the probability of surgery is 100% (1.000), and the probability of death (the negative utility value) from complications of surgery is 0.04% (0.004, or 1 of every 250 patients undergoing surgery). If the clinician decides to wait, there are four possible outcomes, each with a different probability and negative utility value: (1) 81.5% (0.815) probability of remaining asymptomatic, in which case the probability of dying from gallstones would be 0% (0.000); (2) 15% (0.150) probability of developing biliary pain, which would lead to surgery and a 0.4% (0.004) risk of death; (3) 3% (0.030) probability of biliary complications (e.g., acute cholecystitis, common duct obstruction), with a 10% (0.100) risk of death; or (4) 0.5% (0.005) probability of gallbladder cancer, with a 100% (1.000) risk of death. The probabilities of the possible outcomes at the chance node add up to 1 (here, 0.815 + 0.150 + 0.030 + 0.005 = 1.000). (From Rose DN, Wiesel J: Letter to the editor. *N Engl J Med* 308:221–222, 1983. © Massachusetts Medical Society. All rights reserved. Adapted with permission in 1996, 1999, 2006, 2011.)

clinicians need to make decisions) are represented by squares or rectangles. **Chance nodes** (i.e., points where clinicians need to wait to see the outcomes) are represented by circles. Time goes from left to right, so the first decision is at the left, and subsequent decisions are progressively to the right. In Fig. 13.3 the beginning point is the presence of asymptomatic gallstones and the primary decision at the decision node is whether to operate immediately or to wait.[18]

3.1.c. Obtain Information on Each Option

First, the **probability of each possible outcome** must be obtained from published studies or be estimated on the basis of clinical experience. In Fig. 13.3, if the clinician waits rather than operates, the probability is 81.5% (0.815) that the patient will remain asymptomatic, 15% that the patient will have periodic biliary pain, 3% that the patient will develop complications such as acute cholecystitis or common duct obstruction from gallstones, and 0.5% that the patient eventually will develop cancer of the gallbladder. The probabilities of the possible outcomes for a chance node must add up to 100%, as they do in this case.

Second, the **utility of each final outcome** must be obtained. In decision analysis the term *utility* is used to mean the value of a chosen course of action. Utility may be expressed as a **desirable outcome** (e.g., years of disease-free survival), in which case larger values have greater utility, or it may be expressed as an **undesirable outcome** (e.g., death, illness, high cost), in which case smaller values have greater utility. Clinical decision analysis seeks to show which clinical decision would maximize utility. In Fig. 13.3, each final outcome is expressed in terms of a negative utility (i.e., probability of death). If surgery is performed now, the probability of death is 0.4% (0.004). If the surgeon waits, and the patient remains asymptomatic for life, the probability of a gallbladder-related death is 0%. The probabilities of death for biliary pain, complications, and cancer are 0.4%, 10%, and 100%, respectively.

3.1.d. Compare Utility Values and Perform Sensitivity Analysis

The decision tree can show how a given set of probabilities and utilities would turn out. If the decision tree shows that one choice is clearly preferable to any other, this would be strong evidence in favor of that choice. Often, however, the decision analysis would give two or more outcomes with similar utilities, which means that better data are needed or that factors other than the decision analysis should be used to make the clinical decision.

In addition to comparing the utility values, it is sometimes helpful to perform a sensitivity analysis. This is done to see if the results of the analysis are fairly stable over a range of assumptions. It might consist of varying the estimated probabilities of occurrence of a particular outcome at various points in the decision tree to see how the overall outcomes and clinical decisions would be affected by these changes. This helps the clinician and the patient to see which assumptions and decisions have the largest impact on the outcomes

through a reasonable range of values. Fig. 13.3 can be used to show how to compare utility values and to discuss the rationale for performing a **sensitivity analysis**. (Note that the use of the word *sensitivity* here is quite different from the way the term was used up to this point. This use of the term was probably developed because the objective of the analysis is to see how sensitive the conclusions are to changes in assumptions.)

In the decision tree in Fig. 13.3, there are two branches from the decision node, one labeled "operate now" and the other labeled "wait." As discussed earlier, the probability of death from operating immediately is 0.004, whereas there are four different probabilities of death from waiting, depending on what happens during the waiting period (the patient remains asymptomatic or develops pain, complications, or cancer). Before the utility of operating now versus waiting can be compared, it is necessary to **average out** the data associated with the four possible outcomes of waiting. First the probability of each outcome from waiting is multiplied by the probability that death would ensue following that particular outcome. Then the four products are summed. In Fig. 13.3, for the choice to wait, the calculation for averaging out is $(0.815 \times 0.000) + (0.150 \times 0.004) + (0.030 \times 0.100) + (0.005 \times 1.000) = 0.0086 = 0.009$, or slightly more than twice the risk of operating now. This probability of death from the gallbladder and its treatment results from the decision to wait.

Based on the previous calculations, the best option would seem to be to operate now. Because these two outcome probabilities are fairly close to each other (0.004 vs. 0.009, a difference of only 0.005, which equals 0.5%, or 1 in 200 cases), however, the decision analysis does not lead strongly to either conclusion and the balance might be changed by newer assumptions. It would be a good idea to perform a sensitivity analysis on these data. If the same conclusion remains for a wide range of data assumptions, the clinician would be relatively confident in the decision. If small changes in the data changed the direction of the decision, the decision analysis is probably unhelpful. However, other issues must be considered as well.

Factors other than probability of death influence patient preference in the real world. Most of the deaths that occur from surgery in the decision tree under discussion would occur immediately, but deaths caused by cancer of the gallbladder or other complications usually would occur many years later. Given the timing of the deaths, many patients would choose to avoid immediate surgery (e.g., because they are feeling well or have family responsibilities), preferring to deal with complications if and when they arise. Some patients, however, who are willing to risk everything for the sake of a cure, might express a preference for the most aggressive treatment possible.

Although this was a simple example, other decision trees have multiple decision nodes that involve complicated issues and factors such as the passage of time. Decision trees need to be redone as time passes, and new data and assumptions arise. In these more complex decision analyses, the objective is to find decisions that are clearly less satisfactory than others and to cut off or "prune" these branches because they are not rational alternatives. The process of choosing the best branch at each decision node, working backward from right to left, is called **folding back**. Decision trees can be used only in problems that do not have a repetitive outcome, such as recurring embolic strokes in patients with atrial fibrillation. Such problems are better evaluated with Markov models or Monte Carlo simulations, which are beyond the scope of this text.[19,20]

3.2 APPLICATIONS OF DECISION TREES

Decision trees can be used in the clinical setting, as discussed earlier in the case of patients with asymptomatic gallstones, but are increasingly being applied to public health problems. When considering what strategy would be most cost effective in eliminating the problem of hepatitis B virus (HBV), some authors used a decision tree to analyze data concerning several possible options: no routine HBV vaccination, a screening program followed by HBV vaccination for persons meeting certain criteria, and HBV vaccination for specific populations (newborns, 10-year-olds, high-risk adults, general adult US population).[2]

4. SUMMARY

Several statistical methods can be used to improve clinical decision making. Systematic review and quantitative meta-analysis aggregate the findings of multiple studies to enhance statistical power and support external validity (generalizability or applicability). When study findings are aggregated using clearly defined methods to assess inclusion and quality, the approach is a systematic review. A meta-analysis statistically aggregates quantitative results to calculate a mean effect size. Among the tools available for decision analysis are Bayes theorem and decision trees. These tools can be applied to individual patient care and to community health programs. Bayes theorem can be used to calculate positive predictive values and posterior probabilities. Decision trees can help health care workers pursue a logical, step-by-step approach to exploring the possible alternative clinical decisions, the sequence in which these decisions must be made, and the probabilities and utilities of each possible outcome.

REFERENCES

1. Koplan JP, Schoenbaum SC, Weinstein MC, Fraser DW. Pertussis vaccine—an analysis of benefits, risks and costs. *N Engl J Med.* 1979;301:906-911.
2. Bloom BS, Hillman AL, Fendrick AM, Schwartz JS. A reappraisal of hepatitis B virus vaccination strategies using cost-effectiveness analysis. *Ann Intern Med.* 1993;118:298-306.
3. Knowler WC, Barrett-Connor E, Fowler SE, et al. Reduction in the incidence of type 2 diabetes with lifestyle intervention or metformin. *N Engl J Med.* 2002;346:393-403.
4. Howard BV, Van Horn L, Hsia J, et al. Low-fat dietary pattern and risk of cardiovascular disease: the Women's Health Initiative Randomized Controlled Dietary Modification Trial. *JAMA.* 2006; 295:655-666.
5. Higgins JPT, Green S, eds. *Cochrane Handbook for Systematic Reviews of Interventions Version 5.1.0* [updated March 2011]. The Cochrane Collaboration, 2011. Available at: http://handbook. cochrane.org.
6. Irving MJ, Tong A, Jan S, et al. Factors that influence the decision to be an organ donor: a systematic review of the qualitative literature. *Nephrol Dial Transplant.* 2011;27:2526-2533.
7. Lehnert T, Sonntag D, Konnopka A, Riedel-Heller S, König HH. The long-term cost-effectiveness of obesity prevention interventions: systematic literature review. *Obes Rev.* 2012;13:537-553.
8. Man SC, Chan KW, Lu JH, Durairajan SS, Liu LF, Li M. Systematic review on the efficacy and safety of herbal medicines for vascular dementia. *Evid Based Complement Alternat Med.* 2012;2012:426215.
9. Petitti DB. *Meta-Analysis, Decision Analysis, and Cost-Effectiveness Analysis: Methods for Quantitative Synthesis in Medicine.* 2nd ed. New York, NY: Oxford University Press; 2000.
10. Kulinskaya E, Dollinger MB, Bjørkestøl K. Testing for homogeneity in meta-analysis I. The one-parameter case: standardized mean difference. *Biometrics.* 2011;67:203-212.
11. Fortier-Brochu E, Beaulieu-Bonneau S, Ivers H, Morin CM. Insomnia and daytime cognitive performance: a meta-analysis. *Sleep Med Rev.* 2012;16:83-94.
12. Michels KB, Yusuf S. Does PTCA in acute myocardial infarction affect mortality and reinfarction rates? A quantitative overview (meta-analysis) of the randomized clinical trials. *Circulation.* 1995;91:476-485.
13. Copas J, Shi JQ. Meta-analysis, funnel plots and sensitivity analysis. *Biostatistics.* 2000;1:247-262.
14. LeLorier J, Grégoire G, Benhaddad A, Lapierre J, Derderian F. Discrepancies between meta-analyses and subsequent large randomized, controlled trials. *N Engl J Med.* 1997;337:536-542.
15. Bailar III JC. The promise and problems of meta-analysis. *N Engl J Med.* 1997;337:559-561.
16. Jekel JF, Greenberg RA, Drake BM. Influence of the prevalence of infection on tuberculin skin testing programs. *Public Health Rep.* 1969;84:883-886.
17. Weinstein MC, Fineberg HV. *Clinical Decision Analysis.* Philadelphia, PA: Saunders; 1980.
18. Rose DN, Wiesel J. Letter to the editor. *N Engl J Med.* 1983; 308:221-222.
19. Sonnenberg FA, Beck JR. Markov models in medical decision making: a practical guide. *Med Decis Making.* 1993;13:322-338.
20. Hunink M, Glasziou P, Seigel J, et al. *Decision Making in Health and Medicine: Integrating Evidence and Values.* Cambridge: Cambridge University Press; 2001.

SELECT READINGS

Blettner M, Sauerbrei W, Schlehofer B, Scheuchenpflug T, Friedenreich C. Traditional reviews, meta-analyses and pooled analyses in epidemiology. *Int J Epidemiol.* 1999;28:1-9.
Friedland DJ, ed. *Evidence-Based Medicine: A Framework for Clinical Practice.* Stamford, CT: Appleton & Lange; 1998.
Kemper P, Murtaugh CM. Lifetime use of nursing home care. *N Engl J Med.* 1991;324:595-600.
Nelson HD. *Systematic Reviews to Answer Health Care Questions.* Philadelphia, PA: Wolters Kluwer; 2014.
Sackett DL, Straus SE, Richardson WS, et al. *Evidence-Based Medicine: How to Practice and Teach EBM.* Edinburgh, Scotland: Churchill Livingstone; 1997.

Weinstein MC, Fineberg HV. *Clinical Decision Analysis*. Philadelphia, PA: Saunders; 1980.

Whitehead A. *Meta-Analysis of Controlled Clinical Trials*. West Sussex, UK: Wiley & Sons; 2002.

REVIEW QUESTIONS

1. In Bayes theorem, the numerator represents:
   A. False-negative results
   B. Incidence
   C. Prevalence
   D. Sensitivity
   E. True-positive results

2. As clinicians, we are usually interested in using Bayes theorem to determine:
   A. Cost effectiveness
   B. Disease prevalence
   C. False-negative results
   D. Positive predictive value
   E. Test sensitivity

3. When applying Bayes theorem to the care of an individual patient, the prior probability is analogous to:
   A. Prevalence
   B. Sensitivity
   C. Specificity
   D. The likelihood ratio
   E. The odds ratio

4. The application of Bayes theorem to patient care generally results in:
   A. Greater sensitivity
   B. Greater specificity
   C. Higher costs
   D. Improved selection of diagnostic studies
   E. More diagnostic testing

5. A young man complains of reduced auditory acuity on the left side. You take his medical history and perform a physical examination. Before you begin diagnostic testing, you estimate a 74% chance that the patient has a large foreign object in his left ear. This estimate is the:
   A. Likelihood ratio
   B. Odds ratio
   C. Posterior probability
   D. Relative risk
   E. Prior probability

6. To apply Bayes theorem to a screening program to estimate the posterior probability that a patient has a disease, given that the patient has tested positive, which of the following information must be known?
   A. Prior probability, sensitivity, and false-negative error rate
   B. Prevalence, sensitivity, and specificity

C. Prevalence, specificity, and posterior probability
D. Prior probability, false-positive error rate, and incidence
E. False-positive error rate, sensitivity, and false-negative error rate

7. A 62-year-old woman complains that during the past several months she has been experiencing intermittent left-sided chest pain when she exercises. Her medical records indicate she has a history of mild dyslipidemia, with a high-density lipoprotein (HDL) cholesterol level of 38 mg/dL and a total cholesterol level of 232 mg/dL. She says she has a family history of heart disease in male relatives only. Her current blood pressure is 132/68 mm Hg, and her heart rate is 72 beats/min. On cardiac examination, you detect a physiologically split second heart sound (S_2) and a faint midsystolic click without appreciable murmur. The point of maximal impulse is nondisplaced, and the remainder of the examination is unremarkable. You are concerned that the patient's chest pain may represent angina pectoris and decide to initiate a workup. You estimate that the odds of the pain being angina are 1 in 3. You order an electrocardiogram, which reveals nonspecific abnormalities in the ST segments and T waves across the precordial leads. You decide to order a perfusion stress test, the sensitivity of which is 98% and the specificity of which is 85% for ischemia. The stress test results are positive, showing reversible ischemia in the distribution of the circumflex artery on perfusion imaging, with compatible electrocardiogram changes. The prior probability of angina pectoris is:
   A. 2%
   B. 15%
   C. 33%
   D. 67%
   E. Unknown

8. Considering the details from question 7, the posterior probability of angina pectoris after the stress test is:
   A. 10%
   B. 33%
   C. 67%
   D. 76%
   E. Unchanged

9. Based on the previous findings in questions 7 and 8, you decide to treat the 62-year-old female patient for angina pectoris. You prescribe aspirin, a statin, and a beta-adrenergic receptor antagonist (beta blocker) to be taken daily, and you prescribe sublingual nitroglycerin tablets to be used if pain recurs. Pain does recur, with increasing frequency and severity, despite treatment. After you consult a cardiologist, you recommend cardiac catheterization. Assume that the sensitivity of cardiac catheterization for coronary artery disease is 96%, and that the specificity is 99%. When the

procedure is performed, it yields negative results. At this stage of the workup, the prior probability of angina pectoris is:

A. 11%
B. 33%
C. 76%
D. 96%
E. Unknown

10. Considering the previous findings in questions 7 through 9, based on the results of cardiac catheterization, the probability of coronary artery disease is:

A. 11%
B. 33%
C. 76%
D. 96%
E. Unknown

ANSWERS AND EXPLANATIONS

1. **E.** Bayes theorem describes the probability that a patient has the disease, conditional on the diagnostic test for the disease being positive. The theorem is essentially an expression of the positive predictive value (i.e., given a positive test result, how likely the disease is present). The numerator of the formula for the theorem represents true-positive test results (E); the denominator, as in the formula for the positive predictive value, represents all positive test results (i.e., true-positive and false-positive results). Bayes theorem adjusts prior probability: the probability of disease in a patient before running a test, also known as pretest probability. The pretest probability is analogous to the prevalence (C) of the disease in a population (the probability of disease for individuals in that population). Bayes theorem does not comment on sensitivity (D), the probability of a test being positive conditional on the patient having the disease. However, the Bayes theorem numerator of true-positive test results = sensitivity × prevalence. Bayes theorem is not associated with incidence (B; mathematically the prevalence of disease over duration of illness) or false-negative results (A), which relate to sensitivity.

2. **D.** It is necessary to know how likely disease is when the results of testing are positive in a screening program. Bayes theorem is used to establish the positive predictive value of a screening test, based on an estimate of the pretest probability (i.e., underlying population prevalence of disease under investigation). Disease prevalence (B) must be known or estimated to use Bayes theorem; it is not used to determine prevalence. The test sensitivity (E) is an intrinsic property of the test when applied to a population with given characteristics; it is unaffected by prevalence and is not determined by use of Bayes theorem. The cost effectiveness (A) of a screening program is an important consideration but is distinct from the predictive value

of the test. Bayes theorem is based on the proportion of true-positive results to all positive results (true-positive + false-positive results); false-negative results (C) are irrelevant to use of the theorem.

3. **A.** Conceptually, Bayes theorem states that the probability of a disease in an individual with a positive test result depends partly on the prevalence of that disease in the population of whom the individual is a part. For a child with fever in New Haven, Connecticut, the probability of malaria is low. The probability (prior probability or pretest probability) is low in this child because the prevalence of malaria is so low in the population. For a child with fever in a refugee population in Nigeria, the pretest probability of malaria might be high because malaria is prevalent in the population. The prior probability of a disease in an individual is an estimate based on the prevalence of that disease in a population of similar persons.

   In another example to emphasize this point, the prior probability of pregnancy in a male patient presenting with abdominal distention and complaining of nausea in the morning is zero. It is not zero because the status of the individual is known with certainty; rather, it is zero because the prevalence of pregnancy in a population of males is zero. When the prior probability of a condition is either 0 or 100%, no further testing for that condition is indicated.

   Sensitivity (B) and specificity (C) are important performance characteristics of clinical tests, but do not relate at all to prior probability; these measures are completely independent of prevalence. Likewise, likelihood ratios (D) and odds ratios (E) are independent of prevalence.

4. **D.** When Bayes theorem is used appropriately in planning patient care, the result is more careful selection and refined use of diagnostic testing. Even when the theorem is used qualitatively, it suggests that if the prior probability of disease is high enough, no further testing is required, because neither a positive nor a negative test result will substantively modify pretest probability of disease or in any way change clinical decision making. Performing a test in such a scenario is pointless and can only result in unnecessary costs (e.g., time, resources) and possible harm from invasive tests (e.g., biopsy, catheterization). At other times, when successive tests fail to establish a posterior probability that is sufficiently high for decisive action to be taken, the theorem compels the clinician to continue testing. Neither sensitivity (A) nor specificity (B) is enhanced by use of the theorem; both depend in part on the choice of diagnostic test. Using Bayes theorem in planning patient care should result in better use of diagnostic tests—sometimes more frequent use (E), sometimes less frequent use. The overall cost (C) varies accordingly.

   For example, an otherwise healthy 32-year-old man with no significant medical problems visits your office complaining of chronic lower back pain. His symptoms have been fairly constant over the last few months. He works in custodial services but denies any significant trauma or injury on the job or elsewhere. He reports no fever, chills, recent infection, or illicit drug use. He has no night pain or pain that wakes him from sleep. He has no difficulty walking and reports no numbness or tingling or incontinence. He is using no medications. His physical examination reveals tense, tender lumbar paraspinal muscles with no neurologic deficits or functional limitations. In a patient with these findings, you estimate that the prior probability of nonspecific musculoskeletal lower back pain (e.g., lumbar sprain or strain) is greater than 95%. By reflex—the type of reflex acquired only with medical training—you might order some blood tests and a back x-ray film and consider magnetic resonance imaging (MRI). However, you may realize that you have already made up your mind to start with a prescription for back exercises, stretching, and acetaminophen, and see him again in about 6 weeks (or sooner for worsening). When the prior probability is sufficiently high, further diagnostic testing would not, and should not, alter your course of action and is not indicated. Conversely, it may be inappropriate to take immediate action when you have a considerable amount of uncertainty about what to do next for your patient (e.g., a patient of intermediate vascular risk presenting for chest pain that you are unsure whether sounds mostly like angina or esophageal spasm), and further diagnostic studies would help reduce the uncertainty. If you apply the concept of Bayes theorem to your clinical care planning, without even using the actual formula, the standards of your practice are likely to improve.

5. **E.** The prior probability is an estimate of the probability of a given condition in a given patient at a given point in time, before further testing. Posterior probability (C) is the revised probability of a given condition in a given patient at a given point in time, after testing. In actual practice, prior and posterior probabilities flow freely into one another. Estimating the probability of sinusitis after interviewing a patient gives you the prior probability of disease before you examine the patient. The revision in your estimate after the examination is the posterior probability, but this revision is also the prior probability before any diagnostic testing, such as sinus x-ray films, that you may be considering. A likelihood ratio (A) describes performance characteristics of a test, such as the diagnostic test in the question that has not yet been performed. Odds ratios (B) and relative risks (D) are ways of comparing probabilities of conditions between two different groups.

6. **B.** The only choice that includes everything that must be known to use Bayes theorem, in terms appropriate for a screening program, is (B). The prevalence (if discussing a population) or prior probability (if discussing an individual patient) must be known, ruling out (E). Sensitivity must be known, ruling out (C) and (D). Specificity (or 1 – false-positive error rate) must be known, ruling out A. The numerator for Bayes theorem is the sensitivity of the test being used, multiplied by the prevalence. The denominator contains the numerator term plus a term that is the false-positive error rate, or (1 – specificity) $\times$ (1 – prevalence). The numerator of Bayes theorem describes cell *a* in a 2 $\times$ 2 table (see Table 7.1), and the denominator includes the term from the numerator (cell *a*, or true-positive results) and adds to it the term for the false-positive results (cell *b* from 2 $\times$ 2 table). Bayes theorem can be rewritten as $a/(a + b)$, which is the formula for the positive predictive value. This is what Bayes theorem is used to determine, so it is not necessary to know the predictive value before using the theorem.

7. **C.** Prior probability (for an individual) is analogous to prevalence (for a population) and represents an estimate of the likelihood of disease. In this case, the prior probability is your estimate of the likelihood of angina pectoris before any testing. You estimate that the pretest odds of the patient's pain being angina pectoris is 1 in 3, or a 33% (1/3) probability or 33% prior probability. This value is easily calculated and thus not unknown (E). The probability of the pain not being angina pectoris is 1 – (1/3) = (2/3), or 67% (D). The 2% (A) is 1 – sensitivity of the perfusion stress test and represents the false-negative error rate (FNER) for the test; 15% (B) is 1 – specificity of the perfusion stress test and represents the false-positive error rate (FPER) for the test.

8. **D.** Either Bayes theorem or a 2 $\times$ 2 table can be used to calculate the posterior probability.

   Use of Bayes theorem: The sensitivity is provided in the vignette as 98%, or 0.98. The prior probability estimate is substituted for the prevalence and is 33%, or 0.33. The false-positive error rate is (1 – specificity). The specificity is provided as 85%, so the false-positive error rate is 15%, or 0.15. In this case, (1 – prevalence) is the same as (1 – prior probability) and is (1 – 0.33), or 0.67.

$$p(\text{T1}|\text{D1}) = \frac{p(\text{T1}|\text{D1})p(\text{D1})}{\left[p(\text{T1}|\text{D1})p(\text{D1}) + p(\text{T1}|\text{D2})p(\text{D2})\right]}$$

$$= \frac{(\text{Sensitivity})(\text{Prevalence})}{\left[\begin{array}{l}(\text{Sensitivity})(\text{Prevalence}) + \\ (\text{False} - \text{positive error rate})(1 - \text{Prevalence})\end{array}\right]}$$

$$= \frac{(0.98)(0.33)}{\left[(0.98)(0.33) + (0.15)(0.67)\right]}$$

$$= \frac{0.3234}{\left[(0.3234) + (0.1005)\right]}$$

$$= \frac{0.3234}{0.4239} = 0.76 = 7690$$

Use of a 2 × 2 table: To use this method, an arbitrary sample size must be chosen. Assuming that the sample size is 100, the following is true: Cell *a* is the true-positive results, or sensitivity × prevalence. The prior probability becomes the prevalence. Cell *a* is (0.98) (33) = 32.3 (rounded to 32). Cells *a* plus *c* must sum to 33, so cell *c* is 0.7 (rounded to 1). Cell *d* is the true-negative result, which is specificity × (1 – prevalence), or (0.85)(67) = 57. Cells *b* plus *d* must sum to 67, so cell *b* is 10.

TEST RESULT	DISEASE	
	Positive	Negative
Positive	32	10
Negative	1	57

When the 2 × 2 table is established, the formula for positive predictive value, which is *a*/(*a* + *b*), can be used to calculate the posterior probability, as follows:

$$a/(a+b) = 32/(32+10) = 32/42 = 0.76 = 76\%$$

Given either method of reasoning or calculation, we arrive at the same answer choice and all other answer choices—(A), (B), (C), and (E)—can be excluded.

9. **C.** As discussed in the explanation for question 5, prior and posterior probabilities may flow freely into one another in the sequence of diagnostic workups. In this case the disease probability after the stress test (posterior probability) is the pretest or prior probability before the catheterization. For this reason, the explanation for question 9 and its supporting logic are the same as for question 8. After the stress test, the posterior probability of angina is 76%. This is also the probability of angina before any further diagnostic studies, such as catheterization. For these reasons, answer choices (A), (B), (D), and (E) are incorrect.

10. **A.** Up to this point, we have been discussing positive predictive value (PPV; i.e., how likely a disease will be present if a test result is positive). Presented with a negative or normal test result as in this question, however, what we are concerned about is negative predictive value (NPV; i.e., how likely a disease is absent if the test is negative). From the NPV we can calculate the likelihood of coronary artery disease (CAD) given a negative test result (1 – NPV). For NPV we can use the formula *d*/(*c* + *d*). To use this formula, we must first set up a 2 × 2 table (Bayes theorem is not helpful in this situation). Assume a sample size of 100. The prior probability, 76%, becomes the prevalence. Cell *a* is sensitivity × prevalence, or (0.96)(76) = 73. Cells *a* plus *c* sum to the prevalence, so cell *c* is 3. Cell *d* is specificity × (1 – prevalence), or (0.99)(24) = 23.8. Cells *b* plus *d* sum to (1 – prevalence), so cell *b* is 0.2.

TEST RESULT	DISEASE	
	Positive	Negative
Positive	73	0.2
Negative	3	23.8

The NPV is thus:

$$d/(c+d) = 23.8/(3+23.8) = 23.8/26.8 = 89\%$$

This is the probability that the patient does not have CAD. What we are interested in, however, is the probability that the patient actually has CAD, which is 1 – NPV, or 1 – 0.89 (100% – 89%), or 11%. This is the posterior probability (probability after catheterization) given a prior probability of 76% (probability after stress test, but before catheterization). In other words, at the end of the workup (which included a stress test followed by a catheterization), the final likelihood (posterior probability) of ischemic heart disease is relatively small, about a 1 in 10 chance.

Preventive Medicine

14

Introduction to Preventive Medicine

"An ounce of prevention is worth a pound of cure."

Benjamin Franklin

Sections 1 and 2 of this text focus on epidemiology and biostatistics, two basic sciences for preventive medicine and public health. This third section focuses on the theory and practice of preventive medicine, which seeks to enhance the lives of **individuals** by helping them improve their own health. Preventive medicine shares common goals with public health (the topic of Section 4), such as promoting general health, reducing risks, preventing specific diseases, and applying epidemiologic concepts and biostatistical techniques toward these goals. However, public health attempts to promote health in **populations** through the application of organized community efforts, whereas preventive medicine targets the lives of individuals.

Even when dealing with individual patients though, health care clinicians need to be aware that "the conditions in which people are born, grow, live, work, and age"[1] have a profound impact on their health, sometimes more so than the medical care they receive. These conditions are collectively called **social determinants of health**, and no discussion of preventive medicine or public health is complete without a discussion of them. After a discussion of health and its determinants, this chapter discusses the different levels of prevention and how to know if specific preventive measures are effective and a good use of resources. The economics of prevention have become even more germane as practices and health systems bear financial responsibility for the well-being of groups of patients (e.g., in accountable care organizations or patient-centered medical homes) (see Chapter 29). The chapter ends with information on how to obtain postgraduate training in preventive medicine.

1. BASIC CONCEPTS

Western medical education and practice have traditionally focused on the diagnosis and treatment of disease. While these will always be important, equal importance should be placed on the attainment and enhancement of health. Although specialists undertake research, teaching, and clinical practice in the field of preventive medicine, prevention is not the exclusive province of preventive medicine specialists, just as the care of elderly persons is not limited to geriatricians. All clinicians should incorporate prevention into their practice.

1.1. HEALTH DEFINED

Health is more difficult to define than disease. Perhaps the best-known definition of health comes from the preamble to the constitution of the World Health Organization (WHO): "Health is a state of complete physical, mental, and social well-being and not merely the absence of disease or infirmity."[1] This definition is strengthened by recognizing that any meaningful concept of health must include all dimensions of human life; and that a definition must be positive, encompassing more than only the absence of disease.

Nevertheless, the definition has been criticized for two weaknesses: (1) its overly idealistic expectation of complete well-being and (2) its view of health as a static rather than dynamic process that requires constant effort to maintain.

1.1.a. Health as Successful Adaptation

In the 1960s, Dubos defined health as the "success…experienced by the organism in its efforts to respond adaptively to environmental challenges."[2] These environmental challenges are also called stress, which denotes any response of an organism to demands, whether biologic, psychologic, or mental. Stress can be helpful (**eustress**) or harmful (**distress**). Good health requires the presence of eustress in such forms as exercise (for the heart, muscles, and bones) or infant stimulation. An individual in good health also may experience some distress, as long as it is limited to a level to which the organism can adapt. Constant, major adaptation may exact a serious toll on the body, particularly on the lungs and the neural, neuroendocrine, and immune systems. Early trauma in particular seems to have a profound impact on brain function and immunology in later life.[3]

1.1.b. Health as Satisfactory Functioning

To most people, being healthy means they can function in their own environment. Loss of function brings many people to a physician more quickly than the presence of discomfort. Functional problems might impinge on a person's ability to see, hear, or be mobile. As Dubos states, "Clearly, health and disease cannot be defined merely in terms of anatomical, physiological, or mental attributes. Their real measure is the ability of the individual to function in a manner acceptable to himself and to the group of which he is a part."[2] Therefore health can be described as "both (1) the current state of a human organism's equilibrium with the environment, often called health status, and (2) the potential to maintain that balance."[4]

Regardless of how health is defined, it derives principally from forces other than medical care. While biologic factors clearly play a role in health, about half of a person's health status can likely be attributed to the social determinants of health.[5]

1.1.c. Social Determinants of Health

Social determinants have been called the "causes of the causes."[6] They include employment and working conditions, social exclusion, access to housing, clean water and sanitation, social protection systems (such as social security), access to health care, gender equity, early childhood development, globalization, and urbanization (see also Chapter 30).[1] Social determinants matter to everyone, not only to those in developing countries. In all countries, health and illness follow a gradient that correlates with social determinants, and health generally improves stepwise as social status rises. Social determinants impact health through a variety of complex causal pathways, including through direct causation (e.g., higher lead levels in low-income children lead to impaired cognitive development), through changing the likelihood of certain behaviors (e.g., lower availability of fresh produce in disadvantaged neighborhoods makes it harder to provide good nutrition), or by impacting cellular function (e.g., stress leads to increased inflammation, blood pressure, and cholesterol).[6]

Countries that spend more on social services relative to health care may attain better health.[7] A review of effective interventions of social determinants of health found that housing interventions, nutritional support, income support, and community outreach are among the most powerful interventions.[8] To fully address the impact of social determinants of health, providers may need to team up with nontraditional partners such as food banks, schools, and housing authorities.[8]

2. MEASURES OF HEALTH STATUS

Measures of health status can be based on mortality, the impact of a particular disease on quality of life, and the ability to function. Historically, measures of health status have been based primarily on **mortality data** (see Chapter 2). Clearly, a low age-adjusted death rate and a high life expectancy form the basis of good health in a population. Life expectancy is defined as the average number of years remaining at a given age. This measure counts all deaths independently of when they occur.

Several metrics attempt to account for premature mortality. One of the most commonly used is **years of potential life lost** (YPLL). In YPLL, deaths are weighted depending on how many years a person might have lived if he or she had not died prematurely (in the developed world usually defined as death before age 75). This measure gives more weight to deaths occurring in young people.

An increasing proportion of the population lives to old age and accumulates various chronic and disabling illnesses. An appropriate societal goal is for people to age in a healthy manner, with minimal disability until shortly before death. Therefore health care investigators and practitioners now show increased emphasis on improving and measuring the **health-related quality of life**. Measures of the quality of life are subjective and thus more controversial than measures of mortality. However, efforts to improve methods for measuring quality of life are ongoing; and a multitude of age-specific, disease-specific, and general measures have been developed.[9,10]

Examples of quality-of-life measures include a **health status index**, which summarizes a person's health as a single score, and a **health profile** that seeks to rate a person's health on several separate dimensions.[11] Most health indices and profiles require that each subject complete some form of questionnaire. Many health status indices seek to adjust life expectancy based on morbidity, the perceived quality of life, or both. Such indices also can be used to help guide clinical practice and research. For example, they might show that a country's emphasis on reducing mortality may not be producing equal results in improving the function or self-perceived health of the country's population. When clinicians consider which treatments to recommend to patients with a chronic disease, such as prostate cancer, this approach allows them to consider not only the treatment's impact on mortality but also its adverse effects, such as incontinence and impotence. Describing survival estimates in terms of the quality of life communicates a fuller picture than survival rates alone.

The metric of **quality-adjusted life years** (QALY) incorporates both life expectancy and "quality of life"—that is, the perceived impact of illness, pain, and disability on the patient's quality of life.[12] For example, a patient with hemiparesis from a stroke might be asked to estimate how many years of life with this disability would have a value that equals to 1 year of life without the disability (healthy years). If the answer were that 2 limited years is equivalent to 1 healthy year, 1 year of life after a stroke might be given a quality weight of 0.5. If 3 limited years were equivalent to 1 healthy year, each limited year would contribute 0.33 year to the QALY. Someone who must live in a nursing home and is unable to speak might consider life under those conditions to be as bad as, or worse than, no life at all. In this case the weighting factor would be 0.0 for such years.

Healthy life expectancy is a measure that attempts to combine mortality and morbidity into one index.[12] The index reflects the number of years of life remaining that are expected to be free of serious disease. The onset of a serious disease with permanent sequelae (e.g., peripheral vascular disease leading to amputation of a leg) reduces the healthy life expectancy index as much as if the person who has the sequela had died from the disease.

Fig. 14.1 is an illustration of the different health status measures for a hypothetical patient who develops serious symptoms of cardiac disease at age 45, disability at age 55, and dies at age 63. His quality-adjusted life years, his healthy life expectancy and his life expectancy free of disability are less than 63. This is because this hypothetical patient rated his quality of life as less than perfect for his last years.

Other indices combine several measures of health status. The **general well-being adjustment scale** is an index that measures "anxiety, depression, general health, positive well-being, self-control, and vitality."[13,14] Another index is called the **life expectancy free of disability**, which defines itself. The US Centers for Disease Control and Prevention (CDC) developed an index called the **health-related quality of life** based on data from the Behavioral Risk Factor Surveillance System (BRFSS).[15] Using the BRFSS data, CDC investigators found that 88% of US adults considered their health to be "good to excellent" in 2014.[15]

Several scales measure the ability of patients to perform their daily activities. These functional indices measure activities that directly contribute to most people's quality of life, without asking patients to estimate the quality of life compared to how they would feel if they were in perfect health. Such functional indices include the Katz **activity of daily living** (ADL) index and the Lawton-Brody **instrumental activities of daily living** (IADL) scale. These scales have been used extensively in the geriatric population and for developmentally challenged adults. The ADL index measures a person's ability to independently bathe, dress, toilet, transfer, feed, and control his or her bladder and bowels. Items in the IADL scale include shopping, housekeeping, handling finances, and taking responsibility in administering medications. Other scales are used for particular diseases, such as the **Karnofsky index** for cancer patients and the **Barthel index** for stroke patients.

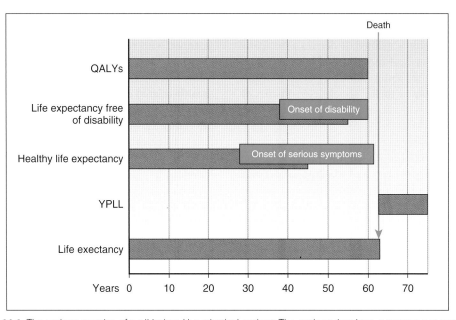

Fig. 14.1 The various metrics of well-being: Hypothetical patient: The patient develops symptoms at age 45, disability at age 55, and dies at age 63. YPLLs: Years of Potential Life Lost (here before age 75), QALYs: Quality-adjusted life years.

3. NATURAL HISTORY OF DISEASE

The natural history of disease can be seen as having three stages: the predisease stage, the latent (asymptomatic) disease stage, and the symptomatic disease stage. Before a disease process begins in an individual—that is, during the **predisease stage**—the individual can be seen as possessing various factors that promote or resist disease. These factors include genetic makeup, demographic characteristics (especially age), environmental exposures, nutritional history, social environment, immunologic capability, and behaviors. Efforts to improve favorable factors and reduce harmful ones may reduce risk for disease during this stage.

Over time, these and other factors may cause a disease process to begin, either slowly (as with most noninfectious diseases) or quickly (as with most infectious diseases). If the disease-producing process is underway, but no symptoms of disease have become apparent, the disease is said to be in the **latent (hidden) stage**. If the underlying disease is detectable by a reasonably safe and cost-effective means during this stage, screening may be feasible. In this sense, the latent stage may represent a **window of opportunity** during which detection followed by treatment provides a better chance of improving outcomes. For some diseases, such as pancreatic cancer, there is no window of opportunity because safe and effective screening methods are unavailable. For other diseases, such as rapidly progressive conditions, the window of opportunity may be too short to be useful for screening programs. Screening programs are detailed in Chapter 16 (see Table 16.2 for screening program requirements).

When the disease is advanced enough to produce clinical manifestations it is in the **symptomatic stage** (see Chapter 1). Even in this stage, the earlier the condition is diagnosed and treated, the more likely the treatment will delay death or serious complications, or at least provide the opportunity for effective rehabilitation.

The **natural history of a disease** is its normal course in the absence of intervention. The central question for studies of prevention (field trials) and studies of treatment (clinical trials) is whether the use of a particular preventive or treatment measure would change the natural history of disease in a favorable direction by delaying or preventing clinical manifestations, complications, or deaths. Many interventions do not prevent the progression of disease, but slow it so that the disease occurs later in life than it would have occurred if there had been no intervention.

In the case of myocardial infarction, risk factors include male gender, a family history of myocardial infarction, elevated serum lipid levels, a high-fat diet, cigarette smoking, obesity, sedentary lifestyle, other illnesses (e.g., diabetes mellitus, hypertension), and advancing age. The speed with which coronary atherosclerosis develops in an individual would be modified not only by the diet, but also by the pattern of physical activity over the course of a lifetime. Hypertension may accelerate the development of atherosclerosis; and it may lead to increased myocardial oxygen demand, precipitating infarction earlier than it otherwise might have occurred and making recovery more difficult. In some cultures, coronary artery disease is all but unknown, despite considerable genetic overlap with cultures in which it is hyperendemic, showing that genotype is only one of many factors influencing the development of atherosclerosis.

4. LEVELS OF PREVENTION

A useful concept of prevention has come to be known as **Leavell levels**.[16] Based on this concept, all the activities of clinicians and other health professionals have the goal of prevention. There are three levels of prevention (Table 14.1). The factor to be prevented depends on the stage of health or disease in the individual receiving preventive care.

Primary prevention keeps the disease process from becoming established by eliminating causes of disease or by increasing resistance to disease (see Chapter 15). **Secondary prevention** interrupts the disease process before it becomes symptomatic (see Chapter 16). **Tertiary prevention** limits the physical and social consequences of symptomatic disease (see Chapter 17). Which prevention level is applicable also depends on which disease is considered. For example, reducing cholesterol levels in an otherwise healthy person can be primary prevention for coronary artery disease (e.g., if the physician treats incidental high cholesterol before the patient has any signs or symptoms of coronary artery disease). However, if hypercholesterolemia is considered a disease itself or a sign of underlying atherosclerotic processes, treating cholesterol levels could be considered secondary prevention (i.e., treating cholesterol levels before critical fatty atheromatous deposits form). Reducing cholesterol levels in a patient after a myocardial infarction to prevent additional cardiovascular disease illustrates tertiary prevention. For hypertension, efforts to lower blood pressure can be considered primary, secondary, or tertiary prevention. Primary prevention includes efforts to treat prehypertension through increasing physical activity and weight loss, secondary prevention involves treating a hypertensive patient, and tertiary prevention involves treating a patient with symptoms from a hypertensive crisis to prevent a stroke.

4.1 PRIMARY PREVENTION AND PREDISEASE STAGE

Most noninfectious diseases can be seen as having an early stage, during which the causal factors start to produce physiologic abnormalities. During the predisease stage, atherosclerosis may begin with elevated blood levels of the so-called bad low-density lipoprotein (LDL) cholesterol and may be accompanied by low levels of the good or scavenger high-density lipoprotein (HDL) cholesterol. The current goal of a health intervention is to modify risk factors in a favorable

TABLE 14.1 Levels of Prevention*

Stage of Disease and Care	Level of Prevention	Appropriate Response	Examples
Predisease Stage			
No known risk factors	Primary prevention	Health promotion	Encourage healthy changes in lifestyle, nutrition, and environment
Disease susceptibility	Primary prevention	Specific protection	Recommend nutritional supplements, immunizations, and occupational and automobile safety measures
Latent Disease			
"Hidden" stage; asymptomatic disease	Secondary prevention	*Screening* (for populations) or *case finding* (for individuals in medical care)	Screening for osteoporosis by measuring bone mineral density in older women; testing bone mineral density in patients on long-term corticosteroids; treating those with low values.
Symptomatic Disease			
Initial care	Tertiary prevention	*Disability limitation**	Institute medical or surgical treatment to limit damage from the disease and institute primary prevention measures
Subsequent care	Tertiary prevention	*Rehabilitation*	Identify and teach methods to reduce physical and social disability

*Although Leavell originally categorized disability limitation under secondary prevention, it has become customary in Europe and the United States to classify disability limitation as tertiary prevention because it involves the management of symptomatic disease.
Modified from Leavell HR, Clark EG: *Preventive medicine for the doctor in his community,* ed 3, New York, 1965, McGraw-Hill.

direction. Lifestyle-modifying activities, such as changing to a diet low in saturated and *trans* fats, pursuing a consistent program of aerobic exercise, and ceasing to smoke cigarettes, are considered methods of primary prevention because they are aimed at keeping the pathologic process and disease from occurring.

4.1.a. Promoting Overall Health (Health Promotion)

Health-promoting activities usually contribute to the prevention of a variety of diseases and enhance a positive feeling of health and vigor. These activities consist of nonmedical efforts such as changes in lifestyle, nutrition, and the environment. Such activities may require structural improvements or societal changes that make healthy choices easier. Dietary modification may be difficult unless a variety of healthy foods are available in local stores at a reasonable cost. Exercise is more difficult if bicycling or jogging is a risky activity because of automobile traffic or social violence. Even more basic to health promotion is the assurance of the basic necessities of life, including freedom from poverty, environmental pollution, and violence (see previous social determinants of health and also Chapter 30).

Health promotion applies to infectious diseases as well. Infectious diseases are reduced in frequency and seriousness where the water is clean, where liquid and solid wastes are disposed of in a sanitary manner, and where animal vectors of disease are controlled. Crowding promotes the spread of infectious diseases, whereas adequate housing and working environments tend to minimize the spread of disease. In the barracks of soldiers, for example, even a technique as simple as requiring soldiers in adjacent cots to sleep with their pillows alternating between the head and the foot of the bed can reduce the spread of respiratory diseases, because it doubles the distance between the soldiers' upper respiratory tracts during sleeping time.

4.1.b. Preventing Particular Diseases (Specific Protection)

Usually general health-promoting changes in environment, nutrition, and behavior are not fully effective for prevention. Therefore it becomes necessary to employ specific interventions to reduce risk and prevent disease (see Table 14.1). This form of primary prevention is targeted to specific diseases or types of injuries. Examples include immunization against poliomyelitis; use of aspirin to prevent cardiovascular disease in high-risk patients; use of ear-protecting devices in loud working environments, such as around jet airplanes; and use of seat belts, air bags, and helmets to prevent bodily injuries in automobile and motorcycle crashes. Some measures provide specific protection while contributing to the more general goal of health promotion. For example, a diet low in refined sugars prevents dental caries, but will also help combat obesity and prevent diabetes. Use of medication to prevent disease is called chemoprevention.

4.2 SECONDARY PREVENTION AND LATENT DISEASE

Sooner or later, depending on the individual, a disease process such as coronary artery atherosclerosis progresses sufficiently to become detectable by medical tests, such as cardiac stress test, although the individual is still asymptomatic. This may be thought of as the latent (hidden) stage of disease.

For many infectious and noninfectious diseases, *screening tests* allow the detection of latent disease in individuals considered to be at high risk. Presymptomatic diagnosis through screening programs, along with subsequent treatment when needed, is referred to as *secondary prevention* because it is the secondary line of defense against disease. Although screening programs do not prevent the causes from initiating the disease process, they may allow diagnosis at an earlier stage of disease when treatment is more effective.

4.3 TERTIARY PREVENTION AND SYMPTOMATIC DISEASE

When disease has become symptomatic and medical assistance is sought, the goal of the clinician is to provide tertiary prevention in the form of disability limitation for patients with early symptomatic disease, or rehabilitation for patients with late symptomatic disease (see Table 14.1).

4.3.a. Disability Limitation

Disability limitation describes medical and surgical measures aimed at correcting the anatomic and physiologic components of disease in symptomatic patients. Most care provided by clinicians meets this description. Disability limitation can be considered prevention because its goal is to halt or slow the disease process and prevent or limit complications, impairment, and disability. An example is the surgical removal of a tumor, which may prevent the spread of disease locally or by metastasis to other sites.

4.3.b. Rehabilitation

Although many are surprised to see rehabilitation designated a form of prevention, the label is correctly applied. Rehabilitation may mitigate the effects of disease and prevent some of the social and functional disability that would otherwise occur. For example, a person who has been injured or had a stroke may be taught self-care in activities of daily living.

Rehabilitation may enable the person to avoid the adverse sequelae associated with prolonged inactivity, such as increasing muscle weakness that might develop without therapy. Rehabilitation of a stroke patient begins with early and frequent mobilization of all joints during the period of maximum paralysis. This permits easier recovery of limb use by preventing the development of stiff joints and flexion contractures. Next, physical therapy helps stroke patients to strengthen remaining muscle function and to use this remaining function to maximum effect in performing ADLs. Occupational and speech therapy may enable such patients to gain skills and perform some type of gainful employment, preventing complete economic dependence on others. It is legitimate, therefore, to view rehabilitation as a form of prevention.

5. ECONOMICS OF PREVENTION

In an era of cost consciousness there are increasing demands that health promotion and disease prevention be proven economically worthwhile. With a shift in health care payment and more health systems bearing financial risk based on health outcomes, the economic impact of preventive and curative efforts becomes increasingly more important. Furthermore, many people in the political arena promote prevention as a means of controlling rising health care costs. This argument is based on the belief that prevention is always cost saving. One way to examine that claim is to look at the cost effectiveness of various preventive measures and compare them to the cost effectiveness of treatment for existing conditions.

As outlined in Chapter 6, **cost-benefit analysis** compares the costs of an intervention to its health benefits. To compare different interventions, it becomes necessary to express the health benefits of different interventions with the same metric, called **cost-effectiveness analysis** (Box 14.1). Examples for such metrics are mortality, disease, and costs, or their

---

BOX 14.1 Cost-Benefit and Cost-Effectiveness Analyses

Cost-benefit analysis measures the costs and the benefits of a proposed course of action in terms of the same units, usually monetary units such as dollars. For example, a cost-benefit analysis of a poliomyelitis immunization program would determine the number of dollars to be spent on vaccines, equipment, and personnel to immunize a particular population. It would determine the number of dollars that would be saved by not having to pay for the hospitalizations, medical visits, and lost productivity that would occur if poliomyelitis were not prevented in that population.

Incorporating concepts such as the dollar value of life, suffering, and the quality of life into such an analysis is difficult. Cost-benefit analysis is useful, however, if a particular budgetary entity (e.g., government or business) is trying to determine whether the investment of resources in health would save money in the long run. It also is useful if a particular entity with a fixed budget is trying to make informed judgments about allocations between various sectors (e.g., health, transportation,

education) and to determine the sector in which an investment would produce the greatest economic benefit.

Cost-effectiveness analysis provides a common measurement unit for comparing different proposed solutions and diseases. This estimate is only useful for health services that are effective in the first place. For example, by measuring lung cancer cases prevented, deaths prevented, and QALYs saved, the incremental cost effectiveness of three different strategies of screening for lung cancer in high-risk patients could be compared:

1. No screening
2. Screening with chest x-ray
3. Screening with chest tomography

For screening with x-ray and chest tomography, actual data on cases of lung cancer and quality of life from the National Lung Screening Trial were used, in which participants were randomly assigned to different screening regimes. Mortality with no screening was estimated from the data in the no screening arm to determine an incremental cost-effectiveness ratio (CER) of $81,000 per QALY.[1]

Continued

BOX 14.1   Cost-Benefit and Cost-Effectiveness Analyses—cont'd

While the researchers in this example mostly used actual trial data, other cost-effectiveness analyses are often based on mathematical models. In these cases, the conclusions may be less robust. Before the National Lung Screening Trial, several cost-effectiveness analyses published widely varying results. In such cases, the most helpful part of the analysis might be the **sensitivity analysis.** In sensitivity analysis, researchers vary the underlying assumptions of their model to explore how the conclusion would change. If a conclusion remains unchanged even with wide ranges in the underlying assumptions, it is more likely to be a true reflection of reality. On the other hand, factors that could greatly change a conclusion may merit additional research.

In addition, the concept of **discounting,** which is important in business and finance, must be used in medical cost-benefit and cost-effectiveness analysis when the costs are incurred in the present but the benefits will occur in the future. Discounting is a reduction in the **present value** of delayed benefits (or increase in present costs) to account for the **time value of money.** If the administrators of a prevention program spend

$1000 now to save $1000 of expenses in the future, they will take a net loss. This is because they will lose the use of $1000 in the interim, and with inflation the $1000 eventually saved will not be worth as much as the $1000 initially spent. The use of discounting is an attempt to adjust for these forces.

To discount a cost-benefit or cost-effectiveness analysis, the easiest way is to increase the present costs by a yearly factor, which can be thought of as the interest that would have to be paid to borrow the prevention money until the benefits occurred. For example, if it costs $1000 today to prevent a disease that would have occurred 20 years in the future, the present cost can be multiplied by $(1 + r)^n$, where r is the yearly interest rate for borrowing and n is the number of years until the benefit is realized. If the average yearly interest rate is 5% over 20 years, the formula becomes $(1 + 0.05)^{20} = (1.05)^{20} = 2.653$. When this is multiplied by the present cost of $1000, the result is $2653. The expected savings 20 years in the future from a $1000 investment today would have to be greater than $2653 for the initial investment to be a net (true) financial gain.

[1]Black CB et al: Cost-effectiveness of CT screening in the National Lung Screening Trial. *NEJM* 371(19):1793–1802, 2014.

inverse: longevity, disease-free time, and savings. A subtype of cost-effectiveness analysis is **cost-utility analysis**, which has the outcome of the cost/quality-adjusted life year, also called the **cost-effectiveness ratio** (CER). The CER allows comparisons of a wide range of interventions for different conditions. A CER will determine that an intervention actually brings more health benefits than it costs (i.e., cost saving), that it is an effective use of funds compared to other commonly funded interventions (i.e., having a favorable cost-effectiveness ratio), or that it costs much more than other interventions (i.e., unfavorable). Both preventive and curative measures can be cost saving, favorable, or unfavorable.[17] Tables of the most valuable clinical services based on these measures are available.[18]

5.1 DEMONSTRATION OF BENEFITS

Measuring the benefits of prevention poses numerous challenges. First there needs to be evidence that an intervention is beneficial. However, scientific evidence of benefits may be limited because it is often impractical or unethical to undertake randomized trials of human subjects. For example, it is impossible to assign people randomly to smoking and nonsmoking groups. Apart from research on animal models, investigators are limited to observational studies, which may be biased and usually are not as convincing as experiments. Life is filled with risks for one disease or another, and many of these operate together to produce the levels of health observed in a population. These risks may be changing in frequency in different subpopulations, making it impossible to infer what proportion of the improvement observed over time is caused by a particular preventive measure. For example, if there is a reduction in the incidence of lung cancer, it is difficult to infer what proportion is caused by smoking

reduction programs for patients, the elimination of smoking in workplaces and public areas, the increase in public awareness of (and action against) the presence of radon in homes, and other factors as yet poorly understood. In addition, clinical research is expensive. Much research on treatment and diagnosis is sponsored by pharmaceutic companies. The money spent by industry to support clinical research is vastly greater than the research funds spent on prevention. Therefore some of the lack of data on the benefits of prevention results from the lack of large-scale, well-funded studies.

5.2 DELAY OF BENEFITS

With most prevention programs, there is a long delay between the time the preventive measures are instituted and the time that positive health changes become discernible. Because the latent period (incubation period) for lung cancer caused by cigarette smoking is 20 years or more, benefits resulting from investments made now in smoking reduction programs may not be identified until many years have passed. There are similar delays for other smoking-related pulmonary problems, such as obstructive pulmonary disease. Most chronic diseases have similarly long latent periods between when the causes start and the disease appears.

5.3 ACCRUAL OF BENEFITS

Even if a prevention program could be shown to produce meaningful economic benefit, it is necessary to know to whom the benefits would accrue (this problem is also called the "wrong pocket problem"). For example, a financially stressed health insurance plan or health maintenance organization might cover a preventive measure if the financial benefit were fairly certain to be as great as or greater than the cost of providing that benefit, but only if most or all of the financial benefit would accrue to the insurance plan in the near future (meaning the savings go into the "pockets" of the insurance plan). If plan members switch insurance plans frequently, or if most of the financial benefit would go to the enrollees or a government rather than to the insurance plan, the prevention program would be seen as only a financial cost by the insurance plan (since the benefits go to the employees' or governments' pockets).

The same principle is true for the financially strapped budgets of local, state, and federal governments. If the savings from prevention efforts would go directly to only a few individuals, rather than to a government budget, the elected representatives might not support the prevention effort, even if the benefits clearly outweighed the costs. Elected representatives may want to show results in their government budget before the next election campaign. Disease prevention may show results only over an extended time and may not lend itself to political popularity. Even so, there is growing political support for prevention as a medical priority reflecting a societal perspective.

5.4 DISCOUNTING

If a preventive effort is made now by a government body, the costs are present-day costs, but any financial savings may not be evident until many years from now. Even if the savings are expected to accrue to the same budgetary unit that provided the money for the preventive program, the delay in economic return means that the benefits are worth less to that unit now. In the jargon of economists, the present value of the benefits must be discounted (see Box 14.1), making it more difficult to show cost effectiveness or a positive benefit-cost ratio.

5.5 PRIORITIES

As the saying goes, "The squeaky wheel gets the grease." Current, urgent problems usually attract much more attention and concern than future, less publicized problems. Emergency care for victims of motor vehicle crashes is easy to justify, regardless of costs. Although prevention may be cost effective, it may be difficult to justify using money to prevent crises that have not yet occurred. The same dilemma applies to essentially every phase of life. It is difficult to obtain money for programs to prevent the loss of topsoil, prevent illiteracy, and prevent the decay of roads and bridges. Even on an individual level, many patients do not want to make changes in their lives, such as eating a healthier diet, exercising, and stopping smoking, because the risk of future problems does not speak to them urgently in the present. As a broader example, even though hurricanes and storms keep degrading the US Gulf coastline, preparations by individuals, cities, and states involved and by the federal government are often inadequate.

6. PREVENTIVE MEDICINE TRAINING

Physicians desiring to become board certified as specialists in preventive medicine in the United States may seek postgraduate residency training in a program approved for preventive medicine training by the **Accreditation Council for Graduate Medical Education**.[19] Certification in preventive medicine must be in one of the following three **subspecialty areas**:

- General preventive medicine and public health
- Occupational medicine
- Aerospace medicine

Occasionally a physician becomes certified in two subspecialties (most often the first and second areas listed). A few medical residency programs offer a combined residency in a clinical specialty (e.g., internal medicine) and preventive medicine. A residency program in medical toxicology is governed by a tripartite board, with representatives from the American boards of preventive medicine, pediatrics, and emergency medicine.

Certification in preventive medicine requires 3 years of residency.

1. The first postgraduate year is called the clinical year. It consists of an internship with substantial patient care responsibility, usually in internal medicine, family practice, or pediatrics, although other areas are acceptable if they provide sufficient patient responsibility. The internship may be done in any accredited, first-postgraduate-year residency program. A few preventive medicine residency programs offer the first postgraduate year, but most do not.
2. The second postgraduate year is called the academic year and consists of coursework to obtain the master of public health (MPH) degree or its equivalent. The coursework may be pursued in any accredited MPH program and need not be done in a formal preventive medicine residency program, although there are some advantages in doing so.
3. The third postgraduate year is called the practicum year, which must be completed in an accredited preventive medicine residency program. It consists of a year of supervised practice of the subspecialty in varied rotation sites, and it is tailored to fit an individual resident's needs. It typically includes clinical practice of the subspecialty; experience in program planning, development, administration, and evaluation; analysis and solution of problems (e.g., problems related to epidemics); research; and teaching. Some residency programs offer preventive medicine training combined with other specialties such as internal medicine, pediatrics, or family medicine. Typically in these cases the training time is shorter in a combined program than if residents did both programs sequentially.

The certification examination has two parts: a core examination and a subspecialty examination. The core examination is the same for all three subspecialties and covers topics included in this textbook, such as epidemiology, biostatistics, environmental health, health policy and financing, social science as applied to public health, and general clinical preventive medicine. Further information for specialty training and board examination is available online (see Websites later in the chapter).

7. SUMMARY

Preventive medicine seeks to enhance the lives of patients by helping them promote their health, reduce risk and prevent specific diseases, diagnose diseases early, improve function, and reduce disability. Preventive medicine also tries to apply the concepts and techniques of health promotion and disease prevention to the organization and practice of medicine (clinical preventive services). Health is an elusive concept, but means more than the absence of disease; it is a positive concept that includes the ability to adapt to stress and function in society. The three levels of prevention define the various strategies available to practitioners to promote health and prevent disease, impairment, and disability at various stages of the natural history of disease. Primary prevention keeps a disease from becoming established by eliminating the causes of disease or increasing resistance to disease. Secondary prevention interrupts the disease process by detecting and treating it in the presymptomatic stage. Tertiary prevention limits the physical impairment and social consequences from symptomatic disease. It is not easy for prevention programs to compete for funds in a tight fiscal climate because of long delays before the benefits of such investments are noted. Specialty training in preventive medicine prepares investigators to demonstrate the effectiveness, cost effectiveness, and cost benefits of prevention.

REFERENCES

1. Commission on Social Determinants of Health. *Closing the Gap in a Generation: Health Equity Through Action on the Social Determinants of Health. Final Report of the Commission on Social Determinants of Health.* Geneva, Switzerland: World Health Organization; 2008.
2. Dubos R: *Man Adapting.* New Haven, CT: Yale University Press; 1965.
3. Danese A, Lewis SJ. Psychoneuroimmunology of early-life stress: the hidden wounds of childhood trauma? *Neuropsychopharmacology.* 2017;42(1):99-114.
4. Breslow L. From disease prevention to health promotion. *JAMA.* 1999;281:1030-1033.
5. Marmot M, Allen JJ. Social determinants of health equity. *Am J Public Health.* 2014;104(4):S517-S519.
6. Braveman P, Gottlieb L. The social determinants of health: it's time to consider the causes of the causes. *Public Health Rep.* 2014;129(2):S19-S31.
7. Bradley EH, Sipsma H, Taylor LA. American health care paradox—high spending on health care and poor health. *QJM.* 2017;110:61-65.
8. Taylor LA, Tan AX, Coyle CE, et al. Leveraging the social determinants of health: what works? *PLoS One* 2016;11:e0160217. doi:10.1371/journal.pone.0160217.
9. Solans M, Pane S, Estrada MD, et al. Health-related quality of life measurement in children and adolescents: a systematic review of generic and disease-specific instruments. *Value Health.* 2008;11(4):742-764.
10. Makai P, Brouwer WB, Koopmanschap MA, Stolk EA, Nieboer AP. Quality of life instruments for economic evaluations in health and social care for older people: a systematic review. *Soc Sci Med.* 2014;102:83-93.
11. McDowell I, Newell C. *Measuring Health: A Guide to Rating Scales and Questionnaires.* 2nd ed. New York, NY: Oxford University Press; 1996.
12. Last JM. *A Dictionary of Epidemiology.* 4th ed. New York, NY: Oxford University Press; 2001.
13. Barendregt JJ, Bonneux L, Van der Maas PJ. Health expectancy: an indicator for change? Technology assessment methods project team. *J Epidemiol Community Health.* 1994;48:482-487.
14. Revicki DA, Allen H, Bungay K, Williams GH, Weinstein MC. Responsiveness and calibration of the General Well-Being Adjustment Scale in patients with hypertension. *J Clin Epidemiol.* 1994;47:1333-1342.
15. Xu F, Mawokomatanda T, Flegel D, et al. Surveillance for certain health behaviors among states and selected local areas—Behavioral Risk Factor Surveillance System, United States, 2011. *MMWR Surveill Summ.* 2014;63(9):1-149.
16. Leavell HR, Clark EG. *Preventive Medicine for the Doctor in his Community.* 3rd ed. New York, NY: McGraw-Hill; 1965.
17. Cohen JT, Neumann PJ, Weinstein MC. Does preventive care save money? Health economics and the presidential candidates. *N Engl J Med.* 2008;358:661-663.
18. Maciosek MV, LaFrance AB, Dehmer SP, et al. Updated priorities among effective clinical preventive services. *Ann Fam Med.* 2017;15(1):14-22.
19. American College of Preventive Medicine. *Residency Programs. Resources for Medical Students.* Available at: https://www.acpm.org/page/pmr. Accessed April 6, 2019.

SELECT READINGS

Bradley EH, Taylor EH. *The American Healthcare Paradox. Why Spending More is Getting us Less.* New York, NY: Public Affairs; 2015.

Muir Gray JA. *Evidence-Based Healthcare: How to Make Health Policy and Management Decisions.* 3rd ed. Edinburgh, Scotland: Churchill Livingstone; 2009.

Stanhope M, Lancaster J. *Public Health Nursing e-Book: Population-Centered Health Care in the Community.* St. Louis, MO, USA: Elsevier Health Sciences; 2015.

WEBSITES

American Board of Preventive Medicine: https://www.theabpm.org/

American College of Preventive Medicine: http://www.acpm.org/?GME_MedStudents

American College of Preventive Medicine: Graduate Training and Careers in Preventive Medicine: http://www.acpm.org/?page=GME_Home

American Medical Student Association; Information on Preventive Medicine: http://www.amsa.org/

Cost-Effectiveness Analysis Registry: http://healtheconomics.tuftsmedicalcenter.org/cear4/Home.aspx

Partnership for Prevention: http://www.prevent.org

REVIEW QUESTIONS

1. Measures of health status traditionally have been based on mortality data. The principal reason this is no longer satisfactory is that:
   A. Changes in diagnostic technology permit earlier detection of disease
   B. The infant mortality rate has declined so much that it no longer serves as a useful index
   C. The population is older and more subject to chronic illness than in the past
   D. There is less risk of fatal infection than in the past
   E. Traditional sources of mortality data have failed to include relevant subpopulations

2. After the onset of blindness resulting from diabetic retinopathy, a 54-year-old man seems depressed. When you question him regarding the quality of life, he dejectedly tells you that 10 years "like this" is not worth 1 year of good health. Before going blind, the patient's physician estimated that his life expectancy was 74 years. Which of the following statements is true for the patient?
   A. His adjusted life expectancy is 76 years
   B. His healthy life expectancy is 76 years
   C. His healthy life expectancy cannot be calculated if he actually is depressed
   D. Each year of his life contributes less than 0.1 QALY
   E. Each year of his life contributes 10 QALY

3. In which of the following ways is health promotion distinguished from disease prevention?
   A. Only health promotion can begin before a disease becomes symptomatic
   B. Only health promotion involves materials and methods that are generally nonmedical
   C. Only health promotion is applied when a disease has developed
   D. Only health promotion is targeted at populations rather than individuals
   E. Only health promotion is targeted at specific diseases

4. Which of the following is an example of secondary prevention?
   A. Cholesterol reduction in a patient with asymptomatic coronary artery disease
   B. Prescription drug therapy for symptoms of menopause
   C. Physical therapy after lumbar disk herniation
   D. Pneumococcal vaccine in a patient who has undergone splenectomy
   E. Thrombolysis for acute myocardial infarction

5. In chemistry, the Le Chatlier principle states that when a system at equilibrium is stressed, the system reacts to counterbalance the stress and reestablish equilibrium. Applied to individual health, this principle might be adapted to state that when a healthy individual experiences distress, successful adaptation to harmful stressors results in restoration of wellness. Unsuccessful adaptation would result in compromised function and would be an indication of:
   A. Eustress
   B. Overwhelming distress
   C. Latent disease
   D. An advanced Leavell level
   E. A low Leavell level

6. Years of potential life lost (YPLL) is a measure of health status that:
   A. Gives more weight to deaths occurring in those older and more experienced
   B. Directly assesses health-related quality of life
   C. Is a health status index
   D. Is equivalent to quality-adjusted life years (QALY)
   E. Can always be calculated using life expectancy and age of death only

7. You are interested in helping a 45-year-old perimenopausal woman avoid osteoporosis. The patient is motivated but has a fixed income, is personally liable for her medical expenses because of lack of health insurance, and is concerned about the expense. Assume that (1) the cost of preventive medical therapy is fixed at $500 per year, (2) this therapy will prevent the development of a hip fracture in the patient at age 65 years, (3) the current cost of surgical fixation of the hip fracture is $12,000, and (4) the yearly rate of inflation is 4%. Disregarding any effects of inflation, how much money would the patient spend to prevent a hip fracture at age 65 years if she started medical therapy now?
   A. $3180
   B. $12,000
   C. $10,000
   D. $22,500
   E. $32,500

8. In regard to question 7, when inflation is taken into account, what is the cost of surgery to repair a hip fracture in the patient at age 65 years?
   A. $(\$10,000)(0.04)^{20}$
   B. $(\$10,000)(1 + 0.04)^{20}$
   C. $(\$12,000)(0.04)^{20}$
   D. $(\$12,000)(1 + 0.04)^{20}$
   E. $(\$12,000)(1 - 0.04)^{20}$

9. In regard to question 7, when true inflation-adjusted costs are considered, you determine that the total cost of medical therapy would be close to $22,000 over 20 years, whereas surgical fixation would cost about $26,000 in 20 years. Given this information, you decide that medical therapy to prevent a hip fracture:
   A. Has a favorable cost-benefit ratio
   B. Has a higher time value of money
   C. Is appropriate for the patient
   D. Is not worth the money for the patient
   E. Is cost effective

10. Vaccinating a health care worker against hepatitis B virus is considered:
    A. Health promotion
    B. Secondary prevention
    C. Specific protection
    D. Tertiary prevention

ANSWERS AND EXPLANATIONS

1. **C.** Until the 20th century, relatively few individuals in most societies lived long enough to die of processes principally related to senescence, or aging. With the advances in medical technology and hygiene of the past decades, life expectancy in the developed world has increased to the point where deaths in adults are mostly related to chronic diseases, many of which compromise the quality of life over many years before causing death. So far, the state of medical care is better suited to stave off death than to prevent disease. Consequently the measurement of quality of life has assumed greater importance as a measure of health status because the burden of chronic disease on an aging population has increased. With the shift to deaths from chronic conditions, infectious diseases now account for smaller percentages of total deaths in the developed world. However, the risk of fatal infections still remains (D). In fact, infections are often the final pathway to death in people whose ability to fight infection is compromised by long periods of suffering with chronic conditions, such as patients with diabetes or chronic obstructive pulmonary disease (COPD) ultimately dying of influenza or bacterial pneumonia. Thus changes in infectious risk have not had much effect on the adequacy of health measures, and neither have changes in diagnostic technology (A); the issue is not detecting disease early but suffering longer before dying. Infant mortality (B) is still a useful marker of the health status of a population, but with general declines in infant deaths, more people surviving into old age, and more people suffering chronic illnesses for long periods before ultimately expiring, infant mortality alone is an inadequate measure of a population's health status. Likewise, other mortality statistics are inadequate, but not because of their inclusiveness (E). Although the quality of different sources of mortality data may vary, especially to the extent to which they represent certain subpopulations, no subpopulations are deliberately and systematically excluded from mortality statistics.

2. **D.** Quality-adjusted life years (QALY) is a measure of the quality and the length of life. Each year of life with a disability represents some portion of the quality of that year of life without disability. In this case, if 1 year of good health is worth more to the patient than 10 years with blindness, the disability results in a quality of life that is less than 10% of the quality the patient would experience with intact health. Thus each year of life with disability contributes less than 0.1 QALY as determined by the patient. If each year of life contributed 10 QALY (E), the patient would be saying life is 10 times better being blind than being sighted. It is unclear how the patients' physician calculated the patient's life expectancy. The question does not provide enough information to calculate a new or adjusted life expectancy (A) in the context of clinically worsening diabetes and now blindness. We can say for certain, however, that his healthy life expectancy (B) has already been achieved. He is now blind, so the number of years of life remaining that are expected to be free of serious disease with permanent sequelae is zero. Whenever his blindness occurred is when he attained his maximal healthy life expectancy, which has now been reduced as much as if he had died. This is not to state that the patient's life from here on out has no quality and is no better than death. Indeed, the patient himself estimates that only 90% of the quality of his life has been lost because of his blindness. Although clinical depression certainly could influence this appraisal, which could change with time (affecting his QALY), resolution of depression or a revised appraisal would not affect his healthy life expectancy (C).

3. **B.** Health promotion and disease prevention share the goal of keeping people well. Disease prevention generally is directed specifically at a disease or a related group of diseases (E); the tools of disease prevention, such as vaccines, are generally medical. Health promotion is not disease oriented, but rather is an effort to enhance overall wellness. The materials and methods of health promotion, such as regular physical activity, proper nutrition, safe sexual practices, and the provision of adequate housing and transportation, are generally related to lifestyle and are nonmedical entities. Although health promotion and disease prevention are closely linked in efforts to enhance public health, they are different in philosophy and application. Both can be applied before a disease becomes symptomatic (A) or after a disease has developed (C) and is apparent. Both are targeted at individuals and populations (D).

4. **A.** Secondary prevention interrupts the disease process before it becomes symptomatic. This definition implies a disease process in the patient for secondary prevention to take place. The reduction of an elevated cholesterol level (a risk factor in this case) in a patient without coronary artery disease (the disease in this case) is an example of primary prevention. Once the disease process has begun, however (e.g., once silent atherosclerotic plaques begin to form), the modification of the cholesterol level to prevent the development of symptoms is secondary prevention. If the disease becomes symptomatic (e.g., if angina pectoris develops due to critical stenosis in coronary arteries), attempts to reduce cholesterol levels would be tertiary prevention (e.g., to prevent ischemic cardiomyopathy). Similarly, drug therapy for the symptoms

of menopause (B) would be tertiary prevention, as would physical therapy after lumbar disk herniation (C) and thrombolysis for acute myocardial infarction (E). All three measures are targeted against disease that is already established and symptomatic. Conversely, pneumococcal vaccine in a patient who has undergone splenectomy (D) is a measure targeted against a disease process that has not yet occurred or begun. This is an example of primary prevention—to prevent the development of pneumococcal disease.

5. **B.** Distress is defined as stressors that negatively impact physical and mental function. When they overwhelm an individual's capacity to adapt or counterbalance the stress, dysfunction and poor health result. In contrast, eustress (A) is generally beneficial to an individual and tends to help protect against dysfunction (e.g., exercise challenges or "stresses" the cardiopulmonary and musculoskeletal systems, resulting in greater conditioning and fitness and resilience to "distress"). Latent disease (C) is by definition "hidden" or asymptomatic. Once compromised function is apparent, such dysfunction would indicate a symptomatic process. Leavell levels (D and E) pertain to stages of prevention. Compromised function would not be an "indication of" but rather an "indication for" the highest Leavell level, an indication for tertiary prevention, or rehabilitation. With rehabilitation, balance and wellness may be restored.

6. **E.** Years of potential life lost (YPLL) is simply a mathematical calculation of the average years an individual would have lived if he or she had not died prematurely (e.g., life expectancy of 75 years – death at age 3 years = 72 YPLL). YPLL is a consideration of lost potential life expectancy only and thus gives more weight to death occurring among young people, not older people (A). Although young people on average generally have better health and less chronic disease than older adults, YPLL does not directly assess health-related quality of life (B). Likewise, YPLL is not a health status index (C), which seeks to adjust life expectancy on the basis of morbidity and quality of life and generally requires completion of a questionnaire. YPLL is not equivalent to QALY (D), which incorporates the perceived impact of illness, pain, and disability on the quality of life and is not merely an adjustment of life expectancy.

7. **C.** The scenario stipulates that the yearly cost of medical therapy (which might entail use of calcium and vitamin D plus a bisphosphonate or other drug) was fixed at $500. To prevent a hip fracture at age 65 years, a 45-year-old patient would need to spend $500 each year for 20 years, or $500 × 20 = $10,000. In reality the calculation of actual projected costs would be much more complex; and preventing a hip fracture would be considered a probability, not a 100% certainty as in this simplified case.

A more sophisticated cost projection would account for changes in the price of prescription medication over time to keep pace with inflation, changes in the type of medications available over time with medical advances, changes in the type of medication the patient takes over time based on the patient's evolving stage of disease, cost of medical care for monitoring (physician visits, lab tests, imaging) while the patient is taking prescription therapies, cost of any side effects (direct medical expenses, lost productivity from missed work), loss of revenue, opportunity costs of money not spent on other items, and so on. Many insurance plans include at least partial coverage of prescription drugs, so the simple direct cost of these drugs is generally not fully borne by an insured patient. The $32,500 (E) is the cost of taking medical therapy for 65 years and $22,500 (D) the cost of taking medical therapy for 45 years. The $12,000 (B) is the cost of the alternative therapy of reactive surgical fixation, and $3180 (A) is the cost saving of medical therapy for 20 years compared to the cost of surgical fixation.

8. **D.** See Box 14.1. The rate of inflation is analogous to the annual interest rate on money borrowed now to prevent a future event. The current cost of surgical fixation of the hip is provided as $12,000. The patient will require this surgery 20 years in the future, unless a fracture is avoided. To obtain the cost of the operation for the patient at age 65 years, the current cost is multiplied by $(1 + \text{inflation})$ raised to the number of years, which is $(\$12,000)(1 + 0.04)^{65 - 45}$. Choice B is the cost of medical management when inflation is taken into account. Choices A, C, and E present the wrong formula for calculating inflation-adjusted costs. As noted in the explanation for question 2, even this more sophisticated inflation-adjusted value is a gross oversimplification, ignoring important considerations in calculating true costs.

9. **A.** Cost-benefit analysis is the process of determining and comparing the cost of an intervention versus an alternative—either a different intervention or doing nothing. In this scenario the financial cost of preventing an inevitable hip fracture is lower than the cost of treating the inevitable fracture once it occurs. Thus the cost-benefit ratio favors preventive medical therapy because the net financial benefit of this course amounts to roughly $4000. The time value of money (B) is considered for both preventive medical therapy and reactive surgical repair as each is inflation adjusted. The value of medical therapy over 23 years is actually lower than the value of surgical repair in 23 years in the scenario. However, we cannot conclude that medical therapy is cost effective (E). Cost effectiveness would require that alternative means of achieving the same goal (prevention of a hip fracture) be compared on the basis of cost; the least costly method would be the most cost effective. If stopping smoking and regularly performing weight-bearing exercise were as effective at preventing hip fracture as medical therapy but less expensive, medical therapy

would not be the most cost-effective option. Determining whether medical therapy is appropriate for the patient (C) and whether it is worth the patient's money (D) are subjective value judgments and depend on the patient's personal preferences for alternative preventive strategies. These preferences may be informed only partially by financial considerations; other considerations include time, inconvenience, and discomfort, which the patient may value more than money.

10. **C.** Vaccinating a health care worker against hepatitis B virus is specific protection. Vaccination prevents the initial establishment of specific disease process in the host. In contrast to health promotion, which is generally nonmedical, specific protection is often medical, as in this case.

15

Methods of Primary Prevention: Health Promotion and Disease Prevention

"One way of preventing disease is worth fifty ways of curing it."

Trevor Howard

CASE INTRODUCTION

In your primary care office, you see a mother and her 12-year old daughter for the daughters well-child visit. After eliciting their concerns, taking a clinical history, and performing a physical examination, you review age-recommended vaccinations, among them human papillomavirus (HPV). While the daughter in the past has had all age-recommended vaccinations, the mother now adamantly refuses any new vaccinations on the grounds that they "cause autism." The daughter states that "she would never get involved with a boy who is not clean and healthy," therefore she does not believe it is necessary to get the vaccine. How would you interpret and address the patient's and her mom's concerns?

Health is the result of people's genetic makeup, their environment, and their behavior interacting over time. Behavior and environment intersect on two factors with profound impact on overall health, namely diet and exercise ("forks and feet"). Whereas public health managers are concerned with the availability of healthy food and the safety of the environment for the population (see Section 4 of this book), the chapters in this Preventive Medicine section expand the discussions to explore how clinicians can intervene with individual patients for better health. Beyond healthy exercise and a good diet, many other interventions can promote health at both patient and population levels. These specific interventions (called specific protection) are usually only indicated in select groups. For example, supplementing the diet with folic acid to prevent spinal cord defects in babies only makes sense in women of child-bearing age. Sometimes it is not as easy as in this example to determine who will benefit from an intervention and who will not. For this reason, sophisticated methods to assess someone's risk for a particular outcome, such as breast cancer or cardiovascular diseases, are often used. After discussing risk assessment, this chapter covers prevention of disease through general health promotion and specific protection. Health promotion and disease protection require effective counseling grounded in sound theories of behavior change. In the second half of the chapter, we discuss vaccines as particularly important instruments of specific protection, as well as a sample of other interventions.

1. SOCIETY'S CONTRIBUTION TO HEALTH

The health care system is of vital importance when it comes to treating disease and injury, but all of society and personal actions provide the basic structure for who becomes ill in the first place. Examples of societal sources of health include socioeconomic conditions, opportunities for safe employment, environmental systems (e.g., water supply, sewage disposal), and regulation of the environment, commerce, and public safety. Society also helps to sustain social support systems (e.g., families, neighborhoods) that are fundamental to health and facilitate healthful behaviors.

Because socioeconomic and other conditions vary greatly from country to country and over time, health problems and the success of health promotion efforts also vary. For example, in wartime conditions, adequate nutrition and medical assistance often do not exist, and international relief efforts may be hindered. As another example, in the aftermath of industrial accidents, such as the chemical disaster in Bhopal, India (1984), or the radiation disaster in Chernobyl, Ukraine (1986), it may be impossible for people in the immediate area to find an environment safe from these toxic exposures. Clearly genetics also play a role in health, but once people have access to adequate nutrition, clean water, and a safe environment, behavior becomes the major determining factor for how genetic risk or protective factors play out (see Chapters 19 and 20).

2. GENERAL HEALTH PROMOTION AND RISK ASSESSMENT

The World Health Organization (WHO) defines health promotion as "the process of enabling people to increase control over their health and its determinants, and thereby improve their health."[1] General health promotion addresses the underpinnings of general health, such as healthy diets, regular exercise, abstaining from tobacco, and avoiding unhealthy stress. Of these underpinnings, the connections between dietary patterns and various diseases are most complex. Numerous diets have been proposed as superior to others, and even long-lived recommendations such as limiting dietary fat have been criticized.[2] While there have been no long-term, rigorous studies comparing various diets, there seems to emerge a set of consistent findings suggesting a "theme" of many healthful diets: Avoid processed foods and eat predominantly plants. This means limiting added sugars, refined starches, processed foods, and certain fats, while consuming mostly whole plant foods, with or without lean meats, fish, poultry, and seafood.[2] In contrast, claims that particular "superfoods" or food groups such as fat or carbohydrates are inherently superior or inferior have not held up well over time.

Guidelines for general health promotion through physical activity recommend at least 150 minutes a week of moderate-intensity exercise, or 75 minutes a week of vigorous-intensity aerobic activity. The individual episodes of exercise should last at least 10 minutes each and should be spread throughout the week. More extensive health benefits can be gained by 300 minutes/week of moderate-intensity exercise or 150 minutes of vigorous-intensity exercise. In addition, muscle-strengthening activities on at least 2 days a week are recommended.[3]

Thanks to many years of research, an individual's risk for various health outcomes can be estimated, often in the form of interactive risk calculators. Risk calculators exist to estimate risk for osteoporotic fractures, certain forms of cancer (mainly breast, ovarian, and colon), and suffering a cardiovascular event such as stroke, myocardial infarction, or death from cardiovascular disease. For patients at elevated risk, certain medications can be used to decrease their chances of developing disease. For example, a patient aged 40 to 75 years with a calculated 10-year cardiovascular event risk over 10% may benefit from taking certain lipid-lowering medications and aspirin[4] (see Chemoprevention later in the chapter).

3. BEHAVIORAL FACTORS IN HEALTH PROMOTION

Human behavior is fundamental to health. The primary causes of death in the United States and most other countries involve modifiable lifestyle behaviors: cigarette smoking, poor diet, and lack of exercise.[5] Therefore efforts to change patients' behavior can have a powerful impact on their short-term and long-term health. Clinicians may not be aware of individual behavioral choices made by their patients, and if they are aware, they may not feel comfortable trying to influence patient choices. Clinicians may also be more likely to counsel patients regarding topics that require medical techniques such as cancer screening or family planning. They are more likely to counsel patients when they discover definite risk factors for disease, such as obesity, hypertension, elevated cholesterol levels, or unprotected sexual activity.

An important window of opportunity for counseling occurs after the development of symptomatic disease, such as an acute myocardial infarction, when a patient's motivation to modify diet, begin exercising regularly, and quit smoking may be at its peak ("**teachable moment**"). Another situation in which many patients are open to behavior change is pregnancy.

Box 15.1 provides specific recommendations for promoting smoking cessation. Also, the US Preventive Services Task Force offers recommendations for clinician counseling on additional prevention topics, including alcohol misuse, physical activity, sexually transmitted diseases, and skin cancer.[6]

3.1 THEORIES OF BEHAVIOR CHANGE

To impact behavior, it is helpful to understand how health behavior is shaped and how people change. Behavior change is usually difficult. Intervening in accordance with a valid theory of behavior change increases the chances of success. Theories also help in targeting interventions, choosing appropriate techniques, and selecting appropriate outcomes to measure.[7] We can only sketch out the basics of the most common health theories here. For further details, readers should

---

BOX 15.1   The Five A's Model for Facilitating Smoking Cessation, With Implementation Suggestions*

1. **Ask about tobacco use during every office visit.**
   Include questions about tobacco use when assessing the patient's vital signs. Placing tobacco-use status stickers on patient charts, noting tobacco use in electronic medical records, or using computer reminder systems also may be helpful.
2. **Advise all smokers to quit.**
   Advice should be:
   Clear: "I think it is important for you to quit smoking now. Cutting down or changing to light cigarettes is not enough."
   Strong: "As your physician, I need to tell you that smoking cessation is one of the most important decisions you can make for your health."
   Personalized: Physicians should talk with patients about how smoking specifically is affecting their health, children, or other family members; the social and economic costs of smoking; and the patient's readiness to quit.
3. **Assess the patient's willingness to quit.**
   Assess the patient's willingness to quit by asking, "On a scale from 0 to 10, with 0 being 'not at all motivated' and 10 being 'extremely motivated,' how motivated are you to quit smoking?" Use the patient's level of motivation to determine the next step:
   If the patient is willing to make a quit attempt, offer medication, brief counseling, and self-help resources and schedule a follow-up visit.
   If the patient is unwilling to quit, identify why the patient is not motivated. Explore what he or she likes and does not like about smoking and the potential advantages and disadvantages of quitting. Identify the patient's core

values (e.g., health, being a role model for children) and how smoking affects these values.
4. **Assist the patient in his or her attempt to quit.**
   Help the patient make a quit plan:
   Set a quit date, ideally within 2 weeks of the office visit.
   Request encouragement and support from family and friends.
   Anticipate triggers and cues to smoking, and identify alternative coping strategies.
   Help the patient change his or her environment:
   Throw away cigarettes, matches, lighters, and ashtrays; launder clothing; and vacuum home and car.
   Avoid smoking in places where the patient spends a lot of time (e.g., home, work, car).
   Avoid other smokers and drinking alcohol.
   Provide basic information about smoking and cessation (e.g., addictive nature of smoking, importance of complete abstinence, possible withdrawal symptoms).
   Recommend pharmacotherapy, unless contraindications exist, and behavior therapy for smoking cessation.
   Provide supplementary self-help materials.
5. **Arrange follow-up contact.**
   Follow-up should occur within the first week after the quit date. A second follow-up contact is recommended within the first month. Further follow-up visits should be scheduled as needed.
   During a follow-up visit, success should be congratulated. If the patient has relapsed, review the circumstances and elicit a new commitment to quit. Consider referral for more intensive treatment.
   Follow-up contact can be by telephone, email, or in person.

*The five *As* are from Fiore MC: *Treating tobacco use and dependence*, Rockville, MD, 2000, US Department of Health and Human Services, Public Health Service.
Modified from National Heart, Lung, and Blood Institute and American Lung Association recommendations. http://www.aafp.org/afp/2006/0715/p262.html#afp20060715p262-b2.

---

consult the pertinent literature. Other theories support the approach to changing group norms and helping communities identify and address health problems (see Chapter 24).

Most health behavior theories have been adapted from the social and behavioral sciences. Therefore they share common assumptions, as follows:

- Knowledge is necessary, but not sufficient, for behavior change
- Behavior is affected by what people know and how they think
- Behavior is influenced by people's perception of a behavior and its risks, their own motivation and skills, and the social environment

An important part of motivation is also their self-perceived ability to influence their life. The degree to which people believe this is most often called **self-efficacy**.

The most common theories for health behavior counseling are the health belief model, transtheoretical model (stages of change), theory of planned behavior, precaution adoption process model, and social cognitive/social learning theory (Table 15.1).

3.1.a. Health Belief Model

The health belief model holds that, before seeking preventive measures, people generally must believe the following[8]:

- The disease at issue is serious, if acquired
- They or their children are personally at risk for the disease
- The preventive measure is effective in preventing the disease
- There are no serious risks or barriers involved in obtaining the preventive measure

In addition, cues to action are needed, consisting of information regarding how and when to obtain the preventive measure and the encouragement or support of other people. This theory has been used to promote screening interventions.

3.1.b. Stages of Change (Transtheoretical Model)

The transtheoretical model was developed first to explain how patients quit smoking. The underlying insight was that people do not change their behavior dramatically in one moment. Change is a process, and patients have different counseling and informational needs depending on where they are in this process. This model addressed both the stages of

TABLE 15.1	**Overview of Common Theories of Behavior Change**	
Theory	**Focus**	**Key Concepts**
Individual Level		
Health belief model	Individuals' perceptions of the threat posed by a health problem, the benefit of avoiding the threat, and factors influencing the decision to act	Perceived susceptibility Perceived severity Perceived benefits Perceived barriers Cues to action Self-efficacy
Stages of change model	Individuals' motivation and readiness to change a problem behavior	Precontemplation Contemplation Preparation Action Maintenance
Theory of planned behavior	Individuals' attitudes toward a behavior, perceptions of norms, and beliefs about the ease or difficulty of change	Behavioral intention Attitude Subjective norm Perceived behavioral control
Precaution adoption process model	Individuals' journey from lack of awareness to action and maintenance	Unaware of issue Unengaged by issue Deciding about acting Deciding not to act Deciding to act Acting Maintenance
Interpersonal Level		
Social cognitive theory	Personal factors, environmental factors, and human behavior exert influence on each other	Reciprocal determinism Behavioral capability Expectations Self-efficacy Observational learning Reinforcements

Modified from Rimer BP, Glanz K: Theory at a glance: a guide for health promotion practice. Downloaded from https://cancercontrol.cancer.gov/brp/research/theories_project/theory.pdf on 575/2019

change and the process of changing. The stages of change are called precontemplation, contemplation, preparation, action, and maintenance.

In **precontemplation**, the patient is not convinced there is a problem and is unwilling to consider change. In **contemplation**, the patient has some ambivalence about the behavior but is not ready to take direct action. Acceptance of the need to act and preparation for action follow. In the **action** stage, people actually make changes. This phase is followed by **maintenance** (and often, relapse). People may cycle through the process many times before they make sustained changes. This theory has informed efforts to change addictive behaviors.

3.1.c. Theory of Planned Behavior and Theory of Reasoned Action

Both the theory of planned behavior and the associated theory of reasoned action explore how people form intentions for behavior change and how beliefs and attitudes play a role in those intentions. **Behavioral intentions** are the most important factor in predicting behavior. In turn, behavioral intentions are influenced by a person's attitude and the presumed attitudes of other important individuals (subjective norms). In addition to this construct, theory of planned behavior includes perceived behavioral control. This concept is similar to self-efficacy and describes how much people believe they can control their behavior. Both theories have been used to target a wide range of behaviors, such as dieting, questioning genetically engineered food, and limiting sun exposure.

3.1.d. Precaution Adoption Process Model

The precaution adoption process model distinguishes seven steps, from unawareness of a problem to behavior change. People progress from ignorance or unawareness (stage 1) via un-engagement (stage 2) through contemplating the decision to act (stages 3 and 4). If a decision to act has been made (stage 5), the next steps involve implementing change (stage 6) and maintenance (stage 7) of behavior change. Although it has some similarities to the stages of change model, this model assumes that the development is linear (i.e., people cannot go back to stage 1 and become unaware of an issue). The precaution adoption process model is particularly suited for newly recognized hazards, such as radon exposure or newly diagnosed osteoporosis, and provides guidance on how to impact people in stages before they make decisions.

3.1.e. Social Learning Theory and Social Cognitive Theory

Behavior and behavior change do not occur in a vacuum. For most people, their social environment is a strong influence to change or maintain behaviors. Social learning theory asserts that people learn not only from their own experiences but also from observing others. Social cognitive theory builds on this concept and describes reciprocal determinism; the person, the behavior, and the environment influence each other. Therefore recruiting credible role models who perform the intended behavior may be a powerful influence. This theory has been successfully used to influence condom use to reduce the risk of human immunodeficiency virus (HIV) transmission.[9]

3.2 BEHAVIORAL COUNSELING

Patients often want and need counseling, particularly those with risk factors for significant diseases. Still, if medications can be prescribed, it is tempting for the physician to provide these as the first line of treatment for pain, obesity, smoking, hypertension, and elevated cholesterol levels. Nevertheless, unless the problem is severe when the patient is first seen, generally the best approach is to try first to modify diet, exercise, or other aspects of lifestyle. Only if these approaches to reducing risk factors are refused or are unsuccessful within a reasonable time, or if the risk to the patient is high, medications can be considered as an addition to counseling.

Many clinicians are uncomfortable counseling patients, thinking they lack skills or time. However, good data show that even brief interventions can have a profound impact on patients. Each year, millions of smokers quit smoking because they want to, because they are concerned about their health, and because their providers tell them to quit. At the same time, even more individuals begin smoking worldwide. Box 15.1 summarizes the approach that the National Heart, Lung, and Blood Institute and the American Lung Association recommend for use by clinicians in counseling their patients.

Across a broad area of behavior, patient adherence is based on a functioning physician-patient relationship and skilled physician communication.[10] Beyond a good relationship, it matters *how* clinicians counsel. Despite its venerable tradition, simply giving advice is rarely effective.[11] Given the importance of social determinants of health, physician counseling is only one, often minor, influence. Even though insufficient to cause change in itself, however, counseling can provide motivation and support behavior change.

3.2.a. Motivational Interviewing

Motivational interviewing is a counseling technique aimed at increasing patients' motivation and readiness to change. It has been shown to be effective across a broad range of addictive and other health behaviors[12] and outperforms traditional advice giving.[11] Motivational interviewing fits well with the transtheoretical model of change and provides concrete strategies on how to increase people's motivation toward change. The model rests on three main concepts:

1. Patients with problem behaviors are ambivalent about their behavior.
2. "I learn what I believe as I hear myself talk." It is important to let the patient explore the advantages of changing and allow the patient to do most of the talking.[13]
3. Change is motivated by a perceived disconnect between present behavior and important personal goals and values (cognitive dissonance).

Therefore successful counseling involves increasing patients' cognitive dissonance and directing the dissonance toward behavior change. These steps are achieved by the following four strategies:

1. Expressing empathy
2. Developing cognitive dissonance
3. Rolling with resistance (resistance is a signal for the counselor to respond differently)
4. Supporting self-efficacy

Table 15.2 gives some examples of how a skilled counselor might encourage a patient to "talk change."

Regardless of the extent of the clinician's activity in behavior change, the clinician is responsible for monitoring the progress of the patient on a regular basis and for changing the approach if sufficient progress is not being made. If necessary, the clinician can assist the process of risk factor modification by recommending appropriate medications, such as nicotine patches for cessation of smoking or statins for reduction or modification of blood lipid levels.

3.2.b. Shared Decision Making

Shared decision making describes a process by which patients and providers consider outcome probabilities and patient preferences and reach a mutual decision. This method is best used for areas of uncertainty regarding risk versus benefit,[14] such as prostate cancer screening or ages to initiate or discontinue breast cancer screening. For problems such as these, which treatment or screening option is preferable depends on how patients view risks and benefits and their own values and preferences. During shared decision making, provider and patient together explore options, expected benefits and harms, and patient preferences. Many computerized decision aids have been developed to help this process. Examples include aids regarding screening decisions, use of aspirin for chemoprevention, and obtaining genetic testing for hereditary cancers.[15]

3.3 TALKING ABOUT HEALTH WITH UNDERSERVED PATIENTS

Ample data sources show that important health care disparities exist and persist in the United States and other countries. Racial minorities receive lower quality care and have less access to interventions.[16] Such disparities result from different underlying rates of illness because of genetic predisposition, social determinants of health, local environmental conditions, inadequate care, unhealthy lifestyles, different care-seeking

TABLE 15.2 Specific Motivational Interviewing Techniques for Early Stages of Change

Stage	Technique	Example
Precontempla-tion	Eliciting self-motivational statements	What concerns do you have about your drinking?
	Provide only objective assessment	Your liver function indicates some damage, likely from your drinking. I don't know whether this is of any concern to you or not. . . .
	Reflective listening and affirmation	You have expressed a lot of concerns to me, and I respect you for that. Let me try to put all of these together. . . .
Contemplation	Increasing cognitive dissonance	I can see how this might be confusing to you. On the one hand, you see there are serious problems around your alcohol use. And on the other hand, it seems like the label "alcoholic" doesn't quite fit.
	Paradoxical interventions	There are many advantages you see from drinking. It is possible that you will never be able to change.
	Education	Providing pamphlets or links to websites patients trust
Action	Providing information on treatment options Continued affirmation	You have taken a big step today, and I respect you for it. Here is some information on how to stay on track.
Maintenance	Providing information and support Continued affirmation	What do you remember as the most important reason to quit drinking?
Relapse	Increasing self-efficacy	You've been through a lot, and I admire you for the commitment you've shown to stay sober for so long.

Modified from Miller WR: Motivational interviewing with problem drinkers. *Behav Psychother* 2:147–172, 1983; Miller WR et al: *Motivational enhancement therapy manual,* Rockville, MD, 1995, US Department of Health and Human Services.

behaviors, linguistic barriers, and lack of trust in health care providers.[17] The impact of these disparities on health, life, and well-being are profound, and most disparities in care have persisted in spite of numerous efforts to correct them.[16] One strategy to decrease such disparities is to provide **culturally and linguistically appropriate services (CLAS)**, which encompass cultural competency and health literacy.

3.3.a. Cultural Competency

Cultural competency is defined as health care services delivered in a way that is respectful of and responsive to the health beliefs, practices, and needs of diverse patients.[18] This concept posits that cultural issues and communication about culture underlie all clinical and preventive services. Cultural competency usually includes language-access services and translated patient education materials, but also requires providers to be familiar with the cultural perspectives and beliefs more prevalent in certain groups. For example, individuals in some cultures believe that the mention of an illness will cause the illness; and some ethnic groups expect family members to have an important role in treatment decisions and believe telling terminally ill patients about their condition is uncaring. Such beliefs may or may not be true for the individual whom the provider is treating. Cultural competency requires providers to reflect on their own attitudes, beliefs, biases, and behaviors that may influence care, and to explore with their patients how they see their illness.[19]

Suggested questions to explore the cultural context of a disease include the following[20]:

What do you call your problem? What name does it have?

What do you think caused your problem?

What do you fear most about your disorder?

What kind of treatment do you think you should receive?

What are the most important results you hope to receive from the treatment?

What do friends, family, or others say about these symptoms?

What kind of medicines, home remedies, or other treatments have you tried for this illness?

Is there anything you eat, drink, or do/avoid on a regular basis to stay healthy?

Have you sought any advice from alternative/folk healer, friend, or other people (nondoctors) for help with your problem?

3.3.b. Health Literacy

Health literacy refers to "an individual's ability to read, understand, and use healthcare information to make effective healthcare decisions and follow instructions for treatment."[21] Low health literacy is common, with up to 50% of the US population unable to comprehend and act on basic medical information. For example, many individuals do not understand the terms *polyp, tumor,* or *screening test.* Providers must realize that native speakers of English may not understand the information presented and may be ashamed to speak up about problems or lack of understanding. Differences in health literacy level are consistently associated with increased hospitalizations and emergency department visits, lower use of preventive services, poorer ability to interpret labels and health messages, and among seniors, poorer overall health status and higher mortality. Health literacy level potentially mediates health care disparities between blacks and whites.[21] Improving consumer health literacy is one of the US *Healthy People* goals.

Several factors account for low health literacy, but it is probably best to assume that no patient will understand information presented at a reading level higher than sixth grade ("universal health literacy precautions"). Recommended interventions to improve information uptake for patients with low health literacy include the following[22]:

- Redesigning patient information at lower reading levels and simplifying the content and design
- *Teach-back:* Asking the patient to teach the information back to the provider to confirm understanding
- *Ask me 3:* Promoting three simple but essential questions that patients should ask their providers in every health care interaction:
  1. What is my main problem?
  2. What do I need to do?
  3. Why is it important for me to do this?[23]

Other types of literacy also impact how people access health information, such as media literacy (i.e., the ability to accurately assess and evaluate information found in media) and health numeracy (i.e., the ability to understand numbers, probability, and mathematical evidence). Interested readers should consult the current literature for further information (see Websites later in the chapter).

4. PREVENTION OF DISEASE THROUGH SPECIFIC PROTECTION

The major goals of primary prevention by specific protection involve prevention in the following three areas:

- Specific diseases (e.g., by using vaccines or chemoprevention)
- Specific deficiency states (e.g., by using iodized salt to prevent iodine deficiency goiter; by using fluoride to prevent dental caries)
- Specific injuries and toxic exposures (e.g., by using helmets to prevent head injuries in construction workers, goggles to prevent eye injuries in machine tool operators, or filters and ventilation systems to control dust; see Chapters 22 and 23)

Oral health is a special case, where general health promotion (mainly diet) combines with specific interventions (e.g., fluoride, dental hygiene, regular dental visits) to improve the health of a specific body area. This section that follows in this chapter discusses vaccinations, prevention of deficiency, chemoprevention, and oral health. Chapter 22 discusses occupational and environmental injury prevention and toxic exposures in detail.

4.1 PREVENTION OF DISEASE BY USE OF VACCINES

An intact immune system in a well-nourished and otherwise healthy individual provides basic protection against infectious diseases. Intact immunity implies that the immune system was normal at birth and has not been damaged by a disease, such as infection with HIV or side effects from medications (e.g., anticancer drugs, long-term steroid use).

4.1.a. Types of Immunity

Passive immunity is protection against an infectious disease provided by circulating antibodies made in another organism. Newborn infants are protected by maternal antibodies transferred through the placenta before birth and through breast milk. If recently exposed to hepatitis B virus (HBV) and not immunized with HBV vaccine, a person can be given human immune globulin, which confers passive immunity and protects against HBV infection. In an emergency a specific type of antitoxin, if available, can be used to confer passive immunity against bacterial toxins, such as diphtheria antitoxin in the patient with clinical diphtheria or trivalent botulinum antitoxin for botulism. Passive immunity provides incomplete protection and usually is of short duration.

Vaccines confer **active immunity**. Some types of vaccines, such as the inactivated polio vaccine, do this by stimulating the production of humoral (blood) antibody to the antigen in the vaccine (see Chapter 1). Other types, such as the live attenuated polio vaccine, not only elicit this humoral antibody response but also stimulate the body to develop cell-mediated immunity. This tissue-based cellular response to foreign antigens involves mobilization of killer T cells. Active immunity is much superior to passive immunity because active immunity lasts longer (a lifetime in some cases) and is rapidly stimulated to high levels by a reexposure to the same or closely related antigens. All approved vaccines provide most immunized persons with some level of individual immunity to a specific disease (i.e., they themselves are protected).

Some vaccines also reduce or prevent the shedding (spread) of infectious organisms from an immunized person to others, which contributes to herd immunity (see Fig. 1.2).

4.1.b. Types of Vaccines

Some vaccines are inactivated (killed), some are live attenuated (altered), and others are referred to as toxoids (inactivated or altered bacterial exotoxins). To reduce the likelihood of negative side effects, the antigens are prepared in a cell-free (acellular) manner. Other vaccines consist of only antigenic fragments from the organisms of concern (e.g., polysaccharides), usually conjugated to a harmless biologic substance. Genomic methods permit the identification and replication of antigenic sequences of base pairs (epitopes) that are recognized by T or B lymphocytes, which then produce antibodies.

The older pertussis and typhoid vaccines are examples of inactivated bacterial vaccines, and injected influenza vaccine and the inactivated polio vaccine are examples of inactivated viral vaccines. The bacille Calmette-Guérin (BCG) vaccine against tuberculosis (which is no longer used in the United States) and the oral typhoid vaccines are examples of live attenuated bacterial vaccines, whereas the measles and oral polio vaccines are examples of live attenuated viral vaccines. Live attenuated vaccines are created by altering the organisms so that they are no longer pathogenic, but still have antigenicity.

Diphtheria and tetanus vaccines are the primary examples of toxoids (vaccines against biologic toxins). *Clostridium tetani,* an organism that is part of the normal flora of many animals and is found frequently in the soil, can cause tetanus in unimmunized individuals with infected wounds. This is because *C. tetani* produces a potent toxin when it grows under anaerobic conditions, such as are often found in wounds with necrotic tissue.

4.1.c. Immunization Recommendations and Schedules

Active immunization of adults. The need for adequate immunization levels in adults is illustrated again and again by outbreaks of vaccine-preventable disease in under-vaccinated groups. For example, a dramatic epidemic of diphtheria occurred in the independent states of the former Soviet Union, where more than 50,000 cases, with almost 2000 deaths, were reported between 1990 and 1994. In 70% of the cases, diphtheria occurred in persons 15 years or older.[24] Most of these individuals had been immunized against diphtheria as children, but the immunity had waned. Other instances include measles outbreaks in Amish communities in Ohio in 2014; a measles outbreak in Berlin, Germany, in 2015, which affected 574 patients and caused the death of one unvaccinated infant; a pertussis outbreak in Denmark in 2016 (likely from waning herd immunity); and a measles outbreak in a Somali community in the Midwest in 2017 due to declining vaccination rates. Globally the most common vaccine-preventable diseases are measles, mumps, and whooping cough.[25]

The immunization schedules for children and adults are maintained by the CDC Advisory Committee on Immunization Practices (ACIP) and updated regularly.[26] Readers should consult the appropriate websites for current recommendations. The immunization of adults builds on the foundation of vaccines given during childhood. If an adult is missing diphtheria and tetanus vaccines, these should be started immediately. Many adults need boosters because their immunity levels have declined since they were immunized. For protection against tetanus, several combination preparations are available; however, adults usually are given the combined tetanus and diphtheria (Td) vaccine, which contains a reduced amount of diphtheria antigen to decrease the number of reactions.

International travelers should ensure that all their basic immunizations are up to date (e.g., poliomyelitis, tetanus, diphtheria, measles). Before traveling to less developed countries, it may be necessary or desirable to receive other immunizations, such as hepatitis A, hepatitis B, typhoid, cholera, yellow fever, rabies, and other diseases. For recommendations and help in determining requirements, individuals planning to travel abroad should consult a local clinician who specializes in international travel, their local or state health department, or the CDC. The CDC website has country-specific information regarding preventive measures needed for travel there, such as vaccines, immune globulins, and chemoprophylaxis.

4.1.d. Passive Immunization

The medical indications for passive immunization are much more limited than the indications for active immunization. For immunocompetent individuals who are at high risk for exposure to hepatitis A, usually because of travel to a country where it is common, hepatitis A vaccine can be administered if there is time, or immune globulin can be administered before travel as a method of **preexposure prophylaxis**. For individuals recently exposed to hepatitis B or rabies and not known to have a protective antibody titer, a specific immune globulin can be used as a method of **postexposure prophylaxis** (see also Chapter 20). For immunocompromised persons who have been exposed to a common but potentially life-threatening infection such as chickenpox, immune globulin can be lifesaving if given intravenously soon after exposure.

4.2 VACCINE SURVEILLANCE AND TESTING

As discussed in Chapter 3, the rates and patterns of reportable diseases are monitored and any cases thought to be vaccine associated are investigated. The goals are to monitor the effectiveness of vaccines and to detect vaccine failures or adverse effects.

4.2.a. Randomized Field Trials

The standard way to measure the effectiveness of a new vaccine is through a randomized field trial, the public health equivalent of a randomized controlled trial. In this type of trial, susceptible persons are randomized into two groups and are given the vaccine or a placebo, usually at the beginning of the high-risk season of the year. The vaccinated subjects and unvaccinated controls are followed through the high-risk season to determine the **attack rate** (AR) in each group.

$$AR = \text{Number of persons ill/} \\ \text{Number of persons exposed to the disease}$$

Here, AR among the vaccinated is the number of vaccinated persons ill with the disease divided by the total number vaccinated. For the unvaccinated, AR is the number of unvaccinated persons in the study group who are ill divided by the total number of unvaccinated persons in the study group.

Next, the **vaccine effectiveness** (VE) (sometimes called protective efficacy), when calculated as a percentage, is:

$$VE = AR_{(unvaccinated)} - AR_{(vaccinated)} \times 100/AR_{(unvaccinated)}$$

In the VE equation, the numerator is the observed reduction in AR as a result of the vaccination and the denominator represents the total amount of risk that could be reduced by the vaccine. The VE formula is a specific example of the general formula for **relative risk reduction**.

Field trials were used to evaluate inactivated polio vaccine, oral polio vaccine, measles vaccine, influenza vaccine, varicella vaccine, human papillomavirus, and HIV vaccines.

4.2.b. Retrospective Cohort Studies

The antigenic variability of influenza virus necessitates frequent (often yearly) changes in the constituents of influenza vaccines to keep them up to date with new strains of the virus (see Chapter 1). This requires constant surveillance of the disease and the protective efficacy of the vaccine. Because there are insufficient resources and time to perform a randomized controlled field trial of each new influenza vaccine, retrospective cohort studies are done sometimes during the influenza season to evaluate the protective efficacy of the vaccines.

In these studies, because there is no randomization, investigators cannot ensure that no selection bias occurred on the part of the clinicians who recommended the vaccine or the individuals who agreed to be immunized. If selection bias were present, the participants who were immunized might be either sicker or more interested in their health than those who were not immunized. The CDC publishes yearly estimates of influenza vaccine efficacy. Depending on the year and the vaccine, the effectiveness varies between 40% and 60%, but has been as low as 13% for some influenza A strains.[27]

4.2.c. Case Control Studies

Because randomized field trials require large sample sizes, they are usually impossible to perform for relatively uncommon diseases such as *Haemophilus influenzae* infections or pneumococcal pneumonia. To overcome this problem some investigators have recommended using case control studies.[28] This is based on the fact that when the risk of disease in the population is low, the vaccine effectiveness formula, expressed as a percentage, may be rewritten as follows:

$$VE = 1 - [AR_{(vaccinated)}/AR_{(unvaccinated)}] = (1 - RR) \approx (1 - OR)$$

The risk ratio (RR) is closely approximated by the odds ratio (OR) when the disease is uncommon, as in the cases of *H. influenzae* infections in children and pneumococcal infections in adults.

4.2.d. Incidence Density Measures

The questions that vaccine research and surveillance are designed to answer include the following:

- When should a new vaccine be given?
- What is the duration of the immunity produced?

How to solve these questions can be illustrated with a historical example. In the case of measles vaccine, initial surveillance studies suggested that when the vaccine was given to infants before 12 months of age, often it was ineffective presumably because the vaccine antigen was neutralized by residual maternal antibody.

To determine answers to both these questions, one group of investigators performed a study in which they monitored the incidence density of measles cases in Ohio over a full winter and spring season.[29] To adjust for the duration of exposure to measles, which varied between individuals, they used the incidence density as their measure of measles incidence (Box 15.2) (see also description in Chapter 2). The formula for **incidence density** (ID) is as follows:

$$ID = \text{Number of new cases of a disease/Person-time of exposure}$$

The denominator (person-time) can be expressed in terms of the number of person-days, person-weeks, person-months, or person-years of exposure to the risk.

The results in Box 15.2, along with other studies, suggested that measles vaccine should be postponed until children are approximately 15 months old. One concern in delaying the vaccine is that measles is more severe in newborns than in older infants. Partly to reduce the risk that new schoolchildren

---

BOX 15.2   Data Showing Why Measles Vaccine Is Postponed Until Children Are 15 Months Old

Part 1 Relationship between the age at measles vaccination and (1) measles incidence density (incidence of disease per 1000 person-weeks) and (2) relative risk of measles per 1000 person-weeks of exposure at different ages of vaccination compared with children vaccinated at 15 months old

Age at Vaccination	Measles Incidence per 1000 Person-Weeks	Relative Risk Compared With Risk in Children Vaccinated at 15 Months Old
Never	155.3	33.0
<11 months	39.6	8.5
11 months	15.0	3.2
12 months	7.1	1.5
13 months	5.2	1.1
14 months	4.7	1.0

Part 2 Relationship of time elapsed since measles vaccination and (1) measles incidence density (incidence of measles per 1000 person-weeks) and (2) relative risk of measles compared with children vaccinated recently (0–3 years)

Time Since Vaccination	Measles Incidence per 1000 Person-Weeks	Relative Risk
0–3 years	4.0	1.0
4–6 years	4.2	1.1
7–9 years	5.4	1.4
10–12 years	11.7	2.9

Data from Marks J, Halpin TJ, Orenstein WA: Measles vaccine efficacy in children previously vaccinated at 12 months of age. *Pediatrics* 62:955–960, 1978.

will be exposed to measles and bring the disease home to younger siblings, experts recommend that all children be re-vaccinated with measles vaccine before they enter school, at age 5 or 6 years. This also serves as a booster dose to protect the children as they enter school.

Another concern has been the duration of immunity. As shown in the second part of Box 15.2, the measles vaccine lost its protective ability slowly during the first 6 years, but the relative risk of acquiring measles had almost tripled by 10 to 12 years after immunization. This was another line of evidence that led to the recommendation that children be revaccinated before entering school, at age 5 or 6 years.

4.3 IMMUNIZATION GOALS

The strategy of developing disease control programs through the use of vaccines depends on the objectives of the vaccine campaign. The goal may be **eradication** of disease (as has been achieved for smallpox), regional **elimination** of disease (as has been achieved for poliomyelitis in the Western Hemisphere), or **control** of disease to reduce morbidity and mortality (as in chickenpox). Global efforts to eradicate poliomyelitis have been underway for several decades. Total eradication appeared close several times, yet achieving it has remained—so far—elusive.[30] Disease eradication by immunization is feasible only for diseases in which humans are the sole reservoir of the infectious organism. Although vaccines are available to prevent some diseases with reservoirs in other animals (e.g., rabies, plague, encephalitis) and some diseases with reservoirs in the environment (e.g., typhoid fever), these infections are not candidates for eradication programs. The surveillance systems to achieve eradication or regional elimination must be excellent, and any eradication or elimination program requires considerably more resources and time and general political and popular support than a disease control program. For these reasons, immunization strategies are frequently the subject of much scrutiny and debate.

4.3.a. Vaccine-Related Supplies and Lawsuits

Since the very beginnings of vaccinations with Jenner's discovery of the smallpox vaccine, there have been recurring problems with secure funding mechanisms, streamlining of manufacturing, sufficient supplies, safety concerns, and deep-seated public fears.[31] In response to these problems, the US federal government instituted the National Vaccine Injury Compensation Program, which covers almost all routinely administered vaccines. The program essentially protects vaccine manufacturers from liability lawsuits, unless it can be shown that their vaccines differed from the federal requirements. It also simplifies the legal process and reduces the costs for people making a claim, and almost all the costs of the program and payouts to patients are borne by the federal government (and by taxpayers).

Even though this program has significantly reduced the liability costs to for-profit vaccine producers, the vaccine market remains fragile and prone to mismatches between demand and supply. A consequence of fewer companies being willing to make vaccines is the impact on the ability to respond to emergencies. In the case of pandemics, large amounts of vaccines are needed in a short time, and the capacity to do this might be waning. Specifically, it would take at least 6 months from the time an influenza H5N1 pandemic strain of virus is isolated until significant amounts of the vaccine can be produced.[32] This difficulty was brought into stark reality in 2009 when a novel H1N1 strain with characteristics of an epidemic strain appeared, and there were substantial difficulties in distributing vaccines to high-risk groups.[32]

4.3.b. Missed Opportunities for Immunizations

Many children and adults have not received all vaccinations they need. Often clinicians do not vaccinate children who have mild upper respiratory tract infections, even though the office visit was scheduled to include a vaccination. Guidelines emphasize that children should receive the appropriate vaccines despite having mild infections. Also, the parent often brings the child's siblings, who should receive vaccinations if their immunization records are not up to date; however, this is seldom done. These two scenarios are common in outpatient clinics and especially emergency departments, where opportunities may be missed because providers lack records, time, and a relationship with patients. Hospitalized children and adults whose immunization records are not up to date should be given the appropriate vaccines unless contraindications exist.

The list of true contraindications to vaccinations is short, and many contraindications are temporary:
- Moderate to severe acute illness
- History of severe allergic reaction to previous immunizations (e.g., anaphylaxis)
- Severe immunodeficiency (for live virus vaccines)
- Pregnancy (for live virus vaccines).[33]

However, most missed immunizations are not because of the presence of contraindications. Both patients and clinicians are often poorly informed about contraindications. The following factors are not considered contraindications to immunizing children or adults:
1. Mild reaction to a previous DTP or DTaP dose, consisting of redness and swelling at the injection site or a temperature less than 40.5°C (<105°F) or both
2. Presence of nonspecific allergies
3. Presence of a mild illness or diarrhea with low-grade fever in an otherwise healthy patient scheduled for vaccination
4. Current therapy with an antimicrobial drug in a patient who is convalescing well
5. Breastfeeding of an infant scheduled for immunization
6. Pregnancy of another woman in the household.[33]

Strategies to increase vaccination rates in medical practices include:
- Assessing every patient's immunization record regularly, even when they come in for other reasons
- Provide clear and forceful recommendations for vaccination and the need for follow-up
- Use reminder systems for patients
- Provide standing orders

- Address incorrect perceptions of contraindications
- Track vaccination rates as part of continuous quality improvement.[34]

4.4 CHEMOPREVENTION

Chemoprevention includes all instances where medications are taken to prevent a disease. The most common forms of chemoprevention include antimicrobial prophylaxis, use of aspirin and lipid-lowering agents to prevent cardiovascular disease, and the use of selective estrogen receptor modulators to prevent breast cancer in high-risk women.

For travelers to countries where malaria is endemic, antimicrobial prophylaxis against the causative organism *Plasmodium* is desirable. Oral chemoprophylaxis for adults should be performed depending on local resistance rates, which vary greatly and change over time. Because resistance rates change rapidly and new regimens become available, travelers should consult CDC websites or travel medicine clinics.

The natural history of tuberculosis (TB) is discussed in Chapter 20. Patients with latent TB should be treated to prevent active TB. Latent TB is diagnosed through a positive purified protein derivative (PPD) skin test or interferon-gamma release blood assay. The cutoff of the PPD test depends on the risk to the patient (Table 15.3). The different cutoff points reflect different relative risks of developing disease.

PPD tests may provide false-positive and false-negative results. Reasons for *false-positive results* may be caused by:
- Infection with non-TB mycobacteria
- Previous BCG vaccination
- Incorrect administration method
- Incorrect interpretation of reaction
- Incorrect use of antigen[35]

False-negative test results may occur in case of:
- Inability to react to skin tests because of a weakened immune system (also called cutaneous anergy)
- Recent TB infection (within 8–10 weeks of exposure)
- Very old TB infection (many years)
- Very young age (<6 months old)
- Recent live virus vaccination (e.g., measles and smallpox)
- Overwhelming TB disease
- Some viral illnesses (e.g., measles and chickenpox)
- Incorrect administration
- Incorrect interpretation of the test[35]

While the PPD test is still widely used in the United States and worldwide, blood tests for TB (interferon gamma release assays [IGRA]) are also available. These blood tests are more popular with clinicians, because they are more specific and do not require a return visit.

Apart from prophylactic therapy of latent TB, other examples for antimicrobial prophylaxis include short-term antibiotics before procedures for patients with some cardiac defects, antibiotics to prevent meningococcal disease in outbreaks, and use of antiretroviral drugs in health care workers after needlesticks to prevent HIV transmission.

4.5 PREVENTION OF DEFICIENCY STATES

When specific vitamin and mineral deficiencies were identified in the past, food or water was fortified to ensure that most people would obtain sufficient amounts of nutrients of a specific type. Iodine in salt has essentially eliminated goiter; vitamin D in milk has largely eliminated rickets; and fluoridated water has greatly reduced dental caries in children. Cereal grain products enriched with folic acid prevent folic acid deficiencies in newly pregnant women, which in turn can lead to neural tube defects. This fortification has led to a 23% decrease in neural tube defect–affected births.[36]

4.6 ORAL HEALTH

Oral health means much more than healthy teeth. Good oral health is essential to general health and quality of life and should therefore be included in health care and the provision of community programs.[37] In addition to preventing dental cavities and gum disease, oral health also addresses oral cancer and oral infectious diseases. Strategies that

Reaction	Groups at Risk
≥5 mm	Human immunodeficiency virus (HIV)–positive patients Recent contacts of tuberculosis (TB) case patients Fibrotic changes on chest radiograph consistent with prior TB Patients with organ transplants and patients receiving immunosuppressant medications such as prednisone
≥10 mm	Recent immigrants (≤5 years) from high-prevalence countries Injection drug users (if HIV negative) Residents and employees of high-risk settings (e.g., correctional institutions, long-term care facilities, homeless shelters) Patients with high-risk clinical conditions (e.g., silicosis, diabetes mellitus, chronic renal failure, some hematologic disorders [e.g., carcinoma of head/neck or lung], weight loss [≥10% of ideal body weight], gastrectomy, jejunoileal bypass, malignancies) Children under 4 years of age or infants, children, and adolescents exposed to adults at high risk
≥15 mm	Persons with no known risk factors for TB

TABLE 15.3 Criteria for Tuberculin Positivity, Millimeters of Induration (mm), by Risk Group

Modified from Papadakis MA, McPhee SJ, eds: *2018 current medical diagnosis and treatment*, ed 57, New York: 2017, McGraw Hill. Adapted from CDC factsheet https://www.cdc.gov/tb/publications/factsheets/testing/skintesting.htm.

decrease both the burden of oral diseases and other chronic diseases include:

- Decreasing sugar intake and maintaining a well-balanced diet
- Consuming fruit and vegetables
- Stopping tobacco use
- Decreasing alcohol consumption
- Ensuring proper oral hygiene
- Using protective sports and motor vehicle equipment to reduce the risk of facial injuries
- Maintaining a safe physical environment[38]

CASE RESOLUTION

Throughout this chapter we have discussed multiple theories that would aid in interpreting the patient's and mother's comments and concerns. If viewed through the lens of the health belief model, the child does not believe she is herself at risk for HPV-induced cancer, whereas the mother is convinced of serious risks of the vaccine. Therefore they are both in the precontemplation phase of the stages of change model. In the precaution adoption model, both would be considered to be in the unawareness stage; proponents of the social learning/social cognitive theory would ask what credible role models exist for mother and child in the area of sexual health and vaccines. Lastly, a provider trained in cultural competency would ask what norms exist around young girls and sexual health, and what thoughts mother and daughter have about vaccinations in general and this one in particular.

To discuss with your patients the benefits of the vaccine, it helps to know the salient medical facts: The vaccine is made from purified viruslike particles and is a noninfectious recombinant vaccine. It is most effective in girls who have never been exposed to the virus and therefore should be given *before* girls become sexually active. HPV infection in males is usually asymptomatic; a man "looking clean" is therefore no indication that he does not carry the virus. The vaccine reduces infection rates by about two-thirds.[39] As for potential adverse effects, since the HPV vaccine was introduced in 2006, more than 270 million doses have been given. Several high-ranking studies about adverse effects have been conducted and the only side effects associated with receipt of the vaccine were syncope related to anxiety and anaphylaxis at a frequency of one case in 1.7 million doses.[40] Since the daughter received all her earlier vaccines without major side effects, she is unlikely to have a bad reaction now. These facts alone, however, will certainly not convince either patient or her mother. (Remember, a common assumption of most behavior change theories is that knowledge is necessary, but not sufficient, for behavior change!) Therefore, following both the theory of motivational interviewing and cultural competence, you should work on building an empathic relationship and understanding both the cultural and individual concerns, values, and preferences involved.

Once an empathic relationship has been developed, and since both patient and mother are in the precontemplation phase, you would use interventions suited to that stage of change, exploring important personal goals and values, and examining if the decision to forego vaccination would be in line with these goals. You would endeavor to help mother and daughter explore the pros and cons of the vaccination, so they "hear themselves talk change." That way, even if they decide against a vaccination today, you have a better chance of a productive encounter the next time this question comes up.

---

5. SUMMARY

Primary prevention begins with general health promotion, which aims to improve the nutritional, environmental, social, and behavioral conditions in which people are conceived, born, raised, and live. Primary prevention also includes specific interventions to prevent certain diseases (specific prevention). Specific prevention interventions are often based on calculating a patient's risk for developing certain diseases such as cardiovascular disease. The clinician's role in counseling patients regarding personal habits is underused. Theories of behavior change are important to design and evaluate health promotion efforts and include the health belief model, stages of change model, theory of reasoned action, and precaution adoption process model. Motivational interviewing is a counseling method that encourages the patient to "talk change" and outperforms traditional advice-giving for many addiction and health behavior problems. To decrease health care disparities among their patients, providers need to provide culturally and linguistically appropriate services. Cultivation of widespread health literacy is a social and public health priority as well.

Many biologic, nutritional, pharmaceutical, or environmental interventions exist to protect individuals against certain diseases, deficiency states, injuries, or toxic exposures. The prototype of specific protection is the vaccine, which is directed against one disease and prevents the disease by increasing host resistance. Host resistance can be temporarily increased by passive immunization or sometimes by prophylactic antibiotic therapy. Other types of specific prevention include adding nutrients to common foods (e.g., adding iodine to salt) to prevent a particular disease (e.g., goiter) and chemoprevention with medication to prevent cardiovascular disease or certain cancers. Oral health is an underappreciated topic where providers can greatly impact patients' quality of life and reduce the risk of chronic diseases.

REFERENCES

1. Health Promotion Unit, Department of Chronic Diseases and Health Promotion, World Health Organization, Switzerland. A charter to achieve health for all. *Health Promot J Austr*. 2005;16(3):171. Available at: http://www.who.int/healthpromotion/conferences/HPJA_2005-3Tang.pdf.
2. Katz DL, Meller S. Can we say what diet is best for health? *Annu Rev Public Health*. 2014;35:83-103.
3. U.S. Department of Health and Human Services. *2008 Physical Activity Guidelines for Americans*. Hyattsville, MD: US DHHS; 2008.
4. U.S. Preventive Services Task Force. *Draft Recommendation Statement: Statin Use for the Primary Prevention of Cardiovascular Disease in Adults: Preventive Medication*. 2016. Available at: https://www.uspreventiveservicestaskforce.org/Page/Document/draft-recommendation-statement175/statin-use-in-adults-preventive-medication1.
5. Mokdad AH, Marks JS, Stroup DF, Gerberding JL. Actual causes of death in the United States, 2000. *JAMA*. 2004;291:1238-1245.
6. U.S. Preventive Services Task Force. *Recommendations for Primary Care Practice*. 2017. Available at: https://www.uspreventiveservicestaskforce.org/Page/Name/recommendations.

7. Rimer BP, Glanz K. *Theory at a Glance: A Guide for Health Promotion Practice*. 2005. Available at: https://cancercontrol.cancer.gov/brp/research/theories_project/theory.pdf.

8. Rosenstock IM. Historical origins of the health belief model. *Health Educ Monogr*. 1974;2:328-335.

9. Carlos JA, Bingham TA, Stueve A, et al. The role of peer support on condom use among Black and Latino MSM in three urban areas. *AIDS Educ Prev*. 2010;22:430-444.

10. Zolnierek KB, Dimatteo MR. Physician communication and patient adherence to treatment: a meta-analysis. *Med Care*. 2009;47:826-834.

11. Rubak S, Sandbaek A, Lauritzen T, Christensen B. Motivational interviewing: a systematic review and meta-analysis. *Br J Gen Pract*. 2005;55:305-312.

12. Lundahl B, Moleni T, Burke BL, et al. Motivational interviewing in medical care settings: a systematic review and meta-analysis of randomized controlled trials. *Patient Educ Couns*. 2013;93(2):157-168.

13. Miller WR. Motivational interviewing with problem drinkers. *Behav Cogn Psychother*. 1983;11:147-172.

14. Edwards A, Elwyn G, eds. *Shared Decision Making in Health Care: Achieving Evidence-Based Patient Choice*. Oxford, UK: Oxford University Press; 2009.

15. Stacey D, Légaré F, Col NF, et al. Decision aids for people facing health treatment or screening decisions. *Cochrane Database Syst Rev*. 2014;1:CD001431. doi:10.1002/14651858.CD001431.pub4.

16. Agency for Healthcare Research and Quality. *2016 National Healthcare Quality and Disparities Report*, Pub. No. 17-0001. Rockville, MD: AHRQ; 2017.

17. Institute of Medicine (US) Committee on the Review and Assessment of the NIH's Strategic Research Plan and Budget to Reduce and Ultimately Eliminate Health Disparities. Health disparities: concepts, measurements, and understanding. In: Thomson GE, Mitchell F, Williams MB, eds. *Examining the Health Disparities Research Plan of the National Institutes of Health: Unfinished Business*. Washington, DC: National Academies Press; 2006. Available at: https://www.ncbi.nlm.nih.gov/books/NBK57052/.

18. Office of Minority Health. *Think Cultural Health. A Physician's Practical Guide to Culturally Competent Care*. Available at: http://cccm.thinkculturalhealth.hhs.gov. Accessed April 24, 2018.

19. Williamson M, Harrison L. Providing culturally appropriate care: a literature review. *Int J Nurs Stud*. 2010;47(6):761-769.

20. Office of Minority Health. *A Physician's Practical Guide to Culturally Competent Care*. Available at: http://cccm.thinkculturalhealth.hhs.gov.

21. Berkman ND, Sheridan SL, Donahue KE, Halpern DJ, Crotty K. Low health literacy and health outcomes: an updated systematic review. *Ann Intern Med*. 2011;155(2):97-107.

22. Institute of Medicine. *Health Literacy: A Prescription to End Confusion*. Washington, DC: National Academies Press; 2004.

23. Institute for Healthcare Improvement/National Patient Safety Foundation. *Ask Me 3: Good Questions for Your Good Health*. Available at: http://www.ihi.org/resources/Pages/Tools/Ask-Me-3-Good-Questions-for-Your-Good-Health.aspx. Accessed May 5, 2019.

24. Centers for Disease Control and Prevention. Diphtheria epidemic: new Independent States of the former Soviet Union, 1990-1994. *MMWR*. 1995;44:177-181.

25. Vaccines work. *Vaccine-Preventable Disease Outbreaks*. Available at: http://www.vaccineswork.org/vaccine-preventable-disease-outbreaks/. Accessed May 5, 2019.

26. Centers for Disease Control and Prevention. *Immunization Schedules*. Available at: https://www.cdc.gov/vaccines/schedules. Accessed May 5, 2019.

27. Paules CI, Sullivan SG, Subbarao K, Fauci AS. Chasing seasonal influenza—the need for a universal influenza vaccine. *N Engl J Med*. 2018;378(1):7-9.

28. Clemens JD, Shapiro ED. Resolving the pneumococcal vaccine controversy: are there alternatives to randomized clinical trials? *Rev Infect Dis*. 1984;6:589-600.

29. Marks JS, Halpin TJ, Orenstein WA. Measles vaccine efficacy in children previously vaccinated at 12 months of age. *Pediatrics*. 1978;62:955-960.

30. World Health Organization. *Report by the Director-General. Eradication of poliomyelitis. Report at the Seventy-First World Health Assembly*. 2018. Available at: http://apps.who.int/gb/ebwha/pdf_files/WHA71/A71_26-en.pdf.

31. Stern AM, Markel H. The history of vaccines and immunization: familiar patterns, new challenges. *Health Aff (Millwood)*. 2005;24(3):611-621.

32. SteelFisher GK, Blendon RJ, Bekheit MM, Lubell K. The public's response to the 2009 H1N1 influenza pandemic. *N Engl J Med*. 2010;362:e65.

33. Centers for Disease Control and Prevention. *Vaccine Recommendations and Guidelines of the ACIP*. Available at: https://www.cdc.gov/vaccines/hcp/acip-recs/general-recs/contraindications.html. Accessed May 5, 2019.

34. Centers for Disease Control and Prevention. *Epidemiology and Prevention of Vaccine-preventable diseases. Immunization Strategies for Healthcare practices and Providers*. 13th ed. 2015. Available at: https://www.cdc.gov/vaccines/pubs/pinkbook/strat.html.

35. Centers for Disease Control and Prevention. *Tuberculosis Fact Sheets*. Available at: https://www.cdc.gov/tb/publications/factsheets/testing/skintesting.htm. Accessed May 5, 2019.

36. Erickson JD. Folic acid and prevention of spina bifida and anencephaly. 10 years after the U.S. Public Health Service recommendation. *MMWR Recomm Rep*. 2002;51(RR-13):1-3.

37. National Institutes of Health. *Oral Health in America: A Report of the Surgeon General 2000. (Executive Summary)*. 2000. Available at: https://www.nidcr.nih.gov/research/data-statistics/surgeon-general.

38. World Health Organization. *Oral Health: Sugars and Dental Caries*. 2017. Available at: https://www.who.int/oral_health/publications/sugars-dental-caries-keyfacts/en/. Accessed May 5, 2019.

39. Drolet M, Bénard É, Boily MC, et al. Population-level impact and herd effects following human papillomavirus vaccination programmes: a systematic review and meta-analysis. *Lancet Infect Dis*. 2015;15(5):565-580.

40. World Health Organization. *Vaccine safety updates. Extract from report of GACVS meeting of 7-8 June 2017, published in the WHO Weekly Epidemiological Record of 14 July 2017*. Available at: http://www.who.int/vaccine_safety/committee/topics/hpv/June_2017/en/.

SELECT READINGS

Berkman ND, Sheridan SL, Donahue KE, Halpern DJ, Crotty K. Low health literacy and health outcomes: an updated systematic review. *Ann Intern Med*. 2011;155(2):97-107.

Chin MH, Clarke AR, Nocon RS, et al. A roadmap and best practices for organizations to reduce racial and ethnic disparities in health care. *J Gen Intern Med*. 2012;27(8):992-1000.

Glanz K, Rimer BK. *Theory at a Glance: A Guide for Health Promotion Practice*. NIH Pub. No. 97-3896. Washington, DC: National Cancer Institute, National Institutes of Health, U.S. Department of Health and Human Services; 1997.

Institute of Medicine. *Health Literacy: A Prescription to End Confusion*. Washington, DC: National Academies Press; 2004.

Institute of Medicine. *Unequal Treatment*. Washington, DC: National Academies Press; 2002.

Katz DL, Friedman R, Lucan SC. *Nutrition in Clinical Practice. 3rd ed*. Philadelphia, PA: Lippincott Williams & Wilkins; 2014.

Stern AM, Markel H. The history of vaccines and immunization: familiar patterns, new challenges. *Health Aff (Millwood)*. 2005;24(3):611-621.

WEBSITES

Infectious Disease Society: www.idsociety.org

Resources to treat tobacco use and dependence: https://www.ahrq.gov/professionals/clinicians-providers/guidelines-recommendations/tobacco/index.html

Robert Wood Johnson Foundation (regarding health care disparities): https://www.rwjf.org/en/our-focus-areas/topics/health-disparities.html

Think Cultural Health: A Physician's Practical Guide to Culturally Competent Care: https://cccm.thinkculturalhealth.hhs.gov/

US Preventive Services Task Force Recommendations (regarding primary prevention): https://www.uspreventiveservicestaskforce.org/BrowseRec/Index/browse-recommendations

Vaccinations and antimicrobial prophylaxis: https://www.cdc.gov/vaccines/index.html

REVIEW QUESTIONS

1. Which of the following is a relatively minor contributor to individual health?
   A. Household income
   B. Personal education
   C. Clean water
   D. Adequate food
   E. Health care

2. A 63-year-old man has high blood pressure, high cholesterol, and poorly controlled diabetes. His physician is concerned that he is at high risk for a heart attack and counsels him to quit smoking. According to the health belief model, for the patient to change his behavior and quit smoking, he must believe:
   A. Smoking is a disease
   B. He can easily survive a heart attack
   C. Quitting will be difficult
   D. Quitting can prevent a heart attack
   E. The physician has the patient's best interests in mind

3. The patient from question 2 considered his physician's advice and purchased nicotine gum. By the transtheoretical model, the purchase of the gum represents what stage of change?
   A. Precontemplation
   B. Contemplation
   C. Preparation
   D. Action
   E. Maintenance

4. Mother cows (*vacca* in Latin) pass protection from disease to their calves through breast milk. Similarly, human mothers can pass protection from disease to their infants through breast milk. Both such transfers of immunity are examples of:
   A. Vaccination
   B. Passive immunity
   C. Active immunity
   D. Herd immunity
   E. Cell-mediated immunity

5. A population's risk of disease unvaccinated is 90%. With vaccine that risk falls to 10%. The vaccine's effectiveness is thus $(0.9 - 0.1)/0.9 = 88.9\%$. This quantity is equivalent to the:
   A. Attack rate (AR)
   B. Number needed to treat (NNT)
   C. Relative risk (RR)
   D. Relative risk reduction (RRR)
   E. Absolute risk reduction (ARR)

6. Which of the following is a valid medical reason not to immunize a child (or an adult)?
   A. Redness and swelling at the injection site following a previous vaccination
   B. Fever from a previous vaccination
   C. Fever at presentation for vaccine
   D. Current therapy with antibiotic
   E. Encephalopathy of unknown cause within 7 days of previous vaccination

7. After a lecture on diabetes management, a medical student tells a patient, "Your hyperglycemia is well above the normal range. The indicated treatment at this time is insulin." The patient stares blankly. When the attending physician enters the room, she asks the patient, "What do you call your problem? What do you think causes it, and how do you think we should treat it?" The patient replies, "I have 'the sugar.' I think it's because I eat too many sweets. I think I need to cut back on sweets." The physician nods and says, "You're right in that you have too much sugar in the wrong places, and your body is not handling it well. Certainly the foods you choose to eat, including sweets, are an important part of getting your sugar under control. Let's talk about how we can improve your sugar by changing the kinds of foods you eat, then about other ways we may need to consider to get the problem under control." In this scenario, the attending physician's approach is sensitive to:
   A. Cultural competency and health literacy
   B. Cultural competency but not health literacy
   C. Health literacy but not cultural competency
   D. Neither health literacy nor cultural competency
   E. Only to the medication agenda of the medical student

8. A woman has taken an online calculator to estimate her risk for developing breast cancer. It has shown an increased

risk, and she is now asking about using selective estrogen receptor modulators. This process is an example of:
A. General health promotion
B. Specific protection
C. Risk assessment and specific protection
D. Chemoprevention, but not risk assessment
E. Prevention of deficiency states

ANSWERS AND EXPLANATIONS

1. **E.** Health care is a relatively minor contributor to individual health. The most fundamental contributors to individual health have nothing to do with health care delivery, quality, or access. Far more basic and more important are social determinants. Socioeconomic conditions such as household income (A) and personal education (B) provide examples. These factors partially determine whether people have the means and knowledge necessary to engage in the types of prudent behaviors that will support health (e.g., eating well and exercising). Other social determinants include discrimination, persecution, segregation, and the inequitable distribution of money, power, and resources. The distribution of resources to meet basic human needs is especially important. The availability of adequate food (C) and clean water (D) provide examples.

2. **D.** According to the health belief model, patients must believe that the preventive measure is effective in preventing the disease. Patients should also believe that there are no serious barriers to obtaining the preventive measure. In this case, the patient would need to believe that there are no significant barriers to quitting, not that quitting will be difficult (C). The physician's motivations (E) are not a factor in the model. However, the information the physician provides may be a factor; the patient must believe that he is at risk for the possible outcome (heart attack) and that this outcome is serious, not that he can easily survive (B). Smoking in this scenario is the behavioral risk factor, not the disease (A).

3. **C.** Preparation is the stage of experimenting with small changes, in this case toward quitting smoking. Preceding preparation are precontemplation (A), not yet thinking about quitting, and contemplation (B), weighing the benefits and costs of quitting. Following preparation are action (D), taking the definitive step by quitting, and maintenance (E), taking measures to remain smoke free.

4. **B.** Passive immunity is protection against an infectious disease provided by circulating antibodies made in another organism. In the examples given, there is the passive transfer of antibodies through milk from mother to young. Antibodies are humoral immunity, not cell-mediated immunity (E). Humoral immunity, when passively acquired, is short lived but can also result from active immunity (C), when an organism generates protective antibodies itself, and is longer lasting in this case (often lasting a lifetime). Vaccination (A) is one way to produce active immunity. Natural infection is another way. Herd immunity (D) is a

population concept, describing the reduced ability of a disease to transmit through a population as a result of immunity to the disease in a percentage of individuals.

5. **D.** Mathematically, RRR is the absolute risk reduction (ARR) over the risk of disease in treated people (E). With vaccine effectiveness, ARR = risk in unvaccinated people minus risk in people treated with vaccine, or $0.9 - 0.1 = 80\%$. Thus the vaccine would reduce the risk of disease 80% in absolute terms. The number needed to treat (B) is equal to 1 divided by the ARR, or $1/0.8 = 1.25$. Rounding up to the nearest whole person, this means only 2 people would need to be vaccinated for at least 1 to benefit (or more precisely, only 5 would need to be vaccinated for 4 to benefit). Numerically, the relative risk (C) would be the risk of disease in vaccinated people divided by the risk in unvaccinated people, or $0.1/0.9 = 0.11$. (Note: $1 - RR = RRR$.) The attack rate (AR) is a separate consideration for vaccinated and unvaccinated people (A): Among vaccinated people, AR is the number of vaccinated persons ill with the disease divided by the total number vaccinated; among unvaccinated people, AR is the number of unvaccinated persons ill with the disease divided by the total number of unvaccinated persons. The question does not give enough information to calculate either of these "rates."

6. **E.** The medical contraindications to vaccination are few, mostly limited to very rare, very severe conditions. Examples include unexplained encephalitis (DTAP, Tdap, Td), and pregnancy or immunocompromised status (with live virus vaccines MMR, varicella zoster). Answer choices A and B represent inconsequential and relatively uncommon reactions that can occur with the administration of any injectable product. Choices C and D suggest concurrent illness and are not contraindications to administering any vaccines. Moreover, there is no upper limit of vaccines that can be administered in a single visit, and almost without exception, any vaccine can be administered at the same time as any other vaccine; the exception is that live vaccines should not be administered during the same visit and should be separated by 4 weeks or more.

7. **A.** The attending physician takes an approach that is respectful of and responsive to the health beliefs of the patient (cultural competency) and conveys information at a basic level, without jargon, in a way that can be understood by even someone with limited health literacy. For these reasons, answer choices B, C, and D are incorrect. Although the physician may agree with the medical student that insulin is indicated at this time, she does not let the medication prescribing drive the agenda (E).

8. **C.** This patient is undergoing risk assessment as well as counseling regarding a strategy for specific protection (i.e., estrogen receptor modulators). Using estrogen receptor modulators constitutes chemoprevention. Since this is specific protection, A is wrong. B is correct, but incomplete, since risk assessment is missing. For the same reasons, D is incorrect. Medication use in this case does not correct a deficiency state, such as folic acid supplementation, therefore E is incorrect.

16

Principles and Practice of Secondary Prevention

"Treatment without prevention is simply unsustainable."

Bill Gates

Secondary prevention is based on early detection of disease followed by treatment. **Screening** is the process of evaluating a population of individuals for asymptomatic disease or a risk factor for developing a disease or becoming injured. In contrast to case finding, which focuses on individuals undergoing clinical care, screening applies to populations of individuals eligible for a specific screening test. These include students in a school or workers in an industry, for example, as well as asymptomatic patients in routine clinical practice. Because a positive screening test result usually is not conclusive evidence of a disease or condition, it must be followed by a *diagnostic* test. For example, a positive finding on a screening mammogram examination must be followed by additional diagnostic imaging or a biopsy to rule out breast cancer.

As shown in Fig. 16.1, the process of screening is complex and involves a series of actions. In this regard, initiating screening is similar to boarding a roller coaster: Participants must continue until they reach the end of the process. Many consumers assume that screening will automatically be valuable or cost effective; this explains the popularity of screening tests in general and the direct-to-consumer marketing of tests such as genomic analysis. In contrast, many preventive medicine specialists demand that screening meet the same rigorous standards of evidence and cost effectiveness as therapeutic interventions. A case may be made for even higher standards. Screening means looking for trouble. It involves, by definition, individuals with no perception of disease, most of whom are well. Therefore great potential exists to do net harm if screening is performed inappropriately or if the test produces many false-positive and false-negative results.

Screening is different from **case finding,** which is the process of identifying latent disease among asymptomatic patients in the course of medical care. If a patient is being seen in a medical care setting, clinicians and other health care workers usually take a thorough medical history and perform a careful physical examination and, if indicated, obtain laboratory tests. Establishing baseline findings and laboratory values in this way may produce case finding if diseases and conditions are discovered, and in some situations is considered good medicine, but is not true screening.

A program to take annual blood pressure of employees of a business or industry would be considered screening, whereas performing chest radiography for a patient who was just admitted to a hospital for elective surgery would be called *case finding.* The distinction between screening and case finding is sometimes blurred in practice, and some professional societies do not distinguish between the two in their recommendations regarding screening. Chapter 7 discusses some of the quantitative issues involved in assessing the accuracy and performance of screening, including sensitivity, specificity, and predictive values of tests. In this chapter we assume the reader is comfortable with these concepts. The purpose here is to discuss broader public health issues concerning screening and case finding. Chapter 18 provides an extensive discussion of the development of evidence-based clinical practice guidelines for screening and other prevention services in the clinical encounter.

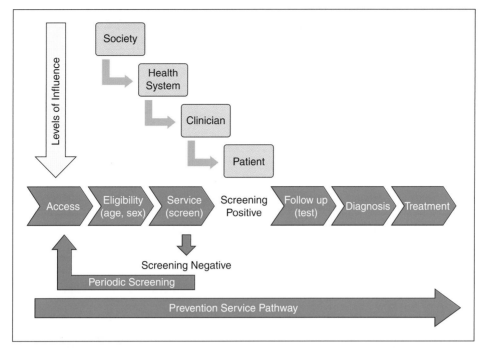

Fig. 16.1 The Process of Screening. Screening involves a series of consecutive steps in a clinical pathway that begins with accessing the health care system, determining eligibility for screening, and obtaining the screening test. Individuals with positive results generally proceed to a follow-up or confirmatory test (e.g., biopsy) that leads to diagnosis and treatment. In the case of periodic screening (e.g., mammography), those with negative results reenter the screening pool for future screening. Several factors influence whether individuals are appropriately screened, including those at societal, health system, clinician, and patient levels. (Nelson HD, Cantor A, Wagner J, et al. Achieving Health Equity in Preventive Services. Comparative Effectiveness Review No. 222. AHRQ Publication No. 20-EHC022-EF. Rockville, MD: Agency for Healthcare Research and Quality; November 2019)

1. POPULATION SCREENING

1.1 OBJECTIVES OF SCREENING

Population screening programs (sometimes also called **community screening**) seek to test large numbers of individuals for one or more diseases or risk factors in various settings (e.g., educational, work, recreational) on a voluntary basis, often with little or no direct financial outlay by the individuals being screened (Table 16.1). For screening in clinical settings, many of the same objectives and requirements apply.

1.2 MINIMUM REQUIREMENTS FOR POPULATION SCREENING PROGRAMS

A screening test is like a smoke detector. If it works well, it can save lives. However, it does not help if it goes off as soon as you fry a pancake (false positives, in statistical terms), or only if the building is already engulfed in flames (false negatives). A smoke detector inside a remote, uninhabitable home makes no sense; neither should it be put somewhere where nobody can or wants to extinguish the fire. Similarly, there are minimum requirements for establishing safe, ethical, and

cost-effective screening programs. They fall into the following three areas:
1. Disease requirements (for smoke detector: What kind of building are we protecting?)
2. Screening test requirements (corresponds to smoke detector responding to frying pancakes or burning building)
3. Health care system requirements (What is the response to the smoke alarm?)

If any of the requirements are not at least partially met, an extensive population-wide screening program may be inappropriate. Table 16.2 outlines these requirements in four common screening programs, for hypertension, high cholesterol, cervical cancer, and ovarian cancer, as discussed in Section 1.2.d.

1.2.a Disease Requirements

- The disease must be *serious* (i.e., produce significant morbidity or mortality), or there is no reason to screen in the first place.
- Even if a disease is serious, there must be an *effective therapy* for the disease detected. Screening is of no value unless there is a good chance that detecting the disease in the *presymptomatic stage* would be followed by effective therapy. Furthermore, the benefits of detecting the condition in a few

TABLE 16.1   Objectives of Screening Programs

Screening Target	Objective	Examples
Disease	Treatment to reduce mortality	Cancer
	Treatment to prevent complications	Hypertension
	Treatment to eradicate infection and prevent its spread	Gonorrhea, syphilis, tuberculosis, human immunodeficiency virus (HIV)
	Changes in diet and lifestyle to prevent occurrence of disease	Coronary artery disease, type 2 diabetes mellitus
Risk Factors		
Behavioral	Change in unhealthy behaviors	Cigarette smoking, unsafe sexual practices
Environmental	Change in hazardous occupation	Chronic obstructive pulmonary disease from work in a dusty trade
Metabolic	Treatment or change in diet and increase in physical activity	Obesity

TABLE 16.2   Requirements for Screening Programs and Ratings of Example Methods to Detect Hypertension, Elevated Cholesterol Levels, Cervical Cancer, and Ovarian Cancer

REQUIREMENTS	SCREENING METHOD AND RATING[a]			
	Sphygmomanometer Reading (Hypertension)	Serum Cholesterol Test (Dyslipidemia)	Pap Smear (Cervical Cancer)	Ultrasound and Blood Work (Ovarian Cancer)
Disease Requirements				
Disease is serious.	++	++	++	++
Effective treatment exists.	++	++	+	+/−
Natural history of disease is understood.	++	++	++	+
Disease occurs frequently.	++	++	+	−
Other diseases or conditions may be detected.	−	−	−	+
Screening Test Requirements				
Test is quick to perform.	++	+	+	−
Test is easy to administer.	++	++	+	−
Test is inexpensive.	++	+	+	−
Test is safe.	++	++	+	+/−
Test is acceptable to participants.	++	++	+	+/−
Sensitivity, specificity, and other operating characteristics are acceptable.	++	++	+	−
Health Care System Requirements				
Method meets the requirements for screening in a community setting.	++	++	+	−
Method meets the requirements for case finding in a medical care setting.	++	++	++	+/−

[a]Ratings are applied to four conditions for which community screening has often been undertaken: hypertension, tested by a sphygmomanometer reading of blood pressure; elevated cholesterol levels, with total cholesterol measurement based on a rapid screening of blood; cervical cancer, tested by Papanicolaou (Pap) smear; and ovarian cancer, tested by ultrasound and blood work. Ratings are as follows: ++, good; +, satisfactory; −, unsatisfactory; +/−, depends on disease stage.

people should outweigh the harms that occur (and accrue) to people with a false-positive test, including unnecessary, invasive workups and treatment. For example, at present, there is no value in screening for pancreatic cancer because the chance of cure by standard medical and surgical methods is extremely small.

- The natural history of a disease must be understood clearly enough to know that there is a significant window of time between when the disease is detectable and effective treatment can occur. For example, colon cancer follows an established disease mechanism from small polyps in the colon to a colon cancer. Early detection and surgical removal of a polyp prevents the development of cancer, and likely is curative. On the other hand, treatment of the disease in earlier stages must produce better outcomes than later treatment. This is relevant to breast cancer screening: A large portion of the mortality gains in the past years may have come from improvements in the treatment of breast cancer rather than early detection from screening.[1]
- The disease or condition must not be too rare or too common. Screening for a rare disease usually means that many false-positive test results would be expected for each true finding. This increases the cost and difficulties of discovering individuals who truly are ill or at high risk, and it causes anxiety and inconvenience for those who must undergo more testing because of false-positive results. Unless the benefits from discovering one case are very high, as in treating a newborn who has phenylketonuria or congenital hypothyroidism, it is seldom cost effective to screen general populations for a rare disease.

Screening for common conditions may produce such a large proportion of positive results that it would be too expensive to provide effective follow-up. It is possible, however, that screening for some common risk factors, such as elevated cholesterol levels, may provide opportunities for education and motivation to seek treatment and change behavior.

1.2.b Screening Test Requirements
- The screening test must be reasonably quick, easy, and inexpensive, or the costs of large-scale screening in terms of time, effort, and money would be prohibitive.
- The screening test must be safe and acceptable to the persons being screened and to their clinicians. If the individuals to be screened object to a procedure (as frequently occurs with colonoscopy), they are unlikely to participate.
- The sensitivity, specificity, positive predictive value, and other operating characteristics of a screening test must be known and acceptable. False-positive and false-negative test results must be considered. An additional difficulty in using screening tests in the general population is that the characteristics of the population screened may be different than the population for whom the screening was developed. For example, if the prevalence of a particular cancer is much lower in the general population than in the screening group initially studied when the test was developed, the predictive value of a positive screening test in the general population will be much lower (see Chapter 7).

1.2.c Health Care System Requirements
- People with positive test results must have access to follow-up. Because screening tests are usually not conclusive, persons who have positive results must receive further diagnostic testing to rule in or rule out actual disease. Follow-up testing may be expensive, time consuming, or painful, and could cause harm. With many screening programs, most of the efforts and costs are in the follow-up phase, not in the initial screening (see upcoming discussion on ovarian cancer). These costs are not trivial (e.g., for breast cancer, yearly outlays for false-positive mammograms and overdiagnoses have been estimated to be around $4 billion).[2]
- Before a screening program for a particular disease is undertaken, treatment already should be available for people known to have the disease. If there are limited resources, it is not ethical or cost effective to allow persons with symptoms of the disease to go untreated and yet screen for the same disease in apparently well persons.
- Individuals who are screened and diagnosed must have access to treatment, or the process is ethically flawed. In addition to being unethical, it makes no medical sense to bring the persons screened to the point of informing them of a positive test result and then abandoning them. This is a major problem for population screening efforts because many people who come for screening have little or no medical care coverage. Therefore the cost for the evaluation of the positive screening tests and the subsequent treatment (if disease is detected) are often borne by a local hospital or other institution. In designing a population screening program, it is vital to consider beforehand who will bear the cost of further diagnosis and treatment, especially for false-positive results.
- The treatment should be acceptable to the people being screened. Otherwise, individuals who require treatment would not undertake it, and the screening would have accomplished nothing. For example, some men may not want treatment for prostate cancer because of possible incontinence and impotence resulting from treatment.
- The population to be screened should be clearly defined so that the resulting data are epidemiologically useful. Although screening at health fairs and in shopping centers provides the opportunity to educate the public about health topics, the data obtained about their effectiveness are mixed.[3]
- It should be clear who is responsible for the screening and its follow-up, which cutoff points are to be used for considering a test result "positive," and how the findings will become part of participants' medical record at their usual place of care.

1.2.d Application of Minimum Screening Requirements to Specific Programs
Table 16.2 applies the previously described criteria to the following four conditions for which community screening has been undertaken:
1. Hypertension, tested by a sphygmomanometer reading of blood pressure.

2. Elevated cholesterol levels, based on a screening of blood.
3. Cervical cancer, with Papanicolaou smear.
4. Ovarian cancer, for which yearly ultrasound and blood testing was considered but rejected.

As shown in Table 16.2, screening for hypertension, hyper-cholesterolemia, and cervical cancer generally fulfill the minimum requirements for a population screening program. However, a screening program using yearly ultrasound scans and a blood test (cancer antigen 125 [CA-125]) to detect ovarian cancer in the general population fails at three critical points. First, the yield of detection is low. Second, there are too many false positive results. Because abnormal results require invasive workup, the harm of false-positive tests is substantial. Third, as numerous studies have shown, only a small proportion of ovarian cancers can be cured by the time they are detected.[4] Because of these problems, community screening of the general population for ovarian cancer is not recommended.

For many screening programs, uncertainty surrounds general screening issues such as what age to start the screening, when to stop, how often to repeat the screening, and whether the methods yield accurate results. The age at which to begin screening women for breast cancer is particularly controversial because breast cancer is less common in younger women, but often more aggressive than later in life, and the harms of screening (e.g., false positives) are higher.[5]

1.3 ETHICAL CONCERNS ABOUT POPULATION SCREENING

The ethical standards are important to consider when an apparently well population of individuals who have *not* sought medical care is screened. In this case, the professionals involved have an important obligation to show that the benefits of being screened outweigh the costs and potential risks. The methods used in performing any public screening program should be safe, with minimal side effects.

1.4 POTENTIAL BENEFITS AND HARMS OF SCREENING PROGRAMS

The potential benefits of screening include reduced mortality, reduced morbidity, and reassurance. With the goal of screening programs to identify disease in the early, presymptomatic stage so that treatment can be initiated, the main potential benefit is reduced mortality for many programs. However, some screening programs have a goal of identifying the disease in the early stages, when less invasive treatment is possible and effective (e.g., taking a small piece of breast tissue rather than removing the entire breast). Another potential benefit of screening is the reassurance to both individuals and providers in the case of a negative result.

The potential adverse effects (harms) of all screening programs also need to be considered. Some screening procedures may be uncomfortable, such as mammography, or require preparation, such as colonoscopy (colon cleansing).

Colonoscopy also carries procedural risks such as bleeding and perforation. Other harms of screening include anxiety from false-positive results, harm from further diagnostic testing (e.g., from biopsies in lung cancer screening), false reassurance for patients with false-negative tests, overdiagnosis, and costs to individuals and society from lost work and productivity.

Test errors are a major concern in screening (see Chapter 7). **False-positive test results** lead to extra time and costs and can cause anxiety and discomfort to individuals whose results were in error. When screening tests are repeated every 1 to 2 years, the cumulative impact on those undergoing the screening needs to be considered (see upcoming discussion). In the case of screening for breast cancer, the more screening mammograms a woman undergoes, the more likely she is to experience a false-positive result. False-positive rates of screening mammography vary by age and population screened but can be substantial. When screening begins at age 40, the probability of a woman having at least one false-positive scan may be close to 60%.[6,7]

False-negative test results can be even worse. An implied promise of screening is that if individuals are screened for a particular disease and found to have negative results, they need not worry about that disease. However, no screening test is perfect: The rate of false-negative mammograms has been estimated at 1 to 1.5 per 1000 women.[8] In the case of genetic screening, things are even more complicated because testing negative for a particular gene does not mean that you cannot develop disease via other pathways. For example, women without deleterious mutations in the *BRCA* cancer genes can still develop ovarian cancer via other pathways. False-negative results may lead people with early symptoms to be less concerned and thus lead to delayed medical visits that might otherwise have been made promptly. False-negative results also may falsely reassure clinicians. False-negative results can be detrimental to the health of the people whose results were in error, and if test results delay the diagnosis in people who have an infectious disease, such as tuberculosis or human immunodeficiency virus (HIV), the screening tests can be dangerous to the health of others as well.

Overdiagnosis is another potential harm of screening programs. For example, screening mammography may lead to a diagnosis of a breast cancer that would never cause symptoms or death during the woman's lifetime. Actions taken in response to such findings, including surgery, may result in a scenario where the ostensible "cure" is in fact worse than the disease. In addition, studies are now identifying a rise in early stage invasive breast cancer after the introduction of screening mammography with no resultant drop in late stage breast cancer. Data such as this suggest that about 2 of 10 women with a new diagnosis of invasive breast cancer may have the true disease, yet it would not have ever bothered them or have presented clinically in their lifetime in the absence of screening.[8]

1.5 BIAS IN SCREENING PROGRAMS

It is not easy to establish the effectiveness of a population screening effort unless a randomized controlled trial (RCT) is conducted, which reduces the potential for bias. In cancer, an association between screening and longer survival does not prove a cause-and-effect relationship because of possible problems such as selection bias, lead-time bias, and length bias.

Selection bias may affect a screening program in different directions, all of which may make it difficult to generalize findings to the overall population. On one hand, individuals may want to participate because they have a family history of the disease or are otherwise aware that they are at higher risk of contracting the disease. In this case, the screening program would find more cases than expected in the overall population, exaggerating the apparent utility of screening. On the other hand, individuals who are more "health conscious" may *preferentially* seek out screening programs or may be less likely to drop out.

Lead-time bias occurs when screening detects disease earlier in its natural history than would otherwise have occurred, so that the period from diagnosis to death is increased. However, the additional *lead-time* (increased time during which diagnosis is known) may not have changed the natural history of the disease or extended the longevity of life. This lead-time bias tends to operate in screening for cancers, no matter how aggressive the tumors (Fig. 16.2).

Length bias occurs when the full spectrum of a particular tumor, such as prostate cancer, includes cancers that range from very aggressive to very slow growing. Individuals with slow-growing tumors live longer than individuals with the aggressive tumors, so they are more likely to be discovered by screening. Screening programs often select for the less aggressive, slower growing tumors, and these patients are likely to survive longer after detection, regardless of the treatment given (Fig. 16.3).

Selection, lead-time, and length biases apply to both case finding and population screening. Given the potential problems in showing the true effectiveness of screening, great care must be exercised to ensure a screening program is worthwhile.

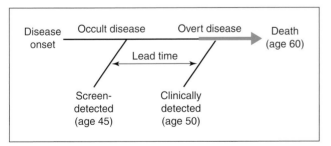

Fig. 16.2 Lead-Time Bias. Overestimation of survival among screen-detected cases (relative to those detected by signs and symptoms) when survival is measured from diagnosis. This patient survives for 10 years after clinical diagnosis and survives for 15 years after the screening-detected diagnosis. However, this simply reflects earlier diagnosis, because the overall survival time of the patient is unchanged. (From Black WC, Welch HG: Advances in diagnostic imaging and overestimates of disease prevalence and the benefits of therapy. *N Engl J Med* 328:1237–1243, 1993.)

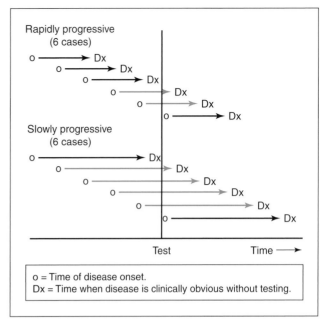

Fig. 16.3 Length Bias: Overestimation of Survival Duration among Screening-Detected Cases. The probability of detecting cases is directly proportional to the length of time during which they are detectable. Therefore more slowly progressing cases are found by screening. In this example of 12 patients, 2 of 6 rapidly progressive cases are detected, whereas 4 of 6 slowly progressive cases are detected. (From Black WC, Welch HG: Advances in diagnostic imaging and overestimates of disease prevalence and the benefits of therapy. N Engl J Med 328:1237–1243, 1993.)

1.6 REPETITION OF SCREENING PROGRAMS

There are pitfalls in not carefully considering the details of repeat screening efforts. This is particularly true if an initial major screening effort is considered a great success, and enthusiasm may lead the organizers to repeat the screening too soon (e.g., 1 year later). Unless the population screened the second time is very different from the one screened the first time, results of a screening effort repeated after a short interval are likely to be disappointing. This is because the initial screening would have detected **prevalent cases** (cases accumulated over many years), whereas the repeated screening would detect only **incident cases** (new cases since the last screening), making the number of cases detected in the second screening effort smaller.[9]

Again, the more screening tests done on an individual, the more likely positive findings will occur, both true positive and false positive.

1.7 SIMULTANEOUS SCREENING FOR MULTIPLE DISEASES (MULTIPHASIC SCREENING)

Multiphasic screening programs involve screening for a variety of diseases in the same individual at one point in time. There are some advantages to simultaneous screening (e.g., during pregnancy visits or when screening for sexually transmitted infections). Some investigators have argued that multiphasic screening makes community efforts more efficient. When a sample of blood is drawn, for example, it is easy to perform a variety of tests using automated laboratory equipment.

However, in many situations, the yield of multiphasic screening is doubtful. One problem is that multiphasic screening can detect diseases or abnormal conditions that were already found earlier and are already being treated, in which case funds are being used for unnecessary testing. Another problem is that multiphasic screening results in a relatively high frequency of false-positive results, which requires many participants to return for more expensive follow-up tests.

For each disease-free person screened with a battery of **independent tests** (tests that measure different values), the probability that at least one of the screening tests would yield a false-positive finding can be expressed as $(1 - [1 - alpha]^n)$, where alpha is the false-positive error rate (see Chapter 7) and n is the number of screening tests done. If two screening tests are performed and alpha is 5% (making the test specificity 95%), the probability of a disease-free person being recalled for further testing is $(1 - [0.95]^2) = (1 - [0.9025]) =$ almost 10%. If four tests are performed, the probability is $(1 - [0.95]^4) = (1 - [0.8145]) = 18.5\%$. As Table 16.3 shows, if 25 tests are performed, more than 70% of disease-free individuals would return for unnecessary but often costly follow-up testing.

1.8 GENETIC SCREENING

Advances in genetic testing have made it more feasible to screen individual patients and populations for many different diseases. Indications for genetic testing may include **presymptomatic testing,** such as a patient tested for Huntington disease. If the test is positive, patients are virtually certain of developing the disease over their lifetime. Alternatively, testing might be done to establish the predisposition for a disease, called **susceptibility testing.** This is an emerging form of testing for a variety of diseases, such as BRCA-associated cancers.

BRCA1 and *BRCA2* are cancer susceptibility genes that increase a person's risk for various cancers, including breast, ovarian, and fallopian tube cancers. Deleterious mutations in the *BRCA* genes can increase a woman's lifetime risk to 45% to 65% for breast cancer and 10% to 39% for ovarian cancer.[10] However, not everyone who has the gene mutations will develop cancer. The BRCA mutations occur in the general population in 0.2% to 0.3% of women, but are more common in some groups, such as Ashkenazi Jews (2%).[10] The US Preventive Services Task Force (USPSTF) recommends that women with a family history of BRCA-associated cancers receive genetic counseling and testing.[10] Women with a mutation may choose to take medications to reduce their risk for cancer or undergo risk-reducing surgery of breasts, ovaries, and fallopian tubes to prevent cancer from developing in these sites.

However, the psychologic impact of genetic test results on patients is often counterintuitive and poorly understood. Significant harms as well as benefits can come from genetic testing,[11] which is why genetic counseling is recommended before testing. Genetic testing in the setting of a health care encounter needs to be distinguished from direct-to-consumer marketing of genetic testing at home, which has no such safeguards and is discouraged by most professional societies.[12]

In contrast, **prenatal screening** has made a significant impact on population health for certain groups. This is particularly well established for individuals of Jewish Ashkenazi heritage, who have high carrier rates for some otherwise rare genetic disorders (e.g., Tay-Sachs disease). For this group, genetic testing combined with careful pretest and posttest counseling has helped couples make informed decisions regarding family planning. Such testing has also led to a decrease in the incidence of screened diseases.[13]

Several quality requirements beyond the accuracy of the test are specific to genetic screening tests. The genetic abnormality found must also correspond to a specific disease or increased risk for disease (**clinical validity**). Even if the test detects a genetic abnormality that meaningfully predicts disease, the information may not be useful to the patient (**clinical utility**).[14,15] For most genetic tests, there is little evidence of clinical utility, and the standards for analytic and clinical validity are still evolving.[15] What is clear, much more than for other diagnostic tests, the effects of the test on both the individual tested and the family need to be considered. Lastly, genomic screening seems to be predicated on the idea that the only way to change genetic vulnerability is through changing genes. In fact, gene expression is influenced by multiple other factors, some of which may be affected by lifestyle interventions.

TABLE 16.3 Correlation Between Number of Screening Tests and Persons With False-Positive Result	
No. of Screening Tests Performed[a]	Percentage of Persons With at Least One False-Positive Test Result[b]
1	50%
2	9.8%
4	18.5%
5	22.6%
10	40.1%
20	64.2%
25	72.3%

[a]It is assumed that the tests measure different values (i.e., the tests are independent).
[b]Percentages are based on tests that each has a 5% false-positive error rate.
Data from Schoenberg BS: The "abnormal" laboratory result. *Postgrad Med* 47:151–155, 1970.

2. INDIVIDUAL SCREENING AND CASE FINDING

2.1 WELL CHILD/WELL VISITS

The yearly well visit has emerged as the clinical setting for primary care providers to discuss health maintenance with patients and to screen for disease. This visit provides a context in which most of the knowledge and skills discussed in this book come together. The content of the visit is guided by clinical prevention recommendations that vary by age, sex, pregnancy status, and risk factors. In the United States, these include recommendations from the USPSTF,[16] Women's Preventive Services Initiative (WPSI),[17] and Bright Futures for children.[18] The USPSTF provides an online tool and app to determine which prevention services are appropriate for individual patients, and the WPSI and Bright Futures provide age-based charts listing recommended services.

Multiple tools can help the provider elicit family history of the patient as well as individual risk factors (see risk assessment discussion in Chapter 15). A useful approach is to calculate a person's risk score, such as the "risk age." In addition to data such as height, weight, blood pressure, cholesterol level, and previous and present diseases, a person's lifestyle and family history are integrated to determine the risk age. The underlying algorithms are derived from large cohort studies, such as the Framingham Heart Study. The **risk age** is defined as the age at which the average individual would have the same risk of dying as the person being assessed. If the assessed person's risk age is older than his or her chronologic age, that means he or she has a higher risk of dying than the average individual of the same chronologic age. Likewise, if the assessed person's risk age is younger than the chronologic age, the person has a lower risk of dying than the average individual of the same chronologic age. Another clever application of the same tool is *lung age* (i.e., the age that

corresponds to a patient's spirometry findings). This has been found to be effective in encouraging smoking cessation.[19]

With increasing information on genomic, biologic, behavioral, environmental, and other data on individual drivers of health, the field of **precision medicine** aims to support personalized health care decision making. In the future, this approach may also utilize personal electronic devices to deliver feedback and behavioral intervention in real time.[20]

3. SCREENING GUIDELINES AND RECOMMENDATIONS

Many of the organizations that issue screening guidelines and recommendations include the following:
- Specialty organizations (e.g., American Urological Association)
- Primary care specialties (e.g., American College of Physicians, American Academy of Family Physicians)
- Foundations for the treatment and prevention of particular diseases (e.g., American Cancer Society)
- Organizations dedicated to developing recommendations for screening and prevention (e.g., USPSTF [see Chapter 18], American College of Preventive Medicine [ACPM], Canadian Task Force on the Periodic Health Examination)

In many cases, these organizations agree on their screening recommendations. However, certain diseases and screening methods have led to major controversies, such as breast and prostate cancer screening (Box 16.1). In general, the specialty organizations are more likely to recommend screening for conditions related to their field. In contrast, the ACPM and USPSTF tend to only recommend screening programs for which there is unequivocal evidence of benefits in patient outcomes (Box 16.2 discusses lung cancer screening). The research field that studies how best to deliver evidence-based interventions is called **health care delivery research** (or **health services research**).

BOX 16.1 Breast and Prostate Cancer Screening Recommendations: "How much worry and lost quality of life is one life saved worth?"

Breast and prostate cancer illustrate the challenges of weighing evidence of small reductions in mortality against adverse effects of screening and treatment. Because of the impact of screening biases, reductions in mortality in the screened population provide the strongest evidence of effectiveness for cancer screening. Past debates about changes in the US Preventive Services Task Force (USPSTF) recommendations from universal to selective screening for breast and prostate cancer demonstrate different perceptions of benefits and harms among the public, politicians, and health care professionals.[21]

Breast Cancer

Many women die prematurely of breast cancer, and mammography screening is intended to detect and treat cancer in early stages to prevent death. However, mammography is an imperfect screening test. Many women whose cancers are detected by screening mammography die of their disease despite early detection. Also, only a fraction of breast abnormalities detected

on a screening mammogram actually lead to a saved life. Most abnormalities are false-positive findings or lesions that would not lead to death (i.e., overdiagnosis). These lesions include ductal carcinoma in situ (DCIS), which is associated with an increased risk for invasive breast cancer but is not harmful itself. No one can predict which women with DCIS will eventually develop invasive breast cancer. Thus women diagnosed with DCIS after screening mammography often undergo breast surgery, chemotherapy, and radiation treatment that is burdensome and costly.

If screening mammography actually saves lives, both breast cancer–associated mortality and total mortality should decrease in screened populations. This hypothesis has been tested in multiple randomized controlled trials of screening. However, breast cancer mortality was not reduced for women in their 40s or above age 75 years in trials, and only modestly reduced for women in their 50s (8 deaths prevented per 10,000 women over 10 years) and 60s (21 deaths prevented per 10,000

Continued

BOX 16.1   Breast and Prostate Cancer Screening Recommendations: "How much worry and lost quality of life is one life saved worth?"—cont'd

women over 10 years).[22] False-positive results were common in screening studies, approximately 50% over 10 years of screening,[6,7] and often led to additional imaging and biopsies.[5,23] Consequently, many women express distress and discomfort during the course of their screening experiences.[5]

In 2009, the USPSTF changed its breast cancer screening recommendations for women in their 40s to reflect updated results of the screening trials indicating lack of mortality benefit. Previously recommending routine screening in this population, the USPSTF argued that the potential improvement in mortality in women between ages 40 and 49 years was small at best, and that possible harms needed to be considered. Instead of screening all women in their 40s, the USPSTF recommended that physicians discuss the individual risks and benefits of screening with women and screen according to their risk/benefit preferences.

While this change was consistent with evidence, it led to a significant public backlash. Many people claimed the decision amounted to care rationing, and that the USPSTF had overstepped its mandate by weighing mortality benefits against anxiety. The USPSTF argued that the evidence did not support a one-size-fits-all recommendation and that their guidelines empowered patients and their physicians to make rational decisions based on evidence and individual values. The 2009[24] recommendations were reaffirmed in 2016, and as of this writing (2018), the USPSTF recommends routine mammography screening for women age 50 to 74 years (B level) and individualized screening for women age 40 to 49 years (C level).[25]

Prostate Cancer

Prostate cancer affects men across a broad age range and its impact on mortality varies widely; some cases are rapidly fatal, whereas others are slow growing and indolent. Screening involves measuring prostate-specific antigen (PSA) in a blood sample. However, false-positive results are common and often lead to prostate biopsies to establish a diagnosis (often without a reliable way to distinguish between indolent and aggressive disease) and treatment (e.g., surgery, radiation, and/or chemotherapy). Treatment can lead to serious harms, including erectile dysfunction, bladder and bowel incontinence, and death. For many men with screen-detected prostate cancer, the existence of prostate cancer may never have been problematic for them (most men die *with* prostate cancer, not *of* prostate cancer).

Similar to breast cancer screening, the benefits and harms of routine screening for prostate cancer are closely balanced.[26] Consequently, in 2018, the USPSTF recommended individualized screening for men age 55 to 69 years and recommended against screening in men age 70 years and older.[27]

Both these examples illustrate the need for **personalizing** screening decisions. The decision to screen for breast or prostate cancer should be based on the patient's risk, preferences, and willingness to have false-positive test results and invasive follow-up testing. While this shared decision-making approach can be complex, decision aids are available that may help individuals make informed screening decisions.

BOX 16.2   Lung Cancer Screening: Simulation Models Versus Randomized Controlled Trials

The development of new diagnostic methods offers new screening possibilities. However, conducting a randomized controlled trial (RCT) of a new screening intervention is expensive and time consuming, particularly when the outcome is a relatively rare event such as cancer or mortality. In the absence of RCTs, single-arm studies or mathematic modeling through cost-utility analysis is sometimes used to determine the effectiveness of a screening intervention (see Chapters 6 and 15). Lung cancer screening illustrates the pitfalls of these approaches.

Lung cancer remains the number-one cause of cancer mortality in the United States. For a long time, there was no effective way to screen for lung cancer. Chest x-ray and sputum examination had been previously evaluated for screening, but only led to more invasive testing with no difference in mortality. Then helical computed tomography (CT) imaging became available and seemed to offer the capacity to find small lung cancer nodules early.[28] Several uncontrolled trials were performed and showed higher cancer detection rates, but did not provide mortality outcomes.[29] Based on the difference in the distribution of cancer stages found in the screened group from that usually found in clinical practice,

several authorities advocated starting screening immediately. In these studies, patients in the screened group were much more likely to be diagnosed with early, small, and potentially curable cancers.[30] Several modeling studies of screening with helical CT were then published, with conflicting results.[31,32]

In 2002, the National Lung Screening Trial was launched. More than 53,000 participants were randomized to either three annual helical CT scans or chest x-ray films. In 2011, results indicated 247 deaths from lung cancer per 100,000 person-years in the low-dose CT group and 309 deaths per 100,000 person-years in the radiography group, representing a relative reduction in mortality from lung cancer with low-dose CT screening of 20%.[33] Although less than expected by proponents, this mortality reduction was clinically significant. A cost-effectiveness analysis was integrated into the trial and showed that screening was cost effective (see Box 14.1).

This example shows that modeling can inform decisions when no evidence is available. However, given the significant biases in uncontrolled studies that tend to overestimate screening benefits, models are often inaccurate alternatives to RCTs.

---

4. SUMMARY

The goal of secondary prevention is the detection of disease or risk factors in the presymptomatic stage, when medical, environmental, nutritional, and lifestyle interventions can be most effective. Preventive medicine specialists distinguish population screening, where all eligible individuals are tested,

from case finding, where individuals are identified with a condition during the course of clinical care. To be beneficial and cost effective, population screening must fulfill various criteria regarding the health problem to be detected, the screening test used, and the system available to provide follow-up health care for those with positive screening results.

Selection, lead-time, and length biases can lead to overestimates of benefit from screening, particularly for cancer detection. Although multiphasic screening seeks to make the process efficient by searching for many conditions at the same time, the high incidence of false-positive results and associated problems have made this technique less successful than was originally anticipated. Genetic screening introduces additional concerns, including clinical validity, clinical utility, and the impact on family members.

In clinical care, the annual well visit provides the setting to promote health maintenance, identify and address risk factors, and engage in age-appropriate screening. Such well visits are guided by clinical recommendations based on a person's individual risk factors as well as prevailing morbidity and mortality of the age group and gender. Calculating a patient's risk age from standardized algorithms can be a useful way to raise awareness of health risks and motivate behavior change.

REFERENCES

1. Welch HG, Prorok PC, O'Malley AJ, Kramer BS. Breast-cancer tumor size, overdiagnosis, and mammography screening effectiveness. *N Engl J Med.* 2016;375(15):1438-1447. doi:10.1056/NEJMoa1600249.

2. Ong MS, Mandl KD. National expenditure for false-positive mammograms and breast cancer overdiagnoses estimated at $4 billion a year. *Health Aff (Millwood).* 2015;34(4):576-583.

3. Escoffery C, Rodgers KC, Kegler MC, et al. A systematic review of special events to promote breast, cervical and colorectal cancer screening in the United States. *BMC Public Health.* 2014;14:274.

4. Henderson JT, Webber EM, Sawaya GF. Screening for Ovarian Cancer: An Updated Evidence Review for the U.S. Preventive Services Task Force. Evidence Synthesis Number 157. Rockville, MD: Agency for Healthcare Research and Quality; 2018. Available at: https://bit.ly/2RPw6Cs.

5. Nelson HD, Pappas M, Cantor A, Griffin J, Daeges M, Humphrey L. Harms of breast cancer screening: systematic review to update the 2009 U.S. Preventive Services Task Force recommendation. *Ann Intern Med.* 2016;164:256-267. doi:10.7326/M15-0970.

6. Elmore JG, Barton MB, Moceri VM, Polk S, Arena PJ, Fletcher SW. Ten-year risk of false positive screening mammograms and clinical breast examinations. *N Engl J Med.* 1998;338(16):1089-1096.

7. Hubbard RA, Kerlikowske K, Flowers CI, Yankaskas BC, Zhu W, Miglioretti DL. Cumulative probability of false-positive recall or biopsy recommendation after 10 years of screening mammography: a cohort study. *Ann Intern Med.* 2011;155(8):481-492.

8. Christopherson WM, Parker JE, Drye JC. Control of cervical cancer: preliminary report on community program. *JAMA.* 1962;182:179-182.

9. Sankaranarayanan R, Budukh AM, Rajkumar R. Effective screening programmes for cervical cancer in low- and middle-income developing countries. *Bull World Health Organ.* 2001;79:954-962.

10. US Preventive Services Task Force. Risk assessment, genetic counseling, and genetic testing for BRCA-related cancer in women: US Preventive Services Task Force Recommendation Statement. *JAMA.* 2019;322(6):652-665.

11. Nelson HD, Pappas M, Cantor A, Haney E, Holmes R. Risk assessment, genetic counseling, and genetic testing for BRCA-related cancer in women: updated evidence report and systematic review for the U.S. Preventive Services Task Force. *JAMA.* 2019;322(7):666-685.

12. Skirton H, Goldsmith L, Jackson L, O'Connor A. Direct to consumer genetic testing: a systematic review of position statements, policies and recommendations. *Clin Genet.* 2012;82(3):210-218.

13. Gross SJ, Pletcher BA, Monaghan KG. Carrier screening in individuals of Ashkenazi Jewish descent. *Genet Med.* 2008;10:54-56.

14. Katsanis SH, Katsanis N. Molecular genetic testing and the future of clinical genomics. *Nat Rev Genet.* 2013;14(6):415-426.

15. ACMG Board of Directors. Clinical utility of genetic and genomic services: a position statement of the American College of Medical Genetics and Genomics. *Genet Med.* 2015;17(6):505-507.

16. U.S. Preventive Services Task Force. *Recommendations for Primary Care Practice.* 2018. Available at: https://www.uspreventiveservicestaskforce.org/Page/Name/recommendations.

17. Women's Preventive Services Initiative. *Recommendations.* 2018. Available at: https://www.womenspreventivehealth.org/recommendations/screening-for-urinary-incontinence/.

18. Bright Futures/American Academy of Pediatrics. *Recommendations for Preventive Pediatric Health Care in Practice.* 2018. Available at: https://brightfutures.aap.org/Pages/default.aspx.

19. Parkes G, Greenhalgh T, Griffin M, Dent R. Effect on smoking quit rate of telling patients their lung age: the Step2quit randomised controlled trial. *BMJ.* 2008;13;336(7644):598-600.

20. Chambers DA, Feero WG, Khoury MJ. Convergence of implementation science, precision medicine, and the learning health care system: a new model for biomedical research. *JAMA.* 2016;315(18):1941-1942.

21. When evidence collides with anecdote, politics, and emotion: breast cancer screening. *Ann Intern Med.* 2010;152(8):531-532.

22. Nelson HD, Fu R, Cantor A, Pappas M, Daeges M, Humphrey L. Effectiveness of breast cancer screening: systematic review and meta-analysis to update the 2009 U.S. Preventive Services Task Force recommendation. *Ann Intern Med.* 2016;164:244-255. doi:10.7326/M15-0969.

23. Nelson HD, O'Meara ES, Kerlikowske K, Balch S, Miglioretti D. Factors associated with rates of false-positive and false-negative results from digital mammography screening: an analysis of registry data. *Ann Intern Med.* 2016;164:226-235. doi:10.7326/M15-0971.

24. US Preventive Services Task Force. Screening for breast cancer: U.S. Preventive Services Task Force recommendation statement. *Ann Intern Med.* 2009;151:716-726.

25. Siu AL, U.S. Preventive Services Task Force. Screening for breast cancer: U.S. Preventive Services Task Force recommendation statement. *Ann Intern Med.* 2016;164:279-296. doi:10.7326/M15-2886.

26. Fenton JJ, Weyrich MS, Durbin S, Liu Y, Bang H, Melnikow J. Prostate-specific antigen-based screening for prostate cancer: evidence report and systematic review for the US Preventive Services Task Force. *JAMA.* 2018;319(18):1914-1931. doi:10.1001/jama.2018.3712.

27. US Preventive Services Task Force. Screening for prostate cancer: US Preventive Services Task Force recommendation statement. *JAMA.* 2018;319(18):1901-1913. doi:10.1001/jama.2018.3710.

28. Kramer BS, Berg CD, Aberle DR, Prorok PC. Lung cancer screening with low-dose helical CT: results from the National Lung Screening Trial. *J Med Screen.* 2011;18:109-111.

29. National Lung Screening Trial Research Team. The National Lung Screening Trial: overview and study design. *Radiology.* 2011;258:243-253.

30. Henschke CI. CT screening for lung cancer is justified. *Nat Clin Pract Oncol.* 2007;4:440-441.

31. Bach PB, Jett JR, Pastorino U, Tockman MS, Swensen SJ, Begg CB. Computed tomography screening and lung cancer outcomes. *JAMA.* 2007;297:953-961.

32. Mahadevia PJ, Fleisher LA, Frick KD, Eng J, Goodman SN, Powe NR. Lung cancer screening with helical computed tomography in older adult smokers: a decision and cost-effectiveness analysis. *JAMA*. 2003;289:313-322.

33. National Lung Screening Trial Research Team. Reduced lung-cancer mortality with low-dose computed tomographic screening. *N Engl J Med*. 2011;365:395-409.

SELECT READINGS

Becker DH, Gardner LD. *Prevention in Clinical Practice*. 2nd ed. New York, NY: Springer; 2012.

Goetzel RZ, Staley P, Ogden L, et al. *A Framework for Patient-Centered Health Risk Assessments—Providing Health Promotion and Disease Prevention Services to Medicare Beneficiaries*. Atlanta, GA: US Department of Health and Human Services, Centers for Disease Control and Prevention; 2011. Available at: https://stacks.cdc.gov/view/cdc/23365. Accessed on 10/5/2019.

WEBSITES

Bright Futures: https://brightfutures.aap.org/Pages/default.aspx

Precision Medicine: https://ghr.nlm.nih.gov/primer/precisionmedicine/definition

Tools for obtaining family history: https://www.acog.org/Clinical-Guidance-and-Publications/Committee-Opinions/Committee-on-Genetics/Family-History-as-a-Risk-Assessment-Tool

US Preventive Services Task Force: http://www.uspreventiveservicestaskforce.org/

Women's Preventive Services Initiative: https://www.womenspreventivehealth.org/

REVIEW QUESTIONS

1. Which of the following could be an example of secondary prevention?
   A. Detection and treatment of hypertension
   B. Early treatment of diabetic nephropathy
   C. Folic acid supplementation of foods
   D. Percutaneous transluminal coronary angioplasty
   E. Vaccination against hepatitis B

2. A screening program is designed for the early detection of lung cancer after a clinical study shows promising results. The survival time from diagnosis in individuals whose lung cancer was detected by screening is 3 months longer than that in individuals who did not undergo screening, but rather were diagnosed after presenting with symptoms of lung cancer. This difference is most likely caused by:
   A. Better clinical care of the patients found through screening
   B. Effect modification
   C. Lead-time bias
   D. Length bias
   E. Observer bias

3. A screening program designed to find candidates for liver transplantation would be ill advised because:
   A. False-negative results might occur
   B. The condition is too common
   C. The necessary resources for treatment are in short supply
   D. The population at risk is unknown
   E. The treatment is invasive

4. Data obtained through screening at health fairs are of little epidemiologic value because:
   A. Comorbid conditions may go undetected
   B. False-positive results are common
   C. Follow-up is inadequate
   D. Most conditions are rare in random samples
   E. Self-selection produces a biased sample

5. Current recommendations for the routine use of prostate-specific antigen to screen for prostate cancer are based on individual considerations of risks and benefits (i.e., selective screening) because:
   A. Prostate cancer cannot be detected until it is symptomatic
   B. Prostate cancer is a rare disease
   C. Although uncommon, false-positive results are associated with poor patient outcomes
   D. The appropriate management of asymptomatic prostate cancer is uncertain
   E. There is no effective treatment for prostate cancer

6. Twenty-five tests are being performed together in a multiphasic screening program. If the tests measure different values (i.e., the tests are independent), and if each test has a 5% false-positive error rate, the approximate percentage of healthy participants in whom at least one false-positive result would be found is:
   A. 26%
   B. 33%
   C. 54%
   D. 71%
   E. 82%

7. Health risk assessments (HRAs) are used to determine an individual's "risk age." Which of the following is correct regarding risk age?
   A. If the chronologic age exceeds the risk age, the risk of death is below average
   B. If the risk age exceeds the chronologic age, the risk of death is below average
   C. If the risk age is low, the risk of death is high
   D. The risk age is defined by the age of onset of risk factors for chronic disease
   E. The risk of death is greatest when the risk age equals the chronologic age

8. A professional organization makes a recommendation for universal screening for autism spectrum disorder (ASD) in young children. The recommendation is not based on a

systematic review of the literature but on expert consensus. Critics of the recommendation point out potential financial and emotional conflicts of interest and are concerned about the very low specificity that prior literature reports for the screening test. The critics' concerns about specificity would be most justified if:

A. The prevalence of ASD is low
B. The sensitivity of the screening test is low
C. The harms associated with false-positive screens are unknown
D. Early detection of ASD by screening results in no meaningful long-lasting improvements compared to detection of ASD through routine care
E. Screening does not detect ASD significantly earlier than detection through routine care

9. The process of screening involves multiple steps in the clinical pathway that are subjected to varying levels of influence. What components affect the first step in this pathway, which is *access to screening*?

A. Affordability
B. Availability
C. Accommodation
D. Acceptability
E. All of these

ANSWERS AND EXPLANATIONS

1. **A.** The distinctions between levels of prevention can be vague but have clinical and policy implications, so a clinician must be familiar with them. Hypertension is usually asymptomatic and often detected through screening or case finding; the detection and treatment of an asymptomatic disease constitute secondary prevention. Treating asymptomatic hypertension would likewise be secondary prevention: managing asymptomatic illness to prevent symptomatic disease. If the hypertension had been symptomatic, however (e.g., causing headaches), detecting hypertension in the workup of symptomatic disease would not be prevention but rather diagnosis. Treating symptomatic hypertension would constitute tertiary prevention. Other examples of tertiary prevention include percutaneous transluminal coronary angioplasty (D) and treatment of diabetic nephropathy (B); both actions limit the complications of an established disease (obvious through reported symptoms, physical signs, or diagnostic testing). Vaccination (E), on the other hand, is an effort to prevent disease in an unaffected individual and is an example of primary prevention. Folic acid supplementation of certain foods (C) is also an example of primary prevention: to prevent neural tube defects in newborns.

2. **C.** When a disease is detected by screening at an earlier point in its natural history than it would be if a screening program were not in effect, lead-time bias results. The patient may survive longer after diagnosis only because the diagnosis is made at an earlier stage of the disease, not because detection changes the natural progression of the disease. Although undergoing screening could conceivably be a marker for better clinical care (A), the question provides insufficient information to suggest a difference in the quality or type of care received by those identified by screening and those identified from symptoms. Early detection may allow for disease-modifying therapy that improves the natural history of disease, as in early breast cancer detected by mammography compared with more advanced breast cancer diagnosed through symptoms or signs, however the question does not give information to suggest this might be occurring. Effect modification (B) is when the strength or direction of a presumed causal association is influenced by a third factor. For example, if smoking causes lung cancer, and ionizing radiation increases the carcinogenic effect of tobacco smoke, screening with chest CT scans might modify tobacco's effects on cancer (screening could increase the strength of association between tobacco smoke and development of cancer). Length bias (D) results when cases of relatively indolent disease are preferentially detected by screening, because cases of fulminant disease tend to produce early deaths and are seldom found in the population at screening. In the question scenario, if all patients with aggressive disease had died, only indolent cases would remain to be screened or eventually become symptomatic, and the two groups should be similar (i.e., they should not show a difference as reported). Observer bias (E) involves a systematic human error. Conceivably, if the person who interpreted the screening test diagnosed many healthy people with cancer (generated many false positives), the screening group would have longer survival, because many would not have actually had cancer. However, the question does not provide information to suggest this remote possibility.

3. **C.** Organs for transplantation are generally in short supply, and waiting lists of desperately ill recipients are long. If a treatment for a disease is not available in adequate supply to meet and exceed the needs of symptomatic patients, screening for the disease would be inappropriate because the asymptomatic or less symptomatic patients who were detected through screening would merely be added to the list of patients who could not be treated. False-negative results (A) occur with any screening (or diagnostic) test, depend on sensitivity of the test and prevalence of the condition in the population, and are unavoidable (unless sensitivity is 100%, which is theoretically possible but never achieved in the real world). For a screening test, you want a condition to be fairly common (B), although not so common as to make preemptive treatment the wiser strategy (e.g., rather than screening for dental carries, which is very common in the absence of adequate fluoride, it makes more sense

to supplement fluoride preemptively). Liver failure requiring liver transplantation is not at all common. The population at risk (D) could probably be defined and would probably include people with a liver (i.e., all living people). Screening would mean testing to see whose liver is dysfunctional enough to require transplantation. The treatment (liver transplantation) is invasive (E), but this is not a problem in terms of screening test criteria. We screen for many other conditions that might require invasive treatments (e.g., colon cancer, with possibility of extensive major surgery, including complete colon removal).

4. **E.** For a screening program to have epidemiologic value, the relevant population must be identifiable. Community-based health fairs usually appeal primarily to only select, nonrepresentative members of population (e.g., health-conscious individuals). These individuals are perhaps less likely to have a particular condition (e.g., hypertension) than those who are less interested in attending health fairs. Because of this self-selection bias, the utility of health fairs in screening a community for diseases is highly questionable. False-positive results (B) may or may not be common in such screening efforts, depending on the specificity of the diagnostic test used and the prevalence of the condition. In any screening program, lack of adequate follow-up (C) and inattention to comorbid conditions (A) are potential drawbacks that affect public health utility, not epidemiologic assessment. A given conditions might be common or rare in a random sample (D), but health fair samples are generally not random.

5. **D.** The best way to detect and treat prostate cancer is the subject of ongoing debate in the medical literature. The disease is rapidly progressive and fatal in some men but indolent in others, and there is no reliable way to distinguish between the two types early enough to affect the outcome. Men with rapidly progressive disease would benefit from early detection and aggressive treatment. For most men destined to have indolent disease, however, treatment may do more harm than good. Prostate cancer does not have to be symptomatic (A) to be detected. Initial screening tests include digital rectal examination and prostate-specific antigen assay, although some evidence suggests that these screens do not reduce prostate cancer–specific or all-cause mortality. False-positive results are common (C) and often lead to other, unnecessary invasive testing (e.g., biopsy). This testing can then lead to diagnosis (often without a reliable way to distinguish between indolent and aggressive disease), treatment (e.g., surgery, radiation, chemotherapy), and serious harm (e.g., erectile dysfunction, bladder/bowel incontinence, death) to manage a disease that might otherwise have never been problematic (i.e., most men die *with* prostate cancer, not *of* prostate cancer). In 2018 the USPSTF advised selective prostate cancer screening, but this recommendation may be changed if the performance of screening tests is improved or if

reliable methods to distinguish indolent cancer from aggressive cancer become available. There is effective treatment for prostate cancer (E), depending on the stage of disease. By no means rare (B), prostate cancer is "the most incident cancer" and the second leading cause of cancer death among US men.

6 **D.** For each disease-free person screened, the probability of at least one false-positive result is $(1 - [1 - \text{alpha}]^n)$, where alpha is the false-positive error rate and n is the number of screening tests done. In this case, alpha is 0.05 and n is 2425. Therefore $(1 - [0.95]^{25}) = (1 - [0.27738957]) = 0.72261043 = 70.8723 = $ approximately 72%.

7. **A.** The risk age is not defined by the age of onset of risk factors for chronic disease (D). The risk age is the age of the average individual from a population whose risk of death equals that of the patient in question. If risk age and chronologic age are equivalent, the patient in question has the average risk of death for his or her age group and thus is not at comparatively greater risk of dying (E). Because the risk of death increases with advancing age, if risk age is below chronologic age, the implication is that the patient has the same risk of death as an average younger person. The higher the risk age, the higher the risk of death. In other words, if the risk age exceeds the chronologic age (B), the risk of death is above average. If the risk age is low (C), the risk of death is low.

8 **C.** If a test has low specificity, it will have a high false-positive error rate, and many children will screen positive for ASD when they do not actually have the condition. A high number of false-positive results will be a problem especially if the prevalence of the condition is relatively high, not low (A). The harms of screening positive for ASD when a child does not actually have it could be substantial (e.g., stigma, psychologic distress, additional unnecessary testing), and if these potential harms are unknown, this is a cause for concern. The sensitivity of the screening test (B) is also important but does not relate to the critics' concerns for the specificity of the test. An ideal screening test would have perfect sensitivity (i.e., it would detect ASD 100% of the time when it is there, with no false negatives) and perfect specificity (i.e., it would exclude ASD 100% of the time when it is absent, with no false positives). Answer choices D and E are also critical concerns for the screening test but relate more to whether the test is worth doing given the likely impact on true positives (those identified as having ASD who actually have it) and not to the specificity of the screening test.

9. **E.** Access is affected by the affordability of the preventive service; availability in clinical settings; accommodation for individual circumstances; and acceptability for patients and clinicians. Screening rates increase when barriers related to these components are removed, such as not requiring copay or deductible charges for services, providing tests in close proximity to clinics, and using language translators, for example.

Methods of Tertiary Prevention

"It is not a case we are treating; it is a living, palpitating, alas, too often suffering fellow creature."

John Brown

CASE INTRODUCTION

Mr. M. has worked hard all his life. He left secondary school after 1 year to work in a factory and has rarely taken a vacation since. A massive heart attack at age 53 years suddenly stops him in his tracks. In spite of a timely percutaneous coronary intervention with a stent and the reassurance of his physicians that his heart is "back to pumping at 55% capacity," Mr. M. is no longer working, and he avoids any physical exertion. The slightest twinge in his chest makes him very anxious, and in spite of several attempts to begin work again, he cannot cope with his fear that he might have another heart attack very soon. He mainly stays home, and his daughter tells his primary physician that he has started smoking again.

In practice, tertiary prevention resembles treatment of established disease. The difference is in perspective. Whereas treatment is expressly about "fixing what is wrong," tertiary prevention looks ahead to potential progression and complications of disease and aims to forestall them. Thus, although treatment and tertiary prevention often share methods, their motives and goals diverge. In this chapter, we illustrate the principles of tertiary prevention for several important diseases: cardiovascular disease and major metabolic diseases, as well as musculoskeletal problems. We provide specific clinical examples of disability limitation and rehabilitation. Tertiary prevention of other major chronic diseases is covered in Chapter 19.

Methods of tertiary prevention are designed to limit the physical and social consequences of disease or injury after it has occurred or become symptomatic. There are two basic categories of tertiary prevention. The first category, **disability limitation**, has the goal of halting the progress of the disease or limiting the damage caused by a disease or injury. This category of tertiary prevention can be described as the "prevention of further impairment." The second category, called **rehabilitation**, focuses on reducing the functional disability produced by a given level of impairment. It aims to strengthen the patient's abilities and to help the patient learn to function in alternative ways. Disability limitation and rehabilitation usually should be initiated at the same time (i.e., when the disease is detected or the injury occurs), but the emphasis on one or the other depends on factors such as the type and stage of disease, the type of injury, and available methods of treatment.

1. DISEASE, DISABILITY, ILLNESS, AND DISEASE PERCEPTIONS

Although sometimes used interchangeably, there are important distinctions between disease, disability, and illness. Typically,

disease is defined as the medical condition or diagnosis itself (e.g., coronary artery disease in our case description). **Disability** is the adverse impact of the disease on objective physical, psychologic, and social functioning, such as Mr. M.'s inability to exert himself, walk up stairs, carry heavy grocery bags, etc. Different diseases can result in the same disability, as in the example of stroke and paralytic polio in which both can lead to weakness of one leg and inability to walk. **Illness** is the adverse impact of a disease or disability on how the patient feels, illustrated in our case by Mr. M's fear of having another heart attack and being unable to work. One way to distinguish these terms is to specify that disease refers to the medical diagnosis, disability to the objective impact on the patient, and illness to the subjective impact on the patient.

Disability and illness obviously derive from the medical disease. However, illness is also powerfully influenced by patients' perceptions of their disease, its duration and severity, and their expectations for a recovery; together, these beliefs are called **illness perceptions**. Patients' illness perceptions strongly predict recovery, loss of workdays, adherence, and health care utilization, at least as much as objective measures of impairment.[1–3] To be successful, tertiary prevention and rehabilitation therefore must not only improve patients' physical functioning, but also influence their illness perceptions. For our case example, a successful tertiary prevention has to control Mr. M.'s disease, control his risk factors, and reestablish his trust in himself and his cardiac health.

2. OPPORTUNITIES FOR TERTIARY PREVENTION

The first sign of an illness provides an excellent opportunity to initiate methods of tertiary prevention. The sooner disability limitation and rehabilitation begin, the greater the chance of preventing significant impairment. In the case of infectious diseases, such as tuberculosis and sexually transmitted diseases, early treatment of a disease in one person may prevent its transmission to others, making treatment of one person the primary prevention of that disease in others. Similarly, early treatment of alcoholism or drug addiction in one family member may prevent social and emotional problems, including codependency, from developing in other family members.

3. DISABILITY LIMITATION

Disability limitation includes therapy as well as attempts to halt or limit future progression of the disease, called **symptomatic stage prevention**. Most medical or surgical therapy of symptomatic disease is directed at preventing or minimizing impairment over the short and long term. For example, both coronary angioplasty and coronary artery bypass are aimed at improving function and extending life. These are attempts to undo the threat or damage from an existing disease, in this case, coronary artery disease (CAD). Strategies of symptomatic stage prevention include the following:
1. Modifying diet, behavior, and environment
2. Monitoring frequently for incipient complications
3. Treating any complication that is discovered

In this section, cardiovascular disease (CVD), hyperlipidemia, hypertension, diabetes mellitus, and chronic back pain are used to illustrate how methods of disability limitation can be applied to patients with chronic diseases.

3.1 CARDIOVASCULAR DISEASE

Cardiovascular disease (CVD) encompasses coronary artery disease and strokes.

3.1.a. Assessment

Assessment of CVD includes determining the anatomic function of the affected organs (e.g., what percentage of its volume the left ventricle can eject) and patients' function (as determined by activities of daily living, stress testing, or distance a patient can walk).

3.1.b. Therapy and Symptomatic Stage Prevention

When CVD becomes symptomatic (e.g., with a heart attack), the acute disease needs to be addressed with interventions such as revascularization (opening up blocked arteries) by inserting stents through percutaneous transluminal coronary angioplasty (cardiac catheterization) or by performing surgical bypass. Once the patient is stabilized, further disease progression needs to be prevented. In this effort, the same risk factors to slow or reverse disease progression are targeted as for patients without symptoms, but action is much more urgent.

The following modifiable risk factors are important to address when CVD has already occurred: hypertension, smoking, dyslipidemia, diabetes, diet, and exercise.[4] In practice, which risk factor to address first should be negotiated between clinician and patient. The most important risk factor to modify should be the one the patient is actually motivated and able to change. Any change there will improve risk; and successful behavior change in one area can provide motivation for further change later.

Cigarette smoking. Smoking accelerates blood clotting, increases blood carbon monoxide levels, and causes a reduction in the delivery of oxygen. In addition, nicotine is vasoconstrictive (i.e., it causes blood vessels to tighten). The age-related risk of myocardial infarction (MI) in smokers is approximately twice that in nonsmokers. For individuals who stop smoking, the excess risk declines fairly quickly and seems to be minimal after 1 year of nonsmoking. Smoking cessation is probably the most effective behavioral change a patient can make when CVD is present. Smoking cessation also helps to slow other smoking-induced problems likely to complicate the cardiovascular disease, such as chronic obstructive pulmonary disease (COPD). Strategies for smoking cessation are discussed in Chapters 15 and 21.

Diabetes mellitus. Type 2 diabetes mellitus increases the risk of repeat MI or restenosis (i.e., reblockage) of coronary arteries. Keeping the level of glycosylated hemoglobin (i.e., a measure of blood sugar control [e.g., HbA_{1c}]) at less than 7% significantly reduces the effect of diabetes on the heart, kidneys, and eyes. Many authorities advocate treating diabetes as a coronary heart disease equivalent.[5] The approach should not only focus on blood sugar control, but aim for multifactorial strategy to identify and target patients' broader cardiovascular risk factors, such as treating lipids and controlling blood pressure (BP).

Hypertension. Control of hypertension is crucial at any stage to prevent progression of CVD. For patients with established heart disease, the current hypertension treatment guidelines recommend a target blood pressure below 130/80 mm Hg.[6] In spite of volumes of research on the topic of hypertension and its impact on cardiovascular health, there is still considerable uncertainty about the ideal blood pressure target, and guidelines are conflicting.[7]

Sedentary lifestyle. Exercise at any intensity improves cardiovascular health in a dose-response fashion. Physical activity improves several CVD risk factors, such as blood pressure, blood sugar, and lipid levels. Conversely, there is a growing appreciation for adverse health effects of "sedentariness, independent of physical activity."[8]

Excess weight. In people who are overweight, the risk for CVD partly depends on how the body fat is distributed. Fat can be distributed in the hips and legs (i.e., peripheral adiposity, giving the body a pear shape) or predominantly in the abdominal cavity (i.e., central adiposity, giving the body an apple shape, more common in men than women). Fat in the hips and legs does not seem to increase the risk of cardiovascular disease. In contrast, fat in the abdominal cavity seems to be more metabolically active, thus increasing the risk of cardiovascular disease.

Weight loss ameliorates some important cardiac risk factors such as hypertension and insulin resistance. However, weight loss needs to be sustained, because weight cycling itself is likely detrimental to health.[9]

Dyslipidemia. The risk of progression of CVD is increased in patients with dyslipidemia (i.e., abnormal levels of lipids and the particles that carry them), which can act synergistically with other risk factors (see later discussion; and also see Chapter 5, especially Table 5.2; and Chapter 19). The genetic makeup of populations varies, and with it the risk for CVD. Countries outside the United States have different rates of disease even with identical lipid levels. Therefore risk calculators and treatment decisions need to be made in the context of the treatment population, which may be "high risk" or "low risk" for cardiovascular disease.[4]

Dyslipidemia, sometimes imprecisely called "hyperlipidemia," is a general term used to describe an abnormal elevation in one or more of the lipids or lipid particles found in blood. The complete lipid profile provides information on the following:

- Total cholesterol (TC)
- High-density lipoprotein (HDL) cholesterol (also called good cholesterol because it acts as a scavenger to remove excess cholesterol from the body)
- Low-density lipoprotein (LDL) cholesterol (also called bad cholesterol because it may be a necessary precursor for atherogenesis [i.e., the development of fatty arterial plaques])

- Very-low-density lipoprotein (VLDL) cholesterol, which is associated with triglycerides (TGs)

Low-density lipoprotein is likely the most important predictor of cardiovascular disease. Risk reduction from lowering LDL is linear: the lower the LDL, the lower the cardiovascular risk. However, this protective effect needs to be balanced with considerations of medication side effects and costs.

In the presence of demonstrated atherosclerotic disease or multiple major risk factors, LDL levels should be decreased as much as possible with the use of high-intensity statins. For patients over 75 years of age or those who have contraindications to such tight control, moderate-intensity statins may be used.[10] In addition to lipid levels, the individual patient's values and risk tolerance need to be considered. Here, as in many screening decisions, risk factor treatment for patients should be individualized based on a conversation between providers.[11] Diagnosis and treatment of the many other lipid abnormalities is a rapidly evolving field. Interested readers should consult the resources and websites listed at the end of the chapter for more information.

Other measures. There is a complex interplay between psychosocial stress, anxiety, depression, and cardiovascular disease. Patients benefit from assessing those psychosocial factors, and from interventions that enhance stress management and coping.[4] As in our case example of Mr. M., for highly stressed individuals this may require referral to multispecialty interventions.

3.2 HYPERTENSION

As of 2016, about 75 million people (1 in 3 adults) in the United States live with high blood pressure. Of those, only about half have their blood pressure controlled to recommended levels.[12] Groups at increased risk include pregnant women, women taking estrogens or oral contraceptives, elderly persons, and African Americans.

3.2.a. Assessment

According to the Eight Joint National Committee Report (JNC 8), hypertension is defined as an average systolic BP of 140 mm Hg or greater, or an average diastolic BP of 90 mm Hg or greater, when blood pressure is properly measured on two or more occasions in a person who is not acutely ill and not taking antihypertensive medications. These levels are high enough for treatment to bring proven benefits (Table 17.1).

Hypertension may be detected by community or occupational screening, by individual case finding (e.g., when a person seeks dental care or for medical problems unrelated to hypertension), or when a person develops one or more common complications of hypertension, such as visual problems, early renal failure, congestive heart failure, stroke, or MI. Over the last 20 years, the risk of mortality from coronary artery disease (CAD) and stroke in hypertensive individuals has decreased, in part because of the early detection and improved management of high blood pressure. However, much still remains to be done.

Table 17.1 provides information regarding the evaluation and staging of hypertension, based on average systolic and

TABLE 17.1   Evaluation of Blood Pressure (BP) and Staging of Hypertension, Based on Average Systolic BP and Diastolic BP in Persons over 18, Not Acutely Ill and Not Taking Antihypertensive Medications*

Systolic BP (mm Hg)	Diastolic BP (mm Hg)	Interpretation	Initiate Drug Treatment?
<120	<80	Normal BP	No
120–139	80–89	Prehypertension	No Implement lifestyle modifcation
140–159	90–99	Stage 1 hypertension	Trial of lifestyle Yes; thiazides for most**
≥160	≥100	Stage 2 hypertension	Yes; may need two-drug combination

*The highest stage for which either systolic BP or diastolic BP qualifies is taken as the stage of hypertension. For example, if systolic is 165 mm Hg and diastolic 95 mm Hg, this is stage 2 hypertension.
**JNC 8 recommends treating all patients under age 60. British and Canadian Guidelines differ in their recommendations depending on the age of the patient and the presence of macrovascular target organ damage and cardiovascular risk.
Adapted from Table 11- from: Papadakis MA, McPhee SJ, Rabow MW: Current Medical Diagnosis and Treatment 2018, 57th ed. : McGraw Hill New York, Chicago San Francisco Athens London Madrid Mexico City Milan New Delhi Singapore Sydney Toronto. Page 456,

diastolic BPs. In addition to listing the ranges for normal BP and prehypertension, Table 17.1 shows the ranges for two stages of hypertension. Target blood pressure varies with age: Patients over 60 years of age should be treated less aggressively than younger patients.

3.2.b. Therapy and Symptomatic Stage Prevention

Only half of patients with hypertension are well controlled (up from 29% in 2000). This fact underscores how many lives could be saved and how much disability could be prevented if we were better at delivering consistent care (see Chapter 28).

Treatment of hypertension differs by stage (see Table 17.1). Individuals with normal blood pressure should be monitored at 2-year intervals. Individuals with prehypertension should be counseled about lifestyle changes and monitored at 1-year intervals. Patients with stage 1 hypertension should begin diet and lifestyle changes and should receive one antihypertensive medication, usually a thiazide diuretic. Patients with stage 2 hypertension should begin diet and lifestyle changes and should be treated with two antihypertensive medications. During evaluation, the clinician should check for any evidence of target organ damage, because any stage of hypertension is more severe if there is evidence of such damage.

Most hypertension is classified as essential hypertension, meaning that the specific underlying cause is unknown.

Symptomatic stage prevention and therapy are aimed at reducing systolic BP to less than 140 mm Hg, reducing diastolic BP to less than 90 mm Hg, and monitoring patients to ensure that these levels are maintained. The goal is to prevent damage to the organs at risk from hypertension to prevent disability, organ failure, and death. For patients with any stage of hypertension, the following lifestyle modifications are indicated: weight reduction, tobacco cessation, increased physical activity, and institution of a healthy diet. In the Dietary Approaches to Stop Hypertension (DASH) trials, investigators found that instituting a diet that was rich in fruits,

vegetables, grains, and nonfat dairy products was associated with a reduction in systolic BP, and even greater BP reductions were seen if sodium intake was restricted to no more than 1200 mg/day.[13] Other dietary measures to reduce BP include moderation of alcohol intake and an increase in the intake of potassium, calcium, and magnesium. Smokers should be encouraged to stop smoking, because smoking cessation reduces the risk of damage to many of the same organs as hypertension damages.

For patients whose BP levels remain elevated despite these lifestyle modifications, use of one or more antihypertensive medications is indicated. Because most hypertension is asymptomatic, providers must counsel patients about the importance of taking medications and the risks of stopping treatment. The first line antihypertensive agents in non-black patients include thiazide diuretics, angiotensin-converting enzyme (ACE) inhibitors, angiotensin receptor blockers (ARBs), and calcium channel blockers. For black patients, first line treatment should be with calcium channel blockers or thiazides. Although many antihypertensive medications cause significant side effects, the wide range of choices should be used to develop a treatment plan that is satisfactory to the patient.

3.3 DIABETES MELLITUS

As of 2015, about 30 million people in the United States have diabetes, of which about 7 million are not aware of their diagnosis.[14] Most patients have type 2 diabetes mellitus, usually associated with obesity and insulin resistance. As in dyslipidemia, treatment of diabetes requires balancing the benefits of avoiding diabetic complications against the risks of low blood sugar (hypoglycemia), which are considerable.

3.3.a. Assessment

Diagnosis of diabetes for most patients involves a simple blood test, evaluating the degree of glycosylation of hemoglobin A1c (HbA1c). Once diagnosed with diabetes, patients should undergo a comprehensive evaluation and assessment of their comorbidities. This assessment should include:

- Presence of microvascular and macrovascular complications
- Cardiovascular health and the other components of syndrome X
- Other comorbidities
- Patients' own treatment goals
- Current lifestyle choices
- Mental health
- Psychosocial situation
- Vaccinations (influenza, hepatitis B, pneumococcal polysaccharide vaccine)
- Oral health
- Comprehensive foot examination
- Laboratory evaluation of lipids, liver, kidney function

3.3.b. Therapy and Symptomatic Stage Prevention

Much can be done to prevent target organ damage from diabetes, as shown in the landmark Diabetes Control and Complications Trial (DCCT) and the United Kingdom Prospective Diabetes Study (UKPDS). In patients with type 1 diabetes, DCCT showed that improved control of blood glucose levels significantly reduced the incidence of microvascular disease (retinopathy, nephropathy, neuropathy) and reduced the incidence of macrovascular disease (atherosclerosis of large blood vessels, MI, angina pectoris, stroke, aneurysm, amputations of distal lower extremity).[15,16] Similarly, in patients with type 2 diabetes, UKPDS found that in general the lower the average glycemic level in patients, the fewer the complications.[17]

Patients in the DCCT intervention group had to self-monitor their blood glucose level, keep detailed records of insulin dosage and glucose level, regulate dietary intake and level of insulin based on self-monitoring results, and be actively involved in other aspects of their care. Although the risk of hypoglycemic episodes was three times as high in the intervention group as in the control group, no serious sequelae of hypoglycemia occurred in the intervention group. One death from hypoglycemia occurred in the control group. Weight gain was a common side effect of tight diabetic control.

Based on the results of DCCT, control of HbA1c may benefit patients who are willing to participate actively in their own care. Currently, the most used definition of tight control is HbA1c (glycohemoglobin, or sugar linked to Hb) values less than 7% of total hemoglobin. Many US patients with diabetes may have glycohemoglobins above the recommended level. Tight control should be supplemented with frequent examination of the retina and with laser treatment of microvascular lesions when indicated. The use of ACE inhibitors is valuable not only in controlling hypertension but also in reducing the incidence of microalbuminuria (i.e., albumin protein in the urine), a sign of diabetic kidney damage, and delaying the onset of diabetes-induced renal failure. Guidelines for the care of diabetics have been last updated in 2017 as of this writing.[18] Considerations of psychosocial aspects have been included in the guidelines, and the authors explicitly endorse patient-centered discussion of treatment goals as well as the chronic care model (see Chapter 28).[18]

The cornerstone of diabetes therapy is to support the patient's self-management and to improve lifestyle management. This includes healthy lifestyle choices, self-monitoring of glucose and blood pressure, taking and managing medications, prevention of diabetes complications, and problem solving and coping. All patients with type 1 or type 2 diabetes should be advised of the need for moderate to high levels of physical activity, smoking cessation, and individual counseling about nutrition. Topics that should be covered in individualized nutritional counseling include:

- The role of nutrition
- Energy balance
- Eating patterns and recommended macronutrient intake
- Intake of dietary fat and sodium
- The role of alcohol, sodium, and nonnutritive sweeteners

The goal for most patients would be to achieve a weight loss of at least 5% of their body weight. For most patients, metformin should be the first line agent. Other oral antihyperglycemics are numerous and their respective roles are evolving.

For most patients, a reasonable HbA1c goal is a value below 7%. For selected patients, such as those with short disease duration and long life expectancy, stricter goals such as a HbA1c below 6.5% may be reasonable if it can be achieved without significant hypoglycemia or polypharmacy. Similarly, in patients who have already experienced significant microvascular or macrovascular complications, less stringent treatment goals may be appropriate. Because diabetic patients are at high risk of developing cardiovascular disease, control of blood pressure and lipids is recommended. Many diabetic patients have hypertriglyceridemia, which may require therapy. For patients with diabetes who are aged over 50 years and have at least one additional risk factor for heart disease, aspirin may be recommended for primary prevention of heart disease. Similarly, patients should be closely monitored for the detection of kidney, eye, and foot abnormalities and promptly referred as necessary.

3.4 MUSCULOSKELETAL DISEASES

Chronic low back pain is defined as symptoms for more than 3 months. Low back pain causes more years of disability than any other health condition. For patients and society, the costs of care as well as lost wages, absenteeism, and disability are staggering.[19] Indirect effects also include opiate prescriptions, which in turn can cause addiction and diversion of pain medicines (see Chapter 21). Because of the impact of low back pain on mental health as well as social, recreational, and work life, back pain has been formulated as a biopsychosocial problem, which should be targeted in a comprehensive manner. A key contributor to the burden from low back pain is its recurrence.

3.4.a. Assessment

While most patients with back pain may have mild, self-limited symptoms, those with persistent low back pain should undergo careful history and physical examination to exclude serious pathology such as bacterial infections, malignancy, or vertebral disc protrusions. The majority of patients, however, suffer from nonspecific low back pain. In these patients, those with high levels of anxiety, depression, dissatisfaction with work, and particular disease (e.g., fear-avoidance) beliefs have a high risk of developing long-term disability. Therefore early attention should be given to identifying these patients, although the performance of various screening surveys is mixed.[20]

3.4.b. Therapy and Symptomatic Stage Prevention

Nonpharmacologic treatment options such as exercise, mindfulness-based stress reduction, and relaxation are the first line treatment in chronic low back pain.[21] For those patients who do not respond, analgesics should be considered, as far as possible without opiate pain medications.[22] Patients at high risk for opiate abuse as well as those who do not respond to treatment may benefit from treatment by pain specialists and/or rehabilitation (see upcoming discussion). Interestingly, exercise by itself or in combination with education is more effective than medications at preventing low back pain.[23]

3.5 ORGAN TRANSPLANTATION

In 2016, over 100,000 people in the United States were on a waiting list for organ donation, while almost 16,000 donors provided more than 30,000 transplants.[24] The most commonly transplanted organs are kidney, liver, heart, lung, pancreas, and intestines. While the immediate posttransplant care is provided by specialists, general and preventive medicine providers are involved in the long-term care of patients living with organ transplants, as well as with preventing the transmission of infections through donated organs and tissues.

After transplantation, patients are maintained on strong immunosuppressive medications. Patients need to be monitored and counseled regarding the following common health problems:
- Development of skin cancer (very common)
- Development of other cancers (e.g., head and neck, lung, esophagus)
- Osteoporosis
- Tobacco cessation
- Updated immunizations (no live virus vaccines)
- Interactions of common immunosuppressive medications with organ function (e.g., renal failure) and other common medications (e.g. statins, antibiotics)
- Opportunistic infections
- Transplant rejection or malfunction.[25]

In the past, many infectious pathogens have been unknowingly transmitted through donated organs and tissues, among them HIV, hepatitis C, rabies, tuberculosis, and others. For this reason, the safety of transplants is tightly monitored. Hospitals that transplant organs work with organizations to coordinate organ and tissue recovery and donation.[26] These organizations are required to screen donors for various transmittable diseases such as HIV, hepatitis B and C, syphilis, and cytomegalovirus. The Centers for Disease Control and Prevention (CDC) investigates suspected disease transmission and helps identify transmitted organisms.[26]

4. REHABILITATION

Occurring after disease already has caused damage, rehabilitation may seem to take place when there is nothing left to prevent. However, the **goal of rehabilitation is to reduce the functional and social disability produced by a given level of impairment**, by strengthening the patient's remaining abilities, by helping the patient learn to function in alternative ways, and hopefully by enabling the patient to stay or become employed again.

4.1 GENERAL APPROACH

Rehabilitation must begin in the early phases of treatment if it is to be maximally effective. In patients who have had a stroke, head injury, hip fracture, or other problem that temporarily immobilizes them, it is important to keep joints flexible from the beginning of the illness or injury, so that weakened but recovering muscles do not have to overcome stiffened joints. Early rehabilitation efforts also increase the cooperation of patients and family members by conveying to them that improvement is expected.

The most effective rehabilitation program is tailored to meet the physical, emotional, psychologic, and occupational needs of the individual, including his or her illness perceptions.

Often a *rehabilitation counselor* coordinates the efforts of a team of specialists. *Physical therapists* work to strengthen weakened muscles, increase joint movement and flexibility, and teach patients ways of accomplishing routine tasks despite their disabilities. These tasks, or activities of daily living (see Chapter 14), include feeding oneself, transferring between bed and chair, grooming, toileting, bathing, dressing, walking on a level surface, and using stairs. *Speech therapists* seek to improve the ability of patients to articulate their thoughts after a stroke or head injury that produces aphasia, and they may help to evaluate whether stroke patients can swallow food safely. *Occupational therapists* evaluate the occupational abilities of patients, counsel them regarding suitable types of work, provide them with job training or retraining, and help them find a suitable job. Usually the most cost-effective efforts are those designed to help a patient return to the previous place of employment. Some patients may be able to resume their job, whereas others may obtain a new or modified job. *Psychiatric or emotional counseling* may be important, as may spiritual counseling by a member of the clergy.

4.2 CORONARY HEART DISEASE

Coronary heart disease was one of the first diseases for which rehabilitation programs were developed, and these programs still provide the template for most rehabilitation. Most cardiac rehabilitation programs follow defined components and stages[27] (Table 17.2). Core components of rehabilitation for all cardiac conditions include a comprehensive assessment of

TABLE 17.2 Core Components of Cardiac Rehabilitation

Component	Established/Agreed Issues
Patient assessment	*Clinical history:* review clinical courses of ACS. *Physical examination:* inspect puncture site of PCI and extremities for presence of arterial pulses. *Exercise capacity and ischemic threshold:* Submaximal exercise stress testing by bicycle ergometry or treadmill maximal stress test (cardiopulmonary exercise test if available) within 4 weeks after acute events, with maximal testing at 4–7 weeks.
Physical activity counseling	*Exercise stress test guide:* With exercise capacity more than 5 METs without symptoms, patients can resume routine physical activity; otherwise, patients should resume physical activity at 50% of maximal exercise capacity and gradually increase. *Physical activity:* Slow, gradual, progressive increase of moderate intensity aerobic activity, such as walking, climbing stairs, and cycling, supplemented by an increase in daily activities (e.g., gardening, housework).
Exercise training	Program should include supervised, medically prescribed, aerobic exercise training: *Low risk patients:* At least three sessions of 30–60 min/wk aerobic exercise at 55%–70% of maximum workload (METs) or HR at onset of symptoms; ≥1500 kcal/wk to be expended. *Moderate-risk to high-risk patients:* Similar to low-risk group, but starting with <50% METs *Resistance exercise:* At least 1 hr/wk with intensity of 10–15 repetitions per set to moderate fatigue.
Diet/nutritional counseling	Caloric intake should be balanced by energy expenditure (physical activity) to avoid weight gain.
Weight control management	Mediterranean diet with low levels of cholesterol and saturated fat.
Lipid management	Foods rich in omega-3 fatty acids. Statins for all patients, intensified to a lipid profile of cholesterol: <175 mg/dL, or <155 mg/dL in high-risk patients. LDL-C: <100 mg/dL, or <80 mg/dL in high-risk patients. Triglycerides: <150 mg/dL.
Blood pressure monitoring	Assess BP frequently at rest and as indicated during exercise. Use lifestyle modification and drugs if necessary to treat to optimal BP.
Smoking cessation	Ask about tobacco and intervene according to stage of change.
Psychosocial management	Screen for distress and intervene if necessary.

ACS, Acute coronary syndrome; *HR,* heart rate; *LDL-C,* low-density lipoprotein cholesterol; *METs,* metabolic equivalent tasks; *PCI,* primary percutaneous coronary intervention.[27]

the patient's clinical and functional status. This information provides the basis for a rigorous program aimed at gradually improving physical functioning, risk factor profile, and psychosocial status. Criteria for core requirements to use in low-resource settings have been defined.[28]

4.2.a. Blood Pressure Monitoring

- If resting systolic BP is 130 to 139 mm Hg or diastolic BP is 85 to 89 mm Hg, recommend lifestyle modifications, exercise, weight management, sodium restriction, and moderation of alcohol intake (<30 g/day in men; <15 g/day in women), according to the DASH diet.
- If resting systolic BP is 140 mm Hg or greater or if diastolic BP is 90 mm Hg or greater, initiate drug therapy. Expected outcomes are BP less than 140/90 mm Hg.

4.2.b. Smoking Cessation

All smokers should be professionally encouraged to stop using all forms of tobacco permanently. Follow-up, referral to special programs, and pharmacotherapy (including nicotine replacement) are recommended as a stepwise strategy for smoking cessation. Structured approaches are to be used (e.g., five A's: ask, advise, assess, assist, arrange) (see Chapter 15, Box 15.1).

4.2.c. Psychosocial Issues

- Screen for psychologic distress as indicated by clinically significant levels of depression, anxiety, anger or hostility, social isolation, marital/family distress, sexual dysfunction/adjustment, and substance abuse of alcohol and/or other psychotropic agents.
- Offer individual and/or small group education and counseling on adjustment to heart disease, stress management, and health-related lifestyle change (profession, motor vehicle operation, sexual activity resumption).
- When possible, include spouses and other family members, domestic partners, and/or significant others in such sessions.

- Teach and support self-help strategies and ability to obtain effective social support.
- Provide vocational counseling in case of work-related stress.

Cardiac rehabilitation has been shown to be one of the most cost-effective interventions in preventing progression of heart disease. It may be particularly powerful in improving self-management by disadvantaged patients.[29] A good rehabilitation program usually extends into structured programs once the patient is discharged and on lifelong maintenance.

4.3 REHABILITATION FOR OTHER DISEASES

4.3.a. Pulmonary Rehabilitation

Evidence of the positive impact of pulmonary rehabilitation first came from a landmark study on lung reduction surgery[30] and was later confirmed in systematic reviews.[31] Since then, indications for pulmonary rehabilitation have been broadened beyond chronic obstructive pulmonary disease (COPD), and rehabilitation programs are now used for many chronic respiratory diseases. Pulmonary rehabilitation continues to be underutilized despite its considerable symptom-reducing and health economic benefits.[32]

4.3.b. Cancer Rehabilitation

More and more patients experience cancer not as an acute lethal illness but a chronic disease. This trend has engendered an increased interest in the role of cancer rehabilitation. Rehabilitation has been shown to increase quality of life even in patients with advanced cancer.[33] In contrast to patients with most other diseases, cancer patients often suffer as much from complications of therapy as from the disease itself.[34]

4.3.c. Chronic Low Back Pain Rehabilitation

There is moderate quality evidence that multidisciplinary rehabilitation, which addresses social and psychologic issues, decreases pain and disability more than purely physical rehabilitation and at least as well as surgery.[19] Multidisciplinary rehabilitation programs for low back pain pay particular attention to risk factors for chronification of pain, such as depression, anxiety, exercise and relaxation, as well as coping with personal and job-related problems.

4.4 CATEGORIES OF DISABILITY

Disability is a socially defined concept but has practical implications for financial support. Most states delineate several categories for reimbursement of workers who have job-related injuries or illnesses covered under a workers' compensation program, as follows:
- Permanent total disability (e.g., loss of two limbs or loss of vision in both eyes)
- Permanent partial disability (e.g., loss of one limb or loss of vision in one eye)
- Temporary total disability (e.g., fractured arm in truck driver)
- Temporary partial disability (e.g., fractured arm in elementary school teacher)
- Death

In these categories, state statutes stipulate benefits for disabled persons (or for their surviving family in the case of death) according to a fixed schedule. Less well-defined illnesses and injuries, such as repetitive motion or back injuries, are usually compensated by a mixture of financial and vocational rehabilitation benefits, including counseling, retraining, and even job placement.[35]

A disability is considered "temporary" if it is expected that a person will return to his or her job within a time defined by statute. If the disability is job related, the person may be partially reimbursed for lost wages and fully reimbursed for the costs of medical care from the state workers' compensation fund.

In the United States a person with a permanent disability may be reimbursed at a fixed rate for life or for a defined period. The rate varies from state to state (as stipulated by law), but is based on the type of disability and the degree of function lost (as determined by a clinician).

> **CASE RESOLUTION**
> Mr. M. underwent an intensive multidisciplinary rehabilitation program, which included psychologic counseling and relaxation training. He has returned home and is more able to participate in daily life, but he continues to struggle with mood swings and has not been able to return to work. However, after referral to a mental health specialist he is addressing his anxiety and is expected to go back to work eventually.

5. SUMMARY

The goal of tertiary prevention is to limit the physical and social consequences of an injury or disease after it has occurred or become symptomatic. The two major categories of tertiary prevention are disability limitation and rehabilitation. Whereas disease and disability describe objective diagnoses and impairments, illness also encompasses patients' perceptions, assumptions, and expectations about their disease. These illness perceptions strongly predict disease outcomes and patient recovery.

Methods of disability limitation include therapy, which seeks to undo or reduce the threat or damage from an existing disease, and symptomatic stage prevention, which attempts to halt or limit progression of disease. The strategies of symptomatic stage prevention are taken from primary prevention (modification of diet, behavior, and environment) and secondary prevention (frequent screening for complications, treatment for complications). The effective management of chronic diseases, such as coronary artery disease, hypertension, and diabetes mellitus, requires a combination of therapy and symptomatic stage prevention. This approach also can be used in the management of many other diseases, including pulmonary disease, low back pain and cancers, among others.

Rehabilitation should begin in the early stages of treatment. Depending on the needs of the patient, the rehabilitation team may include a rehabilitation counselor;

physical therapist; speech therapist; occupational therapist; and psychiatric, emotional, or spiritual counselor. Under most state laws governing workers' compensation, several categories of job-related illnesses or injuries are recognized: permanent total disability, permanent partial disability, temporary total disability, temporary partial disability, and death. The goal of rehabilitation for workers, whether their impairment is temporary or permanent, is to minimize the social and occupational consequences of the impairment.

Although it might seem that the opportunity for prevention is lost when a disease appears or an injury occurs, this is often not the case. The appearance of symptoms or the threat of severe complications may lead patients to take an active interest in their health status, seek the health care that they need, and make positive changes in their environment, diet, and lifestyle.

REFERENCES

1. Petrie KJ, Jago LA, Devcich DA. The role of illness perceptions in patients with medical conditions. *Curr Opin Psychiatry*. 2007; 20:163-167.
2. Giri P, Poole J, Nightingale P, Robertson A. Perceptions of illness and their impact on sickness absence. *Occup Med (Lond)*. 2009;59:550-555.
3. van der Have M, Fidder HH, Leenders M, et al. Self-reported disability in patients with inflammatory bowel disease largely determined by disease activity and illness perceptions. *Inflamm Bowel Dis*. 2015;21(2):369-377.
4. Piepoli MF, Hoes AW, Agewall S, et al. 2016 European guidelines on cardiovascular disease prevention in clinical practice: the Sixth Joint Task Force of the European Society of Cardiology and Other Societies on Cardiovascular Disease Prevention in Clinical Practice (constituted by representatives of 10 societies and by invited experts) developed with the special contribution of the European Association for Cardiovascular Prevention & Rehabilitation (EACPR). *Atherosclerosis*. 2016;252:207-274.
5. Hajar R. Diabetes as "coronary artery disease risk equivalent": a historical perspective. *Heart Views*. 18(1):34-37, 2017. Available at: http://doi.org/10.4103/HEARTVIEWS.HEARTVIEWS_37_17.
6. Cifu AS, Davis AM. Prevention, detection, evaluation, and management of high blood pressure in adults. *JAMA*. 2017;318(21): 2132-2134. doi:10.1001/jama.2017.18706.
7. James PA, Oparil S, Carter BL, et al. 2014 evidence-based guideline for the management of high blood pressure in adults: report from the panel members appointed to the Eighth Joint National Committee (JNC8). *JAMA*. 2014;311(5):507-520. doi:10.1001/jama.2013.284427.
8. de Rezende LF, Rodrigues Lopes M, Rey-López JP, Matsudo VK, Luiz Odo C. Sedentary behavior and health outcomes: an overview of systematic reviews. *PLoS One*. 2014;9(8):e105620. doi: 10.1371/journal.pone.0105620.
9. Montani JP, Schutz Y, Dulloo AG. Dieting and weight cycling as risk factors for cardiometabolic diseases: who is really at risk? *Obes Rev*. 2015;16(suppl 1):S7-S18.
10. Stone NJ, Robinson JG, Lichtenstein AH, et al. 2013 ACC/AHA guideline on the treatment of blood cholesterol to reduce atherosclerotic cardiovascular risk in adults. *J Am Coll Cardiol*. 2014;63(25 Pt B):2889-2934. doi:10.1016/j.jacc.2013.11.002.
11. Krumholz HM. The new cholesterol and blood pressure guidelines: perspective on the path forward. *JAMA*. 2014;311(14):1403-1405.
12. Centers for Disease Control and Prevention. *High Blood Pressure Facts*. Available at: https://www.cdc.gov/bloodpressure/facts.htm. Accessed May 5, 2019.
13. Svetkey LP, Sacks FM, Obarzanek E, et al. The DASH diet, sodium intake and blood pressure trial (DASH-sodium): rationale and design. DASH-Sodium Collaborative Research Group. *J Am Diet Assoc*. 1999;99(8):S96-S104.
14. Centers for Disease Control and Prevention. *National Diabetes Statistics Report 2017*. Available at: https://www.cdc.gov/diabetes/pdfs/data/statistics/national-diabetes-statistics-report.pdf. Accessed May 5, 2019.
15. The Diabetes Control and Complications Trial. DCCT Research Group. *N Engl J Med*. 1993;329:683-689.
16. Santiago JV. Lessons from the Diabetes Control and Complications Trial. *Diabetes*. 1993;42:1549-1554.
17. Stratton IM, Adler AI, Neil HA, et al. Association of glycaemia with macrovascular and microvascular complications of type 2 diabetes (UKPDS 35): prospective observational study. *BMJ*. 2000;321:405-412.
18. American Diabetes Association. Standards of Medical Care in Diabetes 2017. *Diabetes Care*. 2017;40(suppl 1). Available at: http://care.diabetesjournals.org/content/diacare/suppl/2016/12/15/40.Supplement_1.DC1/DC_40_S1_final.pdf. Accessed May 5, 2019.
19. Kamper SJ, Apeldoorn AT, Chiarotto A, et al. Multidisciplinary biopsychosocial rehabilitation for chronic low back pain: Cochrane Systematic Review and Meta-analysis. *BMJ*. 2015;350:h444.
20. Karran EL, McAuley JH, Traeger AC, et al. Can screening instruments accurately determine poor outcome risk in adults with recent onset low back pain? A systematic review and meta-analysis. *BMC Med*. 2017;15(1):13.
21. Qaseem A, Wilt TJ, McLean RM, Forciea MA. Noninvasive treatments for acute, subacute, and chronic low back pain: a clinical practice guideline from the American College of Physicians. *Ann Intern Med*. 2017;166:514-530. doi:10.7326/M16-2367.
22. Dowell D, Haegerich TM, Chou R. *CDC Guideline for Prescribing Opioids for Chronic Pain*. Atlanta: Centers for Disease Control and Prevention; 2016. In: JAMA. 2016 Apr 19;315(15):1624-1645. doi: 10.1001/jama.2016.1464.
23. Steffens D, Maher CG, Pereira LS, et al. Prevention of low back pain: a systematic review and meta-analysis. *JAMA Intern Med*. 2016;176(2):199-208.
24. U.S. Department of Health and Human Services. *Organ Donation Statistics*. Available at: https://www.organdonor.gov/statistics-stories/statistics/data.html. Accessed May 5, 2019.
25. Starr SP. Immunology update: long-term care of solid organ transplant recipients. *FP Essent*. 2016;450:22-27.
26. Centers for Disease Control and Prevention. *Transplant Safety: Frequently Asked Questions*. Available at: https://www.cdc.gov/transplantsafety/overview/faq.html. Accessed May 5, 2019.
27. Piepoli MF, Corrà U, Benzer W, et al. Secondary prevention through cardiac rehabilitation: from knowledge to implementation. A position paper from the Cardiac Rehabilitation section of the European Association of Cardiovascular Prevention and Rehabilitation. *Eur J Cardiovasc Prev Rehabil*. 2010;17:1-17.
28. Grace SL, Turk-Adawi KI, Contractor A et al. Cardiac rehabilitation delivery model for low-resource settings: an International Council of Cardiovascular Prevention and Rehabilitation consensus statement. *Prog Cardiovasc Dis*. 2016 Nov - Dec;59(3):303-322. doi: 10.1016/j.pcad.2016.08.004. Epub 2016 Aug 17.
29. Mead H, Andres E, Ramos C, Siegel B, Regenstein M. Barriers to effective self-management in cardiac patients: the patient's experience. *Patient Educ Couns*. 2010;79:69-76.

30. Fishman A, Martinez F, Naunheim K, et al. A randomized trial comparing lung-volume-reduction surgery with medical therapy for severe emphysema. *N Engl J Med.* 2003;348:2059-2073.

31. Puhan MA, Gimeno-Santos E, Scharplatz M, Troosters T, Walters EH, Steurer J. Pulmonary rehabilitation following exacerbations of chronic obstructive pulmonary disease. *Cochrane Database Syst Rev.* 2011;(10):CD005305.

32. Rochester CL, Vogiatzis I, Holland AE, et al. An official American Thoracic Society/European Respiratory Society policy statement: enhancing implementation, use, and delivery of pulmonary rehabilitation. *Am J Respir Crit Care Med.* 2015;192(11):1373-1386.

33. Salakari MR, Surakka T, Nurminen R, Pylkkänen L. Effects of rehabilitation among patients with advances cancer: a systematic review. *Acta Oncol.* 2015;54(5):618-628.

34. Spence RR, Heesch KC, Brown WJ. Exercise and cancer rehabilitation: a systematic review. *Cancer Treat Rev.* 2010;36:185-194.

35. LaDou J. *Occupational and Environmental Medicine.* 3rd ed. Stamford, CT: Appleton & Lange; 2004.

SELECT READINGS

The Diabetes Control and Complications Trial. DCCT Research Group. *N Engl J Med.* 1993;329:683-689.

Franklin DJ. Cancer rehabilitation: challenges, approaches, and new directions. *Phys Med Rehabil Clin N Am.* 2007;18:899-924.

Petrie KJ, Jago LA, Devcich DA. The role of illness perceptions in patients with medical conditions. *Curr Opin Psychiatry.* 2007;20:163-167.

WEBSITES

Joint National Committee Guideline on Prevention, Detection, Evaluation, and Treatment of High Blood Pressure (JNC 8): https://jamanetwork.com/journals/jama/fullarticle/1791497

National Cholesterol Education Program: https://www.nhlbi.nih.gov/health-topics/management-blood-cholesterol-in-adults

REVIEW QUESTIONS

1. Which is an example of tertiary prevention?
   A. Hospice care (end-of-life palliative care)
   B. Occupational therapy after a stroke
   C. Postexposure prophylaxis for rabies
   D. Treatment of essential hypertension
   E. Using nasal steroids with topical decongestants to prevent rebound congestion

2. Under what circumstances can primary and tertiary prevention of medical disease most obviously be achieved concurrently in different individuals through the treatment of one patient?
   A. Never, because primary and tertiary prevention are mutually exclusive
   B. When a patient is treated for a hip fracture
   C. When a patient is treated for active tuberculosis
   D. When a patient is treated for cystitis (an uncomplicated urinary tract infection)
   E. When a patient is treated for a heart attack

3. How much higher is the age-specific risk of myocardial infarction (heart attack) in smokers than in nonsmokers?
   A. No higher
   B. 1.33 times as high
   C. Twice as high
   D. 10 times as high
   E. 100 times as high

4. A disadvantage of using only the total cholesterol (TC) level to predict the risk of cardiovascular disease is that:
   A. HDL is included in the measure
   B. The ratio of LDL to VLDL is unknown
   C. TC levels are estimated rather than measured
   D. TC levels fluctuate wildly
   E. In contrast to triglyceride levels, TC levels vary with meals

5. According to the Eighth Report of the Joint National Committee on Prevention, Detection, Evaluation, and Treatment of High Blood Pressure (JNC 8), which of the following medication classes has a compelling indication to be given for all these conditions associated with hypertension: high cardiovascular disease risk, treatment after heart attack, treatment after stroke, treatment for heart failure, chronic kidney disease, and diabetes?
   A. Alpha blockers
   B. Angiotensin-converting enzyme (ACE) inhibitors
   C. Calcium channel blockers
   D. Thiazide diuretics
   E. Beta blockers

6. The Diabetes Control and Complications Trial (DCCT) showed that:
   A. Microvascular complications of diabetes are independent of glycemic control
   B. Monitoring the urine glucose level is more cost effective than monitoring the blood glucose level
   C. Only macrovascular complications of diabetes are preventable
   D. The risk of hypoglycemia outweighs the benefit of tight glycemic control
   E. Tight glycemic control delays the onset of microvascular complications

7. Kidney damage in diabetes, as revealed by microalbuminuria (i.e., inappropriate appearance of protein in urine), is best treated with:
   A. A sulfonylurea
   B. An ACE inhibitor
   C. Dialysis
   D. Insulin
   E. Lifestyle modifications

8. An elderly man has his first stroke (cerebrovascular accident). In the United States, tertiary prevention of a first stroke:
   A. Includes the restoration of functional ability through physical therapy

B. Is generally ineffective because the incidence of first stroke is rising

C. Is generally ineffective because risk factors for a first stroke are largely unknown

D. Relies predominantly on pharmacotherapy for hyperlipidemia

E. Relies predominantly on screening for carotid stenosis

9. Two soldiers are severely burned in an explosion during combat. They have minimal loss of physical function but comparably disfiguring facial and body burns. After the war, one soldier becomes a confident motivational speaker, whereas the other becomes chronically depressed and avoids leaving the house. The two soldiers have:

A. Different disease, different disability

B. The same disease, different disability

C. Different disease, different illness

D. The same disease, different illness

E. The same illness, different disability

ANSWERS AND EXPLANATIONS

1. **B.** Tertiary prevention is the prevention of disease progression and complications that might result in further impairment, and it comprises rehabilitation to reverse impairment and disability. Occupational therapy is a form of rehabilitation directed at preventing disability after a stroke and is an example of tertiary prevention. The treatment of essential hypertension (D) is best considered a form of secondary prevention, although arguably might constitute primary prevention of ischemic heart disease or cardiomyopathy. Postexposure prophylaxis (C) for rabies is secondary prevention, preventing possibly contracted disease from becoming manifest. Using nasal steroids with topical decongestants (E) is a method for primary prevention of rebound congestion. Hospice care (A) is intended to provide comfort during the late stages of terminal illness and does not specifically have the goal of preventing disease progression.

2. **C.** The management of communicable diseases such as tuberculosis offers a unique opportunity for prevention. When a patient with active disease is treated, the progression of disease and impairment are prevented in the patient; this is tertiary prevention. At the same time, the spread of disease to the patient's various social contacts is prevented; this is primary prevention in a different individual. Thus primary and tertiary prevention are not mutually exclusive (A) and, in fact, can even occur in the same person. For instance, dietary measures used to prevent the progression of coronary artery disease after a heart attack (E) might serve as primary prevention for the development of diabetes for the same person. Likewise, giving antibiotics for cystitis (D) could conceivably prevent other infections, and rehabilitating a broken hip (B) could increase balance, flexibility, strength, and agility to prevent other musculoskeletal injuries from developing.

3. **C.** Multiple sources suggest that smoking increases the risk of age-specific cardiovascular mortality by a factor of approximately 2. Cigarette smoking is generally considered the most important preventable cause of death and disease in the United States. The risk of myocardial infarction is certainly higher (A) with smoking, and definitely more than a third higher (B), but probably not 10 (D) or 100 (E) times as high.

4. **A.** High-density lipoprotein levels are inversely associated with the risk of cardiovascular disease (although emerging evidence challenges causality). All other lipid fractions contributing to the total cholesterol level have been associated directly, to varying degrees, with cardiovascular disease risk. The TC level includes several generally positive correlates and one generally negative correlate (HDL) of heart disease risk, and this mix of "bad" and "good" reduces the utility of the total. The ratio of TC to HDL purifies the measure somewhat, so that a positive correlate of cardiovascular disease risk is produced. Total cholesterol can be easily measured (C) and is part of the reason for the original association between TC and heart disease (a weak association). The levels of TC do not fluctuate wildly (D) or vary much with meals (E); in fact, contrary to popular belief, dietary cholesterol has almost no impact on serum cholesterol. The ratio of LDL to VLDL (B) highlights that oversimplifying associations based on single categories of lipids almost always misses the mark; the more we understand about the heterogeneity within categories, the more the difference and relative proportions seem to matter a great deal.

5. **B.** The one class of drugs that has a compelling indication for all the listed conditions is ACE inhibitors. Generally, angiotensin receptor blockers (ARBs) are acceptable alternatives when ACE inhibitors are not tolerated, although the evidence supporting this drug class for most conditions is not as robust as for ACE inhibitors. Alpha blockers (A) do not have a compelling indication for any of the listed conditions. Calcium channel blockers (C) have compelling indications for high cardiovascular disease risk and diabetes, but side effects (leg swelling, constipation) often limit their utility, particularly in older patients. Thiazide diuretics (D) are recommended expressly for all listed conditions except chronic kidney disease and treatment after heart attack. Thiazides are effective, affordable, and a usual part of the antihypertensive regimen for most people. Beta blockers (E) have a compelling indication for heart failure, treatment after heart attack, and diabetes. In people without compelling indication, beta blockers are falling out of favor for first line treatment of high blood pressure (meta-analyses suggest they may be associated with an increase in risk of cardiovascular events and death).

6. **E.** In the 1990s the DCCT was designed specifically to test the hypothesis that tight glycemic control could

forestall microvascular complications of diabetes. The trial showed that the closer to normal that serum glucose and glycohemoglobin levels were maintained, the less the progression of microvascular complications such as retinopathy (eye damage) and nephropathy (kidney damage). Thus microvascular complications of diabetes do not seem to be independent of glycemic control (A) and do seem to be preventable (C). Greater effort is now devoted to achieving near-normal control of serum glucose levels when feasible, although this increases the risk of hypoglycemia. The risk of hypoglycemia may not outweigh the benefit of tight glycemic control (D). In fact, striving for tighter control of blood sugar is associated with increased mortality in some populations (e.g., intensive care unit patients, patients at high risk for CVD). Monitoring the urine glucose level is not more cost effective than monitoring the blood glucose level (B). In fact, monitoring urine glucose is useless in cases of tight control, because glucose generally does not appear in the urine until blood level exceeds about 200 mg/dL (200 mmol/L), levels far above what would be considered tight control.

7. **B.** Before renal function begins to decline as a result of diabetic nephropathy, there is a period during which glomerular filtration increases because a high osmotic load is delivered to the glomerulus. Renal hyperfunction is associated with microalbuminuria and presages a decline in creatinine clearance (an accepted measure of kidney function and filtering capacity). Evidence is now substantial that ACE inhibitors attenuate renal hyperfunction in diabetic patients, mitigate the associated microscopic proteinuria, and slow the subsequent decline in glomerular filtration (i.e., slow the progression of diabetes-related kidney damage). Sulfonylureas (A) and insulin (D) may indirectly slow the progression of nephropathy by providing tight glycemic control, but the mechanisms through which diabetes produces kidney damage likely involve factors other than just blood sugar. Dialysis (C) is life-sustaining therapy after renal failure has occurred, but has no role in the management of early microalbuminuria, when kidney function is still mostly preserved. Lifestyle modification (E) may contribute to better glycemic control and management of the metabolic derangements associated with diabetes, but there is no evidence that lifestyle measures will be as effective in preserving renal function as ACE inhibitors.

8. **A.** Tertiary prevention consists of rehabilitation and efforts to prevent disease progression after an injury or event has occurred. After the event of a stroke, physical therapy is a form of rehabilitation and a means of preventing further impairment and disability. In the United States the incidence of strokes has been decreasing for several decades, not increasing (B). More importantly, however, whether strokes occur more often in a population is not a concern to a person who has already had a stroke; tertiary prevention occurs after an injury (stroke in this case). Incidence of a first stroke would be a concern for primary and secondary prevention, not tertiary prevention. Likewise, whether the risk factors for a first stroke are known is not related to tertiary prevention, because the event has already occurred and the focus is now on limiting disability, maximizing function, and preventing recurrence. To prevent recurrence, understanding risk factors is important, but the risk factors for a primary event may be different than those for a repeat event, so the risk factors of concern in this case are not those for a first stroke (C), which has already occurred, but those for a second stroke. For stroke though, the risk factors for first and subsequent events are similar and well established, including hyperlipidemia and carotid stenosis. Treatment of hyperlipidemia (D) certainly may be a component of tertiary prevention but would not be predominant (e.g., treating blood pressure would be more important). Screening for carotid stenosis (E) is secondary prevention by definition (detection of asymptomatic disease). Once a stroke has occurred though, it is impossible to screen; one could look for carotid stenosis, but this would now be a diagnostic evaluation.

9. **D.** Disease refers to a medical diagnosis, or an objective description of a condition. Disability refers to the impact a condition has on a patient in objective terms. Illness is the subjective impact of a disease or condition on a patient—that is, how patients perceive themselves and their disease and disability. These two soldiers have the same disease or condition (facial and body burns). They also have the same disability (comparable disfigurement). The difference is their illness, or their perceptions and how their disease and disability is affecting them. Given these considerations, answer D is the only choice that is correct. The expectations surrounding the impact of the illness, its impact on functioning, and its duration are mediated through illness perceptions. Impacting illness perceptions is crucial for successful rehabilitation.

Developing Recommendations for Clinical Preventive Services

"Primum non nocere (first, do no harm)." Attributed to

Thomas Sydenham

Delivering preventive health services to patients is an essential part of clinical practice in the United States. However, preventive services subject otherwise healthy individuals to screening tests and other interventions for the purpose of improving future health conditions, not current ones. Consequently, clinical preventive services must be thoughtfully administered, and are only appropriate when two conditions are met: (1) The preventive service is effective in improving important health outcomes for specific patients, and (2) the preventive service causes no harm. Of these, avoiding harm is the most important.

The successful delivery of preventive medicine depends on the following two goals:

1. Preventive services are only provided if they demonstrate more benefit than harm.
2. The preventive service can be realistically integrated in clinical practice environments.

The US Preventive Services Task Force (USPSTF) was founded to address these goals. This chapter focuses on why its work is important, how it develops evidence-based recommendations, and how busy clinicians can keep up to date with and incorporate the USPSTF recommendations in their practices. Recommendations for clinical preventive services change frequently with emerging evidence. For more details and updated recommendations, readers should consult the USPSTF website.[1] Note that other groups, such as the National Institute for Health and Care Excellence (NICE) in the United Kingdom, also use evidence-based methods to determine clinical practice recommendations. Clinicians outside the United States should be familiar with local guidelines.

1. UNITED STATES PREVENTIVE SERVICES TASK FORCE

1.1 MISSION AND SCOPE

When the USPSTF was first convened by the US Public Health Service in 1984, it was modeled on an earlier Canadian task force to serve as an independent panel of nongovernmental experts on prevention and evidence-based medicine (EBM). Sixteen members serve on the USPSTF at any given time. Members are nominated in a public process and are chosen based on their expertise in the subject matter, primary health care, disease prevention, research methods, and application of synthesized evidence to clinical decision making. In addition, they are carefully vetted for important conflicts of interest. Members are chosen through a rigorous process and serve staggered 4-year terms on the committee.

Since 1995, the work of the USPSTF has been supported by the **Agency for Healthcare Research and Quality** (AHRQ). The scope of the USPSTF includes primary and secondary preventive services, including screening, counseling, and prevention medication.[2] The USPSTF aims to provide accurate and objective evidence-based recommendations across a spectrum of populations, types of services, and health conditions. Its mission is to:

1. Assess the benefits and harms of preventive services for individuals asymptomatic for the condition being prevented based on age, gender, and risk factors.
2. Recommend which services should be incorporated into routine primary care practice.

The USPSTF only considers preventive services for **asymptomatic** patients, it only deals with preventive services delivered within the scope of **primary care** or referred from primary care, and it requires evidence of effectiveness in improving health outcomes. Notably, the USPSTF considers the delivery of preventive services across a variety of clinical settings. Occasionally USPSTF recommendations diverge from those developed by specialist organizations with different perspectives than primary care. For example, specialists may see predominantly high-risk patients or preselected patients with subtler symptoms that were missed earlier. Screening decisions for these patients might differ from those for the general population because the pretest probability of disease is much higher.

Recommendations from the USPSTF not only guide clinical practice, but also affect insurance coverage. The USPSTF A-level and B-level recommendations are included in the preventive services mandate for insurance coverage under the US Patient Protection and Affordable Care Act of 2010 (ACA).[3] This means that most patients with private or public health insurance must receive the recommended preventive services without copay or deductible insurance charges. The ACA reduces the financial barrier for preventive services and has resulted in increased access to preventive services since implementation.[4] In contrast to the *Community Preventive Services Guide* (see Chapter 26), the USPSTF does not take cost effectiveness or financial impact into consideration when determining recommendations.

1.2 UNDERLYING ASSUMPTIONS

When the USPSTF was founded, its principles were revolutionary: that preventive care should be rigorously evaluated for effectiveness, not every preventive service was worth doing, and some may be harmful. In the past, the USPSTF recommended against or did not endorse preventive services that were established practices or recommended by other organizations. The reasons for these discrepancies may be based on several assumptions of the USPSTF.

As outlined in Chapter 16, screening studies are subject to biases that can result in an **overestimate of benefits.** Therefore the USPSTF places a higher burden of evidence for benefits than for evidence of harms, usually requiring rigorous studies of effectiveness. The hierarchy of evidence considers studies with less risk of bias (randomized controlled trials [RCTs]) as the most rigorous, followed by observational studies with comparison groups and other study designs (Fig. 18.1). The USPSTF often considers additional sources of evidence to determine harms of preventive services, including drug registries, for example, because most studies of effectiveness are not well designed to detect harms.

Controlled trials of the effectiveness of a preventive service usually describe the **upper bounds of efficacy.** In other words, controlled trials describe a best-case scenario because the study design creates conditions that are better than real-world practice. The USPSTF assumes that in actual clinical practice settings, with unselected providers and general populations, the effectiveness of a screening service will be lower.

Effectiveness is determined by improving health outcomes, not by delivering a service or diagnosing a condition. **Health outcomes** are changes in a patient's health that the

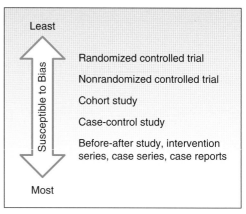

Fig. 18.1 Hierarchy of evidence. The hierarchy of evidence considers studies with the least risk of bias as the strongest (randomized controlled trials), followed by observational studies with comparison groups and other study designs.

patient experiences, such as pain, shortness of breath, or death. In contrast to health outcomes, **intermediate outcomes** are measurements of pathology or physiology that can lead to health outcomes (e.g., high blood pressure). The USPSTF primarily considers studies of health outcomes rather than intermediate outcomes, although these studies may provide corroborative evidence.

Benefits of the preventive service must outweigh harms. Since preventive care involves subjecting healthy patients to health services that could be harmful, the numbers of patient lives potentially saved are weighed against the risks of subjecting healthy patients to potential harms, such as consequences of false-positive tests and benign biopsies. Because this standard is so high, the USPSTF may, for some topics, not endorse preventive services that are recommended by other organizations.

2. EVIDENCE REVIEW AND RECOMMENDATIONS

2.1 THE USPSTF PROCESS

Developing a USPSTF recommendation is a complex process that adheres to procedures that have been developed over 20 years[5] and are consistent with established standards.[6,7] The two main phases include reviewing the evidence and formulating recommendations. Although the USPSTF makes the recommendations, independent researchers at **evidence-based practice centers** (EPCs) systematically review the evidence. The systematic review and recommendation process is highly structured and includes several measures to safeguard the USPSTF's integrity and to improve transparency, accountability, consistency, and independence.[5] These include stringent criteria for selection of USPSTF members; policies regarding conflicts of interest; and expert and public review of research plans, reports, and draft recommendations.

The steps of the recommendation process begin with topic selection, development of a research plan for the systematic review, and creation of the draft evidence review (Table 18.1).

TABLE 18.1   Steps in Making a USPSTF Recommendation

Step	Description
1. Topic selection	Identification of topics to be considered from an open nomination process.
2. Work plan development	Initial work plan developed by designated topic team, including USPSTF topic leads, AHRQ medical officer, and EPC investigators.
3. Work plan external review	Work plans for new topics are reviewed by experts in the field.
4. Research plan development	Based on the full final work plan, a research plan containing the analytic framework, key questions, and inclusion/exclusion criteria is created for public comment.
5. Draft research plan	The draft research plan is posted on the USPSTF website for public comment for a period of 4 weeks.
6. Finalization and approval of work plan	The work plan is revised based on public and partner comments and peer review.
7. Draft evidence review	Based on the final work plan, EPC investigators conduct a systematic evidence review to address the key questions.
8. Review of draft evidence review by USPSTF leads and external experts	Draft evidence reviews are sent to a limited number of experts in the field, USPSTF topic leads, and AHRQ medical officers for comments.
9. Development of draft recommendation statement	USPSTF topic leads discuss specific recommendations and draft the recommendation statement with the AHRQ medical officer for presentation at the USPSTF meeting.
10. USPSTF vote on draft recommendation statement	At the USPSTF meeting, EPC investigators present the evidence review and the USPSTF topic leads discuss the evidence and present the draft recommendation statement. The full USPSTF discusses the evidence and recommendation statement, revising it if needed, before voting.
11. Public comment on draft evidence review and draft recommendation statement	Drafts of the evidence review and recommendation statement are posted on the USPSTF website for public comment for 4 weeks.
12. Final evidence review	After receiving all comments on the draft evidence review from experts, partners, the public, the USPSTF, and the AHRQ medical officer, the EPC revises the evidence review and prepares a manuscript for publication in a peer-reviewed medical journal.
13. Development of final recommendation statement	USPSTF topic leads propose revisions to the recommendation statement based on discussions and comments.
14. Approval of final recommendation statement	The final recommendation statement is sent to all USPSTF members for ratification.
15. Release of final recommendation statement and final evidence review	The final recommendation statement and evidence review are published in peer-reviewed medical journals and posted to the USPSTF website (www.uspreventiveservicestaskforce.org).

AHRQ, Agency for Healthcare Research and Quality; *EPC,* evidence-based practice center; *USPSTF,* US Preventive Services Task Force. (From U.S. Preventive Services Task Force. *U.S. Preventive Services Task Force Procedure Manual.* Rockville, MD: USPSTF; 2017. Available at: https://www.uspreventiveservicestaskforce.org/Page/Name/procedure-manual.)

Evidence reviews typically address key questions essential to supporting a clinical recommendation, such as:

- Does screening for X reduce morbidity and/or mortality; or improve other health outcomes?
- Can a group at high risk for X be identified for screening on clinical grounds?
- What is the accuracy of screening tests for use in routine clinical practice?
- What is the effectiveness of treatments when the condition is detected early?
- What are the harms of the screening test?
- What are the harms of treatment?

Members of the USPSTF use the evidence review to draft a proposed recommendation statement for a vote at a meeting of the entire USPSTF. The recommendation and evidence review are then further reviewed and revised, and the final versions are published on the USPSTF website and in peer-reviewed medical journals. The entire process often spans the course of 2 years, and the research literature is continually monitored for newly published studies throughout this time.

2.2 APPRAISING EVIDENCE

The process of evidence appraisal begins with the evaluation of individual studies by the Evidence-based Practice Center

Level of appraisal	Type	Definition	Rating
Evidence-based Practice Center		
Individual study	Quality/risk of bias (internal validity)	Validity of the study results based on predefined design-specific criteria.	Good Fair Poor
	Applicability (external validity)	Clinical relevance of study participants, settings, and providers to primary care practice in the U.S.	Good Fair Poor
Key question	Strength of evidence	Estimate of confidence in results based on study design; numbers of studies and participants; consistency/precision; reporting bias; limitations; overall quality/risk of bias.	High Moderate Low Insufficient
	Overall applicability	How well the overall body of evidence would apply to the U.S. population based on settings, populations, and intervention characteristics.	High Moderate Low Insufficient
U.S. Preventive Services Task Force		
Key question	Adequacy of evidence	Aggregate internal and external validity of all studies across the key question.	Convincing Adequate Inadequate
Linkage coherence	Adequacy of evidence for benefits	Includes adequacy of evidence for the key questions as well as the six critical appraisal questions, coherence of evidence, and other considerations.	Convincing Adequate Inadequate
	Adequacy of evidence for harms		
Magnitude of effect	Benefits	Estimates of the reductions in disease-related outcomes that could be expected to be prevented by the prevention intervention.	Substantial Moderate Small Zero Negative Cannot be determined
	Harms	Estimates of the increases in harms that could be expected to be caused by the prevention intervention.	
Overall certainty	The likelihood that the assessment of the net benefit of a prevention service is correct	Based on adequacy, coherence, and applicability of existing evidence, and may include extrapolation and conceptual bonding to address gaps.	High Moderate Low
Magnitude of net benefit	Net benefit = benefits – harms	Combines estimates of magnitude for benefits and harms from existing studies and may include extrapolation and conceptual bonding to address gaps.	Substantial Moderate Small Zero Cannot be determined
Grade	Final recommendation	Based on overall certainty and magnitude of net benefit.	A, B, C, D, I

Fig. 18.2 Appraisal of evidence leading to a USPSTF recommendation. The process of evidence appraisal begins with the evaluation of individual studies and results in the determination of letter grades for each recommendation. (From U.S. Preventive Services Task Force. *U.S. Preventive Services Task Force Procedure Manual.* Rockville, MD; 2017. https://www.uspreventiveservicestaskforce.org/Page/Name/Procedure-Manual.)

(EPC) investigators and results in the determination of letter grades for each recommendation by the USPSTF (Fig. 18.2).[5,8] Essential questions underlying criteria for evidence appraisal include:

- Do the studies have the appropriate research design to answer the key questions?

- What is the internal validity?
- What is the external validity?
- How many studies have been conducted that address the key question, and how large are the studies?
- How consistent are the results?
- Are there additional factors that raise confidence in the results (e.g., dose-response effects, consistency with biologic models)?

2.3 GRADING RECOMMENDATIONS

Once USPSTF members have answered these questions, they assign a certainty level (high, moderate, or low) based on the overall evidence available. The certainty level is used to assess the net benefit of a preventive service (substantial, moderate, small, zero, or harms outweigh benefits) (Table 18.2).[5,8] The **net benefit** is defined as benefit minus harm of the preventive service as implemented in a general, primary care

population. This forms the basis of the final letter grades (A, B, C, D, or I) (Table 18.3). In addition to letter grades, the USPSTF provides rationale and clinical considerations to provide additional guidance to clinicians who are their primary audience.

After assigning a tentative grade, the USPSTF discusses the recommendations with federal and primary care partners. Federal partners include the Centers for Disease Control and Prevention (CDC), Center for Medicare and Medicaid Services (CMS), Health Resource and Services Administration (HRSA), National Institutes of Health (NIH), Veterans Administration (VA), and Food and Drug Administration (FDA). Examples of primary care partners include the American College of Physicians, American Academy of Family Practice, American College of Obstetricians and Gynecologists, American Pediatrics Association, and American College of Preventive Medicine.

In clinical practice, services with grade **A** and **B** recommendations are strongly encouraged. Services with grades of **C, D,** and **I** are not routinely provided. However, it is important to understand the difference between these grades. For grades A, B, and D, the USPSTF is reasonably certain it understands the balance of benefits and harm. For services graded C, benefits are considered to be small in a population. For example, breast cancer screening for women in their 40s is a service with a C recommendation (see Chapter 16). However, preventive services with C grades could be beneficial for some, and decisions to use them should be individualized. This is referred to as **shared decision making** because the clinician and patient discuss individual benefits and harms of

TABLE 18.2 Using Certainty and Magnitude of Net Benefit to Make USPSTF Recommendations

CERTAINTY OF NET BENEFIT[a]	MAGNITUDE OF NET BENEFIT			
	Substantial	Moderate	Small	Zero or Harms Outweigh Benefits
High	A	B	C	D
Moderate	B	B	C	D
Low	Insufficient			

[a]The USPSTF assigns a certainty level based on the overall evidence available to assess the net benefit of a preventive service. The net benefit is defined as benefit minus harm of the preventive service as implemented in a general, primary care population.
Modified from Krist AH, Wolff TA, Jonas DE, et al: Update on the methods of the US Preventive Services Task Force: methods for understanding certainty and net benefit when making recommendations. *Am J Prev Med* 54:S11–S18, 2018.

TABLE 18.3 USPSTF Recommendation Grades and Clinical Practice

Grade	Definition	Net Benefit	Suggestions for Practice
A	USPSTF recommends the service.	High certainty that the net benefit is substantial.	Offer or provide this service.
B	USPSTF recommends the service.	High certainty that the net benefit is moderate, or moderate certainty that the net benefit is moderate to substantial.	Offer or provide this service.
C	USPSTF recommends selectively offering or providing this service to individual patients based on professional judgment and patient preferences.	Moderate or high certainty that the net benefit is small.	Offer or provide this service for selected patients depending on individual circumstances.
D	USPSTF recommends against the service.	Moderate or high certainty that the service has no net benefit or that the harms outweigh the benefits.	Discourage the use of this service.
I	The USPSTF concludes that the current evidence is insufficient to assess the balance of benefits and harms of the service.	Evidence is lacking, of poor quality, or conflicting, and the balance of benefits and harms cannot be determined.	Read the clinical considerations section of USPSTF Recommendation Statement. If the service is offered, patients should understand the uncertainty about the balance of benefits and harms.

USPSTF, US Preventive Services Task Force.
Modified from Krist AH, Wolff TA, Jonas DE, et al: Update on the methods of the US Preventive Services Task Force: methods for understanding certainty and net benefit when making recommendations. *Am J Prev Med* 54:S11–S18, 2018; US Preventive Services Task Force: https://www.uspreventiveservicestaskforce.org/Page/Name/grade-definitions.

testing versus not testing and consider patient preferences in the screening decision. For example, women in their 40s with strong family histories of breast cancer may benefit from initiating mammography screening before age 50. In contrast, for services graded D, there is clear evidence that there is *no* net benefit, or that there is net harm, such as screening for ovarian cancer. These D services should be avoided.

For services with an I grade, evidence is lacking or conflicting, and the USPSTF has determined that they can neither recommend for or against the service. For example, as of 2018, services with an I grade include skin cancer screening, screening for adolescent idiopathic scoliosis, and screening for atrial fibrillation with electrocardiography.[9] Many services rated I have not been adequately studied because of lack of research funding, difficulties in measuring and evaluating effectiveness, emphasis on specialty populations, and other limitations of research.

2.4 LIMITS OF EVIDENCE

An important aspect of USPSTF recommendations is that they can be, and often are, *noncommittal*. When evidence is lacking or inconsistent, the USPSTF may conclude that neither a recommendation for nor against a practice is justified. This has two important implications. First, judgment remains a vital element in clinical practice even in the EBM era. Although it may be reasonable to recommend neither for nor against a practice on a population level, a given patient might benefit based on individual considerations, such as important risk factors for the condition. Consequently, many topics addressed by the USPSTF require a process of dialogue and shared decision making between clinician and patient. Such decisions are influenced by individual priorities, preferences, and at times economics; practices not formally recommended may not be routinely covered by third-party payers.

The second implication of USPSTF's noncommittal approach is that "no evidence of benefit" is not the same as "evidence of no benefit." A practice that may ultimately prove to be of decisive benefit may not be recommended because the relevant evidence is not yet available. The same is true of a practice that may ultimately prove to confer net harm. Practice must evolve in tandem with an evolving base of evidence.

3. IMPLEMNTATION OF RECOMEMNDATIONS IN CLINICAL PRACTICE

3.1 OVERUSE, UNDERUSE, AND MISUSE

The process of delivering clinical preventive services to individual patients is complex. Successful delivery of each preventive service requires multiple steps in a clinical pathway that are subjected to varying levels of influence at societal, health system, clinician, and patient levels (Chapter 16, Fig. 16.1).[10–12] In clinical practice, it is difficult to deliver all effective preventive services consistently, avoid the less effective ones, and deliver services only to patients who will derive benefit. This is even more difficult in the context of inequities

and barriers in accessing preventive health services.[13–15] Also, patients have preferences and priorities often driven by passions, convictions, anxieties, and marketing that may conflict with evidence-based guidelines. Additionally, in a typical clinical practice, urgent problems and symptomatic conditions easily supersede preventive health care.[16] In general, preventive services are underused and only half of patients receive all recommended preventive services.[17]

The USPSTF recommends that clinicians track delivery of services with A or B grades for every patient to ensure that they receive them. Some services have become quality measures that gauge the performance of health systems and clinicians.[18] Many electronic health records feature reminders at the point of care to help providers integrate preventive services into their practices. Alternatively, and for paper charts, an assistant can check whether the patient is due for recommended services and can prepare screening instruments and materials in advance. In either case, the time required is considerable. Estimates indicate that it would take 7.4 hours per workday over 1 year to deliver all recommended services to a typical primary care panel of 2500 patients.[19]

It is even more difficult to have meaningful conversations about services that depend on patient preferences or detailed risk assessment, such as those graded C (and some graded B, such as medications to reduce breast cancer risk), or services with conflicting evidence (graded I). Many patients demand services based on anecdotal evidence from friends, family members, or the media. For these services, the USPSTF recommends community education, use of shared decision-making aids, and trained assistants.[20] However, such a sophisticated and personnel-intensive approach is probably not feasible for many primary care clinicians.

Barriers in delivering effective preventive services are not only related to lack of time, but also to overuse and misuse. The challenge for clinicians is therefore twofold: (1) Find more efficient ways to deliver preventive services to patients who need them, and (2) discuss goals of care and expected benefits with patients who are unlikely to benefit.

3.2 DELIVERY AND COMPLIANCE OF CLINICAL PREVENTIVE SERVICES

The USPSTF offers resources to help clinicians stay current and access recommendations at the point of care. These include a pocket guide to the preventive services, a dedicated searchable website with an electronic preventive services selector based on age and gender of patients,[1] and a subscription to email updates from the USPSTF. An approach to delivery of preventive services is illustrated by the case example in Box 18.1.[21]

An important concept in the field of clinical preventive service delivery is that compliance should not be measured for a given service, but rather for a "bundle of services" recommended for an individual based on age and gender. Several such bundled metrics have been proposed, based on Behavioral Risk Factor Surveillance System (BRFSS) data[22] or computerized records.[23] Such packaging of metrics

BOX 18.1 Individualizing Preventive Service Recommendations in Clinical Practice

The USPSTF lists nearly 100 preventive service recommendations on their website.[1] Sifting through this extensive list of topics to identify appropriate services for an individual is not practical for clinicians, patients, or other users. To assist users, the website also provides search capabilities based on specific patient characteristics, including age, sex, pregnancy status, tobacco use, and sexual activity. A similar search screen is available for patient use, and both versions can be downloaded. The USPSTF recommendations are updated on an ongoing basis and real-time searches are the best way to identify current practices.

Using the search screen on the website, a clinician can identify preventive services to address during the course of an individual patient's visit. For example, a 62-year-old man who is sexually active and a nonsmoker would generate a list of 16 preventive services with A-grade or B-grade recommendations indicating that they should be offered (box table).[20] However, of this list, five may not be needed if the patient is not at high risk for syphilis, human immunodeficiency virus (HIV) infection, other sexually transmitted diseases, hepatitis B, or latent tuberculosis infections. Other recommended preventive services may have been provided during previous visits and are not due again, such as screening for abnormal lipids, HIV infection,

colorectal cancer, and hepatitis C. The remaining services that should be addressed at this visit include unhealthy alcohol use screening and behavioral counseling, blood pressure screening, depression screening, and obesity screening and counseling. Blood pressure and weight are usually obtained as part of the check-in process, and screening for depression and alcohol misuse can begin with brief self-administered questionnaires before the clinic visit begins.

Two additional preventive services could be offered selectively if the patient has increased risks for specific conditions. For example, screening for abnormal blood glucose as part of cardiovascular disease (CVD) risk assessment is recommended for adults aged 40 to 70 years who are overweight or obese. If the patient was identified with obesity when his weight was obtained during check-in, then he would be offered blood glucose screening as well. If he has one or more CVD risk factors, and a calculated 10-year CVD event risk of 10% or greater, then a healthful diet and physical activity would be recommended.

Five additional C-grade recommendations could be provided (see box table), but only if the balance of benefits and harms is favorable for this particular patient and he is willing to accept potential risks. These would involve a shared decision-making approach.

USPSTF Recommended Preventive Services for a 62-Year-Old Man (Sexually Active, Nonsmoker)[a]

Service	Description	Grade
PROVIDE PREVENTIVE SERVICE		
Unhealthy alcohol use: screening and behavioral counseling	Screen adults age 18 years or older for unhealthy alcohol use in primary care settings and provide persons engaged in risky or hazardous drinking with brief behavioral counseling interventions to reduce alcohol misuse.	B
Blood pressure screening	Screen for high blood pressure in adults age 18 years or older; obtain measurements outside of the clinical setting for diagnostic confirmation before starting treatment.	A
Colorectal cancer screening	Screen for colorectal cancer starting at age 50 years and continuing until age 75 years using one of several effective methods.	A
Depression screening	Screen for depression in the general adult population, including pregnant and postpartum women. Screening should be implemented with adequate systems in place to ensure accurate diagnosis, effective treatment, and appropriate follow-up.	B
HCV screening	Screen for HCV infection in persons at high risk for infection. The USPSTF also recommends offering one-time screening for HCV infection to adults born between 1945 and 1965.	B
HIV screening	Screen for HIV infection in adolescents and adults age 15–65 years at least once.	A
Obesity screening and counseling	Screen all adults for obesity and offer or refer patients with a body mass index of ≥ 30 kg/m^2 to intensive, multicomponent behavioral interventions.	B
Lipid screening and statin preventive medication	Adults without a history of CVD use a low-dose to moderate-dose statin for the prevention of CVD events and mortality when all the following criteria are met: (1) age 40–75 years; (2) one or more CVD risk factors (i.e., dyslipidemia, diabetes, hypertension, or smoking); and (3) a calculated 10-year risk of a cardiovascular event of 10% or greater. Identification of dyslipidemia and calculation of 10-year CVD event risk require universal lipid screening in adults age 40–75 years.	B
PROVIDE PREVENTIVE SERVICE ONLY IF THE PATIENT HAS INCREASED RISK AS DEFINED FOR EACH CONDITION		
Diabetes screening	Screen for abnormal blood glucose as part of cardiovascular risk assessment in adults age 40–70 years who are overweight or obese. Clinicians should offer or refer patients with abnormal blood glucose to intensive behavioral counseling interventions to promote a healthful diet and physical activity.	B

Continued

BOX 18.1	**Individualizing Preventive Service Recommendations in Clinical Practice—cont'd**	
Service	**Description**	**Grade**
Healthy diet and physical activity counseling to prevent CVD	Offer or refer adults who are overweight or obese and have additional CVD risk factors to intensive behavioral counseling interventions to promote a healthful diet and physical activity.	B
HBV screening	Screen for HBV infection in persons at high risk for infection.	B
HIV PrEP	Provide preventive medication for persons at high risk of HIV acquisition	A
Sexually transmitted infections counseling	Provide intensive behavioral counseling for all sexually active adolescents and adults at increased risk for sexually transmitted infections.	B
Syphilis screening	Screen for syphilis in persons who are at increased risk for infection.	A
Tuberculosis screening	Screen for latent tuberculosis infection in populations at increased risk.	B
PROVIDE PREVENTIVE SERVICE ONLY IF THE BALANCE OF BENEFITS AND HARMS IS FAVORABLE ON AN INDIVIDUAL BASIS AND IT CONCURS WITH THE PATIENT'S PREFERENCES		
Aspirin use to prevent CVD and colorectal cancer	Offer low-dose aspirin for adults age 60–69 years with a ≥10% 10-year CVD risk.	C
Behavioral counseling for skin cancer prevention	Provide counseling about minimizing exposure to ultraviolet radiation to reduce risk of skin cancer to adults older than 24 years with fair skin types.	C
Healthy diet and physical activity counseling to prevent CVD	Offer or refer adults without obesity who do not have known CVD risk factors to intensive behavioral counseling interventions to promote a healthful diet and physical activity.	C
Prostate cancer screening	Periodic prostate-specific antigen–based screening for prostate cancer for men age 55–69 years.	C
Statin preventive medication	Adults without a history of CVD, do not have CVD risk factors, or a calculated 10-year risk of a cardiovascular event of 10% or greater use a low-dose to moderate-dose statin for the prevention of CVD events and mortality.	C

aThis table reflects active recommendations at the time of the USPSTF website search for text publication (2019). The USPSTF recommendations are updated on an ongoing basis and real-time searches are the best way to identify current practices.
CVD, cardiovascular disease; *HBV*, hepatitis B virus; *HCV*, hepatitis C virus; *HIV*, human immunodeficiency virus; *USPSTF*, US Preventive Services Task Force.
Adapted from US Preventive Services Task Force: Search for recommendations. https://epss.ahrq.gov/ePSS/GetResults.do?method=search.

(1) improves accountability, raising the bar for performance, and (2) directs the focus to underserved patients, because the metric only improves if most patients receive all services. For this reason, a packaged measure of up-to-date preventive services was added to the *Healthy People 2020* indicators.[22]

4. SUMMARY

The US Preventive Services Task Force follows an explicit and standardized process to assess the benefits and harms of delivering preventive services to asymptomatic individuals. Five letter grades summarize the evidence for net benefits or harm for services, including screening, counseling, and prevention medication:

A—High certainty the service is beneficial
B—Moderate certainty service is beneficial
C—At least moderate certainty that net benefit is small
D—At least moderate certainty of no net benefit or net harm
I—Evidence is lacking or conflicting

In clinical practice, preventive services are underused, overused, and misused. USPSTF A-level and B-level recommendations are included in the preventive services mandate for insurance coverage under the Affordable Care Act. For these services, most patients with private or public health insurance can receive the recommended preventive services without copay or deductible insurance charges, improving access to care. Considerable clinical judgment is required in the delivery of clinical preventive services for which evidence remains equivocal. Clinicians must deliver recommended services consistently across their clinical practices, and delivery of some services has been established as quality measures. For services with lower grades, clinicians should engage patients in meaningful conversations about the evidence and their risk and preferences enlisting a shared decision-making approach.

REFERENCES

1. U.S. Preventive Services Task Force. *Recommendations for Primary Care Practice*. 2018. Available at: https://www.uspreventiveservicestaskforce.org/Page/Name/recommendations.
2. U.S. Preventive Services Task Force. *Methods and Processes*. 2018. Available at: https://www.uspreventiveservicestaskforce.org/Page/Name/methods-and-processes.

3. HealthCare.gov. *Read the Affordable Care Act.* 2018. Available at: https://www.healthcare.gov/where-can-i-read-the-affordable-care-act/.

4. Blumenthal D, Abrams M, Nuzum R. The Affordable Care Act at 5 years. *N Engl J Med.* 2015;372:2451-2458.

5. U.S. Preventive Services Task Force. *U.S. Preventive Services Task Force Procedure Manual.* Rockville, MD: USPSTF; 2017. Available at: https://www.uspreventiveservicestaskforce.org/Page/Name/procedure-manual.

6. Institute of Medicine. *Clinical Practice Guidelines We Can Trust.* Washington, DC: National Academies Press; 2011.

7. Agency for Healthcare Research and Quality. *Methods Guide for Effectiveness and Comparative Effectiveness Reviews.* Rockville, MD: AHRQ; 2017. Available at: https://effectivehealthcare.ahrq.gov/products/cer-methods-guide/overview.

8. Krist AH, Wolff TA, Jonas DE, et al. Update on the methods of the U.S. Preventive Services Task Force: methods for understanding certainty and net benefit when making recommendations. *Am J Prev Med.* 2018;54:S11-S18.

9. U.S. Preventive Services Task Force. *Published Recommendations.* 2018. Available at: https://www.uspreventiveservicestaskforce.org/BrowseRec/Index.

10. Donabedian A. *Aspects of Medical Care Administration: Specifying Requirements for Health Care.* Cambridge, MA: Harvard University Press; 1973.

11. McLaughlin CG, Wyszewianski L. Access to care: remembering old lessons. *Health Serv Res.* 2002;37:1441-1443.

12. Nelson HD, Cantor A, Wagner J, et al. *Achieving Health Equity in Preventive Services—Systematic Evidence Review Protocol.* Rockville, MD: Agency for Healthcare Research and Quality; 2018.

13. Hou SI, Sealy DA, Kabiru CW. Closing the disparity gap: cancer screening interventions among Asians—a systematic literature review. *Asian Pac J Cancer Prev.* 2011;12:3133-3139.

14. Jones TP, Katapodi MC, Lockhart JS. Factors influencing breast cancer screening and risk assessment among young African American women: an integrative review of the literature. *J Am Assoc Nurse Pract.* 2015;27:521-529.

15. Martinez ME, Ward BW. Health care access and utilization among adults aged 18-64, by poverty level: United States, 2013-2015. *NCHS Data Brief.* 2016;262:1-8.

16. Crabtree BF, Miller WL, Tallia AF, et al. Delivery of clinical preventive services in family medicine offices. *Ann Fam Med.* 2005;3:430-435.

17. McGlynn EA, Asch SM, Adams J, et al. The quality of health care delivered to adults in the United States. *N Engl J Med.* 2003;348:2635-2645.

18. National Committee for Quality Assurance. *Healthcare Effectiveness Data and Information Set (HEDIS) and Performance Measurement.* Available at: http://www.ncqa.org/hedis-quality-measurement.

19. Yarnall KS, Pollak KI, Østbye T, Krause KM, Michener JL. Primary care: is there enough time for prevention? *Am J Public Health.* 2003;93:635-641.

20. Sheridan SL, Harris RP, Woolf SH. Shared decision making about screening and chemoprevention: a suggested approach from the U.S. Preventive Services Task Force. *Am J Prev Med.* 2004;26:56-66.

21. Agency for Healthcare Research and Quality. *Search for Recommendations.* 2018. Available at: https://epss.ahrq.gov/ePSS/GetResults.do?method=search.

22. Shenson D, Bolen J, Adams M, et al. Receipt of preventive services by elders based on composite measures, 1997-2004. *Am J Prev Med.* 2007;32:11-18.

23. Vogt TM, Aickin M, Ahmed F, Schmidt M. The prevention index: using technology to improve quality assessment. *Health Serv Res.* 2004;39:511-530.

SELECT READINGS

Nelson HD. *Systematic Reviews to Answer Health Care Questions.* Philadelphia, PA: Lippincott Williams & Wilkins; 2014.

Nelson HD, Fu R, Cantor A, Pappas M, Daeges M, Humphrey L. Effectiveness of breast cancer screening: systematic review and meta-analysis to update the 2009 U.S. Preventive Services Task Force recommendation. *Ann Intern Med.* 2016;164:244-255.

Nelson HD, Pappas M, Cantor A, Griffin J, Daeges M, Humphrey L. Harms of breast cancer screening: systematic review to update the 2009 U.S. Preventive Services Task Force recommendation. *Ann Intern Med.* 2016;164:256-267.

Siu AL, U.S. Preventive Services Task Force. Screening for breast cancer: U.S. Preventive Services Task Force recommendation statement. *Ann Intern Med.* 2016;164:279-296.

REVIEW QUESTIONS

1. Which of the following is *not* a goal of the US Preventive Services Task Force?
   A. Provide accurate and objective evidence-based recommendations
   B. Recommend which services should be incorporated into routine primary care practice
   C. Consider the cost effectiveness or financial impact of a recommendation
   D. Assess the benefits and harms of preventive services

2. The US Preventive Services Task Force considers preventive services:
   A. For asymptomatic patients
   B. Delivered within the scope of primary care or referred from primary care
   C. With evidence of effectiveness in improving health outcomes
   D. Delivered across a variety of clinical settings
   E. For all of these

3. The US Preventive Services Task Force considers the effectiveness of preventive services on improving health outcomes when determining clinical practice recommendations. Which of the following is an intermediate outcome?
   A. Myocardial infarction
   B. Total cholesterol level
   C. Death
   D. Pain level

4. The US Preventive Services Task Force considers the strength of evidence when determining clinical practice recommendations. Rank the following study designs from the least (1) to the most (5) susceptible to bias:
   A. Case control study
   B. Before-after study

C. Nonrandomized controlled trial
D. Randomized controlled trial
E. Cohort study

5. The US Preventive Services provides a B-level recommendation when:
A. The magnitude of net benefit is substantial, and the certainty of net benefit is moderate
B. The magnitude of net benefit is moderate, and the certainty of net benefit is high
C. The magnitude of net benefit is moderate, and the certainty of net benefit is moderate
D. A and B
E. A, B, and C

6. Which statement regarding US Preventive Services Task Force recommendations is *false*?
A. A-level and B-level recommendations are covered under the Affordable Care Act with no copay or deductible charges for most patients
B. A D-level recommendation means there is moderate or high certainty that the service has no net benefit or that the harms outweigh the benefits
C. An I-level recommendation means that the preventive service can be offered to individual patients based on professional judgment and patient preferences
D. A C-level recommendation means that there is moderate certainty that the net benefit is small

7. What is the most important consideration when issuing a clinical practice recommendation for a preventive service across a large population?
A. The preventive service is effective in improving important health outcomes
B. The preventive service can be realistically integrated in clinical practice environments
C. The preventive service is cost effective
D. The preventive service causes no harm
E. Patients are willing to use the preventive service

8. The US Preventive Services Task Force issued a C-level recommendation for routine mammography screening for breast cancer for women in their 40s in 2016. What does this mean to patients?
A. No women in their 40s should get mammography screening
B. All women in their 40s should get mammography screening
C. Clinicians can decide whether women in their 40s get mammography screening, depending on how they interpret the screening studies
D. Some women in their 40s can get mammography screening, depending on whether their insurance will pay or not

E. Some women in their 40s can get mammography screening, depending on their individual risks and preferences

ANSWERS AND EXPLANATIONS

1. **C.** The USPSTF does not consider the cost effectiveness or financial impact of a recommendation, but bases its recommendations for routine primary care practice on the strength of evidence and balance of benefits and harms.
2. **E.** All of these answers describe characteristics of preventive services that are considered by the USPSTF.
3. **B.** Total cholesterol level is an intermediate outcome. **A, C,** and **D** are health outcomes. Health outcomes are changes in a patient's health that the patient experiences, such as myocardial infarction, death, or pain, while intermediate outcomes are measurements of pathology or physiology that can lead to health outcomes, such as total cholesterol level or bone mineral density measurement.
4. Study designs from least to most susceptible to bias are randomized controlled trial (D), nonrandomized controlled trial (C), cohort study (E), case control study (A), and before-after study (B). In general, results from studies that are less susceptible to bias provide stronger strength of evidence than studies that are more susceptible to bias, assuming that they are powered and conducted appropriately.
5. **E.** The USPSTF assigns a certainty level based on the overall evidence available to assess the net benefit of a preventive service. The net benefit is defined as benefit minus harm of the preventive service as implemented in a general, primary care population. A B-level recommendation is provided when the conditions in answers A, B, or C are met.
6. **C.** An I-level recommendation means that evidence is insufficient (it is lacking, of poor quality, or conflicting), and the balance of benefits and harms cannot be determined.
7. **D.** Preventive services subject otherwise healthy individuals to screening tests and other interventions for the purpose of improving future health conditions and should cause no harm in the process.
8. **E.** A C-level recommendation indicates selectively offering or providing a preventive service to individual patients based on professional judgment and patient preferences. This decision can be guided by a shared decision-making aid or process that involves the clinician and patient. This is referred to as shared decision making because the clinician and patient discuss individual benefits and harms of testing versus not testing and consider patient preferences in the screening decision.

Chronic Disease Prevention

CHAPTER OUTLINE

"Declare the past, diagnose the present, foretell the future."

Hippocrates

1. OVERVIEW OF CHRONIC DISEASE

While infectious diseases posed the biggest threat to the quality and length of human life in the past, the burden of worldwide morbidity and premature mortality has shifted dramatically over the past century to so-called chronic diseases. The term *chronic disease* is less useful than in the past because even infectious diseases such as human immunodeficiency virus (HIV) have become "chronic" with the advent of effective treatments. In essence, any disease that can be effectively managed over years or decades, but not cured, is chronic. The term is applied preferentially, however, to conditions described as follows:

- Not directly transmissible person to person
- Routinely span years and often decades
- Degenerative in some way, relating to aberrant or declining function of some body part or system
- Often propagated by fundamental physiologic imbalances or disturbances, such as inflammation

The conditions of greatest concern—contributing most to years lost from life, lost quality of life, and costs—are cardiovascular diseases (including stroke), cancer, pulmonary diseases, and diabetes and related metabolic derangements. These conditions now constitute the leading causes of mortality worldwide. In addition, conditions such as osteoarthritis, chronic pain syndromes, and dementia exact a high toll in morbidity and cost, generally without causing direct mortality.

Of particular interest to epidemiologists is the strong body of evidence suggesting that fully 80% of premature chronic disease is potentially preventable by means already available.[1]

In this chapter, we will review the prevention of several important chronic diseases. The tertiary prevention of some of these (such as diabetes, cardiovascular disease, hypertension, and dyslipidemia) has already been covered in Chapter 17. For most of these diseases, the medical field progresses rapidly, and new recommendations arise constantly. We concentrate here on major principles of prevention. For more details about treating these conditions, readers should consult the primary literature. Some helpful websites are listed at the end of the chapter.

1.1 THE HUMAN TOLL

A short list of chronic diseases—ischemic heart disease, cancer, stroke, diabetes, and chronic lung disease—constitute the leading force of worldwide mortality.

In some ways, the mortality toll of chronic diseases exaggerates their harms. Chronic degeneration of vitality and function is, to one degree or another, the human fate. As life expectancy rises, so does the opportunity for time-dependent degeneration of organ systems. Chronic, degenerative disease is simply a point along this spectrum and thus inescapable under prevailing conditions: if we escape dying from accidents or infectious disease, we must eventually die of something. To the extent chronic diseases merely represents this inevitable "something," the attributed death toll can inflate their impact. The importance of causes of death earlier in life is best captured not by the number of deaths but by the number of *years of potential life lost*.

In another important way, however, the mortality toll of chronic diseases greatly underestimates their human cost. Long before taking years from life by causing premature death, chronic diseases take *life from years* by reducing ability, function, vitality, and quality of life. This is an ever more salient concern because chronic diseases, driven largely by a short list of lifestyle factors, including obesity,[2] occur at ever younger ages. What was called "adult-onset diabetes" only a generation ago is now called type 2 diabetes and routinely diagnosed in children.

The burden of chronic disease affects some population groups more than others and results from a small number of key risk behaviors that include high blood pressure, tobacco smoking and second-hand smoke exposure, high body mass index (BMI), physical inactivity, alcohol use, and unhealthy diets.[3] Addressing these risk behaviors, as well as the social determinants underlying them, contributes to a more equitable distribution of health.

Collectively, these trends indicate the importance of factoring the chronicity of chronic disease into any assessment of its human cost. As serious and potentially disabling disease begins at ever-younger ages, mortality becomes an increasingly less useful measure of the total impact of these conditions, and measures such as quality-adjusted life years or disability-adjusted life years become more suitable. By such metrics, the human cost of chronic disease is enormous, and it continues to rise.[4]

1.2 THE FINANCIAL TOLL

There are glib expressions in the halls of medicine about the relative financial costs of life and death. Death is cheap, in financial terms, as expenditures related to treatment and preservation of life cease. Life, burdened by chronic disease, can be enormously expensive. As we grow ever more adept at forestalling death through the application of pharmacotherapy, procedures, and medical technology, the costs of living with chronic disease are rising.[4]

As with the mortality statistics, these costs represent several mixed messages. The positive message is that costs of chronic disease care rise as care becomes more effective. When treatments are ineffective, death comes earlier. More effective treatment is unquestionably good, but it means a longer treatment period before death and thus higher costs. Advances in pharmacotherapy and technology tend to improve treatment and function (favorable) but generally involve higher costs (unfavorable). The positive message lost in gloomy statistics about cost is that we "get what we pay for": longer lives despite the high and rising prevalence of chronic disease.

Other messages related to the financial costs of chronic disease are decidedly less positive. As addressed later, chronic diseases are substantially preventable by means already available. The reliance on high-cost treatment is to some degree testimony to the failure to make better use of lower cost prevention. There is also widespread failure to treat risk factors such as high blood pressure, high blood sugar, and dyslipidemia to optimal levels.[5]

Also the *direct* financial costs of chronic disease care do not fully capture the economic toll. Reduced productivity, absenteeism, presenteeism (attending work while sick), and related effects, known in economic terms as *externalities* or *indirect costs*, are high and may even exceed the direct costs.[6]

Projections about the financial costs of chronic disease are genuinely alarming and constitute nothing less than a crisis. If accurate, they question the fundamental solvency and economic viability of the US health care system beyond the middle of the 21st century should current trends persist. As a result, there is increasing awareness about the importance of chronic disease prevention and the strategies that will convert what is known in this area into what is done, as well as increased attention to better management of chronic disease with patient-centered medical homes and the chronic care model. Professionals directly involved in public health and preventive medicine have a clear opportunity to advance the mission of prevention in this chronic disease crisis.

1.3 COMMON ELEMENTS IN PATHOGENESIS

There is increasing appreciation for a unifying constellation of processes that underlie most if not all chronic degenerative diseases.[7,8] These pathways and their details will spawn discussion and debate for years. A case may be made, however, for a short list of common pathways, as shown in Box 19.1.

Of particular relevance in the context of epidemiology is that a common constellation of factors underlying most or all chronic diseases suggests the presence of common pathways to prevention as well.[9]

BOX 19.1 Four Pathophysiologic Pathways in Chronic Disease[a]

1. Cellular Senescence

Aging, or *senescence,* at the organ system and cellular levels encompasses gradual attenuation of function (e.g., age-related decline in glomerular filtration rate) and ultimately a termination of cellular renewal and the loss of formerly functional cells through *apoptosis* (programmed cell death). Chronologic and biologic aging are related but different. *Chronologic aging* refers to a measure in units of actual time; *biologic aging* refers to

function relative to age-standardized norms. By either measure, the time-dependent attenuation of functional capacity is a common element in the development and progression of chronic diseases.

2. Degeneration

Degeneration can occur as a time-dependent process but can also occur independently. Cumulative injury to the vascular

2. PREVENTION OF CHRONIC DISEASE

Literature spanning at least the past two decades makes a compelling case that the leading causes of premature death—and thus the leading causes of chronic morbidity, because they are the same—are overwhelmingly preventable by means already available. A seminal 1993 (updated in 2004) paper first highlighted that chronic diseases leading to premature death were not meaningfully "causes" of death but rather "effects."[10] These effects—the chronic diseases—were the result of 10 factors, mostly behaviors that individuals can control. This analysis found that about 80% of all premature deaths were attributable to the first three factors: tobacco, diet, and physical activity. In other words, we die prematurely because of, alternatively, "how we use our feet, our forks, and our fingers."[11] Subsequent studies updated and supported the same fundamental conclusions.[1, 12] In addition, recent and accumulating evidence indicates that lifestyle interventions can modify gene expression and thus alter the risk for chronic disease development and progression at the genetic level.[13,14] In the aggregate, this literature belies the importance of the nature/nurture debate by highlighting the hegemony of "epigenetics" and the apparent human potential to "nurture nature."

3. CONDITION-SPECIFIC PREVENTION

3.1 OBESITY

More than one-third of the US population is considered obese (Fig. 19.1 and Table 19.1).[15] Obesity is clearly established as a risk factor for most major chronic diseases. Obesity raises the risk for hypertension, dyslipidemia, type 2 diabetes, coronary heart disease, stroke, gallbladder disease, osteoarthritis, sleep apnea and respiratory problems, and some cancers.[16] Whether obesity itself qualifies as a disease is important in several ways. First, obesity bias is a prevalent and pernicious influence, and the establishment of obesity as a true medical condition defends against this in the form of legitimacy. The codification of obesity as a disease implies that, as with other diseases, it is (at least relatively) inappropriate to "blame the victim."

There is a potential liability, however, in cataloging obesity as a disease. Diseases are states of aberrant body function generally amenable to medical treatments (e.g., pharmacotherapy, surgery). If obesity constitutes such an aberrant state, it invites a focus on such treatments as bariatric surgery and antiobesity drugs. This focus might distract attention and divert resources from policies and programs that facilitate better use of feet and forks. In other words, by *blaming* obesity on a diseased state of the body, the potential to address the *diseased* state of the **obesigenic** (obesity-causing) environment may be diminished.

An analogy well suited to clarify this perspective is drowning. Drowning is a legitimate medical condition for which medical care is warranted. However, no one mistakes the propensity to drown as an "aberrant state of the body." Rather, a perfectly normal and healthy body is simply not suited to breathing under the water. Drowning occurs when a normal body spends too much time in an environment (underwater) to which it is poorly suited. The importance of this perspective is in how it relates to prevailing societal responses. The treatment of drowning after it occurs is relatively rare and far from optimal. Many routine steps are taken—from posting lifeguards at beaches, to teaching children how to swim, to putting fences around pools—to prevent drowning from occurring. Only when the clear emphasis on environmental approaches to prevention fails does the treatment of drowning become germane, as a last resort.

Throughout most of human history, calories have been relatively scarce, and physical activity has been an unavoidable requirement for survival. Modern society has devised an environment in which physical activity is scarce and often difficult to maintain, and calories are unavoidable. Homo sapiens are endowed with no native defenses against caloric excess and the tendency toward "sedentariness." The result is the modern obesity trend. In essence, we are *drowning* in calories. This perspective might promote an emphasis on environmentally based approaches (policies and programs that facilitate healthful eating and routine physical activity) to obesity prevention and control, even while establishing the medical legitimacy of obesity as a condition deserving treatment. This fact also explains the epidemic of obesity—that is, the environment has changed, whereas genes have not. A summary of obesity risk factors and prevention activities is listed in Box 19.2

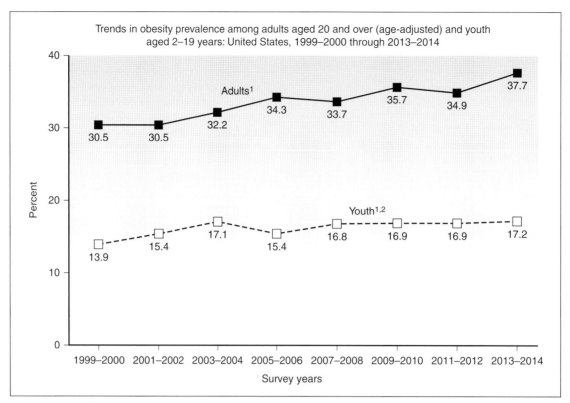

Fig. 19.1 Obesity trends among US adults: 1999–2014.
[1]Significant increasing linear trend from 1999-2000 through 2013-2014.
[2]Test for linear trend for 2003-2004 through 2013-2014 not significant (*p*>0.05)
Note: All adult estimates are age-adjusted by the direct method to the 2000 U.S. census population using the age groups 20-39, 40-59, and 60 and over.
Source: CDC/NCHS, National Health and Nutrition Examination Survey.

TABLE 19.1 **Classification of Weight Status Based on Body Mass Index (BMI)**	
BMI[a]	**Classification**
<18.5	Underweight
18.5–24.9	Normal weight
25–29.9	Overweight
30–34.9	Stage I obesity
35–39.9	Stage II obesity
>40	Stage III (severe) obesity

[a]Expressed as weight in kilograms divided by the square of the height in meters (weight [kg]/height[2] [m]). From Papadakis MA, McPhee SJ, Rabow MW (eds): *Current Medical Diagnosis and Therapy 2018*, ed 57, McGraw Hill, 2017, New York/Chicago/San Francisco.

Nonmodifiable risk factors for obesity include low resting energy expenditure, genetic polymorphisms that predispose to weight gain and impede weight loss, and an ethnic heritage that increases the propensity for obesity. *Modifiable* risk factors relate principally to the quality and quantity of dietary intake and energy expenditure through exercise. Lean body mass can be increased through exercise and thus also constitutes a modifiable risk factor. Insomnia increases obesity risk by several mechanisms, and thus impaired sleep is a potentially modifiable risk factor as well.

The primary and secondary preventions of obesity principally involve appropriate diet and physical activity. Secondary prevention includes screening, which means clinical assessment of weight and height to calculate BMI as well as waist circumference, and for children the plotting of BMI on appropriate growth charts.[17] The US Prevention Services Task Force (USPSTF) recommends that clinicians regularly screen all patients from age 6 onwards for obesity.[18]

Many diets are effective at inducing weight loss as long as they restrict total energy intake, are based mainly on plants, and use mostly unprocessed foods.[19] However, most diets are only modestly effective, if at all, at inducing long-term weight loss. While most patients do not succeed in sustaining weight loss, a small group does. Patients with a weight loss of 33 kg and more for over 5 years reported engaging in high levels of physical activity (around 60 min/day); maintaining a low-calorie, low-fat diet; eating breakfast regularly; performing constant self-monitoring of weight; and maintaining consistent eating patterns throughout the week.[20]

Tertiary prevention, to prevent complications of established obesity, often involves pharmacotherapy for metabolic complications and bariatric surgery. The utility of bariatric surgery is well established and leads to an average of 20% to 35% weight loss.[16] Pharmacotherapy for obesity is, to date, of limited utility and prone to unintended consequences. The

BOX 19.2 Summary of Obesity Risk Factors and Prevention[a]

RISK FACTORS
Nonmodifiable
Resting energy expenditure/basal metabolic rate
Genetics
Ethnicity

Modifiable
Energy consumption
Energy expenditure
Lean body mass
Sleep quality and quantity
Chronic stress
Low socioeconomic status

PREVENTION
Primary Prevention
Dietary management: improved quality, control of quantity
Physical activity

Secondary Prevention
Screening: assessing body mass index (BMI) and waist circumference in clinical practice; plotting pediatric BMI on growth charts
Dietary management
Physical activity promotion
Possible use of pharmacotherapy

Tertiary Prevention
Bariatric surgery
Pharmacotherapy
Dietary management and physical activity promotion as important adjuncts

[a]Managing Overweight and Obesity in Adults. *Systematic Evidence Review from the Obesity Expert Panel.* 2013. Available at: https://www.nhlbi.nih.gov/sites/default/files/media/docs/obesity-evidence-review.pdf.

use of medications for the metabolic complications of obesity, such as prediabetes, is more clearly supported by high-quality evidence.[16]

3.2 TYPE 2 DIABETES MELLITUS

In developed countries, about 95% of patients with diabetes mellitus have type 2. Type 2 diabetes mellitus, formerly called *adult-onset diabetes,* is usually preventable, both by treating the insulin resistance that often precedes it and, more fundamentally, by preventing the accumulation of excess visceral fat that is an important root cause, if not the cause, in most patients.

The Centers for Disease Control and Prevention (CDC) projects that as many as one in three Americans will have diabetes by the mid-21st century if current trends persist,[21] putting the fate of the US health care system in doubt. Many other countries are not far behind. Fortunately, type 2 diabetes is overwhelmingly preventable by available interventions. A fasting glucose between 100 and 125 mg/dL is indicative of

prediabetes. Diagnosing diabetes requires a fasting glucose of more than 126 or a hemoglobin A1c of more than 6.5 (if confirmed by repeat testing). The USPSTF recommends diabetes screening in all patients aged 40 to 70 years who are overweight or obese, as well as those with hypertension or risk factors for obesity such as certain racial/ethnic groups, a family history of diabetes, and a history of gestational diabetes or polycystic ovarian syndrome.[22]

Risk factors for type 2 diabetes overlap substantially with risk factors for obesity. Rates of diabetes are considerably higher in some ethnic groups than others, and there is a known genetic predisposition. The principal driver of the epidemiology of type 2 diabetes, however, and its progression from a disease of adults into a disease of children and adults alike, is **epidemic** (or hyperendemic) **obesity** (see earlier discussion). In particular, central adiposity and the accumulation of excess visceral fat in the liver are causally implicated. Diabetes can be prevented with lifestyle interventions that foster moderate weight loss (a weight loss of 2.5–5.5 kg decreases the risk of developing type 2 diabetes by 30–60%), with pharmacotherapy, and with bariatric surgery. Medical management of diabetes to prevent progression and complications constitutes tertiary prevention (see Chapter 17). Box 19.3 summarizes diabetes risk factors and prevention strategies.

BOX 19.3 Summary of Type 2 Diabetes Risk Factors and Prevention

RISK FACTORS
Nonmodifiable
Genetics
Ethnicity

Modifiable
Obesity, in particular abdominal (visceral) adiposity

PREVENTION
Primary Prevention
Weight loss/management
Dietary management
Physical activity
Pharmacotherapy
Bariatric surgery

Secondary Prevention
Screening: fasting glucose; glucose tolerance testing
Dietary management
Physical activity
Pharmacotherapy
Bariatric surgery

Tertiary Prevention
Pharmacotherapy
Medical assessment for potential complications (e.g., eye and foot examinations)
Bariatric surgery
Weight loss/management
Dietary management
Physical activity

3.3 CARDIOVASCULAR DISEASE

Cardiovascular disease includes coronary artery disease, as well as congestive heart failure, peripheral artery disease, and aortic aneurysms. Risk factors for heart disease vary by culture and circumstance. The focus here is preferentially on the epidemiology of heart disease, specifically **coronary artery disease** (CAD), or ischemic heart disease, in the United States and comparably developed nations. Chronic inflammation is now known to propagate the progression of atherosclerotic plaque, implicating such conditions as periodontal disease.

The principal determinants of cardiovascular risk tend to be lifestyle behaviors. In particular, tobacco use, dietary pattern, and physical activity level are of considerable importance and greatly influence the probability of future cardiac events (e.g., unstable angina, heart attacks, sudden cardiac death). To some extent, however, such effects are indirect. Poor diet and lack of physical activity tend to contribute to dyslipidemia and hypertension, which in turn raise cardiovascular risk. It is these "downstream effects" of diet and physical activity patterns that are incorporated into quantified estimates of future risk, such as the Framingham cardiac risk score.[23]

Box 19.4 summarizes cardiovascular risk factors and prevention strategies. Many risk factors contribute to cardiovascular disease, including age, gender, hypertension, smoking, and dyslipidemia.[24] Treatment and prevention of coronary artery disease are discussed extensively in Chapter 17.

Stroke, or cerebrovascular accident (CVA), is the fourth leading cause of death in the United States after heart disease, cancer, and lung disease[1] and a major cause of long-term morbidity. The incidence rate of stroke in those age 50 and older has declined in the United States, principally because of better detection and treatment of hypertension, the major risk factor.[25]

Risk factors for stroke overlap substantially with risk factors for cardiovascular disease. Medical conditions (e.g., diabetes) that increase the risk of heart disease similarly increase the risk of stroke. Atrial fibrillation, rapid irregular beating of the atria, is a risk factor for stroke, generally managed with anticoagulation. The main modifiable risk factor for stroke is **hypertension.** Patient adherence to management guidelines for blood pressure reliably translates into reduced stroke risk and, at the population level, reduced stroke incidence.

Revascularization, such as carotid endarterectomy after a transient ischemic attack, constitutes secondary stroke prevention. Thrombolytic and anticoagulant therapies to limit stroke-related injury to the brain, and rehabilitation programs to preserve and restore function, constitute the mainstays of tertiary prevention. Updated information about stroke management and prevention is available from the CDC and the National Stroke Foundation (see Websites). As of 2018, the USPSTF recommends against screening for carotid stenosis in asymptomatic individuals.[26]

The USPSTF currently recommends routine screening for hypertension and dyslipidemia, as well as use of statins and aspirin for primary prevention of CAD in patients meeting eligibility criteria.[27] The USPSTF does not recommend population screening with electrocardiogram (EKG) or stress tests.[28]

3.4 CHRONIC LUNG DISEASE

Chronic lower respiratory tract disease, including chronic obstructive pulmonary disease (COPD), emphysema, bronchitis, and pneumoconiosis, constitutes the third leading cause of death in the United States after heart disease and cancer.[1] An enormous portion of this toll is directly related to tobacco and is thus preventable with tobacco avoidance. Pneumoconioses are generally work-related diseases, and prevention is thus an occupational health issue (see Chapter 22).

BOX 19.4 Summary of Cardiovascular Disease Risk Factors and Prevention

RISK FACTORS	PREVENTION
Nonmodifiable	**Primary Prevention**
Age	Tobacco avoidance
Gender	Healthful eating
Family history/genetics	Physical activity
	Stress management
Modifiable	Weight control
Dyslipidemia	Pharmacotherapy for risk factor modification (e.g., hypertension, diabetes, dyslipidemia)
Hypertension	
Diabetes/prediabetes (including insulin resistance)	Risk factor screening (e.g., cholesterol, blood pressure)
Obesity, in particular abdominal (visceral) adiposity	Chemoprophylaxis with low-dose aspirin for high-risk patients
Poor diet	
Lack of physical activity	**Secondary Prevention**
Smoking	Risk factor management, as for primary prevention
Stress	Revascularization (angioplasty; coronary artery bypass surgery)
	Tertiary Prevention
	Risk factor management as for primary prevention to prevent recurrence/ progression
	Revascularization to preserve/restore function
	Cardiac rehabilitation

Asthma, an important chronic condition of the upper airway, is a relatively uncommon cause of mortality but an important cause of morbidity.

Nonmodifiable risk factors for chronic pulmonary disease include age and certain genetic disorders, such as α_1-antitrypsin deficiency and cystic fibrosis. Modifiable risk factors include exposure to airborne toxins caused by pollution, occupation, or tobacco smoke.

Tobacco avoidance and smoking cessation are top priorities in the prevention and treatment of chronic pulmonary diseases. There is no standard screening for pulmonary disease. The USPSTF recommends against screening for COPD,[29] but recommends screening for lung cancer in high-risk patients.[30] Secondary prevention relates to management of early-stage disease to prevent progression. Pharmacotherapy is prominent in such efforts, notably inhaled medications and antiinflammatory drugs (e.g., steroids) for asthma, COPD, and chronic bronchitis. Tertiary prevention may include home oxygen for patients functionally limited by hypoxemia, along with medications to manage symptoms and prevent progression, and pulmonary rehabilitation after decompensation.

3.5 CANCER

Most chronic diseases affect a particular organ system (e.g., heart disease, stroke, pulmonary disease, arthritis, diabetes). In contrast, cancer—the second leading cause of death in the United States—can affect any organ or tissue in the body and is relatively common and potentially lethal. From the preventive medicine standpoint, the most important facts about cancer include the following[31]:

- Cancer is acknowledged to be substantially (up to 60%) preventable by addressing lifestyle behaviors
- Cigarette smoking is the most important preventable cause of cancer
- Cancer is not the unpredictable threat that the public tends to believe it is
- Healthy diet, weight control, and exercise reduce the risk of many cancers, such as breast and colon cancer
- Vaccines can prevent some cancers, such as the human papillomavirus (HPV) vaccine (cervical cancer and possibly some head and neck cancers) and hepatitis B and C vaccine (hepatocellular cancer)
- For many cancers, it is not clear that screening is beneficial (see upcoming discussion and Chapter 16)

The development of some cancers over time is analogous to the progression of atherosclerotic plaque leading to clinically significant coronary disease. The steps of that process span years to decades, sometimes providing opportunities for effective prevention (Table 19.2). *Initiation* refers to the development of a potentially carcinogenic (cancer-causing) mutation. *Promotion* refers to the growth of cancer cells, before any clinical symptoms or signs develop. *Expression* refers to the first clinical evidence of the presence of cancer.

Nonmodifiable risk factors for cancer include age and predisposing genetic mutations, some of which are important

TABLE 19.2 **Steps in Development and Progression of Cancer and Opportunities for Prevention**	
Stage	**Relevant Prevention Methods**
Initiation	Toxin avoidance, particularly tobacco smoke and excess alcohol Healthful diet Weight control Physical activity Immunization, in some cases
Promotion	Early detection and treatment through screening Other methods as for initiation
Expression	Diagnosis and treatment Other methods as for initiation

and well known (e.g., breast cancer susceptibility genes or BRCA; see Chapter 16). Modifiable risk factors include diet, physical activity, body weight, tobacco use, exposure to infectious agents, and toxins.

The primary prevention of cancer mostly involves the avoidance of relevant pathogens, including the following:
- HPV, implicated in cervical cancer, anal and penile cancers, and head and neck cancers.
- Hepatitis B virus (HBV), implicated in hepatocellular carcinoma.
- Toxins, such as tobacco and excess alcohol.
- Industrial chemicals at the worksite that potentially contaminate the environment and food supply.

Healthful eating, moderate physical activity, and weight control offer important defenses at all stages of cancer. As noted in the previous discussion of obesity, the link between excess body fat and cancer risk is well established and of general importance. For patients at high risk of developing certain cancers, such as colorectal cancer, aspirin may be used for primary prevention. The use of selective estrogen receptor modulators to prevent breast and ovarian cancer in high-risk patients is another example.

The secondary prevention of cancer principally involves making use of effective screening protocols. The USPSTF recommends screening specific populations for cervical, breast, colon, and lung cancer. For most other common cancers, the USPSTF concludes that the decision to screen should be individualized to the specific patient (prostate cancer), that there is insufficient evidence for or against screening (skin cancer, bladder cancer, oral cancer), or recommends against screening (thyroid cancer, ovarian cancer, testicular cancer, pancreatic cancer). Screening in women with high-risk mutations such as BRCA are covered in Chapter 16. Readers are encouraged to keep current with these often-changing topics by visiting the USPSTF website (see also Chapter 18).

Tertiary cancer prevention involves effective treatment and a range of strategies aimed at preventing recurrence and progression, as well as strategies to restore function or appearance, such as rehabilitation and reconstructive cosmetic surgery.

3.6 ORAL HEALTH, VISION, AND HEARING

Dental caries are one of the few conditions so common that screening is inappropriate. Instead, prophylaxis in the form of routine dental visits for cleanings and fluoride application is the standard of care.

In addition to caries, periodontal disease is an important form of pathology in the oral cavity. Research over recent decades has highlighted the importance of oral health to general health and the link between gingivitis and periodontitis to a variety of systemic diseases.[32] The following primary strategies help prevent chronic disease of the oral cavity:

- Good oral hygiene (routine brushing and flossing)
- Adequate intake of fluoride from water or dental treatment
- Routine dental visits
- Avoidance of excess alcohol
- Avoidance of toxins, such as tobacco

In many underserved areas, there are even fewer dentists than medical practitioners. Efforts are underway to train related health care fields to incorporate oral health in their efforts.

For glaucoma, hearing loss in the elderly, and vision impairment in the elderly, the USPSTF provides I-recommendations as of 2018.[33]

3.7 DEMENTIA, CHRONIC PAIN, AND ARTHRITIS

Dementia is a diverse category of conditions; some are preventable by means as simple as nutrient supplementation, and others are not preventable at all. Alzheimer's disease is of particular interest in this regard. Because of its rising prevalence and its enormous human and economic costs, Alzheimer's disease is receiving increasing attention and resources related to prevention, early diagnosis, treatment, and cure. However, it is not clear to which degree dementia can be prevented and which screening instruments are suitable for population screening. As of the writing of this text, the USPSTF has concluded that the evidence is insufficient to recommend for or against screening for cognitive impairment.[34]

Conditions of **chronic pain,** especially arthritis, are prevalent and important contributors to morbidity,[1] as well as indirectly to mortality. For example, the physical inactivity leading to progression of obesity and development of diabetes may be a major determinant of a fatal myocardial infarction. With the potential interplay of chronic conditions, each compounding the other, chronic pain may foster physical inactivity, which may lead to weight gain, which may exacerbate the pain. Such complexity occurs in many older patients with chronic disease, warranting meaningful applications of *holistic care.*

Osteoarthritis (OA) may be the quintessential example of a degenerative disease attributable to "wear and tear." Symptoms develop and progress as friction erodes articular cartilage in the knee, hip, hand, and other joints. Some degree of secondary inflammation may occur, but inflammation is relatively unimportant in OA, in contrast to rheumatologic diseases such as rheumatoid arthritis. Strategies for the primary prevention of OA include avoiding excessive stress to joints and exercising to keep muscles well conditioned. Secondary prevention directed at symptom control and preservation of function involves analgesics, supplements, and modalities such as massage, as well as regular physical activity. Tertiary prevention—restoration of function impaired by disease progression and prevention of complications—includes physical therapy and rehabilitation, strategies to reconstitute eroded cartilage, and surgery, especially joint replacement.

4. BARRIERS AND OPPORTUNITIES

4.1 IMPEDIMENTS TO CHRONIC DISEASE PREVENTION

The toll of chronic disease and its well-established preventability by available means make a compelling case for action, especially considering the personal nature of public health statistics. Almost every family in modern society has faced some chronic disease and knows someone with heart disease, cancer, lung disease, stroke, or diabetes. Here, as in many other instances, we do not lack knowledge about what to do, but skills on how to convert what we know consistently to action. If we were to find the means to turn what we know about prevention into what we practice routinely, many persons directly affected by premature chronic disease would not have been affected by the disease.[3] We as a society have the opportunity to bequeath the avoidance of that suffering and loss to our children. One barrier that might be readily overcome is the failure to part the veil of statistical anonymity and recognize the familiar faces on the other side.

4.1.a Personal Barriers

Some barriers to fulfilling the promise of chronic disease prevention relate to lifestyle behaviors. Most of us struggle with eating better or exercising enough. Our patients are no different. As the focus of prevention moves outside the clinical domain and into lifestyle, health professionals have less direct control. Chronic disease prevention increasingly must be a personal endeavor, and many people lack the required skill or the will, or both. Clinical training in lifestyle medicine aims to provide clinicians with more skills to intervene here (see Websites).

4.1.b Systemic Barriers

Many aspects of modern living conspire directly against chronic disease prevention efforts. Overconsumption of calories is routine for many reasons, including federal subsidies that foster the propagation of processed foods, the intentional hyperpalatability of these foods, assertive and creative food-marketing efforts (especially to children), and the ubiquity of food (especially fast food). Lack of physical activity is explained in part by an ever-expanding array of devices that perform tasks once done by muscles, at work and at play, with schedules that make the allocation of time for exercise difficult and excuses easy. In essence, almost everything about modern living that makes it modern is obesigenic, and much is **morbidigenic** (disease causing).[35]

4.2 OPPORTUNITIES FOR CHRONIC DISEASE PREVENTION

Opportunities, however, are as great and numerous as barriers and challenges. There is increasing attention to the importance of prevention for both the public health and the health of national economies. Federal regulations, such as reimbursement for lifestyle counseling by physicians, are evolving. A medical specialty devoted to lifestyle approaches has emerged, and "new age" tools provide novel means to engage health care professionals in effective behavior modification efforts.[36]

Given the traditional focus of formalized medicine on *disease care*, it is not surprising that much of the emphasis on prevention in the health care context relates to better screening, early treatment, and better management of established chronic disease. Two examples for better screening and management are the patient-centered medical home and the chronic care model (see Chapters 28 and 29). Although laudable and important, these models emphasize the delivery of clinical services and define the recipient as a patient. The greatest opportunities for chronic disease prevention (1) involve changing lifestyle behaviors in ways that are acceptable to most people, (2) reside largely outside the clinical setting, and (3) relate to the preservation of health in people who have no cause to be "patients" (see also "Social Determinants of Health" in Chapters 14 and 30).

Clinicians can learn to be more effective agents of change, but only to a certain degree. Environment and various health-related policies can be adopted to facilitate favorable "defaults" (see Chapter 29). Expert guidance may be provided at decision points, such as the purchase of food.[37] Financial incentives may be used to motivate achievement of health goals[38] or to reward healthful choices.[39]

A shining example of the power of comprehensive prevention of chronic disease is the North Karelia Project in Finland. The North Karelia Project was started in 1972 as a national pilot and demonstration program for cardiovascular prevention in Finland, which had then very elevated rates of cardiovascular disease. A comprehensive community-based intervention involving health services, nongovernmental organizations (NGOs), industry, media, and public policy was used to address smoking, hypertension, and elevated cholesterol. Subsequently, mortality from cardiovascular disease among males age 30 to 64 was reduced by 73%, and all-cause mortality and reduced mortality from several cancers followed.[40] The promise of drastic reductions in the human and financial costs of chronic disease beckons and is achievable by means already in hand.

4.3 COMPLEMENTARY AND ALTERNATIVE MEDICINE

Trends in survey data indicate that the use of **complementary and alternative medicine** (CAM) is increasing in the United States, with more than one-third of adults using some form of CAM.[41]

The boundaries of what constitutes CAM are not clearly defined. Some disciplines generally considered alternative, such as chiropractic and acupuncture, are increasingly embraced by allopathic medicine and may eventually become standard in the care of certain medical problems. Other controversies relate to nomenclature and scientific evidence. Neither *alternative* nor *complementary* is thought to be an optimal designation for the field, and actually the terms are contradictory.

Efforts are ongoing to improve the evidence base for CAM.[42] Concerns persist that much of CAM lacks a rigorous evidence base, but most authorities agree that the effectiveness of nearly half of conventional medical practice is similarly unsubstantiated by the modern standards of evidence. Whether CAM use improves outcomes, reduces or increases the costs of care, or improves patient satisfaction is largely uncertain. Currently, there are increasing efforts toward a creative and responsible synthesis of conventional medicine and CAM, which is often called **integrative medicine.**

5. SUMMARY

The human and financial tolls of chronic disease in modern society present many opportunities for prevention, particularly regarding the short list of factors responsible for most chronic diseases, directly or indirectly. This same list indicates the degree to which all or most chronic diseases could be prevented through one common, health-promoting approach, a promise borne out by population studies. As much as an 80% reduction in the mortality and morbidity of heart disease, stroke, and diabetes could be achieved with improvements in dietary and physical activity patterns and tobacco avoidance. Complementary and alternative medicine is increasingly used in the United States, but the evidence base for it is still emerging. Efforts to synthetize complementary and alternative medicine with conventional medicine comprise integrative medicine.

REFERENCES

1. Daar AS, Singer PA, Persad DL, et al. Grand challenges in chronic non-communicable diseases. *Nature.* 2007;450:494-496.
2. Egger G. Obesity, chronic disease, and economic growth: a case for "big picture" prevention. *Adv Prev Med.* 2011;2011: 149-158.
3. Bauer UE, Briss PA, Goodman RA, Bowman BA. Prevention of chronic disease in the 21st century: elimination of the leading preventable causes of premature death and disability in the USA. *Lancet.* 2014;384:45-52.

4. US Burden of Disease Collaborators, Mokdad AH, Ballestros K, et al. The state of US health, 1990-2016: burden of diseases, injuries, and risk factors among US States. *JAMA*. 2018;319:1444-1472. doi:10.1001/jama.2018.0158.

5. Yoon S, Fryar C, Carroll M. *Hypertension Prevalence and Control Among Adults*: United States, 2011–2014. NCHS Data Brief, No. 220. Hyattsville, MD: National Center for Health Statistics, Centers for Disease Control and Prevention, US Dept of Health and Human Services; 2015.

6. Thrall JH. Prevalence and costs of chronic disease in a health care system structured for treatment of acute illness. *Radiology*. 2005;235:9-12.

7. Probst-Hensch NM. Chronic age-related diseases share risk factors: do they share pathophysiological mechanisms and why does that matter? *Swiss Med Wkly*. 2010;140:w13072. doi:10.4414/smw.2010.13072.

8. Diomedi M, Leone G, Renna A. The role of chronic infection and inflammation in the pathogenesis of cardiovascular and cerebrovascular disease. *Drugs Today (Barc)*. 2005;41:745-753.

9. Sagner M, Katz D, Egger G, et al. Lifestyle medicine potential for reversing a world of chronic disease epidemics: from cell to community. *Int J Clin Pract*. 68:1289-1292, 2014.

10. McGinnis JM, Foege WH. Actual causes of death in the United States. *JAMA*. 1993;270:2207-2212.

11. Meeting News American Association of Diabetes Educators Annual Meeting. *The Real Secret Behind Healthy Eating: Feet, Forks and Fingers*. 2018. Available at: https://www.healio.com/endocrinology/diabetes-education/news/online/%7Bf58eeece-351a-4090-9579-5f1631cd69a5%7D/the-real-secret-behind-healthy-eating-feet-forks-and-fingers.

12. Mokdad AH, Marks JS, Stroup DF, Gerberding JL. Actual causes of death in the United States, 2000. *JAMA*. 2004;291:1238-1245.

13. Ornish D, Magbanua MJ, Weidner G, et al. Changes in prostate gene expression in men undergoing an intensive nutrition and lifestyle intervention. *Proc Natl Acad Sci USA*. 2008;105:8369-8374.

14. Ornish D, Lin J, Daubenmier J, et al. Increased telomerase activity and comprehensive lifestyle changes: a pilot study. *Lancet Oncol*. 2008;9:1048-1057.

15. Centers for Disease Control and Prevention. *Adult Obesity Facts*. August 13, 2018. Available at: https://www.cdc.gov/obesity/data/adult.html. Accessed July 16, 2019.

16. Managing Overweight and Obesity in Adults. *Systematic Evidence Review from the Obesity Expert Panel*. 2013. Available at: https://www.nhlbi.nih.gov/sites/default/files/media/docs/obesity-evidence-review.pdf.

17. Centers for Disease Control and Prevention. *Growth Charts*. September 9, 2010. Available at: http://www.cdc.gov/growthcharts/. Accessed July 16, 2019.

18. U.S. Preventive Services Task Force. *Final Recommendation Statement*: *Obesity in Adults: Screening and Counseling*, 2003. 2019. Available at: https://www.uspreventiveservicestaskforce.org/Page/Document/RecommendationStatementFinal/obesity-in-adults-screening-and-counseling-2003. Accessed July 16, 2019.

19. Katz DL, Meller S. Can we say what diet is best for health? *Annu Rev Public Health*. 2014;35:83-103.

20. Wing RR, Phelan S, Long-term weight loss maintenance. *The American Journal of Clinical Nutrition*. 2005;82(1):222S–225S..

21. *Number of Americans with Diabetes Projected to Double or Triple by 2050* [press release]. Atlanta, GA: Centers for Disease Control and Prevention; October 22, 2010. Available at: http://www.cdc.gov/media/pressrel/2010/r101022.html. Accessed July 16, 2019.

22. U.S. Preventive Services Task Force. *Final Update Summary*: *Obesity in Adults: Screening and Counseling*, 2012. Available at: https://www.uspreventiveservicestaskforce.org/Page/Document/UpdateSummaryFinal/obesity-in-adults-screening-and-counseling-2003. (Accessed June 5, 2018.).

23. Framingham Heart Study: Cardiovascular Disease (10 year Risk); available at: https://www.framinghamheartstudy.org/fhs-risk-functions/cardiovascular-disease-10-year-risk; accessed 10/6/2019

24. D'Agostino RB, Vasan RS, Pencina MJ, et al. General cardiovascular risk profile for use in primary care. *Circulation*. 2008;117:743-753.

25. Laino C. Stroke Rates Are Rising for Young Americans. *WebMD*. February 9, 2011. Available at: http://www.webmd.com/stroke/news/20110209/stroke-rates-are-rising-for-young-americans.

26. U.S. Preventive Services Task Force. *Final Recommendation Statement*: *Carotid Artery Stenosis Screening*. 2016. Available at: https://www.uspreventiveservicestaskforce.org/Page/Document/RecommendationStatementFinal/carotid-artery-stenosis-screening. Accessed June 5, 2018.

27. U.S. Preventive Services Task Force. *Final Recommendation Statement*: *Aspirin to Prevent Cardiovascular Disease and Cancer*. 2019. Available at: https://www.uspreventiveservicestaskforce.org/Page/Document/RecommendationStatementFinal/aspirin-to-prevent-cardiovascular-disease-and-cancer. Accessed June 5, 2018.

28. U.S. Preventive Services Task Force. *Final Update Summary*: *Coronary Health Disease Screening with Electrocardiography*. 2018. Available at: https://www.uspreventiveservicestaskforce.org/Page/Document/UpdateSummaryFinal/coronary-heart-disease-screening-with-electrocardiography. Accessed June 5, 2018.

29. U.S. Preventive Services Task Force. *Final Update Summary*: *Chronic and Obstructive Pulmonary Disease Screening*. 2016. Available at: https://www.uspreventiveservicestaskforce.org/Page/Document/UpdateSummaryFinal/chronic-obstructive-pulmonary-disease-screening. Accessed June 5, 2018.

30. U.S. Preventive Services Task Force. *Final Update Summary*: *Lung Cancer Screening*. 2015. Available at: https://www.uspreventiveservicestaskforce.org/Page/Document/UpdateSummaryFinal/lung-cancer-screening. Accessed June 5, 2018.

31. Papadakis MA, McPhee SJ, Rabow MW, eds. *Current Medical Diagnosis and Therapy 2018*. 57th ed. New York/Chicago/San Francisco; McGraw Hill; 2017:13.

32. Teng YT, Taylor GW, Scannapieco F, et al. Periodontal health and systemic disorders. *J Can Dent Assoc*. 2002;68:188-192.

33. U.S. Preventive Services Task Force. *Published Final Recommendations*. Available at: https://www.uspreventiveservicestaskforce.org/BrowseRec/Index. Accessed June 5, 2018.

34. U.S. Preventive Services Task Force. *Final Recommendation Statement*: *Cognitive Impairment in Older Adults: Screening*. 2014. Available at: https://www.uspreventiveservicestaskforce.org/Page/Document/RecommendationStatementFinal/cognitive-impairment-in-older-adults-screening. Accessed June 5, 2018.

35. Katz DL. Obesity…be dammed! What it will take to turn the tide? *Harvard Health Policy Rev*. 2006;7:135-151.

36. Academy of Communication in Healthcare. Webinars. Accessed at: https://www.achonline.org/Resources/Webinars on 10/6/2019

37. The NuVal Attribute Program. Available at: www.nuval.com.

38. IncentaHealth. Available at: http://www.incentahealth.com/; KrowdFit. Available at: http://www.kardio.com/.

39. Katz D. Should Food Stamp Nutrition Be Mandated? *Huffington Post.* September 29, 2011. Available at: http://www.huffingtonpost.com/david-katz-md/food-stamps-healthy-food_b_984684.html.

40. Pekka P. Successful prevention of non-communicable diseases: 25 year experiences with North Karelia Project in Finland. *Public Health Med.* 2002;4(1):5-7. Available at: http://www.who.int/chp/media/en/north_karelia_successful_ncd_prevention.pdf.

41. Barnes PM, Bloom B, Nahin R. *CDC National Health Statistics Report #12. Complementary and Alternative Medicine Use Among Adults and Children: United States,* 2007. December 2008. Available at: https://nccih.nih.gov/research/statistics/2007/camsurvey_fs1.htm#use.

42. Kantor M. The role of rigorous scientific evaluation in the use and practice of complementary and alternative medicine. *J Am Coll Radiol.* 2009;6:254-262.

WEBSITES

American College of Lifestyle Medicine: https://www.lifestyle medicine.org/

Centers for Disease Control and Prevention: http://www.cdc.gov/chronicdisease/

National Stroke Association: www.stroke.org

Robert Wood Johnson Foundation: www.stateofobesity.org

US Preventive Services Task Force: http://www.uspreventiveservicestaskforce.org/uspstf/uspsobes.htm

World Health Organization: http://www.who.int/topics/chronic_diseases/en/

REVIEW QUESTIONS

1. The elimination of as much as 80% of chronic disease could most reliably be achieved with advancements in:
   A. Surgical options for curative procedures
   B. Drug therapies toward better treatment
   C. Vitamin supplementation toward more efficient prevention
   D. Imaging modalities toward more accurate screening
   E. Behavior modification toward healthier lifestyles

2. Other than advances in infectious disease treatment (transforming once rapidly fatal scourges such as HIV into chronic conditions), what other, relatively recent change has challenged historic definitions of chronic disease?
   A. Chronic diseases can now span years or even decades
   B. Chronic diseases are degenerative in some way
   C. Chronic diseases relate to aberrant or declining function of some body part or system
   D. Chronic diseases propagate by fundamental physiologic imbalances or disturbances, such as inflammation
   E. Chronic diseases now occur at younger ages

3. Which of the following pairs are best considered the leading *root* causes of death in the United States?
   A. Cardiovascular disease and cancer
   B. Obesity and diabetes
   C. Cellular senescence and degeneration
   D. Oxidation and inflammation
   E. Diet and exercise

4. With regard to obesity, plotting height and weight on pediatric growth charts represents:
   A. Mandatory disease reporting
   B. Nonmodifiable risk assessment
   C. Primary prevention
   D. Secondary prevention
   E. Tertiary prevention

5. The best example of a degenerative "wear and tear" disease is:
   A. Osteoarthritis
   B. Coronary artery disease
   C. Gastric cancer
   D. Ischemic stroke
   E. Alzheimer disease

6. Should current trends persist, the CDC projects that by the middle of the 21st century, diabetes could affect how many Americans?
   A. Virtually all
   B. 1 in 3
   C. 1 in 5
   D. 1 in 10
   E. 1 in 20

7. A decline in the rate of stroke among older adults is most reliably associated with better detection and treatment of:
   A. Hypertension
   B. Dyslipidemia
   C. Obesity
   D. Coagulopathies
   E. Vascular malformations

8. An example of primary cancer prevention is:
   A. Colonoscopy as recommended by USPSTF
   B. Mammography as recommended by USPSTF
   C. Lumpectomy
   D. HPV vaccination
   E. PSA testing

9. A process common to most if not all chronic diseases is:
   A. Neovascularization
   B. Apoptosis
   C. Fibrosis
   D. Inflammation
   E. Hypertrophy

10. Dietary intake of which of the following substances is inversely associated with blood pressure?
    A. Alcohol
    B. Calcium
    C. Insoluble fiber
    D. Polyunsaturated fat
    E. Sodium

ANSWERS AND EXPLANATIONS

1. **E.** Chronic diseases are intimately linked to lifestyle behaviors, especially diet, exercise, tobacco use, and alcohol consumption. Changing lifestyle behaviors could prevent or eliminate as much as 80% of chronic disease. Surgical options (A) are effective for eliminating certain conditions (e.g., bariatric surgery for obesity and weight-related diabetes), but do not have the impact on chronic diseases as do broader behavioral modifications. Drug therapies (B) help manage chronic conditions but do little to eliminate them; lifestyle modification (e.g., for diabetes prevention vs drug therapy with metformin) are more effective. Vitamin supplementation (C) may only be good for correcting vitamin deficiency. Vitamin D may be an exception, but currently no strong evidence supports its use for any chronic diseases other than bone disease. Healthy diet, more exercise, and tobacco cessation would have greater impact on chronic diseases in general. Imaging modalities and screening (D) are important for the early identification of many chronic diseases but would do little to eliminate them.

2. **E.** Called *adult-onset* diabetes only a generation ago, type 2 diabetes is now routinely diagnosed in children. The proliferation of cardiac risk factors in younger children is well documented, and a marked increase in stroke among patients 5 to 14 years old has been reported. Likewise, the occasional lifestyle-related cancer is diagnosed in surprisingly young persons. Chronic diseases once only seen in adults now often occur in children. Regardless, these diseases are still degenerative in some way (B), are related to aberrant to declining function (C), and propagate by fundamental physiologic disturbances such as inflammation (D). Chronic diseases also still span years or even decades (A), but because they start earlier in life, they may ultimately cause earlier morbidity and mortality.

3. **E.** Along with other lifestyle behaviors (e.g., smoking cessation, alcohol moderation) diet and exercise are fundamental to health promotion and disease prevention. Lifestyles defined by poor diets and physical inactivity lead to oxidation and inflammation within the body (D), cellular senescence and degeneration (C), often obesity and diabetes (B), and then, too often, cardiovascular disease, cancer (A), and death.

4. **D.** Plotting height and weight allows for calculation of body mass index (BMI) and other clinical measures of obesity risk; this is screening, a secondary prevention. Height and weight plotting can identify overweight children and children at risk for obesity so that interventions can be put in place to prevent obesity from occurring. Primary prevention (C) for obesity would be directed at normal-weight children, to prevent the dietary imbalances and hormonal abnormalities that lead to overweight and obesity. Tertiary prevention (E) is directed at obese children and focuses on limiting disability, stopping weight gain, and promoting fat loss. Pediatricians are encouraged to track their patients' BMI; this is not mandatory disease reporting (A). Body weight is modifiable, not nonmodifiable (B).

5. **A.** OA is a degenerative condition defined by the breakdown of the smooth cartilage covering contact surfaces of bone ends within many of the body's large joints. The "wear and tear" process of OA occurs over decades from mechanical stress and is accelerated by factors that make joint friction more severe (e.g., knee arthritis in morbidly obese individuals from increased mechanical load) and/or more frequent (e.g., shoulder arthritis in baseball pitchers from repetitive use). Some degree of secondary inflammation, oxidation, and cellular senescence may occur in patients with OA, but these are not the predominant pathways leading to this chronic disease. Conversely, these pathways play much greater roles in coronary artery disease (B), gastric cancer (C), ischemic stroke (D), and Alzheimer disease (E) in which the wear-and-tear degeneration pathway is not as prominent.

6. **B.** The CDC projects that as many as one in three Americans (a full third of the population) will have diabetes by the mid-21st century should current trends persist.

7. **A.** The incidence rate of stroke in those age 50 and older had declined in the United States, due principally to better detection and treatment of hypertension, stroke's major risk factor. Dyslipidemia (B), obesity (C), coagulopathies (D; blood-clotting disorders), and vascular malformations (E) are also risk factors for stroke.

8. **D.** Human papillomavirus (HPV) is linked to cervical cancer, anal and penile cancers, and cancers of the head and neck. Vaccination may serve for primary cancer prevention by inducing immunity and preventing cancer-initiating infections. Colonoscopy (A), mammography (B), and prostate-specific antigen (PSA) testing (E) are methods of cancer screening and constitute secondary cancer prevention (although, notably, some experts now recommend against PSA as a means of cancer screening). Lumpectomy (C; surgical removal of a "lump" or tumor from breast) is tertiary prevention, intervening after a malignant tumor has become clinically obvious to prevent subsequent spread and progression.

9. **D.** The action of various immune cells and immune substances appropriately defend the body against pathogens but can also be misdirected. An immune system misdirected through various environmental stresses, pathogenic exposures, and dietary imbalances causes chronic inflammation (redness, swelling, warmth, and pain) at various sites throughout the body and has been implicated in the propagation of most chronic diseases. Fibrosis (C; scar formation) may result when inflammation is severe and is often seen in pneumoconioses, with scar tissue forming in the lung as a result of severe inflammation in response to toxic exposures.

Neovascularization (A; new blood vessel formation) is often seen in cancer, as the expanding tumor mass of abnormally dividing cells recruits a blood supply to support its growth. Apoptosis (B; programmed cell death) is one bodily defense against cancer, causing a mutated cell to die rather than replicate. Hypertrophy (E; growth in size) is not necessarily pathogenic and is not a feature of most chronic diseases. Hypertrophy may be physiologic, such as skeletal muscle enlarging in response to weight-bearing exercise.

10. **B.** Alcohol (A) and sodium (E) intake have been positively associated with hypertension. However, moderate alcohol intake is associated overall with improved cardiovascular mortality despite this hypertensive effect, and dietary sodium may largely be a bystander in serum sodium and fluid retention, driven largely by consumption of refined carbohydrates. Insoluble fiber (C) and polyunsaturated fat (D) seem to have no appreciable association with blood pressure. The intake of calcium has been inversely associated with hypertension in some studies, as has the intake of potassium, magnesium, and soluble fiber. However, "association does not equal causation," and although there is some biologic plausibility to consider, reductionist associations with isolated nutritive components is always limited, because people eat many foods in complicated combinations, not as single constituents in isolation.

20

Prevention of Infectious Diseases

With Patricia E. Wetherill

"Infectious disease exists at this intersection between real science, medicine, public health, social policy and human conflict."

Andrea Barrett

CASE INTRODUCTION

In May 2018 Dr. Smith, an internal medicine resident, is coming off her shift in the emergency room. As she mentally plays back all the patients she has seen, she notices that there seemed to be many with diarrhea, more so than the days before. They all seemed to have severe diarrhea, too, with stomach cramps and bloody stools. One of them even had to be admitted to the hospital with acute renal failure. Dr. Smith wonders if there is something going on. It's a good thing she sent off stool cultures!

The next morning, the stool cultures are back showing infection with *Escherichia coli*. Dr. Smith remembers that a particular strain of *E. coli* has been in the news because of a multistate outbreak.

---

1. OVERVIEW OF INFECTIOUS DISEASE

Humans have coexisted with microbes since the beginning of the human race. The foundations of the discipline of epidemiology were also laid by analyzing and controlling cholera, a bacterial disease caused by *Vibrio cholerae*. Even now, after almost 100 years of effective antibiotics, infectious diseases such as human immunodeficiency virus (HIV)/acquired immunodeficiency syndrome (AIDS), malaria, and diarrheal diseases remain major public health challenges; new diseases such as Middle East respiratory syndrome (MERS) and severe acute respiratory syndrome (SARS) evolve, and old diseases such as Ebola and tuberculosis (TB) continue to evolve. Immunity to infection is influenced by a person's genetic background, overall health, access to good sanitation and nutrition, and even social status. Therefore the prevalence of infectious diseases is a good proxy for disenfranchisement and poverty in a population. Poverty plays multiple roles in the cycle of infectious diseases. Poverty can contribute to infectious diseases by making the environment more suitable for disease transmission; poverty can also be a consequence of infectious diseases. Causal pathways include complications of pregnancy, repeated episodes of diarrheal illness in children leading to slowed mental and physical development, and the death of broad swaths of a parent generation (e.g., from AIDS).[1]

In this chapter we discuss several important infectious diseases and their control. Important diseases and control mechanisms are discussed elsewhere (e.g., see Chapter 3 for influenza and outbreak investigation).

Control of infectious disease is challenging because of the adaptive capabilities of microbes. Microbes have inhabited the earth far longer than humans and have successfully adapted to all evolutionary challenges. Several recent developments fuel a global environment in which new infectious

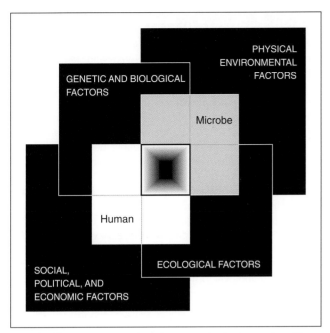

Fig. 20.1 Convergence model of human-microbe interaction. (From Smolinski MS, Hamburg MA, Lederberg J [eds]: *Microbial Threats to Health: Emergence, Detection, and Response,* Washington, DC, 2003, National Academies Press.)

diseases emerge and become rooted in society, as summarized by the **convergence model**[2] (Fig. 20.1). The convergence model is centered on the human-microbe interaction. The black box in the center of the figure indicates that these interactions can be difficult to predict in an emerging disease. More importantly, a microbe is *a necessary but not sufficient*

cause of ill health. Humans constantly encounter millions of potentially harmful microbes without falling ill. Four domains of factors impact humans and microbes or their interactions: (1) genetic and biologic factors, (2) physical environment factors, (3) ecological factors, and (4) social, political, and economic factors. Each of these factors provides a starting point for thinking systematically about pathways of prevention (Box 20.1).

Understanding and controlling infectious diseases requires integrating many different preventive and public health skills. These include obtaining accurate history on sensitive topics such as sexual behaviors, geographic epidemiology, outbreak investigation, analysis of disease rates by different variables (e.g., age, gender, race, socioeconomic status) to detect high-risk groups, successful outreach to public and health professionals, screening, contact tracing, immunization, school health, counseling, sanitation, waste and wastewater management, food protection, disease registries, and prophylactic drugs. Diseases vary, but the epidemiologic skills are similar for different diseases, independent of their mode of transmission (e.g., sexually transmitted disease [STD] vs vectorborne disease). Public health programs have a goal of controlling disease through prevention efforts in three broad categories[2]:

1. **Improving resistance of the host:** Hygiene and nutrition, as well as vaccination, postexposure prophylaxis, and chemoprophylaxis.
2. **Improving environmental safety:** Includes sanitation, air quality control, water and food safety, and control of vectors and animal reservoirs. Public sanitation has been crucial in controlling infectious disease.

BOX 20.1   Four Domains of Human-Microbe Interaction: Pathways in Prevention of Infectious Disease

1. Genetic and Biologic Factors

In human-microbe interaction, genetic and biologic factors include the makeup of the human body, with its physical, cellular, and molecular barriers to infection **(human susceptibility to infection).** Many of these factors are amenable to prevention efforts; exercise and a healthy diet contribute to intact barriers to infection. Biologic factors that **increase infectivity** of the microbe include its prevalence, stability, infectious dose, latency phase, and induction of shedding in the host. The noroviruses, the most common cause of diarrheal illness, exemplify the highly infectious microbe: Viral particles are highly prevalent and can survive for a long time outside the human body; even a few viruses are enough to induce illness, and they are mainly transmitted from people who do not feel ill (viral shedding). **Microbial adaptation and change** also affects the interplay. Many microbes have successfully adapted to their environments through millions of years and continue to evolve. Their constant, rapid pace of mutation helps them develop resistance to potent antibiotics (e.g., vancomycin intermediate *Staphylococcus aureus* [VISA]) and complicates attempts to find vaccines (e.g., malaria, HIV).

Pathways to prevention in this domain include decreasing host susceptibility through better nutrition and vaccines, as well as constant vigilance for emerging resistance patterns.

2. Physical Environment Factors

Physical environment factors include the **climate and latitude** of an environment, which affect a location's conduciveness to microbe or vector survival. Climate can directly impact disease transmission through replication and survival of pathogens and vectors, as well as through its effects on ecology. Landslides, earthquakes, and other **natural disasters** also create conditions conducive to the spread of infectious disease, such as overcrowding, lack of sanitation, and malnutrition.

Prevention efforts in this domain include improved food safety and sanitation, as well as focused surveillance on areas conducive to emerging infections.

3. Ecologic Factors

Changes in ecosystems can affect the transmission of microbes through water, soil, air, food, or vectors. Such alterations also affect microbes with animal reservoirs. Examples include the changes of malaria prevalence in response to a warming climate and the increase in prevalence of Lyme disease because of more deer in expanding New England woods. Also important are changes in land use. A growing number of emerging infectious diseases arise from increased human contact with animal reservoirs **(disruption/destabilization** of

Continued

BOX 20.1 Four Domains of Human-Microbe Interaction: Pathways in Prevention of Infectious Disease—cont'd

natural habitats). An example is the Nipah virus, which was endemic to Southeast Asian fruit bats. When pig farms grew in size and density and expanded into fruit orchards in the late 1990s, the virus was transmitted to the pigs and then their handlers, causing encephalitis outbreaks. Pathways to prevention in this domain can be again found mainly through surveillance.

4. Social, Political, and Economic Factors
Human demographics and behavior involve international travel and commerce that can lead to rapid dissemination of infectious diseases (e.g., SARS) or produce-borne diseases. **Advances in technology** and industry open up new transmission modes (e.g., blood transfusion, use of antibiotics in farm animals). Furthermore, **disruptions of peace** and public health services as well as **income inequality** all worsen infectious

disease transmission. For example, war and famines are closely linked to the spread of infectious diseases, and mortality from infectious diseases is closely correlated with global poverty. **Lack of political will** has also contributed to delayed control. For example, the widespread perception in the second half of the 20th century was that infectious diseases were under control and no longer posed a public health threat. This complacency probably contributed to delays in detecting and controlling multidrug-resistant TB as well as foodborne outbreaks. A relatively new factor here is also the **intent to harm** through the release of microbial agents as an act of aggression.

Pathways for prevention through social, economic, and political factors lie in taking a comprehensive view of health, advocating for improvements to the underlying determinants in populations, and helping create the political will to strengthen public health and overcome health disparities.

TABLE 20.1 Transmission of Infectious Diseases

Transmission Mode	Examples of Diseases	Control Measures
Close personal contact	Upper respiratory infections Tuberculosis STDs, HIV	Practice use of barriers (e.g., handwashing, masks, barrier methods [condoms]) Find and treat/isolate carriers Improve host resistance
Food/water	Norovirus Cholera Legionellosis Giardiasis	Improve sanitation, ensure food safety, improve water quality, improve hygiene, cook meat properly
Soil-transmitted helminths	Ascariasis Hookworm Strongyloidiasis	Improve sanitation Ensure treatment of excreta
Arthropods	Malaria Lyme Dengue Zika	Control/eliminate vectors Eliminate reservoir Use repellents/insecticides
Zoonoses	Rabies Anthrax Tularemia Toxoplasmosis	Eliminate carriers Monitor pet health Control rodents

HIV, Human immunodeficiency virus; *STDs,* sexually transmitted diseases (STIs).
From Wallace RB (ed): Communicable diseases. In: *Maxcy-Rosenau-Last: Public Health and Preventive Medicine,* ed 15, vol II, New York, 2008, McGraw-Hill Medical.

3. **Improving public health systems:** Improved contact tracing, education, containment, herd immunity, and quality of care given. Even for diseases for which there is no known treatment, such as Ebola, different countries with similar resources have stark differences in mortality from these diseases.[3]

Mastering infection control requires a thorough understanding of the various infectious diseases, and an in-depth discussion is beyond the purview of this textbook. However, disrupting the propagation of an infectious disease outbreak often *only* requires understanding how it is transmitted (see Chapter 3). For example, John Snow determined that water from a particular well caused most of the cholera in London. Armed with this understanding and the supporting data, he was able to convince the local council to disable the well. Breaking the chain of transmission helped end the outbreak. Diseases can be usefully grouped according to transmission[4] (Table 20.1), and method of infection control follows transmission.

1.1 BURDEN OF DISEASE

Infectious diseases affect all countries, but the burden of disease is different in developed and developing countries. In the United States, infectious disease mortality has for the most part steadily declined since the early 1900s.[5] Most of this decline *preceded* the availability of antibiotics or vaccines and was likely the result of better hygiene, sanitation, and chlorination of drinking water.

Since the 1980s, the burden of infectious disease in the United States again increased, largely because of emerging or reemerging infections, such as multidrug-resistant *Staphylococcus aureus*, *Clostridium difficile*, hepatitis C, and *Mycobacterium tuberculosis*. Globally, deaths due to communicable diseases declined from 2005 to 2015. This decrease is largely attributable to decreases in mortality rates due to HIV/AIDS and malaria. The impact remains high in sub-Saharan Africa, but inroads have been made even there with decreased death rates due to diarrheal diseases and most other infectious diseases.[6] Still, not all infectious diseases are in retreat: Dengue, Chagas disease, and the Ebola virus disease outbreaks in 2015 and 2018 all testify to the continued threat from infectious diseases. Infectious diseases especially impact children; much of childhood mortality is attributable to acute respiratory infections, measles, diarrheal illnesses, malaria, and HIV/AIDS.

To weigh the effects of disease on life span, many global health experts measure the impact of infectious disease in **disability-adjusted life years (DALY),** which takes into account premature mortality and years of life lived in less than full health (see Chapter 24). Five of the 10 leading diseases for global disease burden are infectious: HIV/AIDS, lower respiratory infections, diarrheal illnesses, malaria, and TB.[7] More importantly, many of the infectious diseases causing a large disease burden (HIV/AIDS, respiratory diseases) disproportionately impact the lowest-income countries.

1.2 OBTAINING AN ACCURATE HISTORY

Transmission of major infectious diseases often results from a person's *behavior,* including eating and hygiene habits, pets in residence, illicit drug use, and sexual partners. Therefore caring for a patient with an infectious disease requires taking a careful behavioral history. The behaviors resulting in transmission can be mainstream and unrelated to any social taboos, such as the restaurant visited before a diarrheal illness.

More often, patients may be embarrassed by behavior that induced the infectious disease. Examples range from people kissing their pets (leading to transmission of *Pasteurella* species)[8] to sexual behaviors and use of illicit drugs (leading to transmission of sexually transmitted and bloodborne diseases). Patients may not be comfortable sharing such information unless the clinician is skilled at putting people at ease and asks about intimate details in a nonjudgmental way. Taking such a history is crucial for understanding how the patient contracted the infectious disease and who else may have been infected. Superior relationship and communication skills are needed, since typically those most burdened by infectious diseases also suffer stigma and disempowerment in their communities (e.g., commercial sex workers, intravenous [IV] drug users).

Additional information on effective STD counseling and behavioral interventions can be found online (see Websites).

2. PUBLIC HEALTH PRIORITIES

2.1 HIV/AIDS, TUBERCULOSIS, AND MALARIA

HIV/AIDS, malaria, TB, neglected tropical diseases, and viral hepatitis together cause about 4 million deaths each year worldwide[9] and seriously impact on health outcomes in every region of the world. These illnesses decrease health and constrain growth and development of many of the poorest nations. In general, they also impact developed countries, either internally through income inequality or externally through immigration and international travel. All these diseases have important lessons to offer for successful infectious disease prevention. Prevention efforts for some of these diseases are often implemented together, as through the Global Fund to Fight AIDS, Tuberculosis, and Malaria.[10] The Global Fund follows an innovative model, targeting all three diseases through partnerships among government, civil society, the private sector (including businesses and foundations), and affected communities, combined with meticulous attention to data and evaluation. Accelerating progress on AIDS, malaria, and TB is also one of the sustainable development goals of the United Nations (see Websites).

2.1.a Human Immunodeficiency Virus/Acquired Immunodeficiency Syndrome

HIV/AIDS epidemiology. No new disease in modern times has had as severe and global impact as AIDS, which is caused by the human immunodeficiency virus. Although HIV transmission and management are of major concern in the United States, the situation is more serious in sub-Saharan Africa, Asia and the Pacific Latin America, Eastern Europe, and Central Asia. In sub-Saharan Africa HIV remains catastrophic with 66% of all new HIV diagnoses made worldwide. In 2016 an estimated 36.7 million people are HIV infected, of which 25.6 million live in sub-Saharan Africa.[11] Worldwide 1.8 million become infected yearly (~5000 new infections per day). Unfortunately only 60% know their HIV status.[10] Despite these large numbers of new infection, death rates are dropping. Globally, AIDS-related deaths dropped 45% since their peak in 2004,[11] caused by less mother-to-infant transmission, improved access to health care, but most importantly antiretroviral treatment. In 2010, 7.5 million were on treatment. In 2017, great strides have been made with 20.9 million on therapy.[12]

Spread of HIV infection. Human immunodeficiency virus is spread through horizontal transmission (generally adult to adult) by sexual contact (both heterosexual and homosexual) and by sharing needles and other equipment for intravenous drug use (IDU). HIV is also spread through vertical transmission (from parent to child) in utero or through breastfeeding. There is another, less frequent mode of transmission (either vertical or horizontal) that includes health care workers (accidental puncture with contaminated needles), blood product transfusions, and more. Globally, heterosexual intercourse is the most important route of spread. In the United States those with the highest transmission rates are gay, bisexual, and other men who have sex with men.[12]

Prevention of HIV infection and AIDS. Prevention strategies have been the most successful countermeasure to the spread of HIV. Globally, an unprecedented coalition of governments, nongovernmental organizations (NGOs), pharmaceutical companies, and private foundations have worked together. Preventive measures have included[13]:

- Condoms.
- Preexposure prophylaxis (an uninfected person takes anti-HIV medication).
- Treating patients as a means to prevent disease in others (treatment as prevention).
- Preventing infected mothers from transmitting the disease to their babies during delivery or through breastfeeding.
- Male circumcision.
- Strengthening local surveillance.
- Building health care infrastructure and capacity globally.

HIV testing. The Centers for Disease Control and Prevention (CDC) recommends routine, voluntary screening for **all** patients age 13 to 64 in health care settings, unless prevalence of undiagnosed HIV infection has been documented at less than 0.1%. Box 20.2 provides additional CDC guidelines.[14] The US Preventive Services Task Force (USPSTF) recommends clinicians screen patients age 15 to 65 and patients of other ages if they are high risk.[15]

HIV testing is now done as an HIV-1/HIV-2 antigen and antibody combination immunoassay on serum or plasma specimens.

2.1.b Tuberculosis

TB Epidemiology. Before industrialization and urbanization transformed Western civilization, TB was a known problem, but it did not become a scourge in Europe and North America until the 19th century. Although predominantly spread within the home, TB also was frequently spread in crowded working conditions.

Despite the lack of any specific medical prevention or therapy, TB mortality began to decline in the late 19th century and continued to decline steadily until the end of World War II. This probably resulted from improvements in socioeconomic conditions, including better nutrition, less crowding in homes and worksites, and improved sanitation. Although far advanced by the late 1940s, control of TB was improved further with the introduction of streptomycin as a treatment and with the subsequent discovery of additional antimicrobial drugs.

In the United States the incidence of TB continued to decline until 1985, when it resurged because of emerging resistance and HIV infection. Since the peak of TB resurgence in the United States in 1992, the number of TB cases reported annually has decreased to 9272 new cases of TB in 2016.[16]

The global burden of disease in 2016 was 10.4 million new cases and 1.7 million deaths from TB.[16] In the 21st century, treatment for TB has entered a new phase because of the emergence of widespread resistance to multiple antibiotics. Resistance to at least the two major antituberculosis drugs, isoniazid and rifampicin (rifampin) has been termed **multidrug-resistant tuberculosis** (MDR-TB). Treatment of MDR-TB requires prolonged and expensive chemotherapy using second-line drugs that have less efficacy and heightened toxicity. If resistance to these drugs also arises, the disease becomes **extensively drug-resistant tuberculosis** (XDR-TB), which is virtually untreatable. The increase of MDR-TB and XDR-TB is fueled by inadequate chemotherapy (patients stopping their treatment prematurely or receiving an inadequate number or choice of agents).[17]

BOX 20.2   CDC Guidelines for HIV/AIDS Screening

Screening all patients starting treatment for tuberculosis and all patients seeking treatment for sexually transmitted diseases/infections (STDs/STIs).

Repeat screening at least annually of all persons at high risk for human immunodeficiency virus (HIV) infection:
- Injection drug users and their sex partners
- Persons who exchange sex for money or drugs
- Sex partners of HIV-infected persons

Counseling of patients that they and their prospective sex partners be tested before initiating a new sexual relationship.

Routine, voluntary, opt-out testing of all pregnant women.

Repeat testing during the third trimester:
- Women receiving health care in settings with elevated incidence of HIV or AIDS

- Women age 15 to 45 years
- Women who receive health care in facilities in which prenatal screening identifies at least one HIV-infected pregnant woman per 1000 screened
- Women at high risk for acquiring HIV
- Women with signs or symptoms consistent with acute HIV infection

Screening of women with undocumented HIV status at the time of labor with a rapid HIV test unless they decline (opt-out testing).

Rapid testing of newborns is recommended when the mother's HIV status is unknown.

In an era of increased mobility, problems with resistant TB can quickly spread within the United States and between countries. Therefore many experts recommend a global strategy for TB control.

TB stages and natural history. The natural history and pathogenesis of mycobacterial infection makes the control of TB considerably more complex than the control of other bacterial diseases. Most importantly, the manifestations of TB vary greatly among patients. In a small number of newly infected individuals the infection proceeds fairly rapidly either to invade lung tissue or to cause a generalized systemic disease, such as **miliary tuberculosis.**[18] In most persons with normal immune systems, however, lesions develop in the lungs and become contained as cell-mediated immunity develops.

The initial infection is called **primary tuberculosis.** The resolution of the primary infection is only part of the interplay of the host and the disease. The disease remains in a quiet (dormant) state, but never resolves completely. This person is therefore more correctly considered to have *inactive* TB or **latent tuberculosis infection** (LTBI). The interplay of the host and the organism during the initial infection is influenced by multiple factors, including age, immune status, amount of inoculum, nutritional status, and comorbidities. The presence of cell-mediated immunity is revealed by a positive reaction in the tuberculin skin test using purified protein derivative (PPD). A simple blood test, interferon-γ release assays (IGRAs), have emerged as an alternative to diagnose latent TB infections.[19]

The person infected with LTBI or inactive TB, which is noninfectious, will ultimately have two possible courses, as follows:

- The TB infection will remain inactive for the rest of the infected person's life. In developed countries, this is by far the most common course.
- The infected person's own disease may reactivate later in life to become **active tuberculosis.** This occurs in 4% to 8% of infected persons (over lifetime of patient) and is called **reactivation tuberculosis.**

Conversely, TB history needs to be distinguished from patients who become exposed to a new TB infection and develop active disease from their new infection, called **reinfection tuberculosis,** or *exogenous* TB.

TB Prevention. The control of TB has been assisted by the discovery of methods for primary, secondary, and tertiary prevention.

The first discovery was a vaccine derived from a live, attenuated mycobacterium called **bacille Calmette-Guérin** (BCG) vaccine, which provides some protection against a first infection with *Mycobacterium tuberculosis.* Immunization with BCG is a method of primary prevention. It is the least expensive approach to TB control, and although considerable debate surrounds its efficacy[20] BCG is widely used in developing nations that have high rates of TB. In the United States, BCG vaccine is recommended only for children who are likely to be exposed to TB in an environment where cooperation with diagnosis and treatment efforts is unlikely. Other forms of primary TB prevention include reduction of overcrowding in prisons and homeless shelters. Immunocompromised hosts are effective transmitters of TB; therefore identifying HIV coinfection, especially in patients with resistant TB, is important as a primary prevention strategy.

The US Public Health Service recommends the identification of those who have positive results in the tuberculin skin test (particularly recent skin test converters) and the use of antituberculosis agents to treat patients at high risk of developing reactivation TB (HIV-positive patients, children age 2–11 years, pregnant women).[21]

Subsequent discoveries have led to new strategies for secondary and tertiary TB prevention. Tuberculosis control depends on early identification and appropriate treatment to ensure complete treatment and identification of comorbidities such as HIV. The focus of global TB control is **directly observed therapy, short course** (DOTS), comprising the following five components[22]:

1. Political commitment and sustained financing.
2. Case detection through quality-assured bacteriology.
3. Standardized treatment with supervision and patient support.
4. Effective drug supply and management system.
5. Monitoring and evaluation system with impact measurement.

This approach highlights the importance of patient support and monitoring systems.

2.1.c Malaria

Malaria Epidemiology. Worldwide, there were 216 million cases of malaria and an estimated 445,000 deaths in 2016.[23] Most deaths occur among children living in sub-Saharan Africa. Within the last decade, malaria control efforts have succeeded in reducing the caseload as well as malaria mortality.[23]

Malaria is caused by a parasitic protozoan called plasmodium, which is transmitted by insect vector, the female *Anopheles* species of mosquito. Of the five types of plasmodia, *Plasmodium falciparum* is the most deadly; *P. falciparum* and *P. vivax* are most common. All plasmodia multiply inside the red blood cells, which then break open to release more parasites (hemolysis). Malaria transmission depends on a complex interplay between the parasite (e.g., resistance to antimalarials), the vector (e.g., mosquito preference for humans), the host (decreased immunity in young children and pregnant women), and the environment (e.g., increased rainfall and temperatures increasing breeding sites for mosquitoes).[23]

Malaria induces a febrile illness, with fever, chills, and anemia. In severe cases, it can lead to convulsions and widespread organ failure. Malaria is diagnosed by microscopy or rapid diagnostic tests. Patients in endemic regions gradually develop immunity to the disease. However, this immunity may wear off after a few years; thereafter new bouts of malaria are as severe as if the patient had never had the disease.

BOX 20.3 Policies for Malaria Prevention

Primary Prevention
Providing insecticide-treated mosquito bed nets to all persons at risk for malaria.
Indoor residential spraying with pesticides.
Malaria vaccine once available.

Secondary Prevention
Intermittent preventive treatment of vulnerable groups in areas of high transmission.
Rapid parasitologic confirmation before treatment to distinguish fevers caused by malaria from nonmalarial fever.

Tertiary Prevention
Treatment with combination therapy to reduce resistance.

Malaria Prevention. The difficulties of preventing and controlling malaria highlight the challenges inherent in controlling a disease for which the vector's animal reservoir cannot be eradicated and to which patients do not build lasting immunity. Treatment regimens were originally based on *chloroquine*. However, many regions now have chloroquine-resistant malaria. Although many antimalarial drug treatments are available, each region has specific guidelines on drug resistance patterns and potential drug options. Work on a vaccine is ongoing and appears promising, especially in children. In January 2016, the World Health Organization (WHO) published its position paper on RTS,S (a first-generation malaria recombinant vaccine), recommending pilot implementation of the vaccine in African settings of moderate-to-high parasite transmission.[24]

Box 20.3 outlines primary, secondary, and tertiary prevention policies for malaria control.[24]

It is particularly important to sustain the malaria control effort to avoid resurgence; repeated attacks of malaria after years of no disease can be particularly severe.

2.2 DISEASES TRANSMITTED BY CLOSE CONTACT

Diseases transmitted by close contact have sometimes been called **hygiene-related diseases** or "diseases of failure to wash your hands." Although these names oversimplify the complexity of such diseases, they do highlight that many of them can be controlled with interventions as simple as handwashing, respiratory masks, and isolation of sick patients. Many contact diseases are vaccine preventable. Most are highly infectious, so constant vigilance is necessary to maintain herd immunity.

The close-contact disease spectrum ranges from the common cold, which causes some loss of work, to diarrheal illnesses, which kill millions of children in developing countries. Many of these diseases are also seasonal: acute respiratory infections peak in the winter, whereas most acute gastrointestinal illnesses peak in the warmer months.

By surface area, the human respiratory tract is probably the largest area of contact between humans and microbes. It is usually well protected by defense mechanisms (e.g., hairs and mucosal surfaces that prevent bacterial adhesion), as well as the normal flora of microorganisms, which compete with pathogenic bacteria for attachment sites. An important concept in acute respiratory infection epidemiology is the **reproductive number** (R_0), calculated as follows:

$$R_0 = \int_0^\infty b(a)F(a)\,da$$

where $b(a)$ is the average number of people infected by an index case per unit time, $F(a)$ is the probability that a newly infected person remains infectious for at least time a; and da is the period of infectivity.[25] R_0 indicates an agent's transmissibility and helps estimate the vaccine coverage required to induce herd immunity. For example, measles has a very high R_0 of 15 to 17. Although **severe acute respiratory syndrome** (SARS) was the first global epidemic in the 21st century, its R_0 was only 2 to 3, which has limited its spread.

Some assume that the common circulating gastrointestinal, respiratory, and skin infections are a minor concern. However, their health burden is considerable in terms of absence from work and school, together with increased pressure on health services.[26] Table 20.2 summarizes hygiene-related diseases, populations affected, and prevention measures.

Viral hepatitis is an important cause of local and sporadic outbreaks. Hepatitis A, B, and C are the most common. Hepatitis B is associated with chronic sequelae such as chronic hepatitis, liver failure, and liver cancer. For viral hepatitis, serology is important in making the diagnosis. A complex pattern on viral surface antigen and different antibodies indicate acute infections, chronic infection, or resolved infection. The hepatitis B virus (HBV) contains both surface antigen (HBsAg) and core protein (HBcAg). The surface antigen suggests ongoing HBV infection, either acute or chronic. People who have recovered and who are immune or have been successfully vaccinated will have HBs antibodies. Because the vaccine contains only HBsAg, the presence of anti-HBc antibodies distinguishes patients who have had the disease from vaccinated patients.[27]

2.3 FOODBORNE AND WATERBORNE INFECTIONS

Foodborne and waterborne infections are caused by a variety of agents and foods, but all are transmitted by oral/fecal contact. Infections are usually spread through contaminated food and water or by contact with vomit or feces. Every year, millions of cases of foodborne illness and thousands of resulting deaths occur in the United States; 1 in 6 Americans are impacted by a foodborne illness yearly.[28] Therefore this group of diseases often highlights issues in water and food safety. Meat can be contaminated during slaughter, raw produce during harvest and processing, and

TABLE 20.2 Major Diseases Transmitted by Close Contact, Vulnerable Populations, and Prevention

Major Syndromes	Significant Pathogens	Vulnerable Populations	Prevention
Respiratory infections (common cold, sore throat, otitis media, pneumonia, bronchiolitis[a])	Streptococcus pneumoniae	Adults >65, children, patients with chronic medical conditions	Polysaccharide vaccine (e.g., Pneumovax)
	Haemophilus influenzae B (Hib) Bordetella pertussis Corynebacterium diphtheriae	Children	Vaccine combining Hib, pertussis, and diphtheria toxin
	SARS Coronavirus	Animal handlers and health care workers	Early recognition, isolation, stringent infection control
	Influenza	Adults ≥65, pregnant women, children age 6–23 months, patients with chronic conditions	Yearly vaccinations, isolation, early antiviral treatment
	Respiratory syncytial virus[a]	Children, elderly, immuno-compromised patients	Passive immunization in children
Viral hepatitis (acute hepatitis, chronic hepatitis, acute liver failure, liver cancer)	Hepatitis A and E (transmitted fecal-oral, acute infections only)	Crowding, endemic in certain countries, day care centers, MSM, IDU	Personal attention to hygiene and environmental sanitation, active and passive immunization (hepatitis A)
	Hepatitis B, C, D (transmitted by parenteral exposure to blood/body fluids, can cause chronic infections)	Health care workers, IDU, MSM	Active and passive immunization (hepatitis B)
Meningitis (bacterial, viral)	Streptococcus pneumoniae, Hib, Neisseria meningitidis	Infants, adolescents (Hib and meningococci)	Vaccines (pneumococcal, Hib, meningococcal)
	Nonpolio enteroviruses, HSV, WNV, measles, influenza	Children in day care	Isolation; hand hygiene
Acute gastrointestinal infections	Norovirus Rotavirus E. coli spp. Shigella spp. Vibrio cholerae	Young children, people living in crowding, lack of clean water	Isolation, hand hygiene
Sexually transmitted diseases (STDs)[b]	HSV, lymphogranuloma venereum, syphilis Chlamydia, gonococci HPV Scabies, pediculosis pubis	Adolescents, patients engaging in unprotected sex with multiple partners	Early identification and treatment; partner management, vaccine (HPV) Antibiotics and antivirals

HPV, Human papillomavirus; *HSV*, herpes simplex virus; *IDU*, intravenous drug use; *MSM*, men who have sex with men; *SARS*, severe acute respiratory syndrome; *WNV*, West Nile virus.
[a]In children.
[b]Sexually transmitted infections (STIs), including genital, anal, or perianal ulcers; urethritis and cervicitis; genital warts; ectoparasitic infections.

all food from inadequate filtering at water treatment plants. Some bacteria replicate particularly well in particular foods, for example:
- *Salmonella* spp. (eggs)
- *Listeria monocytogenes* (unpasteurized milk, raw cheese, cantaloupe)
- *Vibrio* spp. (shellfish)
- *Cyclospora cayetanensis* (fresh produce)

However, many outbreaks have been caused by raw or undercooked meat, gravies, custards, and any food in contact with contaminated drinking water. Most agents will only cause

diarrhea, vomiting, cramps, and sometimes fever. However, some agents can cause other symptoms, such as the following:
- Clostridium botulinum, causing respiratory paralysis and death
- Enterohemorrhagic *E. coli*, causing kidney failure
- Shiga toxin–producing *E. coli* (STEC), associated with hemolytic-uremic syndrome

The CDC estimates that eight known pathogens account for the vast majority of illnesses, hospitalizations, and deaths each year from foodborne illness (Table 20.3). About half of all foodborne disease outbreaks are caused by *Norovirus*.[29]

TABLE 20.3   Clinical Presentations of Foodborne and Waterborne Infections

Pathogen	Incubation Period	Symptom Duration	Symptoms	Food	Comments
Norovirus	1–2 days	1–3 days	Voluminous D&V	Raw produce, contaminated drinking water, food handled by infected person, vomiting, contamination	Resistant to common cleaning agents
Nontyphoidal *Salmonella* spp.	24 hours	2–4 days	D&V, fever	Eggs, meat, poultry, raw milk or juice, cheese, fruits and vegetables	
Campylobacter spp.	1–7 days	1–7 days	Watery D, fever	Poultry, milk, gravy	
Staphylococcus aureus	1–6 hours	24–48 hours	Sudden onset of severe nausea, V	Improperly refrigerated meat, poultry, potato and egg salads, cream pastries	Caused by preformed toxins
Toxoplasma gondii	Variable	Variable	Enlarged lymph nodes, flulike illness	Undercooked meat, contaminated water	Causes severe disease in pregnancy and for HIV/AIDS patients; can also be transmitted by cats
E. coli (STEC)	3–4 days	5–10 days	Severe, bloody D	Undercooked beef, raw juice and milk, raw fruits and vegetables (sprouts)	Can cause kidney failure
Listeria monocytogenes	9–48 hours	Variable	Fever, muscle aches, nausea, D	Raw milk, cheese, ready-to-eat deli meat	Pregnant women at risk for premature delivery and stillbirth
Clostridium perfringens	4–24 hours	1–3 days	Intense abdominal cramps, watery D	Poultry, meat	

D&V, Diarrhea and vomiting; *STEC*, Shiga-toxin producing *E. coli*.

In developed countries, the single most effective intervention to decrease waterborne diseases has been the widespread chlorination of water supplies and effective sewage collection and treatment. If outbreaks occur, isolation of infected patients and treatment with antibiotics for invasive diseases form effective tertiary prevention. Travelers going to developing countries with uncertain water supply should be encouraged to avoid raw fruits and vegetables, to avoid beverages with ice, and to drink only water that has been boiled or disinfected.

2.4 VECTORBORNE DISEASES AND ZOONOSES

Mosquitoes and ticks are the most important disease vectors. Mosquitoes depend on standing water for replication, benefiting from human-made habitats (e.g., water control ditches, irrigation system runoffs), and can even breed successfully in water in discarded tires. Diseases transmitted by mosquitoes include malaria and hemorrhagic viral fevers (e.g., yellow fever, dengue) and multiple encephalitis (neurotropic) viruses (e.g., West Nile, St. Louis encephalitis, Zika).

Ticks transmit the widest variety of pathogens of any blood-feeding arthropod. Usually, times of heavy rainfall (rainy seasons in tropics, late spring through early fall in temperate zones) coincide with seasonal variations of disease intensity. Ticks transmit many pathogens, including:
- *Rickettsia* (Rocky Mountain spotted fever)
- Spirochetes: *Borrelia burgdorferi* (Lyme disease)
- *Ehrlichia* (human monocytic ehrlichiosis)
- *Anaplasma* (human granulocytic anaplasmosis)

Other vectors include rat fleas (*Rickettsia typhi* and *Yersinia pestis*). Globally, many other vectorborne diseases exist, mostly neglected tropical and zoonotic infections. These disproportionately impact the poorest populations.

2.4.a Prevention

Primary prevention includes using insect repellents, wearing appropriate clothing, and avoiding vector-infested sites. Another option for prevention is changing habitats so that they are less attractive to host animals. Prompt removal of attached ticks also reduces disease transmission.

2.4.b Rabies

Globally, rabies is the most important zoonosis. *Zoonoses* are diseases that normally reside in the nonhuman world. In a sense, zoonoses are also vectorborne diseases, only that most of the vectors here are mammals. (Traditionally, however, only insects and ticks have been classified as "vectors.") Rabies causes a devastating viral infection of the central nervous system. Each year, rabies causes more than 50,000 deaths worldwide.[30] It affects people on every continent except Antarctica. It is mainly preventive medicine physicians who decide who should be immunized against rabies. Rabies reservoirs exist in two major forms:

- Urban rabies in domestic dogs
- Wildlife rabies in many mammals, including foxes, coyotes, skunks, raccoons, and bats

The rabies virus is highly neurotropic (targets nerve cells). In humans, rabies is almost always fatal once clinical signs develop. Suspicion of rabies is based on (1) a history of animal exposure, (2) suggestive clinical signs, and (3) a compatible disease course (rabies will become apparent in an animal within 10 days). Animal exposure does not require a bite mark. For example, bat bites can be small and difficult to detect, so the presence of a bat in a bedroom is enough to require postexposure prophylaxis. Wherever possible, the animal should be observed for 10 days.[31]

Rabies preexposure vaccination is only recommended for persons at risk of exposure to rabies, such as veterinarians, laboratory staff, and animal handlers. *Preexposure vaccination does not eliminate the need for postexposure prophylaxis* but alters the schedule and obviates the need for immune globulin.[32]

3. EMERGING THREATS

3.1 EMERGING INFECTIOUS DISEASES AND BIOWEAPONS

Microbes are continually evolving, so the threat of infectious disease is ever present. We are just now beginning to understand the world of "emerging threats," even though the causative agents have been around for millennia. Emerging threats include *old* diseases, such as bubonic plague or influenza, and newer agents such as the Zika virus, which causes fetal loss and increased incidence of microcephaly in the endemic regions. But these are not the only emerging threats. Our overuse of antibiotics in humans and livestock, resulting in multidrug-resistant microbes, and the use of microbes for bioterrorism present even more challenging threats.

Prevention of emerging infectious diseases requires investment in the capacity of the poorest countries to detect and address diseases as they arise before they become global epidemics and the empowerment of the most vulnerable populations in all countries. Prevention also requires thinking about public health in a continuum with changes in the environment (One Health approach). Most emerging diseases are zoonoses with a wildlife origin. They erupt where human population density increases in areas of high wildlife biodiversity. They also tend to develop in emerging infectious disease (EID) hotspots in tropical Africa, Latin America, and Asia.[33] Recent examples of emergence include Ebola virus disease, Zika virus, and H7N9 (avian influenza). All have their own unique path to infection, species, vectors, and the human role in their life cycle.

One of the most concerning developments is the use of microbes with an intent to harm, such as in biologic warfare (bioweapons) or bioterrorism. Certain organisms are particularly suitable for such use because (1) they can be easily transmitted from person to person or easily disseminated, (2) they can cause significant mortality and morbidity, (3) they

might cause particular panic, and (4) the health care system is poorly prepared to deal with these organisms. Such organisms are called **category A organisms** (e.g., anthrax, botulism, smallpox, and viral hemorrhagic fevers).[34]

3.2 ANTIMICROBIAL RESISTANCE AND HEALTHCARE-ASSOCIATED (NOSOCOMIAL) INFECTIONS

The term **healthcare-associated infection** (HAI) is used for any infection that is transmitted in the health care setting. This includes physicians' offices, dialysis centers, nursing homes, hospitals, among others. All health care environments can put patients at risk for infection. However, in addition to microbial resistance, HAIs are also caused by infections from devices or replacement of the normal microbial flora with pathogenic organisms. Similarly, although antimicrobial resistance can result from antibiotic use in health care, the use of antibiotics in animal farming contributes significantly to resistance patterns.

HAIs can be prevented in many patients. These infections occur because patients' normal defenses are weakened or breached by invasive procedures or devices; normal colonizing flora is altered by antibiotics or chemotherapy, and diseases spread from patient to patient through lack of barriers or insufficient handwashing. The CDC estimates that there are about 700,000 healthcare-associated infections each year in US hospitals.[35] HAIs include the following:

- Surgical site infections
- Central line–associated infections
- Ventilator-associated pneumonias
- Catheter-associated urinary tract infections
- *Clostridium difficile*–associated disease.

Resistant organisms are increasingly found in the community (community-acquired methicillin-resistant *Staphylococcus aureus* [MRSA]), which complicates treatment of outpatients. Importantly, most HAIs have decreased over the last 10 years due to better infection control practices and reduced use of catheters, central lines, ventilators, and such. But some multiresistant organisms, such as vancomycin intermittent-resistant *Staphylococcus aureus* or gonococcal disease, are becoming increasingly difficult to treat. If current trends in these organisms persist, clinicians may not have any effective antibiotics left.[36]

Resistance increases if bacteria are exposed to drugs repeatedly, at suboptimal concentrations, or for inadequate time. Clinical examples include unnecessary use of antibiotics for viral colds or antimalarial agents for nonmalarial fever, patients stopping antibiotics before finishing an entire course, and the continuous low-level use of antibiotics in farm animals.

3.2.a Prevention

Prevention of HAI begins with selective and judicious use of antimicrobials, both inside and outside the health care system. The Union of Concerned Scientists estimated that 70% of all antibiotics go toward nontherapeutic uses in livestock.[37] All clinicians should use antibiotics only when there is a high chance of a bacterial infection. If prescribed, an antimicrobial should be the narrowest antibiotic possible

TABLE 20.4 Isolation Measures for Select Infected Patients

Target Patients	Type of Precaution	Measures
All	Universal precautions	Handwashing before and after every patient contact Gloves, gowns, and eye protection as indicated before exposure to body fluids Safe disposal/cleaning of instruments and linen
Tuberculosis, varicella, measles[a]	Airborne	Private room with negative air pressure Wearing of mask with HEPA filter[b]
Meningococcus, pertussis, pharyngeal diphtheria, pneumonic influenza, rubella, mumps, adenovirus, parvovirus B19[a]	Droplets	Private room Hospital personnel wear mask within 1 meter of patient[b]
Colonization with multidrug-resistant bacteria; enteric infections, scabies, impetigo[a]	Contact	Private room or cohorting Nonsterile gloves for all patient contact Gowns for direct substantial patient contact[b]

HEPA, High-efficiency particulate air; *Hib, Haemophilus influenzae* B.

[a]Known or suspected measles, varicella, and draining TB also require contact precautions.

[b]In addition to universal precautions.

Modified from Wallace RB (ed): Communicable diseases. In: *Maxcy-Rosenau-Last: Public Health and Preventive Medicine,* ed 15, vol II, New York, 2008, McGraw-Hill Medical; Siegel JD, Rhinehart E, Jackson M, Chiarello L, and the Healthcare Infection Control Practices Advisory Committee, 2007 Guideline for Isolation Precautions: Preventing Transmission of Infectious Agents in Healthcare Settings https://www.cdc.gov/infectioncontrol/guidelines/isolation/index.html

and should be used for a full course. Furthermore, people who are sick should be properly isolated (Table 20.4).

Hospitals are also required to have an **infection control program,** which includes the following:

- Active infection surveillance system, with reporting of results to staff members
- Presence of vigorous control measures once hazards are recognized
- Sufficient staff (1 infection control staff per 250 patients)
- Knowledgeable physician who is an active program participant.

Historically, public health agencies have tried to decrease HAI by benchmarking facilities and requiring public reporting. More recently, the trend has been toward the following:

- "Bundle approaches," using multiple interventions based on evidence provided by the infection control community and implemented by a multidisciplinary team
- A culture of "zero tolerance"
- Environmental solutions, such as separate sphygmomanometers and stethoscopes for each room or self-cleaning surfaces.[38]

These prevention efforts have helped to decrease most HAIs over the last 10 years. Progress has been slowest with *Clostridium difficile.*[39] The reasons are multifactorial: the ability of the organism itself (which can build highly resistant spores), colonization of the host, increasing virulence, aging population, and more.

3.3 BARRIERS AND OPPORTUNITIES

In the long history of interactions between humans and microbes, the period in the 20th century where antibiotics easily cured many infectious diseases may have been a short interlude. Poverty, inequality, and disenfranchisement continue to fuel the evolution of new infectious diseases and the reemergence of others. The public health community has had many victories over infectious disease, such as the eradication of smallpox and the gains made in the fight against diarrheal illnesses, HIV/AIDS, and malaria. Continuing these gains and preventing the spread of new infections will likely require continued vigilance and continuous solidarity. Continuing those gains will require bolstering monitoring and surveillance, rapidly expanding high-impact interventions, and focusing efforts on high-risk and vulnerable populations.[40] Beyond these, capacity building is crucial. Disease outbreaks often draw funds and attention to specific disease outbreaks. But having robust elements of public health embedded throughout a system during and between outbreaks can often be more effective than simply focusing only on individual surge elements during crises.[41] However, future gains may require more than only becoming better at fighting "the war" against microbes. Perhaps this war can never be won, but becoming better at coexisting peacefully with microbes might be possible through the use of probiotics, immune stimulation, and support of the natural colonizing flora of the gut.[42]

CASE RESOLUTION

In May 2018, the outbreak of *E. coli* was traced back to contaminated romaine lettuce. Per the final report of the CDC, 62 patients from 16 states fell ill.[43] Fig. 20.2 shows the location of this outbreak, with outbreak strains initially reported by 36 states. This outbreak highlighted the growing importance of precut and bagged greens, which have become a major source of food poisonings. This prepackaging has made it harder to identify the source of outbreaks, and the public health system and food industry are still struggling with the question of how to track these food items.[44]

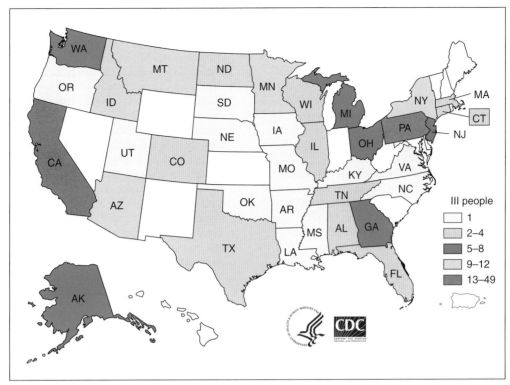

Fig. 20.2 People infected with the outbreak strain of *E. coli* O157:H7, by state of residence (*n* = 210). (https://www.cdc.gov/ecoli/2018/o157h7-04-18/map.html.)

4. SUMMARY

Infectious diseases emerge in a complex interplay between humans and microbes and are affected by physical environmental factors; genetic and biologic factors; ecologic factors; and social, political, and economic factors (convergence model). As described in Box 20.4, the history of medicine includes changing agendas for unraveling the host-microbe relationship. Understanding and controlling infectious diseases requires integrating many different prevention and public health skills. Tasks that preventive medicine physicians may be asked to do include interpreting hepatitis serology patterns and making decisions about rabies vaccination. Infectious disease and poverty reinforce each other. Globally, the burden of infectious disease falls heavily on developing countries and children. In some developing countries, HIV/AIDS, tuberculosis, and malaria together account for more than 50% of deaths. Successful infectious disease prevention strategies include treatment, addressing motivations, social norms, and behavior clusters, and aiming to empower high-risk populations. Of particular public health concern are emerging infectious diseases, multidrug-resistant organisms such as extensively resistant TB, and biowarfare agents. The war against microbes ultimately may be futile, but better coexistence with microbes may be possible.

BOX 20.4	**Barriers and Opportunities in the History of Medicine**
2000 BCE	Here, eat this root.
1000 CE	That root is heathen. Here, say this prayer.
1850	That prayer is superstition. Here, drink this potion.
1920	That potion is snake oil. Here, swallow this pill.
1945	That pill is ineffective. Here, take this penicillin.
1955	Oops . . . bugs mutated. Here, take this tetracycline.
1960–1999	39 more "oops." Here, take this more powerful antibiotic.
2000	The bugs have won! Here, eat this root.

Modified from World Health Organization: Anonymous, 2000. http://books.nap.edu/openbook.php?record_id=11669&page=1

REFERENCES

1. Leyenaar JK. HIV/AIDS and Africa's orphan crisis. *Paediatr Child Health*. 2005;10:259-260.
2. Institute of Medicine, Board on Global Health. *Microbial Threats to Health: Emergence, Detection, and Response*. Washington, DC: National Academies Press; 2003. Available at: https://www.nap.edu/read/10636/chapter/2.
3. Boozary AS, Farmer PE, Jha AK. The Ebola outbreak, fragile health systems, and quality as a cure. *JAMA*. 2014;312:1859-1860.
4. Wallace RB, ed. Communicable diseases. In: *Maxcy-Rosenau-Last: Public Health and Preventive Medicine*. 15th ed., Vol. 2. New York, NY: McGraw-Hill Medical; 2008.
5. Armstrong GL, Conn LA, Pinner RW. Trends in infectious disease mortality in the United States during the 20th century. *JAMA*. 1999;281:61-66. doi:10.1001/jama.281.1.61.

6. Wang H, Naghavi M, Allen C, et al. Global, regional, and national life expectancy, all-cause mortality, and cause-specific mortality for 249 causes of death, 1980-2015: a systematic analysis for the Global Burden of Disease Study 2015. *Lancet.* 2016;388:1459-1544.

7. Vos T, Barber RM, Bell B, et al. Global, regional, and national incidence, prevalence, and years lived with disability for 301 acute and chronic diseases and injuries in 188 countries, 1990-2013: a systematic analysis for the Global Burden of Disease Study 2013. *Lancet.* 2015;386:743-800.

8. Chomel BB, Sun B. Zoonoses in the bedroom. *Emerg Infect Dis.* 2011;17:167-172. doi:10.3201/eid1702.101070.

9. World Health Organization. *Accelerating Progress on HIV, Tuberuclosis, Malaria, Hepatitis and Neglected Tropical Diseases.* 2015. Available at: https://www.who.int/about/structure/organigram/htm/progress-hiv-tb-malaria-ntd/en/. Accessed October 10, 2019.

10. The Global Fund. *Results at a Glance.* 2019. Available at: https://www.theglobalfund.org/en/. Accessed October 10, 2019.

11. *Overview: Data & Trends: Global Statistics.* Available at: https://www.HIV.gov./hiv-basics/overview/data-and-trends/global-statistics.

12. National Institute of Allergy and Infectious Diseases. *HIV/AIDS.* Available at: https://www.niaid.nih.gov/diseases-conditions/hivaids. Accessed October 10, 2019.

13. Centers for Disease Control and Prevention. Revised recommendations for HIV testing of adults, adolescents, and pregnant women in health-care settings. *MMWR Recomm Rep.* 2006;55:1-17.

14. Centers for Disease Control and Prevention. *HIV Testing.* Available at: https://www.cdc.gov/hiv/guidelines/testing.html. Accessed October 10, 2019.

15. U.S. Preventive Services Task Force. *Human Immunodeficiency Virus (HIV) Infection: Screening.* 2019. Available at: https://www.uspreventiveservicestaskforce.org/Page/Document/UpdateSummaryFinal/human-immunodeficiency-virus-hiv-infection-screening.

16. Centers for Disease Control and Prevention. *Tuberculosis (TB): Data and Statistics.* Available at: https://www.cdc.gov/tb/statistics/default.htm. Accessed October 10, 2019.

17. Zager EM, McNerney R. Multidrug-resistant tuberculosis. *BMC Infect Dis.* 2008;8:10. doi:10.1186/1471-2334-8-10.

18. Sharma SK, Mohan A, Sharma A. Miliary tuberculosis: a new look at an old foe. *J Clin Tuberc Other Mycobact Dis.* 2016;3:13-27.

19. Centers for Disease Control and Prevention. *Tuberculosis (TB): Fact Sheets.* Available at: https://www.cdc.gov/tb/publications/factsheets/testing/igra.htm. Accessed October 10, 2019.

20. Clemens JD, Chuong JJ, Feinstein AR. The BCG controversy: a methodological and statistical reappraisal. *JAMA.* 1983;249:2362-2369.

21. Centers for Disease Control and Prevention. *Tuberculosis (TB): Treatment Regimens for Latent TB Infection (LTBI).* Available at: https://www.cdc.gov/tb/topic/treatment/ltbi.htm. Accessed October 10, 2019.

22. World Health Organization. *Pursue High-Quality DOTS Expansion and Enhancement.* Geneva. Available at: http://www.who.int/tb/dots/en/. Accessed October 10, 2019.

23. Centers for Disease Control and Prevention. *Malaria: About Malaria.* Available at: https://www.cdc.gov/malaria/about/index.html. Accessed October 10, 2019.

24. PATH Malaria Vaccine Initiative. *Malaria and Vaccines.* Available at: https://www.malariavaccine.org/malaria-and-vaccines. Accessed October 10, 2019.

25. Heffernan JM, Smith RJ, Wahl LM. Perspectives on the basic reproductive ratio. *J R Soc Interface.* 2005;2:281-293. doi:10.1098/rsif.2005.004. Accessed October 10, 2019.

26. Bloomfield SF, Exner M, Fara GM, Nath KJ, Scott EA, C Van der Voorden. *The Global Burden of Hygiene-Related Diseases in Relation to the Home and Community. An IFH Expert Review.* 2009. Available at: https://www.ifh-homehygiene.org/review/global-burden-hygiene-related-diseases-relation-home-and-community.

27. Centers for Disease Control and Prevention. A comprehensive immunization strategy to eliminate transmission of hepatitis B virus infection in the United States: recommendations of the Advisory Committee on Immunization Practices. Part I. Immunization of infants, children, and adolescents. *MMWR.* 2005;54(RR-16). Available at: http://www.cdc.gov/hepatitis/hbv/PDFs/SerologicChartv8.pdf.

28. Centers for Disease Control and Prevention. *OutbreakNet Enhanced.* Available at: https://www.cdc.gov/foodsafety/outbreaknetenhanced/index.html. Accessed October 10, 2019.

29. Centers for Disease Control and Prevention. *Foodborne Outbreaks: List of Selected Multistate Foodborne Outbreak Investigations.* Available at: https://www.cdc.gov/foodsafety/outbreaks/multistate-outbreaks/outbreaks-list.html. Accessed October 10, 2019.

30. Centers for Disease Control and Prevention. *Rabies in the U.S.* Available at: http://www.cdc.gov/rabies/location/usa/index.html. Accessed October 10, 2019.

31. Centers for Disease Control and Prevention. *Rabies: Domestic Animals.* Available at: http://www.cdc.gov/rabies/exposure/animals/domestic.html. Accessed October 10, 2019.

32. Morbidity and Mortality Weekly Report (MMWR). *Use of a Reduced (4-Dose) Vaccine Schedule for Postexposure Prophylaxis to Prevent Human Rabies: Recommendations of the Advisory Committee on Immunization Practices.* Centers for Disease Control and Prevention. Available at: https://www.cdc.gov/mmwr/preview/mmwrhtml/rr5902a1.htm#tab3. Accessed March 19, 2010.

33. World Health Organization. *Accelerating Progress on HIV, Tuberculosis, Malaria, Hepatitis and Neglected Tropical Diseases. A New Agenda for 2016-2030.* Geneva: World Health Organization; 2015. Available at: https://www.who.int/about/structure/organigram/htm/progress-hiv-tb-malaria-ntd/en/.

34. Centers for Disease Control and Prevention. *Bioterrorism Agents/Diseases.* Available at: https://emergency.cdc.gov/agent/agentlist-category.asp. Accessed October 10, 2019.

35. Centers for Disease Control and Prevention. *Healthcare-Associated Infections: HAI Data.* Available at: https://www.cdc.gov/hai/surveillance/index.html. Accessed October 10, 2019.

36. Centers for Disease Control and Prevention. *Gonorrhea: Antibiotic-Resistant Gonorrhea Basic Information.* Available at: https://www.cdc.gov/std/gonorrhea/arg/basic.htm. Accessed October 10, 2019.

37. Union of Concerned Scientists. *Hogging It!: Estimates of Antimicrobial Abuse in Livestock (2001).* April 2004. Available at: https://www.ucsusa.org/food_and_agriculture/our-failing-food-system/industrial-agriculture/hogging-it-estimates-of.html#.W_SpN9VKiUk.

38. Chemaly RF, Simmons S, Dale Jr C, et al. The role of the healthcare environment in the spread of multidrug-resistant organisms: update on current best practices for containment. *Ther Adv Infect Dis.* 2014;2:79-90.

39. Centers for Disease Control and Prevention. *2014 National and State Healthcare-Associated Infections Progress Report.* March 2016. Available at: www.cdc.gov/hai/progress-report/index.html.

40. Jones KE, Patel NG, Levy MA, et al. Global trends in emerging infectious diseases. *Nature.* 2008;451:990-993. doi:10.1038/nature06536.

41. National Academies of Sciences, Engineering, and Medicine. *Global Health Risk Framework: Resilient and Sustainable Health Systems to Respond to Global Infectious Disease Outbreaks: Workshop Summary.* Washington, DC: National Academies Press; 2016.

42. Institute of Medicine. *"Ending the War" Metaphor: The Changing Agenda for Unraveling the Host-Microbe Relationship. Executive Summary.* 2006. Available at: http://books.nap.edu/openbook. php?record_id=11669&page=1.

43. *E. coli (Escherichia coli): Multistate Outbreak of E. coli O157:H7 Infections Linked to Romaine Lettuce (Final Update).* Centers for Disease Control and Prevention. Available at: https://www.cdc. gov/ecoli/2018/o157h7-04-18/index.html.

44. Belluz J. *How Salad Became a Major Source of Food Poisoning in the US.* Jan 2019. Available at: https://www.vox.com/science-and-health/2018/4/26/17282378/romaine-lettuce-recall-ecoli-yuma.

SELECT READINGS

Farmer P. *Infections and Inequalities: The Modern Plagues.* Oakland, CA: University of California Press; 2001.

Institute of Medicine, Board on Global Health. *Microbial Threats to Health: Emergence, Detection, and Response.* 2003. Available at: http://www.nap.edu/openbook.php?record_id=10636&page=5.

Institute of Medicine, Board on Global Health. *The Causes and Impacts of Neglected Tropical and Zoonotic Diseases: Opportunities for Integrated Intervention Strategies—Workshop Summary.* Washington, DC: National Academies Press; 2011. Available at: https://www.ncbi.nlm.nih.gov/books/NBK62507/.

Ngonghala CN, Pluciński MM, Murray MB, et al. Poverty, disease, and the ecology of complex systems. *PLoS Biol.* 2014;12:e1001827.

Wallace RB, ed. Communicable diseases. In: *Maxcy-Rosenau-Last: Public Health and Preventive Medicine.* 15th ed., Vol 2. New York, NY: McGraw-Hill Medical; 2008.

WEBSITES

Effective Interventions HIV Prevention That Works: https://effectiveinterventions.cdc.gov/

GeoSentinel Network: http://www.istm.org/geosentinel

Global Fund to Fight AIDS, TB, and Malaria: http://www.theglobal-fund.org/en/

Infectious Disease Society of America: http://www.IDSA.org

Joint United Nations Program on HIV/AIDS: http://www.unaids.org/en/

National Public Health Information Coalition: https://www.nphic.org/toolkits/std (a toolkit on communication about sexually transmitted disease)

United Nations: https://www.un.org/sustainabledevelopment/health/ (sustainable development goals on health)

US Centers for Disease Control and Prevention: http://www.cdc.gov

World Health Organization: http://www.who.int

REVIEW QUESTIONS

1. Which of the following best illustrates how modifications to the *physical environment* can help protect against infectious disease?
   A. A college student increases her physical activity to bolster her immunity.
   B. A fast-food chain decides not to contract with beef suppliers who use antibiotics in their feed to promote growth.
   C. An unexpected drop in average temperature leads to a pronounced decrease in the mosquito population around a village.
   D. Housing is built for survivors of an earthquake, gradually reducing an overcrowded tent camp.
   E. New physical changes to a viral surface protein prevent binding to receptors on human mucosa.

2. Which of the following is the most fundamental cause for the decline in infectious disease mortality in the 20th century?
   A. Vaccination
   B. Antibiotic resistance
   C. Having a primary care physician
   D. Having a "medical home"
   E. Socioeconomic conditions

3. A local public health department wants to implement an initiative to control the spread of malaria. Which of the following strategies would be most effective?
   A. Messaging to promote food safety
   B. Educational materials on the importance of hand hygiene
   C. Controlling the local rodent population
   D. Improving sanitation
   E. Making mosquito netting available to residents

4. A country's mortality rate from cardiovascular disease increased precipitously over 20 years. An article in the lay press sounds a clarion cry that something must be done. Responding in a letter to the editor, a public health expert opens with the provocative statement that the increase in cardiovascular mortality is "a good thing." Assuming the expert is credible, what is the most likely reason for his statement?
   A. Cardiovascular deaths are relatively pain free
   B. Cardiovascular deaths are inexpensive and may represent a savings to a country's health care system
   C. Mathematical modeling of the population's cardiovascular risk factors suggests that the cardiovascular mortality rate should actually be worse
   D. Cardiovascular disease and deaths are thought to be driven by an infectious disease in this country, and although the mortality rate has been high initially, those who have not died will develop protective immunity and have extended longevity
   E. The rise in cardiovascular deaths suggests that people are not dying much earlier from infectious diseases

5. Which of the following statements is most accurate regarding the current worldwide spread of HIV infection?
   A. It is most often spread by homosexual contact.
   B. It is most often spread by heterosexual contact.
   C. It is most often spread by intravenous drug use.
   D. When the prevalence of new infections involves more men than women, heterosexual contact is likely to be the dominant route of transmission.
   E. When the prevalence of new infections involves more women than men, homosexual contact is likely to be the dominant route of transmission.

6. Which of the following statements is most accurate regarding HIV prevention?
   A. Condom use represents primary prevention.
   B. Using clean needles represents secondary prevention.
   C. Male circumcision represents tertiary prevention.
   D. Antiretroviral therapy is secondary prevention, not tertiary prevention.
   E. Antiretroviral therapy is secondary prevention, not primary prevention.

7. In general, which characteristic of infectious diseases—as opposed to chronic diseases—might convince policymakers to support interventions toward primary prevention?
   A. Infectious diseases are more serious than chronic diseases.
   B. Infectious diseases cost more to treat than chronic diseases.
   C. Infectious diseases are more difficult to manage than chronic diseases.
   D. Infectious diseases are more often lethal than chronic diseases.
   E. Infectious diseases produce illness more rapidly than chronic diseases.

8. Which of the following statements is most accurate regarding tuberculosis (TB) prevention?
   A. Negative-pressure rooms are primary prevention.
   B. Treatment with antimycobacterial drugs is primary prevention.
   C. Bacille Calmette-Guérin (BCG) vaccine is secondary prevention.
   D. Directly observed therapy, short course (DOTS) is secondary prevention.
   E. There are no prevention strategies for TB.

9. A young girl and her brother object to eating poultry since they learned that their beloved storybook chickens are what wind up in the broiler. Their family eats chicken one night for dinner, and the children satisfy themselves with salad. The brother has just leafy greens, but the little girl slices tomato to add to her greens. Three days later, the little girl develops watery diarrhea and fever and becomes dehydrated to the point that she requires hospital admission. No one else in the family is affected. Stool testing reveals *Campylobacter* infection. What is the most likely explanation for the young girl's illness?
   A. She is likely immunocompromised and therefore had an unusually severe response to *Campylobacter*.
   B. She actually ate some chicken.
   C. The stool test was incorrect and some other organism caused her illness.
   D. The salad was contaminated with *Campylobacter*.
   E. The same knife that cut the raw chicken sliced the tomatoes.

10. A rancher is scratched by a raccoon one night when taking out the trash. He was surprised to find the animal in the dumpster. Usually, raccoons hear him coming and scurry away before he reaches the dumpster. This raccoon was inappropriately unstartled. The rancher is concerned about rabies. He has already received rabies vaccination (preexposure vaccination). Which of the following is most applicable in this situation?
    A. Because the rancher has already been vaccinated, he is protected and safe
    B. Racoons don't transmit rabies, so no therapy is needed
    C. Preexposure vaccination means the rancher only needs the postexposure rabies vaccine now
    D. Preexposure vaccination means the rancher needs both rabies immune globulin and the postexposure rabies vaccine now
    E. Preexposure vaccination does not modify the recommended postexposure treatment regimen

11. Which of the following is likely the most important contributor to emerging antibiotic resistance and multidrug-resistant pathogens in the community?
    A. The prescription of antibiotics for viral syndromes
    B. The prescription of broad-spectrum antibiotic for empirical treatment for presumed bacterial infections
    C. Patients not finishing their course of antibiotics prescribed to treat bacterial infections
    D. Veterinary treatment of infections in livestock
    E. Nontherapeutic uses of antibiotics in livestock

12. A 27-year-old woman wants to be vaccinated against hepatitis B before leaving for Haiti for volunteer work. She comments that she was previously a Peace Corps volunteer and was sent home because of an illness with jaundice. She never sought a cause for the jaundice because it was short lived and resolved shortly after her return home. During a travel medicine consultation, her blood serology shows HBsAg (−), anti-HBc (−), and anti-HBs (+). Which of the following is true regarding this woman's need for a hepatitis B vaccination series?
    A. Because the woman is anti-Hbc (−), she is susceptible and should receive the vaccine
    B. Because the woman is HbsAg (−), she is susceptible and should receive the vaccine
    C. Because the woman is anti-HBs (+), she is chronically infected with hepatitis B. This is the most likely source of her jaundice
    D. The woman has immunity because of a prior hepatitis B vaccination series
    E. The woman has immunity because of a natural infection

ANSWERS AND EXPLANATIONS

1. **D.** The Institute of Medicine's convergence model of human-microbe interaction demonstrates the overlap of four different factors: (1) physical environment, (2) genetic and biologic, (3) social, political, and economic, and (4) ecologic. Moving people out of an overcrowded tent camp best represents a change in the *physical environment*. Changes to individual immunity

(A) or microbial infectivity (E) best represent genetic and biologic factors. Changes in policy or business practice (B) best represent social, political, and economic factors. Changes in temperature or climate (C) best represent ecologic factors. All four domains are interrelated, however, so any given change in affecting the human-microbe interaction might be classified in more than one domain (see Fig. 20.1).

2. **E.** The most fundamental causative factors in health and disease, not just infectious disease mortality, are socioeconomic conditions (also called social determinants of health). These include income and its distribution, education, employment and job security, working conditions, food security, housing, and social exclusion/discrimination. These factors largely determine individual health behaviors and access and utilization of secondary factors related to health, such as different aspects of medical care—having a physician (C), having a "medical home" (D), or receiving vaccinations (A). Antibiotic resistance (B) is a growing problem and cause for concern with emerging bacterial diseases, but its importance is secondary to more fundamental drivers such as agricultural policies and physician prescribing practices.

3. **E.** Malaria is transmitted through an arthropod, the *Anopheles* mosquito. A potentially viable way to reduce the spread of infection would be to provide local residents with mosquito nets, in the hope of preventing contact between the vector (mosquito) and host (local residents). Strategies aimed at foodborne illness (A and D), contact transmission (A and B), and rodent carriers of disease (C and D) would likely be of little use for reducing malaria transmission.

4. **E.** Cardiovascular disease is a chronic disease that results from cumulative insults over a lifetime and therefore usually appears late in life. A surge in the cardiovascular mortality rate may imply that people are no longer dying prematurely from infectious diseases and therefore living long enough to die from cardiovascular disease. A rise in disease-specific mortality is not necessarily concerning, especially when the specific disease is a chronic disease, thus displacing infectious diseases as the cause of death. In this case, although the cardiovascular mortality is on the rise, overall mortality may be decreasing. Fewer early deaths and fewer overall deaths could be interpreted by this public health expert as "a good thing." Cardiovascular deaths are not necessarily pain free (A) or inexpensive (B). In fact, death from congestive heart failure can be preceded by protracted and expensive suffering. Even if mathematical models suggested the situation should be worse (C), this would not make increasing cardiovascular death rates "a good thing" (just a "not as bad as it could be" thing). Although there are infectious diseases (e.g., *Chlamydia*) that have been implicated in cardiovascular disease, choice D is a nonsense answer.

5. **B.** Human immunodeficiency virus (HIV) is spread by heterosexual and homosexual intercourse, by sharing needles and other equipment for intravenous drug use (IDU), and from infected mothers to their children (intrauterine or through breastfeeding). When the rates of new HIV infections are approximately equal in men and women, heterosexual intercourse is the most important route of spread; this is now true in Africa and Southeast Asia, where HIV rates are exploding and account for the greatest prevalence and incidence in the world. Thus HIV is most often spread by heterosexual contact, and choices A and C are incorrect. When the prevalence of new infections involves more men than women, either homosexual intercourse or IDU is likely to be the dominant route, not heterosexual contact (D). Among women, the most frequent route of infection is heterosexual intercourse, not homosexual contact (E).

6. **A.** Using clean needles (B) and male circumcision (C) also represent primary prevention strategies against HIV infection, not secondary and tertiary prevention. Antiretroviral therapy (ART) can be used to prevent the spread of HIV to a seronegative sexual partner (primary prevention for partner). ART can also be used to prevent asymptomatic HIV disease from becoming symptomatic (secondary prevention); the International AIDS Society recommends starting ART in those with asymptomatic HIV disease (CD4 cell counts $<500/mm^3$). Finally, ART can be used to slow, stop, or reverse the progression of HIV disease in those with symptoms (tertiary prevention). Thus ART can be a part of prevention efforts at any stage, so choices D and E are incorrect.

7 **E.** Because of a generally relative short time between contracting the disease and developing of illness, policies to prevent infectious disease are likely to produce a "return on investment" for those instituting the policy. Political leaders and health plan administrators might expect to reap the fruits of their prevention initiatives during their tenure, earning gains in political support and more satisfied and larger client bases, respectively. HIV/AIDS can be a notable exception to the short asymptomatic period for infectious diseases, sometimes with many years between infection and development of symptoms in immunocompetent hosts. This asymptomatic period may have worked against early policy strategies to combat HIV. Infectious diseases are not necessarily more serious (A) or lethal (D) than chronic diseases, or more difficult to manage (D) or more expensive (B). For example, asthma and diabetes are two chronic diseases that are especially serious, often lethal, difficult to manage, and quite costly, especially compared with relatively mild, easy-to-manage, and inexpensive infectious diseases such as viral gastroenteritis, in immunocompetent hosts.

8. **A.** *Mycobacterium tuberculosis* is spread via air-carried droplets, generated when infected patients cough. Negative-pressure rooms keep air flowing inward, preventing the escape of infective droplets outward.

Thus negative pressure limits the spread of TB from a patient being treated to other patients and staff who are not infected (primary prevention). The BCG vaccine is also a strategy for primary prevention, to prevent people uninfected from acquiring TB, not secondary prevention (C). Antimycobacterial medications can be used for secondary prevention (e.g. preventing latent, asymptomatic TB from becoming symptomatic), or tertiary prevention (e.g., stopping, slowing, or limiting the damage done by symptomatic TB), not primary prevention (B). DOTS (D) is only used for treating symptomatic TB. Answer choices A to D are all prevention strategies for TB, making choice E incorrect.

9. **E.** There is no reason to believe the stool test was incorrect and that some other organism was the cause of the girl's illness (C), or that the young girl was immunocompromised (A). *Campylobacter* does generally cause the type of fever and watery diarrhea affecting the girl and can be severe even in immunocompetent hosts. The girl may have eaten some chicken (B), but her stated objection to eating them makes this unlikely. Moreover, although chicken is a common source of *Campylobacter,* cooking the bird thoroughly kills the bug. Notably, no family member who ate the chicken became sick. The raw chicken could have contaminated other, noncooked items, such as the salad (D), but the girl's brother ate salad without getting sick, so such contamination is less likely. A knife used to butcher the raw chicken could have been contaminated with *Campylobacter* and the bacteria passed to the tomatoes if sliced with the same knife. Because the girl was the only one who ate sliced tomatoes, contaminated tomatoes are the most plausible explanation for her illness.

10. **C.** Receiving rabies preexposure vaccination is not sufficient protection after a potential rabies exposure (A), and it does modify the recommended postexposure treatment regimen (E). Raccoons can transmit rabies (B), so treatment is likely necessary. Preexposure prophylaxis (PEP) makes the administration of rabies immunoglobulin (D) unnecessary. All that is necessary is rabies vaccination on two separate occasions (vs four occasions, as required if no PEP was received).

11. **E.** The Union of Concerned Scientists estimated that 70% of all antibiotics go toward nontherapeutic uses in livestock. Specifically, antibiotics are used for growth promotion and prophylaxis against infections likely to result from unhealthy factory farming practices (e.g., feeding cattle corn instead of the grass they evolved to eat, resulting in accelerated growth and frequent infections). Antibiotics are also used to treat infections (D) in livestock, but antibiotics used for this purpose (another 14% of the total) pale in comparison to the volumes used for growth promotion. Likewise, poor antibiotic stewardship in human medicine (A and B) and patients not following medical advice (C) are other important but less dominant drivers of the growing problem of antibiotic resistance and multidrug-resistant pathogens in the community.

12. **D.** Antibody to hepatitis B surface antigen implies immunity when the surface antigen itself is negative. The anti-HBc (+) is associated with natural infection (acute, chronic, or resolved). The absence of this antibody suggests that her immunity is caused by vaccination rather than natural infection (E). The absence of anti-HBc is generally not informative about susceptibility and the need for a vaccine (A). HBsAg is present in acute and chronic infection but disappears once immunity develops. The absence of this antigen does not imply susceptibility and need for vaccine (B) but does imply that she is not chronically infected (C). The cause of her illness with jaundice is unknown.

21

Prevention of Mental Health and Behavior Problems

Elizabeth C. Katz

"Mental health can improve overall well-being and prevent other illnesses. And since mental health problems have a serious economic impact on vulnerable communities, making them a priority can save lives and markedly improve people's quality of life."

Vikram Patel, PhD

1. OVERVIEW

Mental health disorder refers to a set of emotions, cognitions, and/or behaviors that are abnormal from the perspective of society and/or the individual's culture; cause distress to affected individuals and/or their significant others; and result in harm or in functional impairment in one or more life domains (i.e., work, school, home).[1] Many mental health disorders reflect extreme or pathologic manifestations of normal emotions or behaviors (e.g., when social drinking progresses to regular heavy use associated with family or work disruption).

The US Burden of Disease Collaborators[2] published a list of the top 25 contributors to morbidity and mortality in 2016. This chapter will focus on mental health disorders and behavior problems that made it on that list, which include emotional disorders (i.e., depressive disorders, anxiety disorders, and posttraumatic stress disorder), schizophrenia, substance use disorders, and violence (both directed toward the self and others). Research suggests that some of these disorders (e.g., depression) are preventable.[3] However, even disorders that are not preventable (e.g., schizophrenia; an established substance use disorder) can be targeted with interventions that minimize their impact on affected individuals' lives.

1.1 DEFINITIONS

1.1.a Emotional Disorders

Emotional disorders are mental health disorders that have emotion regulation difficulties as a central feature and include depressive disorders, anxiety disorders, and posttraumatic stress disorder (PTSD). Depressive disorders are characterized by feelings of sadness, feeling "blue," or loss of interest in previously enjoyed activities. In addition, affected individuals may experience weight gain or loss, low self-esteem, extreme fatigue and low energy, and suicidal thoughts. Anxiety disorders are characterized by excessive fear and anxiety accompanied by behavioral disturbances, such as hypervigilance, agitation, and avoidance. Each of the anxiety disorders has a different cue, trigger, or target for the individual's anxiety or fear. For example, in social anxiety disorder, the fear or anxiety is triggered by circumstances in which the individual may be judged by others, whereas in specific phobia, the fear is associated with objects (e.g., dogs, needles) or situations (e.g., heights, seeing blood).[1]

The defining feature of PTSD is exposure to a traumatic event involving a threat to an individual's life or physical well-being (e.g., a near fatal car accident, combat experiences, rape). The trauma may be experienced directly (i.e., personally) or indirectly either by witnessing or hearing about the event happening to a loved one or by being repeatedly exposed to distressing details of the event (e.g., first responders who helped recover human remains after the attacks on the World Trade Center and Pentagon on September 11, 2001). After exposure to the traumatic event, the individual begins to experience an array of symptoms, including hypervigilance, an exaggerated startle response, and reexperiencing the traumatic event, among others.[1]

1.1.b Schizophrenia

Schizophrenia involves disturbances of thoughts, perceptions, emotions, and behaviors. Affected individuals experience delusions (i.e., beliefs that conflict with reality, such as the belief that one's thoughts are being controlled by the government), hallucinations (i.e., seeing, hearing, or feeling things that are not there), and disorganized speech and behavior that cause severe functional impairment.[1]

1.1.c Substance Use Disorders

Use of both licit and illicit substances varies along a continuum. The first stage of use is *experimentation* in which an individual tries substances one or more times out of curiosity, to experience their effects or because their friends are doing it. The next stage is *recreational use*. At this stage, individuals use regularly (e.g., on weekends) because of the enjoyment it brings or in social situations. However, use at these early stages is associated with few or no consequences. Individuals who use even more regularly (e.g., daily or almost daily) and experience mild to moderate problems from their use (e.g., engage in behaviors they later regret) have progressed to the stage of *misuse*. In addition, people who misuse substances may do so as a means of coping with stress or negative life events. Misuse is indicative of a risk for more problematic use. The final stage is *pathologic use* when an individual meets diagnostic criteria for a substance-related disorder.[4] This level of use is captured within the *Diagnostic and Statistical Manual of Mental Disorders,* Fifth Edition (DSM5) diagnostic criteria for substance-related and addictive disorders.

The DSM5 substance-related and addictive disorders criteria fall within four broad categories: impaired control

(e.g., the individual is unable to cut down use despite efforts to do so); risky use (e.g., the individual uses in unsafe situations such as while driving); social impairment (e.g., the individual continues to use despite negative impacts in several life domains); and pharmacologic properties (e.g., tolerance, in which the individual must increase use over time to experience the same effect, and withdrawal). The severity of a substance use disorder is determined by the number of criteria met: The level of two to three criteria is considered mild; four to five is considered moderate; six or more is considered severe.[1] The DSM5 includes diagnostic criteria for nine substance-related disorders and gambling disorder.

E-cigarettes. The newest trend in tobacco-delivery products is the e-cigarette. E-cigarettes, which also include hookahs, vape pens, and tank systems, are electronic devices that aerosolize liquid nicotine, flavorings, and other additives that can then be inhaled. Pathologic e-cigarette use would most likely be considered a tobacco use disorder since the addictive substance in both tobacco products and e-cigarettes is nicotine.[5]

The opioid epidemic. Between 1999 and 2011, sales of prescription opioids (e.g., oxycodone) increased dramatically accompanied by substantial increases in both prescription-opioid treatment admissions and opioid-overdose deaths. This increase began in the late 1980s following publication of a paper suggesting that long-term treatment of chronic, noncancer pain with opioids was both safe and effective. It is important to note that this epidemic is not limited to nonmedical (i.e., illegal) use of prescription opioids. Rather, research suggests that deaths due to overdose are higher among individuals using them legitimately (i.e., by prescription) than among nonmedical users (i.e., those obtaining prescription opioids illegally). One stunning example of this involves the late actor Heath Ledger, who died in 2008 at the age of 28. The autopsy concluded that Ledger's death was due to an accidental overdose from a combination of legally prescribed opioids (i.e., oxycodone and hydrocodone), antianxiety medications, and sleep aids.

In addition to substantial increases in overdose deaths, another side effect of this epidemic is the transition from prescription opioid to heroin use. Specifically, research suggests that about 80% of current heroin users reported having switched from legally prescribed opioids because heroin was a less expensive and easier way to sustain their habit.[6]

1.1.d Suicide and Violence

Suicide is defined as a purposeful act directed toward ending one's life. Whereas *suicide* refers to successful completion of the act, the term *suicide attempt* refers to any act of self-harm, including **parasuicidal behavior** such as cutting, regardless of the intent of the behavior or the outcome. **Suicidal ideation** refers to thoughts about killing or harming oneself.[7] Violence refers to any physical act that is intended to inflict harm on another person. While violence is not considered a mental health disorder, and most people with mental health disorders are *not* violent, evidence suggests that the risk of committing a violent act, whether against another person or the self, is elevated among people with mental health disorders.[7]

1.2 PREVALENCE

A recent meta-analysis of studies conducted between 1980 and 2013 found that the global past year prevalence of "common mental disorders" was nearly 18%, and the lifetime prevalence was almost 30%.[8] Among US adults in 2016, rates of any mental illness and of serious mental illness were 18.3% and 4.2%, respectively. Moreover, the past year prevalence of alcohol use and drug use disorders were 2% and 3.2%, respectively, among youth (aged 12–17 years), and 6% and 2.7%, respectively, among adults (aged ≥18).[9] In the same year, the US Surgeon General's office found that past month prevalence of e-cigarette use was 5.3% among middle school students, 16% among high school students, 13.5% among young adults (aged 18–25), and 5.7% among adults aged 25 or older.[10]

The MacArthur Community Violence Study found that more than one-quarter of patients between 1992 and 1995 committed a violent act within 41 weeks of being released from a psychiatric hospital. Among these psychiatric patients, risk was highest when the individual was diagnosed with a major mental health disorder and a comorbid substance use disorder. It is important to note that among people with mental health disorders, the most common form of violence is self-directed (i.e., suicide and self-harm).[7]

1.3 THE HUMAN AND ECONOMIC TOLL

1.3.a Global Burden of Disease Estimates

The 2010 Global Burden of Disease Study found that 2.3% of years of potential life lost (YPLL) and 28.5% of years lived with disability (YLD) were attributable to mental disorders.[11] In 2013, mental illness was ranked as the fifth leading cause of disability adjusted life years (DALYs) after chronic illnesses such as cardiovascular disease (first) and cancer (third).[2] However, it is argued that these numbers grossly underestimate the global impact of mental health disorders because of limitations placed on how they are defined.[12] When expanding the definition to include such things as personality disorders and self-harm, the global disease burden estimate increases to 13% of DALYs, which makes it second only to cardiovascular disease (13.5% of global DALYs).[12] On its own, the opioid epidemic has also had a substantial impact on mortality in the United States. In 2016, opioid use disorders were ranked 15th among all causes of YPLL[2] and accounted for 53,000 deaths.[13] YLD estimates (in thousands) and YLD rank for specific mental health and substance use disorders, including the opioid epidemic, are presented in Fig. 21.1.

In 2016, violence was a major contributor to mortality. Specifically, among all causes of YPLL, self-harm by firearms was ranked 13th (causing approximately 893,000 deaths), self-harm by other means was ranked 12th (causing approximately 981,000 deaths), and violence by firearms was ranked 18th (causing about 660,000 deaths).[2]

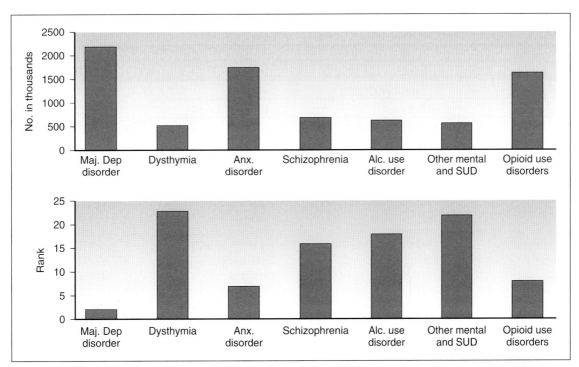

Fig. 21.1 Number of years (in thousands) of years lived with disability (YLD) and rank among the top 25 causes of YLD in 2016. Substance Use Disorder (SUD). (From US Burden of Disease Collaborators, 2018.)

In addition to mortality, there is also an economic toll from mental and behavioral disorders. In 2010, the global cost of mental and behavioral disorders exceeded US $2 trillion, with indirect costs more than double direct costs.[14]Alone, the opioid epidemic was estimated to cost the United States more than $90 billion annually due to overdose deaths, health care costs, lost wages, and incarceration.[13]

1.3.b Other Consequences

In addition to morbidity and mortality, mental health disorders are associated with a variety of social, occupational, and health consequences. For example, mental health disorders may cause impaired social relationships, mental health problems in family members caring for an affected person, and death by suicide or other causes.[15] Substance use disorders are associated with the following:

- Involvement in risky behaviors, such as unprotected sexual intercourse, aggression/violence, and driving under the influence[15]
- Various infectious diseases, such as human immunodeficiency virus (HIV) and hepatitis C virus (HCV)[16]
- Pregnancy complications, such as premature delivery, low birth weight, and neonatal withdrawal syndrome, which contribute to social-emotional deficits, academic problems, and an increased risk of substance use among drug-exposed children[15,17]
- Accidents, injuries and overdoses leading to high levels of hospitalizations[18]
- Increased risk for cardiovascular disease and many different types of cancer.[15]

Following suicide, surviving family members and friends may experience complicated bereavement; feel guilty, confused, depressed, and anxious; and even experience suicidal thoughts or make suicide attempts. Surviving family members often feel socially isolated and stigmatized and may even develop PTSD. Finally, research suggests that direct or indirect exposure to suicide can instigate suicide clusters (or a contagion effect) in which multiple suicides occur either close in time to or physically near (e.g., same town or school) one another. Because this contagion effect can be triggered by media coverage that is seen as glorifying the suicide, the Centers for Disease Control and Prevention (CDC) has developed guidelines for the media about how to portray or discuss suicide.[7]

2. RISK AND PROTECTIVE FACTORS

Mental health disorders as well as behavioral problems share a common set of risk and protective factors at the levels of the individual, family, and community (Table 21.1). It is important to note that the impact of risk and protective factors is cumulative.

2.1 DISORDER-SPECIFIC RISK FACTORS

2.1.a Emotional Disorders

Emotional disorders share a common etiology that includes generalized biologic and psychologic vulnerabilities combined with a specific psychologic vulnerability and/or stress.[19] Genetics are one of the main biologic contributors to the development of emotional disorders accounting for about 30% to 40% of an individual's risk.[20] Inherited traits associated with an increased risk for emotional disorders are *neuroticism*, which is the tendency toward being anxious or fearful; *negative affect*, which is a tendency toward pervasive

---

TABLE 21.1 Individual-Level, Family-Level, and Community-Level Risk Factors and Protective Factors Common to Several Mental Health Disorders and Violence [2,15]

RISK FACTORS			
Individual Level	**Family Level**	**Community Level**	**PROTECTIVE FACTORS**
• Genetics • Insecure attachment • Low self-esteem • Poor impulse control • Racial/ethnic minority status • Bullying or discrimination • Failure to bond with family, school, or community • Involvement with a deviant peer group • Trauma of parental loss due to divorce, incarceration, or death • Gender/sexual minority status • Adverse childhood experiences (e.g., abuse and neglect)	• Maternal substance use (both licit and illicit) during pregnancy • Lack of emotional warmth • Lack of or inconsistent responsiveness to infant's needs leading to insecure attachment • Coercive or aggressive parenting • Parent conflict and domestic violence • Permissive parenting • Inadequate parental supervision of children's behavior	• Poverty • Stress • Inadequate access to mental and behavioral health care • Inadequate transportation, housing, education, employment, and nutrition • Exposure to drugs, crime, and violence within the neighborhood • Social norms supportive of deviant behaviors • Overcrowded schools with insufficient resources and less-qualified teachers	• Secure attachment during infancy and early childhood • Achieving developmental milestones at appropriate times • Being physically healthy • Being physically active • Possessing at least average intelligence • High self-esteem • Good social skills • Adequate coping skills • Strong religious beliefs and affiliation

negative mood; and *behavioral inhibition*, which is a tendency toward shyness and introversion.[19] The generalized psychologic vulnerability is a pervasive belief that one cannot control or cope with negative events (i.e., low self-efficacy). Factors that contribute to this perceived lack of control and low self-confidence include parenting styles characterized by either a lack of responsiveness to children's needs or intrusiveness and overprotection.[19]

Exposure to stress among individuals who possess generalized biologic and psychologic vulnerabilities may cause persistent depressive disorder or generalized anxiety disorder. Other anxiety disorders (e.g., social phobia, specific phobia, PTSD) require a specific psychologic vulnerability, which involves a social or behavioral learning experience. For example, being attacked by a dog (behavioral learning) could lead a vulnerable person to develop a specific phobia, whereas observing a parent behaving fearfully in social situations (social learning) could lead to social phobia.[19] This model also helps explain why some, but not all, individuals who are exposed to traumatic experiences develop PTSD.

Other factors associated with elevated risk for emotional disorders include maladaptive thinking patterns, female gender, younger age, minority status, chronic illness, and presence of other mental health or substance use disorders. Parental depression significantly increases the risk of depression in children.[3] For older adults, additional risk factors for depression include grief and loneliness, sleep disturbances, and a prior history of depression. Postpartum women who have low self-esteem, lack social support, have a history of depression, and lack needed resources (e.g., adequate day care, financial resources) are at elevated risk for a depressive episode with postpartum onset.[21]

2.1.b Schizophrenia

Genetic contributions to schizophrenia have been examined using twin studies that compare concordance rates (i.e., the percentage of times that both members of a twin pair have the disorder) between identical twins (who share 100% of their genes) and fraternal twins (who share about 50% of their genes). These studies have shown that identical twins have concordance rates for schizophrenia that are two to four times higher than fraternal twins. Moreover, individuals with first-degree relatives with schizophrenia have a 6% chance of developing the disorder, which exceeds the rate in the general population (i.e., 1%).[7] Other risk factors for schizophrenia include male gender, maternal stress and flu exposure during pregnancy, and living in an urban environment. For certain vulnerable individuals, marijuana use during adolescence is associated with an increased risk of developing a psychotic disorder later in life.[3]

2.1.c Substance Use Disorders

As with other mental health disorders, risk for substance use disorders may be inherited.[3] Research suggests that genetics account for 50% to 60% of the risk for substance use disorders, although heritability estimates for drug use disorders are more variable than for alcohol use disorders. Several clinical **endophenotypes** have been identified for substance use disorder risk. Endophenotypes are traits that have a high degree of heritability, are associated with the disorder of interest, and are detectable before the disorder is expressed. For example, facial flushing in response to alcohol consumption (which is common among some Asian cultures) is an inherited trait that serves as a protective factor against alcohol use disorders. Endophenotypes that confer a risk for alcohol use disorders include a decreased sensitivity to the effects of alcohol[4] and abnormalities in the brain's electrical activity (i.e., reduced amplitude of the P300 response).[22] Moreover, traits such as behavioral disinhibition, sensation-seeking and impulsivity, as well as the presence of certain psychiatric disorders (e.g., schizophrenia, bipolar disorder) are associated with an increased risk for any substance use disorder.[4]

In addition to genetics, research suggests that there are three main reasons why people use drugs, including mood modification (i.e., to feel good or better), performance enhancement, and social reasons (i.e., to fit in with a peer group). These "reasons" are initially learned vicariously and then stored in memory as outcome expectancies (i.e., if-then statements about the effects of using a substance). For example, prior to any experience with alcohol, a child may develop the belief, "If I drink, I will have fun" (mood modification), by watching his or her parents drink at social occasions. Research has shown that children who hold positive outcome expectancies for alcohol have an earlier onset of drinking than children who do not. Once adolescents begin experimenting, they directly experience the pharmacologic properties of substances. These properties of drugs further reinforce use.[4]

Direct-to-consumer advertising of medications, such as those for attention-deficit hyperactivity disorder (ADHD), may contribute to perceptions that such drugs are not dangerous. Increases in the number of prescriptions written for opioid and stimulant medications, as well as availability for purchase online, increase the accessibility of these drugs.[18]

2.1.d Comorbidity Among Mental Health Disorders

In addition to sharing a common etiology (or likely because they do), research suggests that anxiety and depression are highly comorbid with about 50% of patients meeting criteria for both disorders.[20] Moreover, in some cases, untreated anxiety may become a causal factor in the development of depression.[23] Among individuals with substance use disorders, 60% to 80% of adults and 60% of youth have a comorbid mental health disorder. Some evidence suggests that more than 90% of individuals diagnosed with schizophrenia have a tobacco use disorder. Finally, approximately 25% to 30% of depressed and anxious adults meet criteria for a substance use disorder.[4]

2.1.e Suicide and Violence

The extent to which an individual believes that others would benefit from his or her death (i.e., "perceived burdensomeness") and that an individual's basic needs for affiliation are not being met (i.e., "thwarted belongingness") are risk factors for suicidal ideation.[24] Suicide risk increases when suicidal thoughts are combined with an increased acceptance of suicide as a viable option and feelings of hopelessness. One of the best predictors of future suicide attempts is past suicidal behavior.[25] Beyond distorted thinking styles, other contributors to suicide risk are male gender, ethnic minority status, suicide among family or friends, and serious physical illness.[26]

Violence among individuals with mental disorders has a variety of causes, although risk is highest during the earliest stages of the disorder. PTSD symptoms such as agitation, hypervigilance, and increased sensitivity to threat signals may increase the risk of violent acts. Delusions, especially beliefs that others are bad or dangerous, may lead individuals with schizophrenia toward violence. Depressed individuals' pervasive negative thoughts about the self, world, and future may contribute to an elevated risk for murder/suicide.[7] For example, in 2001, a 37-year-old Texas mother, Andrea Yates, drowned her five children (ages 6 months to 7 years) in a bathtub. At trial, Ms. Yates testified that she had not wanted to hurt her children, but she killed them because she believed she was saving them from going to hell. Prior to this event, Ms. Yates had suffered several episodes of postpartum depression with psychotic features, had made several suicide attempts, and had discontinued taking her medication. Ultimately, Ms. Yates was found not guilty by reason of insanity and sentenced to a mental hospital for the remainder of her life. Events such as this one raised public awareness about the need for early identification and treatment of postpartum depression and psychosis.

3. PREVENTION

3.1 FRAMEWORK FOR PREVENTION

The Institute of Medicine (IOM) developed a typology for prevention of mental health disorders and behavioral problems based on, but different from, the one used for physical health problems. This typology comprises three prevention categories: universal, selective, and indicated. **Universal prevention,** like primary prevention, is targeted toward an entire population, regardless of risk level. The goal of universal programs is either to prevent individuals from developing a disorder or to identify at-risk individuals and refer them for the next levels of care. The other two IOM categories involve secondary prevention, because they are directed toward those at greater risk for mental health disorders. **Selective prevention** is targeted toward individuals who possess risk factors, such as anxious temperament or early childhood adversity, to prevent the onset of a disorder. **Indicated prevention** is intended for individuals who show subclinical signs of a disorder with the goal of preventing progression to clinically significant levels. Selective prevention and indicated prevention are collectively referred to as **targeted prevention.**[3]

3.2 UNIVERSAL PREVENTIVE INTERVENTIONS

3.2.a Media Campaigns

Media campaigns have been evaluated as potential strategies for reducing smoking, alcohol use, driving while intoxicated, illicit substance use, as well as child abuse and violence. Mass media campaigns may impact behavior change in one of two ways. They may work directly by affecting individuals' thoughts and emotions about targeted health behaviors and thereby influence decision making about that behavior.[27] For example, the Legacy Foundation's Truth® campaign links smoking with serious health consequences and death as well as highlights the fact that "big tobacco" selectively targets poor communities with their marketing.[28] The likely intent of this campaign is to influence smokers to quit and to prevent nonsmokers from starting by instigating anger toward the tobacco industry while also triggering negative emotions toward cigarettes. Alternatively, mass media campaigns might work indirectly by encouraging community members to take steps to change social norms (e.g., making them less favorable toward drinking and driving), to assist affected individuals in changing their behavior (e.g., by encouraging them to enter treatment), or to push for policy changes.[27]

Evidence suggests that media campaigns targeting tobacco use have been highly effective in reducing smoking uptake among youth as well as in encouraging adult smokers to quit. Conversely, there is little evidence to support the efficacy of existing media campaigns for alcohol, possibly due to the powerful effects of alcohol advertising and acceptance of drinking as a social norm. In fact, some evidence suggests that mass media campaigns were associated with more positive attitudes toward alcohol and increased intentions to drink. Moreover, mass media campaigns targeting suicide have been largely ineffective, whereas the evidence regarding campaigns targeting mental health, violence, and child abuse is inconclusive. Overall, media campaigns may be most effective when they are accompanied by policies or legislation that increase access to services that support change and penalize continued involvement (e.g., the imposition of sin taxes for cigarettes combined with reductions in health care costs for individuals who engage in treatment).[27]

3.2.b Public Policy

Emotional disorders. Policies that have been shown to improve mental health outcomes include the following:
- Improving nutrition and housing
- Improving access to education and health care
- Improving access to work and reducing poverty.[15]

Substance use disorders. Although legal approaches to substance use (e.g., incarceration of drug users, interdiction efforts) may prevent experimentation or initial use of substances, these efforts have been largely ineffective for stopping established use.[4] The following policies have led to decreases in rates of substance use and related problems:
- Imposing sin taxes (increasing the cost of alcohol and cigarettes)

- Raising the legal age to purchase and drink alcohol
- Reducing the availability of alcohol by regulating number and open hours of places selling alcohol
- Banning advertising and limiting advertising directed at youth
- Banning smoking in public places.[15]

The opioid epidemic. One strategy that may have a beneficial impact on the opioid overdose epidemic is enacting legislation to prevent "doctor shopping." Doctor shopping is the practice of going to multiple doctors to fill prescriptions for opioids. Ideally, doctor shoppers would be identified and then referred for treatment. Three states (Kentucky, Tennessee, and New York) enacted laws that require doctors to use Prescription Drug Monitoring Program (PDMP) data to identify doctor shoppers. The result of this legislation was a reduction in the number of prescriptions written for opioids as well as in rates of doctor shopping in these states.[6]

Suicide and violence. In addition to preventing or treating other mental health disorders and substance use, suicide prevention efforts might also include the following:
- Reducing the toxicity of gasoline and car exhausts
- Minimizing access to high places such as rooftops and bridges
- Enforcing and/or tightening gun control policies
- Controlling the availability of pesticides and prescription medications[15,26]

Given what is known about risk factors for gun violence, it is evident that policies that only target mentally ill patients' access to guns is unlikely to have a meaningful impact. Thus evidence from other countries supports the implementation of stricter gun legislation. A recent systematic review of 130 studies in 10 countries found evidence that enactment of certain types of gun legislation were associated with reductions in gun-related morbidity and mortality (although the authors state that the quality of the research limits confidence in some of the findings).[29] Moreover, following the Port Arthur massacre in 1996, Australia's government enacted strict firearms legislation, which included a buyback program, requirements for owners and dealers to surrender prohibited weapons, requirements for owners to properly store weapons (e.g., in locked gun boxes), and bans on certain types of weapons. A report by the Australian Institute of Criminology found that between 1991 and 2001, gun-related deaths decreased by 47%, and the incidence of firearm-related homicides and suicides decreased by almost half.[30]

3.2.c Other Universal Prevention

Substance use disorders. One of the most well-known universal prevention programs for substance use is Drug Abuse Resistance Education (DARE), which is delivered by police officers in US schools. Despite its popularity, meta-analyses show that DARE produces either no effect or possibly harmful effects on youth drug use.[31] Another program that is being widely implemented is the Life Skills Training (LST) program. LST teaches skills to resist peer pressure and focuses on decreasing motivators for use.

Results of LST evaluations show that it is effective for reducing drug use for up to 3 years following the intervention. As a result, LST has received an endorsement from the US Surgeon General's office.[3]

The opioid epidemic. Universal prevention for the opioid epidemic focuses on reducing medical and nonmedical exposure to prescription opioids. These goals can be accomplished through educating prescribers about the risks associated with long-term use of opioids for noncancer pain as well as about the benefits of using nonopioid analgesics or behavioral approaches to pain management. When patients require opioids, it is recommended that physicians avoid long-acting formulations and limit the amount prescribed to no more than a 3-day supply. In addition, pharmaceutic companies have created delivery methods for prescription opioids that prevent abuse (i.e., cannot be easily snorted or injected). In 2014, the US Drug Enforcement Agency made it legal for patients to return unused doses of prescription opioids to a pharmacy, which decreases the availability of such medications for nonprescribed use.[6]

Suicide. Universal efforts to prevent *suicide* involve psychoeducation programs targeted toward increasing awareness of the symptoms of mental health disorders, their role in suicide, and available resources. In **gatekeeper training,** for example, selected individuals are trained to recognize warning signs of depression and suicide and to intervene with distressed persons. A systematic review found that gatekeeper training improved trainee's knowledge, skills, and attitudes toward intervening and, in specific populations, produced reductions in suicidal ideation and attempts.[32]

3.2.d Screening

Many people with mental health disorders do not receive treatment because their disorder remains undetected. As such, screening can be an effective prevention strategy to identify individuals who would benefit from more targeted prevention efforts. Brief screening tools can be used in a variety of settings (e.g., primary care and other health care settings, schools, emergency rooms) to determine level of risk and type of intervention required. The US Prevention Services Task Force[33] website provides guidelines for screening and prevention of alcohol, tobacco, and illicit drug use; depression; intimate partner violence; abuse of elders and other vulnerable adults; and suicide. Readers may also consult the Substance Abuse and Mental Health Services Administration[34] website for a list of validated screening tools for mental health disorders.

Screening may be useful in efforts to reduce the risks associated with opioid addiction. Specifically, opioid prescribers might require patients to submit routine urine samples for testing to evaluate the level of drug in their system. While this may be effective for individuals prescribed a short course of medication (i.e., to determine if they have, in fact, discontinued use as planned), it can neither provide information about whether individuals are taking more of the medication than prescribed nor indicate whether they have reverted to snorting or injecting their prescribed medication.[6]

3.3 TARGETED PREVENTIVE INTERVENTIONS

3.3.a Emotional Disorders

Few prevention programs specifically target *anxiety.* However, given the shared risk factors between anxiety and other emotional disorders, prevention programs aimed at these disorders will likely have a broad beneficial impact on anxiety.[20] Effective preventive interventions for depressive disorders focus on teaching effective stress-coping skills, modifying negative thinking, and providing support to children of depressed parents.[3] The MacArthur Initiative Depression Toolkit was developed to provide guidelines for primary care physicians and other health professionals about how to manage depression among their patients. The toolkit outlines a four-step process, which begins with assessment. Once a patient is identified as having symptoms of depression, the clinician then provides education about depression and treatment options (e.g., medication and counseling). This second step of the process is collaborative with the patient and clinician working together to develop a care plan. The third step involves selecting and starting the patient's preferred treatment approach; the fourth step involves monitoring patient compliance with treatment as well as the impact of treatment on symptoms.[35]

3.3.b Substance Use Disorders

Targeted brief interventions for substance use include **motivational interviewing,** which is discussed in Chapter 15. In addition to motivational interviewing, research suggests that advice by a physician may be sufficient to enhance motivation to change behavior and to enter treatment.[36,37] The US Public Health Service and National Cancer Institute developed the Five *A*'s model (see Box 15.1) for encouraging smoking cessation.

3.3.c Suicide

A collaborative effort between the Substance Abuse and Mental Health Services Administration (SAMHSA), Screening for Mental Health Inc., and Suicide Prevention Research Center led to the development of the Suicide Assessment Five-Step Evaluation and Triage (SAFE-T) guidelines for mental health professionals. The five steps of SAFE-T are (1) identify risk factors and note any that can be modified to reduce risk; (2) identify protective factors and note any that can be enhanced to reduce risk; (3) conduct a suicide assessment for suicidal thoughts, plans, behaviors, and intent; (4) make a determination about the level of risk and choose the appropriate intervention to reduce risk; and (5) document the interaction. No published evaluations of SAFE-T have been conducted yet, but the recommendations were based on the "American Psychiatric Association (APA) Practice Guideline for the Assessment and Treatment of Patients with Suicidal Behaviors."[38] Research on the efficacy of crisis centers and hotlines, which are widely used, is inconclusive.[15]

4. TREATMENT

As with other diseases, treatment for mental health disorders constitutes both tertiary prevention for patients as well as primary prevention for families and communities. The details of treating individual diseases is beyond the scope of this chapter so interested readers should consult the literature. However, of interest to the public health field are interventions that combine external incentives (i.e., contingency management) or target community involvement (i.e., social network and family interventions).

4.1 CONTINGENCY MANAGEMENT

Contingency management operates on the premise that drug use is highly reinforcing and that motivation for abstinence can be increased when abstinence and participation in nondrug-related activities are reinforced. Contingency management interventions use a variety of reinforcements, including vouchers with monetary value that can be exchanged for goods and services, retail items/gift certificates, and for heroin users, take-home methadone doses. Although contingency management is most effective for promoting drug abstinence when reinforcement is present (with high rates of relapse once the reinforcement is removed), it seems to be an effective approach for improving compliance during treatment (e.g., with counseling session attendance; taking medication as prescribed), which may translate into longer-term posttreatment benefits.[4]

4.2 SOCIAL NETWORK AND FAMILY INTERVENTIONS

Social network and family models are rooted in research showing that social support is critical for increasing the likelihood of treatment entry and engagement, abstinence, and sustained recovery from substance use disorders. In addition to interventions that focus on involving drug-free family members and significant others in treatment, self-help groups (e.g., Alcoholics Anonymous, Narcotics Anonymous, Rational Recovery) are also effective for improving substance use outcomes.[4]

5. HARM REDUCTION

Harm Reduction, as its name implies, is intended to reduce harm associated with established substance use disorders or unremitting mental health disorders. For substance use disorders, harm reduction interventions are designed to prevent disease transmission and overdose or death. For mental health disorders, harm reduction may help prevent worsening of an established mental illness thereby reducing personal and societal costs (e.g., by preventing the need for hospitalizations due to the exacerbation of symptoms).

5.1 OPIOID USE DISORDERS

Harm reduction efforts for opioid use disorders include programs aimed at reducing overdose death rates and spread of infectious diseases associated with injection drug use. For example, programs in which opioid-addicted individuals are prescribed and trained to use naloxone (opioid antagonist) are effective for reversing the effects of opiate overdose in a substantial number of cases. Needle exchange programs, in which injection drug users can safely exchange used for unused hypodermic needles, are designed to prevent transmission of infectious diseases as well as facilitate entry into treatment. Prevention education and HIV testing, providing condoms, and drug substitution therapy may help reduce the spread of HIV and other transmissible infections.[6]

5.2 TOBACCO USE DISORDERS

There is debate about the relative safety of e-cigarettes as compared to other forms of tobacco consumption. Because heavy nicotine consumption among adolescents and young adults can cause deficits in attention, learning, and impulse control; increase the risk for addiction to nicotine and other illicit stimulants (e.g., cocaine); and increase the risk for mood disorders,[10] it seems imprudent to consider e-cigarettes as a treatment for tobacco use disorders. However, it might be reasonable to consider e-cigarette use to be a harm reduction approach given that it may have fewer health consequences than other tobacco products. Moreover, there is at least some evidence to suggest that e-cigarette use may help adults quit smoking.[5] However, this is an area of active investigation and the risks of e-cigarettes need to be better understood. Vaping has been linked to severe lung illnesses, especially among those smoking marijuana. Thus, caution should be used before recommending e-cigarettes or vaping devices as harm reduction measures for cigarette smoking.

5.3 SCHIZOPHRENIA

In recent years, "prodromal clinics" have been established to conduct research on the signs and symptoms of risk for psychosis and to develop and evaluate strategies for preventing conversion from a prodromal to a florid psychotic state. Research suggests that a combination of psychosocial treatment and antipsychotic medication have promise for preventing conversion. Specifically, 36% of untreated prodromal cases, but only 11% of treated cases, subsequently experienced a full-blown psychotic episode.[3]

6. SUMMARY

Emotional disorders (i.e., depression, anxiety, and PTSD), schizophrenia, substance use disorders (including the opioid epidemic), and violence (both self and other directed) are among the top 25 contributors to morbidity and mortality within the United States and worldwide. In addition to morbidity and mortality, these disorders are associated with a myriad of personal (e.g., pregnancy complications, stress on family members caring for an affected individual) and economic costs. Research has identified both shared and disorder-specific risk and protective factors that can help inform pre-

vention programming. While research suggests that some of these disorders are preventable (e.g., depression, substance use disorders, violence), those that are not (e.g., schizophrenia, an established substance use disorder) can be targeted with interventions that reduce the harm they cause to individuals and society. Evidence is accumulating supporting the efficacy of universal prevention programs such as screening for mental health and substance use disorders, mass media campaigns targeting smoking, and public policy changes directed toward substance use disorders, among others. Several brief interventions (e.g., motivational interviewing for substance use disorders and the Five A's Model for smoking cessation) have also been found to be effective as targeted prevention programs. For individuals with established mental health disorders, several treatment and harm reduction approaches have been developed to assist patients in reestablishing mental health and/or preventing harm. Thus resources should be devoted toward ensuring the wide implementation of empirically supported prevention, treatment, and harm reduction programming to reduce the global burden of these disorders while improving quality of life.

ACKNOWLEDGMENT

We appreciate the work of Eugene M Dunne, Samantha Lookatch, and Joshua S Camins on an earlier version of this chapter in the fourth edition.

REFERENCES

1. American Psychiatric Association. *Diagnostic and Statistical Manual of Mental Disorders.* 5th ed. Arlington, VA: American Psychiatric Association; 2013.
2. US Burden of Disease Collaborators. The state of US health, 1990-2016. Burden of diseases, injuries, and risk factors among US states. *JAMA.* 2018;319:1444-1472. doi:10.1001/jama.2018.0158.
3. National Research Council and Institute of Medicine. Preventing mental, emotional, and behavioral disorders among young people: progress and possibilities. In: O'Connell ME, ed. *Committee on the Prevention of Mental Disorders and Substance Abuse Among Children, Youth, and Young Adults: Research Advances and Promising Interventions. Board on Children, Youth, and Families, Division of Behavioral and Social Sciences and Education.* Washington, DC: National Academies Press; 2009.
4. Miller WR, Carroll KM. *Rethinking Substance Abuse: What the Science Shows, and What We Should Do About It.* New York, NY: Guilford; 2006.
5. Kozlowski LT, Warner KE. Adolescents and e-cigarettes: objects of concern may appear larger than they are. *Drug Alcohol Depend.* 2017;174:209-214. doi:10.1016/j.drugalcdep.2017.01.001.
6. Kolodny A, Courtwright DT, Hwang CS. The prescription opioid and heroin crisis: a public health approach to an epidemic of addiction. *Annu Rev Public Health.* 2015;36:559-574. doi:10.1146/annurev-publhealth-031914-122957.
7. Wenzel A. *The SAGE Encyclopedia of Abnormal and Clinical Psychology.* Thousand Oaks, CA: SAGE Publications; 2017.
8. Steel Z, Marnane C, Iranpour C, et al. The global prevalence of common mental disorders: a systematic review and meta-analysis

1980-2013. *Int J Epidemiol.* 2014;43:476-493. Available at: https://academic.oup.com/ije/article/43/2/476/2901736.

9. Center for Behavioral Health Statistics and Quality. *2016 National Survey on Drug Use and Heath: Detailed Tables.* Rockville, MD: Substance Abuse and Mental Health Services Administration; 2017. Available at: https://www.samhsa.gov/data/sites/default/files/NSDUH-DetTabs-2016/NSDUH-DetTabs-2016.pdf.

10. U.S. Department of Health and Human Services. *E-Cigarette Use Among Youth and Young Adults: A Report of the Surgeon General—Executive Summary.* Atlanta, GA: U.S. Department of Health and Human Services, Centers for Disease Control and Prevention, National Center for Chronic Disease Prevention and Health Promotion, Office on Smoking and Health; 2016.

11. Whiteford HA, Ferrari AJ, Degenhardt L, Feigin V, Vos T. The global burden of mental, neurological and substance use disorders: an analysis from the Global Burden of Disease Study 2010. *PLoS One.* 2015;10:e0116820. doi:10.1371/journal.pone.0116820.

12. Vigo DT. Estimating the true global burden of mental illness. *Lancet Psychiatry.* 2016;3:171-178. Available at: http://www.thelancet.com/pdfs/journals/lanpsy/PIIS2215-0366(15)00505-2.pdf.

13. Rhyan CN. *Research Brief. The Potential Societal Benefit of Eliminating Opioid Overdoses, Deaths, and Substance use Disorders Exceeds $95 Billion Per Year.* Ann Arbor, MI: Altarum—Center for Value in Health Care; 2017.

14. Trautmann S, Rehm J, Wittchen HU. The economic costs of mental disorders. Do our societies react appropriately to the burden of mental disorders? *EMBO Rep.* 2016;17:1245-1249.

15. Hosman C, Jané-Llopis E, Saxena S, eds. *Prevention of Mental Disorders: Effective Interventions and Policy Options.* Oxford, UK: Oxford University Press; 2004.

16. Schulte MT, Hser YI. Substance use and associated health conditions throughout the lifespan. *Public Health Rev.* 2014;35(2). Available at: https://www.ncbi.nlm.nih.gov/pmc/articles/PMC5373082/.

17. Substance Abuse and Mental Health Services Administration. Summary of national findings. In: *Results From the 2009 National Survey on Drug use and Health.* Rockville, MD: 2010, NSDUH Series H-38A, HHS Pub No. SMA 10-4856.

18. Manchikanti L. Prescription drug abuse: what is being done to address this new drug epidemic? Testimony before the Subcommittee on Criminal Justice, Drug Policy, and Human Resources. *Pain Physician.* 2006;9:287-321.

19. Suárez LM, Bennett SM, Goldstein CR, Barlow DH. Understanding anxiety disorders from a "triple vulnerability" framework. In: Antony MM, Stein MB, eds. *Oxford Handbook of Anxiety and Related Disorders.* Oxford, UK: Oxford Press; 2012. doi:10.1093/oxfordhb/9780195307030.013.0013.

20. Dozois DJ, Dobson KS, Westra HA. The comorbidity of anxiety and depression, and the implications of comorbidity for prevention. In: Dozois DJ, Dobson KS, eds. *The Prevention of Anxiety and Depression: Theory, Research, and Practice.* Washington, DC: American Psychological Association; 2004.

21. Siu AL, Bibbins-Domingo K, Grossman DC, et al. Screening for depression in adults: US Preventive Services Task Force recommendation statement. *JAMA.* 2016;315:380-387. doi:10.1001/jama.2015.18392.

22. Rangaswamy M, Porjesz B. From event-related potential to oscillations: genetic diathesis in brain (dys) function and alcohol dependence. *Alcohol Res Health.* 2008;31(3):238-242.

23. Barlow DH. Unraveling the mysteries of anxiety and its disorders from the perspective of emotion theory. *Am Psychol.* 2000;55:1247-1263.

24. Joiner T. *Why People Die by Suicide.* Cambridge, MA: Harvard University Press; 2005.

25. Joiner TE. Scientizing and routinizing the assessment of suicidality in outpatient practice. *Prof Psychol Res Pr.*1999;30:447-453.

26. Krug EG, Mercy JA, Dahlberg LL, Zwi AB. The world report on violence and health. *Lancet.*2002;360:1083-1088.

27. Wakefield MA, Loken B, Hornik RC. Use of mass media campaigns to change health behaviour. *Lancet.* 2010;376:1261-1271. doi:10.1016/S0140-6736(10)60809-4.

28. Farrelly MC, Nonnemaker J, Davis KC, Hussin A. The influence of the National truth campaign on smoking initiation. *Am J Prev Med.* 2009;36:379-384. Available at: https://www.thetruth.com/the-facts

29. Santaella-Tenorio J, Cerdá M, Villaveces A, Galea S. What do we know about the association between firearm legislation and firearm-related injuries? *Epidemiol Rev.* 2016;38:140-157. doi: 10.1093/epirev/mxv012.

30. Buchanan K. *Firearms-Control Legislation and Policy: Australia. Report by the Foreign, Comparative and International Law Division I.* Library of Congress; 2013. Available at: https://www.loc.gov/law/help/firearms-control/australia.php#Statistical.

31. Ennett ST, Tobler NS, Ringwalt CL, Flewelling RL. How effective is drug abuse resistance education? A meta-analysis of Project DARE outcome evaluations. *Am J Public Health.* 1994;84:1394-1401.

32. Isaac M, Elias B, Katz LY, et al. Gatekeeper training as a preventative intervention for suicide: a systematic review. *Can J Psychiatry.* 2009;54:260-268.

33. U.S. Preventive Services Task Force. *Published Recommendations.* Available at: https://www.uspreventiveservicestaskforce.org/BrowseRec/Search?s=mental+health.

34. SAMHSA-HRSA Center for Integrated Health Solutions. *Screening Tools.* Available at: https://www.integration.samhsa.gov/clinical-practice/screening-tools#depression.

35. MacArthur Initiative Steering Committee. *Depression Management Tool Kit.* The John D. and Catherine T. MacArthur Foundation Initiative on Depression & Primary Care. 2009. Available at: https://www.integration.samhsa.gov/clinical-practice/macarthur_depression_toolkit.pdf.

36. Fiore MC, Croyle RT, Curry SJ, et al. Preventing 3 million premature deaths and helping 5 million smokers quit: a national action plan for tobacco cessation. *Am J Public Health.*2004; 94:205-210.

37. Fiore MC. Treating tobacco use and dependence: 2008 update U.S. Public Health Service clinical practice guideline executive summary. *Respir Care.* 2008;53:1217-1222.

38. Suicide Prevention Resource Center. *Suicide Assessment Five-Step Evaluation and Triage for Mental Health Professionals (SAFE-T).* SAMHSA-HRSA Center for Integrated Health Solutions. Screening tools; 2009. Available at: https://store.samhsa.gov/system/files/sma09-4432.pdf.

REVIEW QUESTIONS

1. Which of the following is *not* associated with an increased risk for schizophrenia?
   A. Having an identical twin with schizophrenia
   B. Having a first-degree relative with schizophrenia
   C. Maternal stress
   D. Flu exposure during pregnancy
   E. Rural living

2. Which of the following correctly identifies the four stages of substance abuse?
   A. Experimentation, misuse, pathologic use, withdrawal
   B. Experimentation, recreational use, misuse, pathologic use
   C. Experimentation, recreational use, misuse, treatment avoidance
   D. Experimentation, misuse, pathologic use, withdrawal
   E. Experimentation, pathologic use, withdrawal, relapse

3. Substance use disorders are associated with which of the following occupational, social, and health consequences?
   A. Driving under the influence
   B. Low birth weight and neonatal withdrawal syndrome
   C. Hepatitis C infection
   D. Risky sexual behaviors
   E. All of these

4. Which of the following is a common community-level risk factor for mental health disorders?
   A. Poverty
   B. Bullying or discrimination
   C. Failure to bond with school or community
   D. Domestic violence
   E. Involvement with a deviant peer group

5. Following the suicide of a family member or close friend, survivors are most likely to experience which of the following consequences?
   A. Guilt and confusion
   B. Depression, anxiety, and PTSD
   C. Social isolation and stigmatization
   D. Suicidal thoughts and attempts
   E. All of these

6. Which of the following is not considered a protective factor that is common to all mental health disorders?
   A. Secure attachment during infancy and childhood
   B. Being physically healthy and active
   C. Female gender
   D. High self-esteem
   E. Strong religious beliefs and affiliation

7. Which of the following is the definition of selective prevention?
   A. It is targeted toward an entire population, regardless of risk level.
   B. It is targeted toward individuals who possess risk factors to prevent the onset of a disorder.
   C. It is intended for individuals who are showing subclinical signs of a disorder with the goal of preventing progression to clinically significant levels.
   D. It is intended to help the individual resume normal functioning and to prevent relapse.

8. For which behavior problem(s) have media campaigns been found to be effective?
   A. Cigarette smoking
   B. Alcohol consumption

   C. Suicide
   D. Mental health
   E. Child abuse and violence

9. Which of the following is *not* a universal prevention strategy for the opioid overdose epidemic?
   A. Use of Prescription Drug Monitoring Program (PDMP) data to prevent doctor shopping
   B. Sin taxes on prescribed opioid medication
   C. Educating prescribers about the risks of long-term use of opioids for noncancer pain
   D. Educating prescribers about the benefits of using nonopioid analgesics for pain management
   E. Enacting legislation that makes it legal for patients to return unused doses of opioids to a pharmacy

10. Which of the following is a risk factor for violence among individuals with mental disorders?
    A. Being in a later stage of the disorder
    B. Experiencing PTSD symptoms such as agitation, hypervigilance, and increased sensitivity to threat signals
    C. Experiencing delusional beliefs that others are bad or dangerous
    D. Both B and C
    E. All of these

ANSWERS AND EXPLANATIONS

1. **E.** Researchers have found a positive correlation between rural birth and lower rates of schizophrenia. (D) Flu exposure during pregnancy and (C) maternal stress are associated with increased risks for schizophrenia. (A) Identical twins have concordance rates for schizophrenia that are two to four times higher than fraternal twins. (B) Individuals with first-degree relatives with schizophrenia have a 6% chance of developing the disorder.

2. **B.** The first stage of use is *experimentation* in which an individual tries substances one or more times out of curiosity. The next stage is *recreational use*, where individuals use regularly (e.g., on weekends) because of the enjoyment it brings or in social situations. Individuals who use even more regularly and experience mild to moderate problems from their use have progressed to the stage of *misuse*. At this stage individuals also use alcohol or drugs to cope with negative events. The final stage is *pathologic use* when an individual meets diagnostic criteria for a substance-related disorder.

3. **E.** Substance use disorders have been found to be associated with (D) involvement in risky behaviors such as unprotected sexual intercourse and aggression/violence, (A) driving under the influence, (c) various infectious diseases such as HIV and hepatitis C virus, (B) pregnancy complications such as premature delivery, low birth weight, and neonatal withdrawal syndrome, which contribute to social-emotional deficits, academic problems,

and an increased risk of substance use among drug-exposed children. See discussion in text.

4. **A.** Poverty is a common community-level risk factor associated with several mental health disorders and violence. Bullying or discrimination (B), failure to bond with school or community (C), and involvement with a deviant peer group are common individual-level risk factors for mental health disorders. Domestic violence (D) is a family-level risk factor for several mental health disorders.

5. **E.** Following a suicide, surviving family members and close friends experience a wide array of consequences, including (A) guilt and confusion; (B) depression, anxiety, and PTSD; (C) social isolation and stigma; and (D) suicidal thoughts and perhaps even suicide attempts.

6. **C.** Female gender is considered a disorder-specific risk factor for emotional disorders, whereas male gender is a risk factor for schizophrenia and attempted suicide. (A) Secure attachment during infancy and childhood contributes to social/emotional health and (D) high self-esteem and therefore serves as a protective factor against mental health disorders. In addition, (B) being physically active and healthy and (E) having strong religious beliefs and affiliations have also been shown to contribute to good mental health.

7. **B.** Selective prevention is similar to secondary prevention in that it is targeted toward individuals who possess risk factors, but are not yet showing signs of disorder, in an effort to prevent onset of the disorder. (C) Indicated prevention is intended for individuals who have developed subclinical signs of the disorder. The goal of indicated prevention is to prevent symptoms from progressing from subclinical to clinically significant levels. Collectively, selective and indicated prevention are referred to as targeted prevention. (A) Universal prevention is similar to primary prevention in that it is targeted toward an entire population, regardless of risk level, with the goal of preventing onset of a disorder (e.g., the Truth campaign for cigarettes) or to refer individuals for the next levels of care (e.g., vision and hearing screenings for elementary and middle school aged children).

8. **A.** Research has shown that media campaigns targeting tobacco use have been effective in reducing smoking uptake among youth and in encouraging adult smokers to quit. Research suggests that rather than reducing drinking, media campaigns targeting alcohol use (B) were associated with more positive attitudes toward alcohol and greater intentions to drink. This may be due to the powerful effects of alcohol advertising and acceptance of drinking as a social norm. Mass media campaigns targeting (C) suicide were found to be ineffective. Research on media campaigns targeting (D) mental health and (E) child abuse and violence have been inconclusive.

9. **B.** Sin taxes have been effective for reducing alcohol and tobacco use but have not been suggested as an approach to reduce opioid use. Three states have enacted legislation requiring doctors to use Prescription Drug Monitoring Program data (A), which has resulted in a reduction in the number of prescriptions written for opioids as well as in the rate of doctor shopping. Educating prescribers about (C) the risks of long-term use of opioids for noncancer pain and (D) the benefits of using nonopioid analgesics for pain management has been suggested as a means of reducing the number of prescriptions written for narcotic pain killers. When patients do require opioids for pain management, it is recommended that physicians avoid the long-acting formulations and limit the amount prescribed to no more than a 3-day supply. In 2014, the US Drug Enforcement Agency (E) enacted legislation making it legal for patients to return unused doses of prescription opioids to a pharmacy, which reduces the availability of these drugs for nonprescribed use.

10. **D.** Individuals who are (B) experiencing PTSD symptoms, such as agitation, hypervigilance, and increased sensitivity to threat signals, and who are (C) experiencing delusions, such as the belief that others are bad or dangerous (e.g., Andrea Yates who murdered her children to save them from going to hell), are at increased risk of perpetrating violence. (A) Risk for violence is highest during the earliest stages of the disorder.

22

Occupational Medicine and Environmental Health

Mark Russi

"Our technological powers increase, but the side effects and potential hazards also escalate."

Alvin Toffler

Occupational injuries and illnesses substantially impact the health of working adults. In 2016 the US Bureau of Labor Statistics (BLS) reported approximately 2.9 million workplace injuries and illnesses among those employed in the US private sector, an incidence rate of 2.9 cases per 100 full-time workers.[1] More than half of these were serious enough to require days away from work, job transfer, or restriction of work activities. The majority of reported cases were injuries; noninjuries accounted for a smaller proportion, including respiratory and skin conditions, poisonings, hearing loss, and a broad range of other conditions. Annually BLS likely underestimates incidence rates because years of exposure are required for many diseases to develop, and many illnesses caused by work exposures may not be recognized initially as such.

Estimating the frequency of work-related medical conditions is further complicated by the fact that common illnesses such as asthma, bronchitis, hypersensitivity dermatitis, cancers, and musculoskeletal disorders may be caused by workplace exposures, lifestyle factors, or a combination of both. Because clinical manifestations of such diseases are rarely specific to the exposure that caused them, recognizing occupational illness requires a detailed occupational history from the patient, often enumerating decades of workplace exposure. Such detailed occupational history is not consistently incorporated into general medical practice. Other factors that predispose to underreporting include fears among workers of job loss or reprisal, hesitation among medical practitioners to engage with the complexities of workers' compensation insurance, and the lack of a requirement in many states for physicians to report occupational illnesses.

This chapter discusses the hazards of workplaces, the resulting injuries and illnesses, and the role of occupational medicine in assessing and preventing work-related medical conditions. A limited number of environmental exposures and issues related to environmental health are described as well. Hazards can be broadly divided into those resulting from physical, chemical, biologic, and psychosocial factors. Physical hazards include direct trauma, repetitive strain, radiation, noise, and thermal stresses. Chemical hazards include organic solvents and related compounds; metals; mineral dusts such as coal, asbestos, silica, and synthetic vitreous fibers; toxic gases; and a vast array of organic compounds, including pesticides and chemical-manufacturing intermediates. Biologic hazards include the bloodborne pathogens (e.g., human immunodeficiency virus [HIV], hepatitis B and C); pathogens spread by the airborne, droplet, or contact route; pathogens spread by animal contact or arthropod vectors; and allergens. Psychosocial stressors include long hours and fatigue, limited social support, and jobs over which workers have little control.

1. PHYSICAL HAZARDS

One need only consider the range of human activity to imagine ways in which working people may sustain acute traumatic injuries. Industrial accidents, motor vehicle crashes, falls, and trauma involving farming or mining equipment occur frequently. In general, such acute events are addressed immediately and directly, and the link between workplace trigger and health outcome is minimally prone to dispute. When traumas occur more gradually, as from the repetitive strain of lifting, twisting, or manipulating loads in the workplace, establishing a causal link between exposure and health condition may be more challenging. Examples include lumbar disc disease in nurses and nurses' aides from decades of patient lifting, carpal tunnel syndrome among clerical workers, Raynaud disease (vasospasm resulting in reduced blood flow to fingers) in workers who use vibratory tools, and degenerative joint disease in those whose work involves manual lifting or transporting of heavy objects. Such health conditions also occur in individuals without workplace stressors, and a health care practitioner's decision regarding work-relatedness must incorporate a thoughtful approach to the relative importance of various stressors. Generally the receipt of workers' compensation benefits requires that a physician state the condition "more probably than not" ($>50\%$) is related to the workplace.

1.1 RADIATION

As a physical hazard, radiation exposure is widespread. Occupations account for only a small portion of overall population exposures, most of which emanate from radon gas in homes, cosmic rays from the sun, and radioactive elements in the earth's crust. The largest occupational group monitored for radiation is health care workers, although for most, exposures do not exceed typical background levels. Other exposed groups include aircraft pilots and crews, nuclear industry workers, and miners.

Individuals exposed to extremely high levels of radiation, such as in a nuclear accident, may suffer acute radiation sickness with sloughing of the skin, damage and depression of bone marrow, ulceration and bleeding in the gastrointestinal tract, inflammation and scarring of the lungs, and a range of other effects. Survivors of very high acute radiation doses also have elevated risk of blood and solid-organ malignancies. More common radiation exposures may also result in elevated cancer risk; radon exposure in miners is strongly associated with increased risk of lung cancer, and nuclear workers have shown increased rates of leukemia and lung cancer.

1.2 NOISE

Noise is one of the most prevalent physical hazards in workplaces. Decibels (dB), which measure sound intensity, are on a logarithmic scale; hence each 3-dB increase represents an approximate doubling of exposure. More than 10 million US workers may be repeatedly exposed to greater than 80 dB (similar to the noise level of a garbage disposal) and more than 1 million have occupational hearing loss. By age 50, an estimated half of heavily exposed construction workers and 90% of heavily exposed miners will have hearing impairment. Substantial noise exposure occurs in almost every variety of manufacturing; exposures in mining, construction, and transportation may be equally hazardous. The US Occupational Safety and Health Administration (OSHA) requires periodic monitoring of noise levels and periodic audiometry of workers with average exposures over 8 hours/day of 85 dB or higher.[2] Control of noise in the workplace often involves a combination of engineering solutions to reduce noise sources as well as limiting exposure time in noise environments and wearing hearing protection.

1.3 HEAT AND COLD

Thermal stress constitutes another physical stressor in workplaces. Excessive levels of heat are encountered in foundries, smelting operations, firefighting, and in many outdoor settings. Heavy work demands, heavy clothing, lack of air circulation, and high humidity may contribute to heat stress. Health effects may include lightheadedness, swelling of the extremities, muscle cramping, and in more severe cases agitation and delirium, lysing of muscle cells, circulatory collapse, and kidney failure. Workers not accustomed to high-heat environments and those with other medical conditions are at particular risk.

Excessive cold exposure occurs among workers in cold-climate outdoor activities, divers and others in the maritime industry, military personnel, and workers in refrigerated environments. Although the potential for hypothermia (defined as a fall in body temperature to $<35°C$ [$<95°F$]) exists in such settings, localized cold effects are more common, such as frostbite, Raynaud phenomenon, and cold-induced hives.

Cold exposure may also occur in high-altitude environments, although the principal hazard of such settings is reduced oxygen content. High altitude–associated conditions range from acute mountain sickness (AMS) to potentially life-threatening pulmonary and cerebral edema. AMS is characterized by fatigue, malaise, shortness of breath, and disturbances of memory, concentration, and sleep; it generally occurs within 24 hours of arrival at altitudes exceeding ~8000 feet. Pulmonary edema may occur at similar altitudes and is triggered by changes in the pulmonary blood vessels from decreased oxygen, rapid breathing, and the resulting alkalosis and pulmonary hypertension. Edema of the brain may result from hypoxia and may be both insidious and life threatening. Gradual ascent may prevent or moderate altitude-associated illnesses.

2. CHEMICAL HAZARDS

More than 80,000 chemicals are in common use. Although discussion of acute and chronic toxicities is beyond the scope of this chapter, categories of particular interest—due to high frequency of use or significant health impact—are solvents, metals, mineral dusts, polycyclic aromatic hydrocarbons, pesticides, and inorganic gases. Dedicated OSHA standards exist for only a few chemical exposures. For many others, guidance is in place from the National Institute for Occupational Safety and Health (NIOSH), American Conference of Governmental Industrial Hygienists (ACGIH), and other advisory groups. In the absence of a specific standard, OSHA may cite workplaces under the General Duty Clause, which requires employers to provide a workplace free of recognized hazards.

2.1 SOLVENTS

Solvents are widely used in industrial processes. Major classes include aliphatic, aromatic, and halogenated compounds, all of which can cause acute encephalopathy, generally manifested by a sense of lightheadedness, disorientation, and irritability. Exposure occurs primarily by inhalation and skin absorption. Although symptoms generally resolve within hours following exposure, chronic encephalopathic changes, potentially with progression to dementia, may occur after years of heavy exposure. Most solvents may also irritate the skin, cause defatting of dermal tissue, and serve as carriers through the skin of other chemical substances. The following solvents have uniquely toxic properties:

- Both n-hexane and methyl n-butyl ketone may cause a mixed motor and sensory neuropathy

- Benzene is well established as a cause of aplastic anemia and acute myelogenous leukemia
- Carbon tetrachloride is a potent toxin of the liver
- Methylene chloride causes carboxyhemoglobinemia
- Carbon disulfide may cause acute psychosis, optic neuritis, peripheral neuropathy, and over time, atherosclerosis
- Extremely heavy exposure to halogenated solvents has been associated with cardiac arrhythmias and sudden death

Acute encephalopathic effects may result from exposure to a single solvent or a combination of solvents. Assessment of workplace exposure must consider the possibility of combined toxicity and that measured air levels may not adequately account for dermal exposures. Biologic monitoring, generally the measurement of urinary solvent metabolites, has been used to account for body burden from different exposure pathways.

2.2 METALS AND MINERAL DUSTS

Metal exposures occur in a variety of industrial and environmental settings and may trigger a broad range of health effects. Although lead exposure to the general population has been greatly reduced by the removal of lead as a gasoline additive in the 1970s (Fig. 22.1), many occupational groups remain at high exposure risk, including construction workers, welders, solderers, pipe cutters, foundry workers, demolition

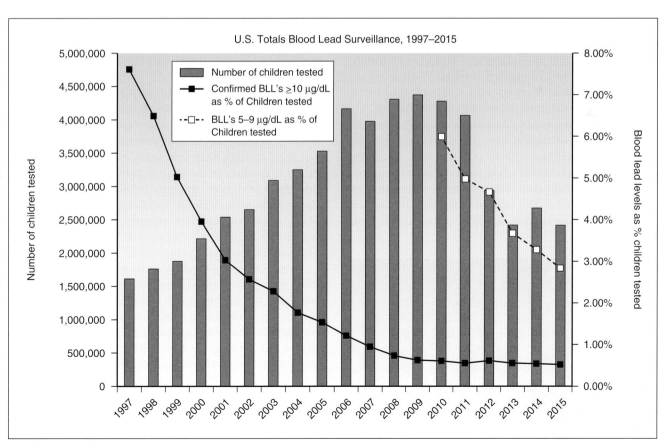

Fig. 22.1 Lead levels in US children, 1997–2015. The proportion of elevated (>10 μg/dL) blood lead levels in sampled children decreased from approximately 7.5% to less than 1%. (From US Centers for Disease Control and Prevention.)

workers, home renovators, and battery makers. Lead has also been found in drinking water in areas where the water has high acidity or low mineral content, which corrodes service pipes and fixtures. Toxicities associated with lead exposure range from subtle behavioral and cognitive effects to hemolytic anemia, peripheral neuropathy, chronic encephalopathy, hypertension, and impotence. The following metals also may cause a variety of acute and chronic effects:

- Arsenic exposure causes hyperpigmented skin lesions, peripheral neuropathy, and peripheral vascular disease and is a well-established risk factor for skin and lung cancer
- Chronic exposure to mercury is linked to tremor, psychologic disturbances, and neuropathy, whereas acute exposure may trigger a severe chemical pneumonitis
- Beryllium may also cause acute pneumonitis and in certain individuals leads to chronic berylliosis, a syndrome similar to sarcoidosis (a systemic disorder often resulting in chronic lung disease)
- Cobalt and cadmium may also affect the lungs. Cobalt causes asthma, giant cell pneumonitis, and scarring of the lungs of certain individuals; acute cadmium exposure is associated with pneumonitis. Cadmium may also severely damage the kidneys
- Chromium and nickel have a number of skin effects and are risk factors for lung cancer

Exposures to metal dusts and fumes in the workplace are better controlled now than in past decades, partly because of the establishment of applicable OSHA standards. For example, the OSHA standard for lead requires both air monitoring in lead-contaminated workplaces and biologic monitoring through blood testing of exposed workers. Workers are required to be removed from exposure without loss of pay if their blood level exceeds the threshold value of 50 μg/dL.[3]

Several widely recognized occupational diseases result from chronic exposures to mineral dusts (Fig. 22.2). Long-term asbestos exposure may cause pleural plaques (areas of scarring along lung lining), as well as asbestosis (a diffuse scarring process in the lungs themselves that may lead to compromise of oxygenation). Chronic silica exposure may also cause diffuse lung scarring (silicosis), which differs pathologically from asbestosis and tends to predominate in the upper lobes. Very heavy exposures to freshly fractured silica have been linked to severe and progressive lung disease (acute silicosis), which may cause death within 1 year of exposure. Coal worker pneumoconiosis leads to scarring and weakening of the lung's connective tissue and formation of carbon-filled nodules, predominantly in the upper lung fields.

Several tumors have been linked with mineral dust exposure. Asbestos is a well-established cause of lung cancer and malignant mesothelioma, a rare tumor of high mortality affecting the pleural lining of the lung. Asbestos is also associated with other malignancies, particularly laryngeal cancer.[4] Silica is a risk factor for lung cancer, whereas coal exposure is not.[5,6]

2.3 HYDROCARBONS AND PESTICIDES

Another established risk factor for lung cancer is exposure to polycyclic aromatic hydrocarbons (PAHs), a diverse group of substances formed from incomplete combustion of coal or oil. Occupational exposures in gas and coke works, iron and steel foundries, aluminum reduction plants, tar distillation facilities, chimney cleaning, and roofing and transportation industries have been linked to increased lung cancer risk. Risk of skin and bladder cancers has also been seen. PAH exposure is widespread in the general environment as well, deriving from tobacco smoke, fire fumes, ambient air pollution, and cooked food. Some studies show an association between lung cancer and urban air pollution, although it is not known whether risk is caused by PAH exposure. Studies in China of cooking and heating fumes have implicated PAH as a lung carcinogen.[7]

Pesticides comprise a broad category of chemicals used to control insect, plant, and fungal species. Exposures occur among farm and orchard workers, greenhouse and nursery workers, landscapers, chemical manufacturers, forestry workers, wood treaters, hazardous waste workers, and a range of others. Exposures to the general public are associated with household and lawn residues, termite control, food and water residues, accidental or intentional ingestions, and spills. Major classes of pesticides include organophosphates and carbamates, pyrethroids, organochlorines, and chlorophenoxy and nitroaromatic compounds.

Organophosphates and carbamates, which are linked with the largest proportion of acute systemic poisonings, act by inhibiting the enzyme acetylcholinesterase, which catalyzes breakdown of the neural transmitter acetylcholine. Depending on dose, the resulting clinical presentation may include nausea and vomiting, diarrhea and cramping, chest tightness, increased tearing and salivation, blurred vision, and profuse sweating. Muscle twitching and weakness, as well as anxiety, tremor, and impaired cognition, may also occur. Long-term effects are controversial; some studies suggest an increased risk of adverse reproductive outcomes. Specific pesticides have also been linked to chronic central and peripheral nervous system effects following heavy exposure. Several studies of farm workers show elevated cancer risk, particularly for

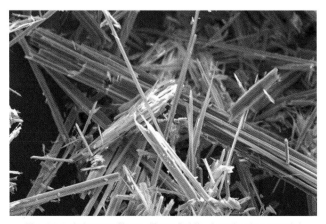

Fig. 22.2 Asbestos fibers. (From Public domain photograph.)

leukemia and lymphoma, but it is not known whether this risk is caused by pesticide exposure.

2.4 INORGANIC GASES

Inorganic gases are encountered in a wide range of industrial settings and are a concern because of their acute toxicity in enclosed environments and long-term sequelae. Simple asphyxiants, such as methane and nitrogen, may dilute oxygen in an enclosed space but do not act as direct toxins. In contrast, cyanide and carbon monoxide interfere with cellular respiration and oxygen transport, respectively, and may be rapidly fatal at sufficient dose. The effects of irritant gases depend on water solubility and the chemical properties of the gas. Ammonia and sulfur dioxide are rapidly absorbed because of high water solubility and exert an irritant effect in the upper respiratory tract. In contrast, low-solubility gases, such as phosgene and nitrogen oxide, may cause profound and delayed effects in the lower respiratory tract, including bronchospasm, pneumonitis, and pulmonary edema. Long-term lung damage may occur in survivors of the acute toxicities of nitrogen oxide, phosgene, or chlorine gas exposures.

3. BIOLOGIC HAZARDS

Occupational biologic hazards are encountered in health care workplaces, areas of contact with animals or arthropod vectors, and locations in the general environment with exposure to an altered range of diseases. In health care facilities the bloodborne pathogens HIV as well as hepatitis B (HBV) and hepatitis C (HCV) viruses are of greatest concern. Other infectious hazards include airborne or droplet-spread organisms (e.g., tuberculosis [TB], varicella, measles, pertussis, parvovirus, influenza) and organisms spread by fecal-oral contact (e.g., enteroviruses, *Salmonella, Shigella*, hepatitis A virus [HAV]) (see Chapter 20). Outside the health care setting, animal breeders and handlers, farmers, and veterinarians are at risk for a range of illnesses that spread from animal to human (zoonoses). Workers in outdoor environments, such as groundskeepers, park rangers, and construction workers, may be at increased risk for diseases spread by arthropod vectors. Workers in the developing world may be at risk for tropical diseases.

3.1 BLOODBORNE PATHOGENS

Bloodborne pathogens are spread in health care settings by needlesticks or by splashes of blood or other infectious body fluids onto mucous membranes or abraded skin. Unfortunately, despite use of safety-engineered sharps, about half a million needlestick injuries still occur each year in the United States. Hollow-bore needles impart higher transmission risk, but exposures with suture needles are more common. One study suggested that needlesticks may occur in up to 15% of surgical procedures.[8] An often-quoted risk for seroconversion after exposure to HIV is 0.3%, although this risk is clearly influenced by the quantity of blood delivered and the

viral load in the source patient. Seroconversion risk after HCV exposure varies from study to study but is likely less than 2%, whereas risk of HBV seroconversion in an unvaccinated individual may be 1% to 6% if the source is e-antigen negative and as high as 22% to 31% from an e-antigen–positive source.[9] The US Centers for Disease Control and Prevention (CDC) is aware of 58 individuals who have become HIV positive after workplace exposure. In the years before broad provision of HBV vaccination, thousands of health care workers, principally surgeons, contracted hepatitis B occupationally.

The OSHA Bloodborne Pathogen Standard requires annual training, engineering controls, personal protective equipment (PPE), and an exposure control plan in work settings with potential bloodborne exposure. Safety-engineered sharps have been shown to reduce needlesticks and must be used where feasible. Also, workers at risk for exposure must be provided hepatitis B vaccine, as well as appropriate medical follow-up after an exposure incident.[10] Such follow-up includes antiretroviral prophylaxis for those with HIV exposure.

3.2 AEROSOL/DROPLET-SPREAD INFECTIONS

Infections spread by aerosols or droplets constitute another risk for health care workers. After years of declining tuberculosis incidence in the United States, a rise in case numbers during the mid-1990s prompted the CDC to issue new guidance for health care settings and the community. Enhanced systems for recognition of potentially infectious patients, construction of negative-pressure isolation rooms, use of fit-tested respirators, and yearly and postexposure monitoring of employees for TB have resulted in minimal rates of new TB infection among US health care workers. Before such measures, several outbreaks were documented, and there continues to be significant risk to health care workers in areas of the world where TB prevalence is high. The presence in many such settings of multidrug-resistant or extensively drug-resistant strains augments the occupational hazard. As with measles and varicella, TB may spread on suspended aerosol particles over longer distances and does not appear to require face-to-face contact for transmission.

In contrast, other infections (e.g., influenza, pertussis, adenovirus, *Neisseria meningitidis*, hemorrhagic fever viruses, severe acute respiratory syndrome [SARS], and Middle Eastern respiratory syndrome [MERS]) generally require closer contact for transmission and may be spread principally by droplets, which fall to the ground more quickly than aerosols. For several apparently droplet-spread infections, however, rare outbreaks suggest transmission over greater distances. Such opportunistic airborne spread may be enhanced by low humidity levels and favorable patterns of air movement. Research is underway to better understand the role of disease spread through suspended aerosol particles. With influenza in particular, polymerase chain reaction (PCR) testing shows virus suspended on small aerosols, and animal studies suggest longer-range transmission. Such issues take on greater importance with the emergence of influenza strains with higher mortality, particularly among young persons (e.g., H1N1, highly pathogenic avian H5N1, Asian lineage avian H7N9).

Policies enacted during the 2009 novel H1N1 influenza pandemic, specifically those addressing protection of health care workers, illustrate an important occupational health principle. As the pandemic began, neither the virulence of the virus nor its transmission characteristics had been fully characterized, and neither the general population nor hospital workers had been vaccinated against it. In the setting of a rapidly spreading virus with particular hazard to younger people, the CDC recommended use of fit-tested N95 respirators for health care workers caring for affected patients. (Such respirators generally are recommended only when caring for patients with diseases spread via the airborne route and are not used by health care workers caring for patients with seasonal influenza.) Although considerable controversy surrounded the policy, and many hospitals did not fully adhere to it, the recommendation was fundamentally grounded in the precautionary principle. The principle states if the level of harm is high, action should be undertaken to prevent or minimize harm even when the absence of scientific certainty makes it difficult to predict the likelihood of harm occurring, or the level of harm should it occur. Under this principle the need for control measures increases with both the level of possible harm and the degree of uncertainty. The precautionary principle relates to a broad range of decisions necessary to protect working populations whenever new and inadequately characterized hazards are introduced. Recommendations for use of airborne precautions when caring for patients with MERS or smallpox are consistent with it, as are recommendations for personal protective equipment use by health care workers caring for victims of biologic weapons when the infectious agent is unknown.

3.3 ANIMAL CONTACT AND ARTHROPOD VECTOR

Outside of hospital settings, major groups at increased risk of occupational infectious diseases include those with frequent animal contact, those likely to have contact with arthropod vectors, and those working in other than their native microbiologic milieu, usually at sites in the developing world. Zoonotic diseases include brucellosis, cat-scratch disease, leptospirosis, plague, psittacosis, tularemia, cryptococcosis, histoplasmosis, ringworm, giardiasis, cryptosporidiosis, hantavirus, monkeypox, and rabies (see Chapter 20). Outside the usual occupational groups at risk for such diseases (farmers, veterinarians, animal handlers, cullers), anyone with regular animal contact, such as pet owners and those who keep livestock species near their home, may be at risk.

Diseases requiring an arthropod vector are a particular risk for those who work in outdoor settings and include West Nile virus, Rocky Mountain spotted fever, Lyme disease, babesiosis, ehrlichiosis, and several viral encephalitides. Malaria, typhoid, dengue, yellow fever, and a broad range of parasitic diseases constitute risks among those who work in the developing world. Important preventive medicine services for those who travel to tropical and subtropical destinations include the provision of vaccines, prophylactic medications, and advice on how to avoid insect vectors and hazardous food or water.

4. PSYCHOSOCIAL STRESS

Long hours, rotating work shifts, demanding jobs, limited decision latitude, competing time demands, repetitive tasks, threat of violence, job insecurity, and poor management contribute to stress in the workplace. Importantly, chronic exposure to such work circumstances may have adverse physiologic effects. Jobs with excessive work hours have been associated with perception of poor health, with increased injury risk, and with increased cardiovascular disease: Cardiovascular risk is also associated with high-demand jobs in which the worker has limited control.[11]

The physiologic connection between stress and adverse health outcomes has not been completely elucidated. Possible etiologic links include elevated catecholamine levels and abnormalities of the pituitary-adrenocortical axis, both components of the body's response to acute and chronic stress. The resulting state may lead over time to increases in blood pressure and heart rate, constriction of blood vessels, increases in circulating lipid levels, and an increased tendency toward blood clotting. Effects on the immune system may occur as well. Animal studies show increased infections under stressful conditions. The International Agency for Research on Cancer (IARC) regards shiftwork involving circadian rhythm disturbance as probably carcinogenic to humans (Group IIA).[12]

5. ENVIRONMENTAL HAZARDS

The key distinguishing characteristic of environmental hazards versus workplace hazards is that although exposure levels are usually lower, environmental hazards may impact all age groups at all times. Environmental exposures result from the following:

- Water contamination from industrial effluents or toxic waste disposal
- Soil contamination from fallout of fumes or particulates released into the air
- Food contamination from compromised soils, water, or processing methods
- Air pollution from industrial or natural sources

Three important examples of environmental hazard with pervasive and significant health impact are domestic radon exposure, ambient air pollution, and global warming (Fig. 22.3).

5.1 RADON EXPOSURE

Radon (Rn) is a product of the radioactive breakdown of uranium. ^{222}Rn has a half-life of approximately 3.5 days and decays by release of an alpha particle to short-lived daughters,

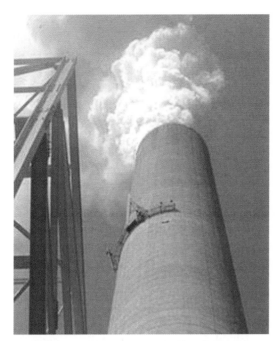

Fig. 22.3 Pollution-emitting smokestack. Air pollution from multiple sources contributes to pulmonary and cardiovascular mortality in the general population. (From US Centers for Disease Control and Prevention.)

which themselves release alpha radiation. Radon is detectable in most environments because of the presence of uranium in rocks and soil and may become concentrated in indoor spaces, particularly in the lower levels of dwellings.

After epidemiologic studies of miners working underground showed elevated lung cancer risk, many studies examined whether exposures to radon in the home may also elevate cancer risk. Most were case control studies comparing measured radon levels in homes occupied over several decades by residents with and without lung cancer. The studies have been challenging because buildings inhabited by subjects may have been torn down or altered over the years in ways that could alter the radon measurement. In addition, because most residents have lived in many places throughout life, cumulative radon exposure tends to become similar from person to person, decreasing the number of study participants who have experienced cumulative exposures in excess of mean population levels. Because of this, and because the relative risk of exposure is small, large numbers of participants have been required to evaluate the impact of domestic radon exposure, necessitating meta-analytic techniques. These meta-analyses demonstrated statistically significant (10%–25%) elevations of lung cancer risk for those exposed to radon levels greater than 4 picocuries per liter (pCi/L), consistent with the risk estimates extrapolated from the studies of radon-exposed underground miners.[13–15]

The US Environmental Protection Agency (EPA) has estimated that more than 20,000 lung cancer deaths per year in the United States may be caused by domestic radon exposure.[16] The EPA recommends retesting and mitigation of homes where basement radon levels exceed 4 pCi/L. From a public health perspective, radon mitigation of such homes is

an important intervention; because of population mobility, much of the mitigation benefit will pass to future residents. Systems to reduce indoor radon levels usually function by establishing a pressure gradient to reduce travel of radon into basements from surrounding soil and rock.

5.2 AMBIENT AIR POLLUTION

Unlike radon, ambient air pollution is derived largely from human activity, principally industrial and vehicular combustion. Pollutants of major concern include sulfur dioxide, nitrogen oxides, acid aerosols, particulates, volatile organic compounds, lead, and ozone. In general, air pollution levels in developed countries have become better controlled in recent decades; in the developing world, however, increased vehicular traffic, industrialization, and in some cases lack of regulation have resulted in less well-controlled levels. The US Clean Air Act of 1970 requires the EPA to set standards to protect the general public, including those predisposed to harm from air pollution, such as asthmatics, the very young, and the very old.[17] National Ambient Air Quality Standards are in place in the United States for carbon monoxide, particulate matter, sulfur dioxide, nitrogen dioxide, lead, and ozone. The World Health Organization (WHO) has set guidance for certain air pollutants as well and challenged governments worldwide to reduce exposures to below recommended levels.[18]

Health outcomes linked to air pollution include increased cardiopulmonary mortality, increased numbers of visits to emergency departments and physician offices, increased rates of hospitalization, exacerbations of asthma, and higher frequency of respiratory infection. Laboratory studies have revealed in response to specific air pollutants increases in airway inflammation, decreases in lung function, and increases in upper respiratory irritation. A study of 100 US counties showed an increase in cardiovascular mortality of 0.24% per 10-µg/m³ increase in inhalable particulate matter (PM10).[19] Effects may be enhanced in elderly persons and those exposed to fine particulate matter (i.e., particles small enough to be inhaled deeply into lungs).[20] The mechanisms by which air pollution may cause increased cardiopulmonary and other mortality remain incompletely understood. Beyond the capacity of respiratory irritants to exacerbate underlying chronic respiratory illness, studies have focused on the role of air pollution in inducing systemic inflammatory mediators, which over time may predispose to cardiovascular disease.[21]

5.3 GLOBAL WARMING

Greenhouse gas emissions from human activity have contributed to a warming of the planet Earth, resulting in increasingly extreme weather events such as floods, droughts, and hurricanes; intense short-term variations of temperature; rising sea levels; and alterations of plant and animal niches. Floods, droughts, and hurricanes threaten sanitation systems, imperil access to clean water and food, disrupt provision of necessary services such as health care, and displace large populations. Such events kill thousands annually and disproportionately affect populations in the developing world. Rapidly fluctuating temperatures may predispose to hyperthermia or hypothermia and may lead to increased death rates from heart and respiratory diseases. According to the WHO, record high temperatures in Western Europe during the summer of 2003 were associated with an estimated 70,000 more deaths than the equivalent period during previous years. With more than half of the world's population living within 60 km of a shoreline, rising sea levels will increasingly predispose to residential damage and displacement of populations, particularly in combination with more volatile coastal weather. Finally, as temperature and rainfall patterns change around the globe, the ranges of arboviral vectors for infectious diseases such as malaria and dengue will likely be increasingly impacted, potentially threatening populations outside current endemic regions. Alteration of animal niches may also increase risk of transmission of zoonotic illness to humans. Impacts of changing weather patterns upon plant proliferation may result in higher airborne pollen and more human allergy and asthma or decreased food supplies when crops fail.

Urgent and global action is necessary to mitigate climate change and its increasing threat to human health and society. Beyond the impacts discussed, the inevitable social upheaval and human conflicts triggered by displacement of populations and imperiled access to resources may constitute the greatest mortality threat from global warming in the coming decades.

6. QUANTIFYING EXPOSURE

The distinguishing challenge of occupational epidemiology is quantifying exposure assessment. Modern workplaces are characterized by rapid turnover of personnel, changes over time in production methods and hygiene, and frequent job switching. Measurement of contaminant levels may be done for specific purposes (e.g., workplace inspection, process change follow-up) and may not adequately represent exposures over time. Such measurements are also carried out relatively infrequently; thus given the multitude of processes in many industrial facilities, such measurements may not reflect exposures of all workers. With the exception of settings in which significant radiation exposure requires daily use of personal dosimeters, there are few workplaces in which widespread and frequent personal exposure monitoring takes place. Such issues become more important when studying exposures linked to diseases of long latency.

Assessing the impact of exposure on a working population also requires a suitable nonexposed group for comparison. The characteristic that working populations are generally healthier than the average population, known as the healthy worker effect, may result from less healthy individuals not entering the workforce, as well as attrition. A demographically similar working population without exposure to the contaminant under study may serve as a better basis for comparison than the general population.

Many smaller epidemiologic studies, such as community-based, registry-based, or hospital-based case control comparisons, have relied on "job title" as a surrogate for exposure. Such an approach offers the advantage of simplicity and low cost. Work records are more often organized by job roles than by the exposures that accompany them, so personnel records or death certificates can be used to ascertain usual or most recent job title. Although occasionally revealing occupations at increased risk, serving as a basis both to target public health interventions and to explore the exposures likely associated with a job title, such studies have several weaknesses. Most reveal large numbers of job titles for comparison, increasing the likelihood of random associations. Jobs may also entail both variety and inconsistency of exposures, making it difficult to identify the specific hazard that may underlie an apparent job-based risk. For studies of cancer, in which decades of workplace exposure must be considered, studies must also tally decades of employment records. Although limited in scope, such investigations have served to develop and refine hypotheses, particularly when several studies have pinpointed the same job title in association with a disease outcome.

Cohort studies, in which hazards of concern are measured over time, can provide a greater detail of information than case control studies. Because complete databases of personal exposure levels rarely exist, investigators use a job-exposure matrix, which relies on measurement of the exposures most likely associated with a job title to assign exposure levels. Although the construction of a job-exposure matrix is a complex task requiring both professional judgment and measurement of contaminants, the exposure information it yields may be quite approximate. Hazards associated with a specific job may be classified merely as present or absent or at low, medium, or high level. Considerable heterogeneity may also exist within a job title, so that two workers assigned the same job in different parts of a factory may have different exposures. Splitting job titles into descriptions of greater specificity may mitigate that problem, but this often leads to more comparisons and fewer individuals in each comparison group and could lead to spurious associations.

As investigators undertake study of lower risk exposures, greater precision of both measurement and estimation may necessitate personal dosimeter measurements of larger samples of a workforce, carried out at greater frequency and at times that best reflect typical hazard levels. Because many studies, particularly those examining long-latency diseases such as cancer, are of retrospective cohort design, reconstructions of past workplace conditions may be undertaken to estimate past exposures more accurately. Many studies have also moved beyond the relatively simple job-exposure matrix to more complex modeling in which exposure levels are tied to specific tasks, production levels, ventilation levels, and other potential predictors.

7. SUMMARY

The practice of occupational and environmental medicine (OEM) exists at an interface of clinical medicine and public health. OEM physicians are required to have knowledge of the broad range of exposures associated with human disease, to understand the toxicologic principles that underlie disease risk for many exposures, to interpret and apply findings of epidemiologic studies to decisions about causality and prevention, and to possess the clinical skills to recognize signs of symptoms of occupational illness. They must engage with public health officials when inspecting workplace hazards, making decisions about removal of a patient or group of workers from exposure, instituting medical screening or surveillance programs, or formulating policies to ensure the safety of a workplace or other environment. Although the OEM field impacts the health of large numbers of workers, it remains grounded in the clinical skills required to care properly for the individual patient: taking a thorough history, performing an appropriate diagnostic workup, and intervening to reduce or eliminate hazardous exposure.

This chapter has outlined physical, chemical, biologic, and psychosocial hazards encountered in workplaces and described a range of clinical conditions associated with them. Prevention principles have been discussed for some exposures, as have specific mechanisms of prevention, such as OSHA standards. Radon, air pollution, and global warming were cited as examples of environmental hazards, which are generally characterized by more widespread exposures than those encountered in workplaces. The challenge of studying links between occupational or environmental exposures and human health is substantial, particularly with respect to quantification of exposures over long-latency periods. However, increasingly sophisticated job-exposure or task-exposure matrices, more frequent and regular hygienic measurements, and complex exposure modeling have enhanced our capacity to perceive effects that may not have been evident in the past, particularly those that may persist despite the workplace hygienic improvements of recent decades.

REFERENCES

1. US Department of Labor, Bureau of Labor Statistics. *Economic News Release: Employer-Reported Workplace Injury and Illnesses*. 2017. Available at: https://www.bls.gov/news.release/osh.nr0.htm.

2. US Department of Labor, Occupational Safety and Health Administration. *1910.95—Occupational Noise Exposure*. 2008. Available at: https://www.osha.gov/pls/oshaweb/owadisp.show_document?p_table=STANDARDS&p_id=9735.

3. US Department of Labor, Occupational Safety and Health Administration. *1910.1025—Lead*. 2012. Available at: https://www.osha.gov/pls/oshaweb/owadisp.show_document?p_table=STANDARDS&p_id=10030.

4. World Health Organization. *Asbestos (Chrysotile, Amosite, Crocidolite, Tremolite, Actinolite, and Anthophyllite)*. IRAC Monograph 100C. 2018. Available at: http://monographs.iarc.fr/ENG/Monographs/vol100C/mono100C-11.pdf.

5. World Health Organization. *Silica, Some Silicates, Coal Dust and Para-Aramid Fibrils*. IARC Monograph 68. 1997. Available at: http://monographs.iarc.fr/ENG/Monographs/vol68/mono68.pdf.

6. World Health Organization. *Silica, Some Silicates, Coal Dust and Para-Aramid Fibrils*. IARC Monograph 68. 1997. Available at: http://monographs.iarc.fr/ENG/Monographs/vol68/index.php.

7. Zhao Y, Wang S, Aunan K, Seip HM, Hao J. Air pollution and lung cancer risks in China—a meta-analysis. *Sci Total Environ*. 2006;366:500-513. Available at: http://www.ncbi.nlm.nih.gov/pubmed/16406110.

8. Quebbeman EJ, Telford GL, Hubbard S, et al. Risk of blood contamination and injury to operating room personnel. *Ann Surg*. 1991;214:614-620. Available at: http://www.ncbi.nlm.nih.gov/pubmed/1953115.

9. US Public Health Service. Updated US Public Health Service guidelines for the management of occupational exposures to HBV, HCV, and HIV and recommendations for postexposure prophylaxis. *MMWR Recomm Rep*. 2001;50(RR-11):1-52. Available at: http://www.ncbi.nlm.nih.gov/pubmed/11442229.

10. US Department of Labor, Occupational Safety and Health Administration. *1910.1030—Bloodborne Pathogens*. 2012. Available at: https://www.osha.gov/pls/oshaweb/owadisp.show_document?p_table=STANDARDS&p_id=10051.

11. Belkic KL, Landsbergis PA, Schnall PL, Baker D. Is job strain a major source of cardiovascular disease risk? *Scand J Work Environ Health*. 2004;30:85-128. Available at: http://www.ncbi.nlm.nih.gov/pubmed/15127782.

12. IARC Working Group on the Evaluation of Carcinogenic Risk to Humans. *Painting, Firefighting, and Shiftwork*. Lyon, FR: International Agency for Research on Cancer; 2010. (IARC Monographs on the Evaluation of Carcinogenic Risks to Humans, No. 98.) Available at: https://www.ncbi.nlm.nih.gov/books/NBK326814/.

13. Darby S, Hill D, Deo H, et al. Residential radon and lung cancer–detailed results of a collaborative analysis of individual data on 7148 persons with lung cancer and 14,208 persons without lung cancer from 13 epidemiologic studies in Europe. *Scand J Work Environ Health*. 2006;32(suppl 1):1-83. Available at: shttp://www.ncbi.nlm.nih.gov/pubmed/16538937.

14. Lubin JH, Boice Jr JD. Lung cancer risk from residential radon: meta-analysis of eight epidemiologic studies. *J Natl Cancer Inst*. 1997;89:49-57. Available at: http://www.ncbi.nlm.nih.gov/pubmed/8978406.

15. Lubin JH, Tomásek L, Edling C, et al. Estimating lung cancer mortality from residential radon using data for low exposures of miners. *Radiat Res*. 1997;147:126-134. Available at: http://www.ncbi.nlm.nih.gov/pubmed/9008203.

16. US Environmental Protection Agency. *Radon*. 2016. Available at: https://www.epa.gov/sites/production/files/2016-12/documents/2016_a_citizens_guide_to_radon.pdf.

17. US Environmental Protection Agency. *Overview of the Clean Air Act and Air Pollution*. 2019. Available at: https://www.epa.gov/clean-air-act-overview.

18. World Health Organization. *News Release: WHO Challenges World to Improve Air Quality*. 2006. Available at: http://www.who.int/mediacentre/news/releases/2006/pr52/en/.

19. Dominici F, Peng RD, Zeger SL, White RH, Samet JM. Particulate air pollution and mortality in the United States: did the risks change from 1987 to 2000? *Am J Epidemiol*. 2007;166:880-888. Available at: http://aje.oxfordjournals.org/content/166/8/880.long.

20. Aga E, Samoli E, Touloumi G, et al. Short-term effects of ambient particles on mortality in the elderly: results from 28 cities in the APHEA2 project. *Eur Respir J Suppl*. 2003;40:28S-33S. Available at: http://www.ncbi.nlm.nih.gov/pubmed/12762571.

21. Thompson AM, Zanobetti A, Silverman F, et al. Baseline repeated measures from controlled human exposure studies: associations between ambient air pollution exposure and the systemic inflammatory biomarkers IL-6 and fibrinogen. *Environ
Health Perspect.* 2010;118:120-124. doi:10.1289/ehp.0900550.
Available at: http://www.ncbi.nlm.nih.gov/pubmed/20056584.

REVIEW QUESTIONS

1. According to the US Bureau of Labor Statistics (BLS),
   approximately what percentage of full-time workers
   sustained work-related injuries or illness in 2016?
   A. 0.5%
   B. 1%
   C. 3%
   D. 10%
   E. 20%

2. An office worker develops carpal tunnel syndrome in both
   her hands that gradually worsens over the year. Generally
   for her to qualify for workers' compensation benefits, it
   would be imperative that her physician state that:
   A. The condition could not have occurred in the absence
      of her job functions
   B. The condition did not result from activities outside of
      work
   C. The woman is not pregnant
   D. The condition more probably than not is caused by her
      job duties
   E. The condition is related to the job beyond a reasonable
      doubt (>95% likelihood)

3. Radiation would be categorized as what type of workplace
   hazard?
   A. Physical
   B. Chemical
   C. Biologic
   D. Psychosocial
   E. Particulate

4. Which organization can cite workplaces under the Gen-
   eral Duty Clause, which requires employers to provide a
   workplace free of recognized chemical hazards?
   A. NIOSH
   B. ACGIH
   C. OSHA
   D. SAMHSA
   E. HRSA

5. The gas that poses the most serious and immediate health
   risk even in relatively low amounts is:
   A. Methane
   B. Cyanide
   C. Ammonia
   D. Sulfur dioxide
   E. Phosgene

6. Which of the following biologic hazards may be con-
   tracted by ingesting food contaminated with feces?
   A. Hepatitis A
   B. Hepatitis B
   C. Hepatitis C
   D. Parvovirus
   E. Pertussis

7. Seroconversion risk after needlestick exposure to HIV,
   HCV, and HBV (e-antigen positive) is best estimated by
   which of the following sets of values, respectively?
   A. 60%, 6%, 0.6%
   B. 6%, 0.6%, 0.006%
   C. 10, 0.1%, 0.001%
   D. 30%, 3%, 0.3%
   E. 0.3%, 3%, 30%

8. Which of the following statements is true?
   A. Radon appears to cause lung cancer in mining popula-
      tions but does not appear to cause lung cancer in the
      general population
   B. Air pollution may exacerbate chronic lung disease but
      is not associated with other health conditions
   C. Asbestos is associated with laryngeal cancer
   D. Lead exposure in the general environment has in-
      creased greatly since the 1970s
   E. Tuberculosis is spread on large respiratory droplets
      that fall quickly to the ground and require close contact
      for transmission to occur

9. A cohort study seeks to determine the chances of develop-
   ing cancer from environmental radiation exposure. The
   exposed group includes commercial airline pilots, who
   have high exposure to cosmic radiation. The best com-
   parison group would be:
   A. Flight attendants
   B. Cancer patients
   C. A random sample from the general population (exclud-
      ing pilots)
   D. Coal miners
   E. Lawyers

ANSWERS AND EXPLANATIONS

1. **C.** According to BLS, workplace injuries and illnesses
   among US private-sector employees occurred at a rate
   of 2.9 cases per 100 full-time workers in 2016 (almost
   certainly an underestimate because years of exposure
   are required for many diseases to develop and because
   many illnesses caused by work exposures may not be
   recognized initially as such). The majority of reported
   cases were injuries, and more than half were serious
   enough to require days away from work, job transfer,
   or restriction of work activities.

2. **D.** Generally the receipt of workers' compensation benefits requires that a physician state the condition is
   "more probably than not" (probability >50%) related

to the workplace. There will often be uncertainty as to how much work and/or nonwork activities are to blame when conditions occur gradually. In many cases, activities both at and away from work may contribute, and it would not be necessary for a physician to state that the condition is impossible in the absence of job-related functions (A); that the job was the principal cause beyond all reasonable doubt (E); or that away-from-work activities were noncontributory (B). Pregnancy (C) is a risk factor for carpal tunnel syndrome, but excluding pregnancy would not be necessary to state that office activities were probably a primary determinant of the condition for the woman. Also, worsening of symptoms over the year makes both known and unknown pregnancy an unlikely cause.

3. **A.** Radiation is a physical hazard. Although some radiation comes in the form of particles (E), some comes in the form of rays. Other physical hazards include direct trauma, repetitive strain, noise, and thermal stresses. Chemical hazards (B) include various metals, organic solvents, mineral dusts, toxic gases, and a vast array of organic compounds, including pesticides and chemical manufacturing intermediates. Biologic hazards (C) include allergens, bloodborne and airborne pathogens, and infectious organisms spread by droplet, contact, or vector mechanisms. Psychosocial stressors (D) include long hours and fatigue, limited social support, and jobs over which workers have little control.

4. **C.** In the absence of a specific standard for chemical exposures, the Occupational Safety and Health Administration may cite workplaces under the General Duty Clause, which requires employers to provide a workplace free of recognized hazards. The National Institute for Occupational Safety and Health (A) and American Conference of Governmental Industrial Hygienists (B) are advisory groups that provide guidance on chemical exposures. The Substance Abuse and Mental Health Services Administration (D) is a constituent agency under the US Public Health Service (PHS) that provides national leadership in preventing and treating addiction and other mental disorders, based on up-to-date science and practices. The Health Resources and Services Administration (E) is another constituent agency under the PHS responsible for developing human resources and methods to improve health care access, equity, and quality, with an emphasis on promoting primary care.

5. **B.** Cyanide potently shuts down cellular respiration and may be rapidly fatal even at a relatively low dose. Methane (A) may also be fatal but only in quantities sufficient enough to displace available oxygen in an enclosed space (i.e., a very large, oxygen-displacing dose); methane is a simple asphyxiant, not a direct toxin. Ammonia (C) and sulfur dioxide (D) exert mostly irritant effects on the upper respiratory tract. Phosgene (E) may cause profound lower respiratory tract toxicities, including bronchospasm, pneumonitis,

and pulmonary edema, which if severe could ultimately be fatal but would not be as rapid as death by cyanide and would require fairly substantial doses.

6. **A.** HAV is spread by the fecal-oral route and reminds us about the importance of thorough handwashing and fully cooking potentially contaminated foods. The other listed hepatitides (HBV [B] and HCV [C]) are bloodborne pathogens spread by needlesticks and splashes of blood in the workplace. Parvovirus (D) and pertussis (E) are spread on respiratory droplets.

7. **E.** The oft-quoted risk for seroconversion after exposure to HIV is 0.3%, although this risk is clearly influenced by the quantity of blood delivered and the viral load in the source patient. Seroconversion risk after HCV exposure varies among studies but is likely 3% or less. HBV seroconversion in an unvaccinated individual may be 1% to 6% if the source is e-antigen negative and as high as 22% to 31% from an e-antigen–positive source.

8. **C.** Although most notable for its link to mesothelioma, asbestos exposure can also cause other aggressive cancers, including those of the larynx and lung. Although the relative risk of exposure is small, there is a 10% to 25% increase in lung cancer risk with exposure to radon above 4 pCi/L in the general population (A). Air pollution is associated with respiratory infections and cardiopulmonary mortality, in addition to exacerbation of asthma and other chronic lung diseases (B). Lead exposure to the general population has been greatly reduced by the removal of lead as a gasoline additive in the 1970s (D). Tuberculosis is aerosolized on fine particles (not large respiratory droplets [E]) that can travel long distances and transmit disease without the close contact generally required for other common respiratory diseases (influenza, pertussis, adenovirus, *Neisseria meningitidis,* hemorrhagic fever viruses).

9. **E.** In a cohort study the objective is to compare a group of "exposed" individuals to a group of "unexposed" individuals, following both groups though time for the development of the outcome. Cancer is the outcome in this case. Thus cancer patients (B) would be a particularly poor comparison group in that they already have the outcome of interest. Cosmic radiation is the exposure in this case. Thus flight attendants (A) would also be a particularly poor comparison group in that they likely have near-identical cosmic radiation exposure as pilots. Coal miners (D) would be about as protected from cosmic radiation as any group on the planet, although they would have higher rates of other radiation exposure from the earth's crust, including radioactive radon gas. Thus miners would not be a good "unexposed" comparison group. A random sample from the general population, excluding pilots (C), seems like a logical choice, but with the "healthy worker effect," pilots may differ systematically from the general population (many of whom will be unemployed) for a variety of reasons

unrelated to radiation exposure, but that could confound study results. For example, the general population would likely have a higher degree of unhealthy habits and poor health than pilots. For these reasons, lawyers would probably be the best comparison group of the choices offered. Lawyers represent a working group, thus diminishing the problem of the healthy worker effect.

They also would tend to have lower radiation exposures than pilots (or flight attendants or miners) and thus would reasonably represent "unexposed." Further, lawyers might be expected to have a similar socioeconomic position as pilots, with fewer confounders from differences in social and educational status or the resulting health opportunities and health behaviors.

Injury Prevention

"What would we do if a plane crashed today and 100 people died?

What would we do if it happened again tomorrow? And the next day? We'd ground air traffic. We wouldn't live with that.

It's been going on every day on our nation's roadways for the last 40, 50, 60 years."

David Teater, NSC Transportation Expert

1. DEFINITIONS

Injury prevention is an effort to prevent or reduce the severity of injuries before they occur. Injuries are a significant source of premature mortality and morbidity. Injury prevention strategies serve as an example of how to think systematically about surveillance and public health prevention efforts.

Injuries can be categorized as follows: motor vehicle crashes, firearms, home incidents (e.g., falls, burns, poisonings, electrocutions, drownings), occupational incidents, homicides, suicides, and miscellaneous injuries (e.g., plane/train crashes, building collapses, natural disasters). This chapter discusses motor vehicle crashes, injuries from firearms, and home incidents. Suicide and occupational incidents are discussed in Chapters 21 and 22.

Specialists in the field of injury prevention do not refer to injuries sustained from motor vehicle crashes or incidents in the home or worksite as "accidents," because the word carries the connotation that they are not predictable. In fact, these injury-producing events are fairly predictable and partially preventable. While the terms *accident* and *accidental injury*

are often used, the word *accident* implies the causes of injuries are random. Instead, injuries are commonly classified based on intentionality, and the terms *intentional injury* and *unintentional injury* are used. **Intentional injury** refers to injuries resulting from purposeful human action, whether directed at oneself or others. Intentional injuries include self-inflicted and interpersonal acts of violence intended to cause harm. Intentional injuries include interpersonal violence (homicide, sexual assault, neglect and abandonment, and other maltreatment), suicide, and collective violence (war). **Unintentional injuries** refer to injuries that are nonvolitional but potentially preventable. Most road traffic injuries, poisoning, falls, fire and burn injuries, and drowning are unintentional. In the field of public health, efforts are made to prevent or reduce intentional and unintentional injuries.

2. BURDEN OF INJURIES

In the United States, injuries are the leading cause of years per life lost (YPLL) before age 65. Fig. 23.1 outlines the 10 leading causes of death by age group, highlighting the public health importance of unintentional and intentional injuries. For people age 1 to 44, unintentional injuries are the leading cause of death. Intentional injuries also exert a major toll on the young. Homicide is the fourth leading cause of death for children age 1 to 9 years, and becomes third for the age group 15 to 34. Suicide is also an important cause of death among young adults, especially for ages 10 to 34.

As shown in Table 23.1, the total number of deaths due to unintentional injuries in the United States in 2016 was

10 Leading Causes of Death by Age Group, United States – 2017

Rank	<1	1–4	5–9	10–14	15–24	25–34	35–44	45–54	55–64	65+	Total
1	Congenital Anomalies 4,580	Unintentional Injury 1,267	Unintentional Injury 718	Unintentional Injury 860	Unintentional Injury 13,441	Unintentional Injury 25,669	Unintentional Injury 22,828	Malignant Neoplasms 39,266	Malignant Neoplasms 114,810	Heart Disease 519,052	Heart Disease 647,457
2	Short Gestation 3,749	Congenital Anomalies 424	Malignant Neoplasms 418	Suicide 517	Suicide 6,252	Suicide 7,948	Malignant Neoplasms 10,900	Heart Disease 32,658	Heart Disease 80,102	Malignant Neoplasms 427,896	Malignant Neoplasms 599,108
3	Maternal Pregnancy Comp. 1,432	Malignant Neoplasms 325	Congenital Anomalies 188	Malignant Neoplasms 437	Homicide 4,905	Homicide 5,488	Heart Disease 10,401	Unintentional Injury 24,461	Unintentional Injury 23,408	Chronic Low. Respiratory Disease 136,139	Unintentional Injury 169,936
4	SIDS 1,363	Homicide 303	Homicide 154	Congenital Anomalies 191	Malignant Neoplasms 1,374	Heart Disease 3,681	Suicide 7,335	Suicide 8,561	Chronic Low. Respiratory Disease 18,667	Cerebro-vascular 125,653	Chronic Low. Respiratory Disease 160,201
5	Unintentional Injury 1,317	Heart Disease 127	Heart Disease 75	Homicide 178	Heart Disease 913	Malignant Neoplasms 3,616	Homicide 3,351	Liver Disease 8,312	Diabetes Mellitus 14,904	Alzheimer's Disease 120,107	Cerebro-vascular 146,383
6	Placenta Cord. Membranes 843	Influenza & Pneumonia 104	Influenza & Pneumonia 62	Heart Disease 104	Congenital Anomalies 355	Liver Disease 918	Liver Disease 3,000	Diabetes Mellitus 6,409	Liver Disease 13,737	Diabetes Mellitus 59,020	Alzheimer's Disease 121,404
7	Bacterial Sepsis 592	Cerebro-vascular 66	Chronic Low. Respiratory Disease 59	Chronic Low. Respiratory Disease 75	Diabetes Mellitus 248	Diabetes Mellitus 823	Diabetes Mellitus 2,118	Cerebro-vascular 5,198	Cerebro-vascular 12,708	Unintentional Injury 55,951	Diabetes Mellitus 83,564
8	Circulatory System Disease 449	Septicemia 48	Cerebro-vascular 41	Cerebro-vascular 56	Influenza & Pneumonia 190	Cerebro-vascular 593	Cerebro-vascular 1,811	Chronic Low. Respiratory Disease 3,975	Suicide 7,982	Influenza & Pneumonia 46,862	Influenza & Pneumonia 55,672
9	Respiratory Distress 440	Benign Neoplasms 44	Septicemia 33	Influenza & Pneumonia 51	Chronic Low. Respiratory Disease 188	HIV 513	Septicemia 854	Septicemia 2,441	Septicemia 5,838	Nephritis 41,670	Nephritis 50,633
10	Neonatal Hemorrhage 379	Perinatal Period 42	Benign Neoplasms 31	Benign Neoplasms 31	Complicated Pregnancy 168	Complicated Pregnancy 512	HIV 831	Homicide 2,275	Nephritis 5,671	Parkinson's Disease 31,177	Suicide 47,173

CDC
Centers for Disease Control and Prevention
National Center for Injury Prevention and Control

Source: National Vital Statistics System, National Center for Health Statistics, CDC.
Produced by: National Center for Injury Prevention and Control, CDC using WISQARS™.

Fig. 23.1 The 10 Leading Causes of Death by Age Group, 2017. Unintentional injury, homicide, and suicide are highlighted. (From Office of Statistics and Programming, National Center for Injury Prevention and Control, National Vital Statistics System, National Center for Health Statistics, Atlanta, 2017, Centers for Disease Control and Prevention.)

TABLE 23.1 Number of Deaths Due to Unintentional Injuries Reported in the United States in 2016[a]

Type of Unintentional Injury	Number of Deaths
Motor vehicle injuries	40,327
Firearms	38,658
Falls	34,673
Other	47,716
TOTAL	161,374

[a]From CDC National Vital Statistics Report, Deaths for 2016. https://www.cdc.gov/nchs/data/nvsr/nvsr67/nvsr67_05.pdf.

161,374, with a large percentage of these deaths related to motor vehicle injuries, firearms, and falls.[1]

Understanding the factors contributing to specific causes of death from injuries can lead to improvements in reducing them. Beyond reducing premature mortality, evaluating causes of injuries also provides a structured way to think about different levers to target to improve public health in general (see discussion on Haddon matrix).

3. THE HADDON MATRIX

Haddon, a founder of the field of automobile injury epidemiology, developed a detailed approach to injury prevention.[2] The **Haddon matrix** classifies the phases of injury and the factors involved (Table 23.2). This approach was originally developed for injury prevention but is also applicable to other fields of prevention.[3–6] The Haddon matrix classifies the *phases* as before or **preinjury** (preevent), during the **injury** (event), and **postinjury** (postevent). The Haddon matrix classifies the *risk factors* involved as **human, vehicle, physical environment,** and **social environment.** By using this framework, investigators can evaluate the relative importance of different factors and design interventions to prevent injuries. Possible ways of preventing injury during the various phases have been suggested and are often called "Haddon's strategies" as described in Box 23.1.

TABLE 23.2 Haddon Matrix of Injury Prevention Applied to Motor Vehicle Crashes

PHASES	HUMAN FACTORS	VEHICLE FACTORS	ENVIRONMENTAL FACTORS	
			Physical	**Social**
Preevent	Attitudes Knowledge Use of alcohol or drugs Driver experience	Vehicle condition Speed	Roadway design Traffic calming Pedestrian facilities	Traffic laws Cultural norms
Event	Use of seat belts Wearing fastened helmet	Seat belts Helmets	Shoulders, medians Guardrails	Helmet and seat belt laws
Postevent	First aid Medical treatment	Fire risk	Availability of trauma care equipment Traffic congestion	Standards of trauma care in hospitals

From Hazen A, Ehiri JE: Road traffic injuries: hidden epidemic in less developed countries. *J Natl Med Assoc* 98:73–82, 2006. http://www.ncbi.nlm.nih.gov/pmc/articles/PMC2594796/pdf/jnma00296-0083.pdf.

BOX 23.1 Haddon's Strategies to Prevent Injury

Preevent (Before the Injury)
1. Prevent the existence of the agent.
2. Prevent the release of the agent.
3. Separate the agent from the host.
4. Provide protection for the host.

Event (Injury)
1. Minimize the amount of agent present.
2. Control the pattern of release of the agent to minimize damage.
3. Control the interaction between the agent and host to minimize damage.
4. Increase the resilience of the host.

Postevent (After the Injury)
1. Provide a rapid treatment response for host.
2. Provide treatment and rehabilitation for the host.

4. MOTOR VEHICLE CRASHES

Because prevention of motor vehicle crashes focuses on human, vehicle, and environmental factors, it requires an understanding of human behavior and the types of behavioral interventions that do and do not work in reducing crashes. Regulations regarding automobile construction have effectively reduced injuries from crashes. Laws regarding human behavior (e.g., requiring drivers to use seat belts) have been less successful, but have resulted in shifting behavior to reduce injuries. Greater controls on behavior of the driver, especially on driving while intoxicated, have been noted as shown by efforts to reduce the allowable blood alcohol level to 0.08%.

4.1 RISK FACTORS IN PREINJURY PHASE

4.1.a Human Factors

Some drivers are at an increased risk for crashes. These include new drivers, young drivers, and drivers with alcohol intoxication, drug intoxication, fatigue, or a combination of these factors. **New drivers** are at increased risk for crashes because they are less able to anticipate and prevent developing hazards, recognize existing hazards, and respond to them quickly and appropriately. For example, inexperienced drivers often do not anticipate the dangers of taking curves at high speeds, particularly when roads are wet, and they often have difficulty coordinating manual actions such as steering and braking suddenly. New drivers are at increased risk, regardless of the age at which they begin driving, but the excess risk decreases with driving experience.

In the United States, the high rates of serious injuries per mile of driving for **young drivers** are generally attributed to a combination of inexperience and immaturity factors, as well as the use of cell phones for talking or texting when driving. This practice distracts drivers and reduces the ability to react quickly in an emergency. Different states have different rules forbidding some or all use of handheld phones while driving.[7]

Most states have specific driving requirements to reduce injuries resulting from teenage driving.[8] *Graduated licensing* requires new teenage drivers to graduate from a provisional or beginner's license to one or more intermediate licenses before receiving an unrestricted license. The major provisions of the restrictive licenses limit how late the driver can operate a vehicle (i.e., impose various curfews) and how many passengers he or she can transport.

Driving while intoxicated with alcohol or drugs interacts with other factors to increase risks late at night, such as fatigue and reduced sensory input. This is one reason for considering a curfew of 11 PM or midnight for new teenage drivers, who are responsible for an excess number of fatal crashes in the United States, particularly single-vehicle crashes.[9] Although some groups advocate driver education programs in all US high schools, a study showed that the rates of teenage crashes and injuries in counties providing in-school driver education were as high as or higher than the rates in counties without such education.[10] Apparently the in-school driver education programs put significant numbers of young drivers on the road at an earlier age.

Laws concerning driving while intoxicated are already in place in the United States, as are regulations on the number of hours that professional drivers can operate trucks, buses, and other vehicles on the road per day and per week. Dozing and fatigue are responsible for numerous vehicle crashes, including those involving trucks.

4.1.b Vehicle Factors

The ability of vehicles to brake, passenger airbags, and other aspects of vehicle design, construction, and maintenance may influence the risk of injuries. A taillight pattern involving two lower red lights at the sides plus one higher red light in the middle of the rearview window catches the attention of drivers best and reduces rear-end collisions.

4.1.c Environmental Factors

Rain, snow, and other adverse weather conditions can decrease visibility for drivers, but not all drivers slow down appropriately or use traction devices when required. Poor design and maintenance of roads and highways also increase the risk of vehicle crashes. Conversely, graded decline between paved roads and edges as well as rumble strips at the center and edges of the road alert drivers who may be inattentive or falling asleep before a crash can happen.[11]

4.2 RISK FACTORS IN INJURY PHASE

4.2.a Human Factors

The ability of humans to resist injury is influenced by the use of specific protection devices, such as seat belts and child seats in automobiles and helmets for motorcycle and bicycle riders. For children age 3 to 9 years, the risk of injury is decreased if booster seats are used and the chest strap of the seat belt is placed so it does not choke.

4.2.b Vehicle Factors

Vehicle design has been steadily improving because of federal regulations. Vehicle safety features include collapsible steering columns, energy-absorbing construction, in-door side protection, seat belts and air bags, and protected gasoline tanks. However, risks keep changing with new technologies such as self-driving cars or different centers of gravity in sports utility vehicles.

4.2.c Environmental Factors

The object into which a vehicle crashes affects the seriousness of the crash. Energy-absorbing barriers on the shoulder of the road reduce the risk that vehicles will go off the road, and median strip barriers reduce injuries from head-on collisions.

4.3 RISK FACTORS IN POSTINJURY PHASE

4.3.a Human Factors

The fate of crash victims may be influenced greatly by the ability of individuals at the crash scene to act quickly in summoning medical help and preventing other vehicles from becoming involved in the crash.

4.3.b Vehicle Factors

The construction of a vehicle, including the protection of the gas tank to prevent post crash fire, may determine whether passengers survive a crash. A strong vehicle frame may reduce crushing and facilitate extraction of passengers by emergency response personnel.

4.3.c Environmental Factors

The extent of injury is influenced by the rapidity and quality of the emergency response. Advanced life support ambulance teams seek to stabilize the condition of injured persons at the crash scene before transport. Helicopter ambulance systems seem to improve outcomes, in part because they carry injured persons to trauma centers rather than to the nearest emergency department, which may not be adequately equipped for serious trauma.

5. FIREARM INJURIES

5.1 FIREARM EPIDEMIOLOGY

Injuries and deaths from firearms are becoming increasingly central to discussions in health, health care, and public health. Media images of gun-related massacres at schools, places of worship, and music venues highlight the loss of innocent life. While mass shootings and terrorist attacks are the most extreme forms of gun violence, they account for only a small fraction of the public health burden of firearm-related morbidity and mortality.[12]

Firearm injuries and deaths are an international concern. Worldwide, it was estimated that 251,000 (95% uncertainty interval [UI], 195,000–276,000) people died from firearm injuries in 2016, with six countries (Brazil, United States, Mexico, Colombia, Venezuela, and Guatemala) accounting for about half of these reported deaths.[13] Globally, most firearm injury deaths in 2016 were homicides (64%), suicide (27%), and unintentional firearm (9%) deaths. Firearm injury deaths in 2016 were highest among persons age 20 to 24 years, and higher among men than women. Countries with the highest number of firearms had the highest rates of firearm suicide and homicide.[13] The age-adjusted death rate for firearm homicide injuries in the United States in 2014 was 3.5 per 100,000, while many developed nations had rates of 2 per million or less, thus placing the United States as an extreme outlier.[14]

Injuries from firearms can be highly lethal in terms of case fatality. Among the firearm-related deaths in the United States in 2016, 59% were recorded as suicide and 37% as assault (homicide). In the United States, patients of firearm injuries are usually treated at level I or II trauma centers, the same centers that also treat patients with motor vehicle injuries. A study of annual mortality trends of patients with firearm or motor vehicle injuries from 2003 to 2013 noted that mortality rates significantly

TABLE 23.3	Application of Haddon Countermeasures to Firearms Injury and Cancer Prevention	
Countermeasure	Preventing Injury by Handguns	Preventing Cancer Associated With Smoking
1. Prevent the creation of the hazard	Eliminate handguns	Eliminate cigarettes
2. Reduce the amount of hazard brought into being	Limit the number of handguns allowed to be sold or purchased	Reduce the volume of tobacco production by changing agricultural policy
3. Prevent the release of the hazard	Install locks on handguns	Limit sales of tobacco to certain age groups; increase taxes on tobacco
4. Modify the rate of release of the hazard from its source	Eliminate automatic handguns	Develop cigarettes that burn more slowly
5. Separate the hazard from that which is to be protected by time and space	Store handguns only at gun clubs rather than at home	Establish shutoff times for vending machines and earlier closings of convenience stores and groceries
6. Separate the hazard from that which is to be protected by a physical barrier	Keep guns in locked containers	Install filters on cigarettes
7. Modify relevant basic qualities of the hazard	Personalize guns so they can be fired only by the owner	Reduce the nicotine content of cigarettes
8. Make what is to be protected more resistant to damage from the hazard	Create and market bulletproof garments	Limit exposure to other potential synergistic causes of cancer (e.g., environmental carcinogens) among smokers
9. Begin to counter the damage done by the hazard	Provide good access to emergency care in the prehospital period	Set up screening to detect cancer in the early stages
10. Stabilize, repair, and rehabilitate the object of damage	Provide high-quality trauma care in hospitals	Provide good-quality health care for cancer patients

Modified from Runyan CW: Introduction: back to the future—revisiting Haddon's conceptualization of injury: epidemiology and prevention. *Epidemiol Rev* 25:60–64, 2003.

declined for motor vehicle crashes in all age groups but not for firearms for any age group regardless of injury intent.[15] These results imply that case fatality trends for injuries resulting from firearms are worsening in severity over time compared with injuries from motor vehicle crashes.

5.2 FIREARM PREVENTION AND POLITICS

Preventing firearm injuries is a challenging goal. Reasonable people often disagree when efforts to reduce injuries and their associated costs necessitate restrictions on behavioral freedoms. This is true for deaths from firearms even more than motor vehicle injuries.

Table 23.3 provides an application of the Haddon countermeasures to firearms injury. For comparison with other public health topics, countermeasures for prevention of cancer from smoking is shown alongside the countermeasures for firearms injury.

The topic of firearm control and safety remains politically volatile in the United States. Medical professionals and the National Rifle Association (NRA) have gone toe-to-toe, the latter telling the former to mind its business; the former reminding the latter that bullet holes through people IS its business.[16–18] Another challenge to establishing firearm safety measures is limited or absent federal funding for research on firearms. Compared with the amount of dollars invested in research on other comparable public health challenges, firearm research is severely underfunded and understudied.

5.3 FIREARM RESEARCH AND POLICY INTERVENTIONS

Effective gun policies require understanding and consideration of many factors, including legal and constitutional rights, the interests of various stakeholders, and information about the likely effects of different laws or policies on a range of outcomes. The RAND Corporation's Gun Policy in America initiative completed its systematic assessment of the available scientific evidence on the effects of firearm laws and policies in 2018.[19] The key findings and recommendations are highlighted in Box 23.2, including many areas with limited and inadequate scientific data. These areas would benefit from rigorous research to inform a more evidence-based policy discussion.

It is our hope that additional research will be forthcoming in this area to help guide policy and public health interventions. Despite research limitations, there is evidence that policies reducing volume and access to firearms can reduce injuries.[20,21] Australia saw a large decrease in mass shootings, suicides, and homicides after a policy intervention removing firearms from public circulation.[20] US states with laws restricting access to firearms for high-risk individuals (e.g., mental illness or violent crime history) show improved injury outcomes.[21] Although more research is needed, policy

---

BOX 23.2 Key Findings and Recommendations of the RAND Corporation's Gun Policy in America Initiative

KEY FINDINGS

Despite Modest Scientific Evidence, the Data Support These Conclusions

- Of more than 100 combinations of policies and outcomes, surprisingly few have been the subject of methodologically rigorous investigation. Notably, research into four of the outcomes examined was essentially unavailable at the time of the review, with three of these four outcomes representing issues of particular concern to gun owners or gun industry stakeholders.
- Available evidence supports the conclusion that child-access prevention laws, or safe storage laws, reduce self-inflicted fatal or nonfatal firearm injuries among youth, as well as unintentional firearm injuries or deaths among children.
- There is moderate evidence that background checks reduce firearm suicides and firearm homicides, as well as limited evidence that these policies can reduce overall suicide and violent crime rates. There is moderate evidence that stand-your-ground laws may increase homicide rates and limited evidence that the laws increase firearm homicides in particular.
- There is moderate evidence that violent crime is reduced by laws prohibiting the purchase or possession of guns by individuals who have a history of involuntary commitment to a psychiatric facility. There is limited evidence these laws may reduce total suicides and firearm suicides.
- There is limited evidence that a minimum age of 21 for purchasing firearms may reduce firearm suicides among youth.

RECOMMENDATIONS

- When considering adopting or refining child-access prevention laws, states should consider making it a felony to violate these laws; there is some evidence that felony laws may have the greatest effects on unintentional firearm deaths.
- States that currently do not require a background check investigating all types of mental health histories that lead to federal prohibitions on firearm purchase or possession should consider implementing robust mental illness checks, which appear to reduce rates of gun violence.
- To improve understanding of the real effects of gun policies, Congress should consider lifting current restrictions in appropriations legislation that limit research funding and access to data. In addition, the administration should invest in firearm research portfolios at the Centers for Disease Control and Prevention, the National Institutes of Health, and the National Institute of Justice at levels comparable to its current investment in other threats to public safety and health.
- To improve understanding of outcomes of critical concern to many in gun policy debates, the US government and private research sponsors should support research examining the effects of gun laws on a wider set of outcomes, including crime, defensive gun use, hunting and sport shooting, officer-involved shootings, and the gun industry.
- To foster a more robust research program on gun policy, Congress should consider eliminating the restrictions it has imposed on the use of gun trace data for research purposes.
- Researchers, reviewers, academics, and science reporters should expect new analyses of the effects of gun policies to improve on earlier studies by persuasively addressing the methodological limitations of earlier studies, including problems with statistical power, model overfitting, covariate selection, and poorly calibrated standard errors, among others.

From RAND Corporation: *The Science of Gun Policy: A Critical Synthesis of Research Evidence on the Effects of Gun Policies in the United States*, Santa Monica, CA, 2018, RAND Corporation. https://www.rand.org/pubs/research_reports/RR2088.html. Also available in print form.

---

solutions hold promise for improving population health in the area of firearm injuries.

6. COMMON INJURIES IN THE HOME

Many preventable injuries occur in the home, including poisoning, fires, falls, and drowning. The victims of **poisoning** are usually toddlers and preschool children, who experiment with tasting or swallowing substances while exploring. Much has been accomplished in recent decades by developing childproof caps for containers of medicines and household products; by counseling parents to keep cleaning solutions, pesticides, medicines, and other hazardous substances out of the reach of their children; and by establishing poison control centers and hotlines.

The risk of **fires** has been reduced by improving building codes, particularly the requirement for hard-wired smoke alarms in houses and sprinkler systems in public buildings. Nevertheless, many older buildings are not retrofitted with these devices. The reduction in the prevalence of cigarette smoking has reduced one source of fires, but arson is still common, either for insurance or revenge purposes.

Although people of all ages can be the victims of **falls,** older people are at greater risk of serious injuries, such as hip fractures. In older people, falls are frequently caused by environmental hazards combined with failing vision, loss of equilibrium or physical strength, and use of medications that decrease stability.[22] A significant reduction in the incidence of hip fractures has been achieved in high-risk elderly persons by safety modification of their home environments, physical therapy, the use of devices such as walkers, and wearing padded hip protectors.[23] In younger persons, falls are likely to be associated with activities such as climbing ladders, shoveling snow, or walking on an ice-covered surface.

Drowning occurs most often among school-age children, especially boys. Swimming lessons and water safety instruction at an early age may reduce the number of deaths and injuries associated with activities that occur in and near pools and other bodies of water.

7. SURVEILLANCE AND PREVENTION OF INJURIES

An important factor in prevention is improved data on the nature of injuries, their rates of occurrence, and their circumstances. The Fatality Analysis Reporting System was developed by the National Highway Traffic Safety Administration and provides valuable epidemiologic data.[24] Other injury surveillance systems depend on the use of the E-codes in the *International Classification of Diseases* (ICD) and the use of hospital emergency department and admission diagnoses.

8. SUMMARY

The goal of injury prevention is to improve population health by preventing injuries and hence improving mortality and quality of life. Injuries are commonly classified as intentional or unintentional. Injuries are the leading cause of years per life lost before age 65. The Haddon matrix classifies the *injury phases* as preevent, event, and postevent and classifies the risk factors involved as human, vehicle, and environment (physical and social).

REFERENCES

1. Xu JQ, Murphy SL, Kochanek KD, et al. *Deaths: Final Data for 2016.* National Vital Statistics Reports 67(5). Hyattsville, MD: National Center for Health Statistics; 2018. Available at: https://www.cdc.gov/nchs/data/nvsr/nvsr67/nvsr67_05.pdf.
2. Haddon Jr W. A logical framework for categorizing highway safety phenomena and activity. *J Trauma.* 1972;12:193-207.
3. Haddon Jr W. The changing approach to the epidemiology, prevention, and amelioration of trauma: the transition to approaches etiologically rather than descriptively based. *Inj Prev.* 1999;5:231-235. doi:10.1136/ip.5.3.231.
4. Haddon Jr W. Advances in the epidemiology of injuries as a basis for public policy. *Public Health Rep.* 1980;95:411-421.
5. Baker SP, Haddon Jr W. Reducing injuries and their results: the scientific approach. *Milbank Mem Fund Q Health Soc.* 1974;52:377-389. doi:10.2307/3349509.
6. Runyan CW. Introduction: back to the future—revisiting Haddon's conceptualization of injury: epidemiology and prevention. *Epidemiol Rev.* 2003;25:60-64.
7. Governors Highway Safety Association. *Distracted Driving.* 2019. Available at: http://www.ghsa.org/html/stateinfo/laws/cellphone_laws.html.
8. Trempel RE. *Graduated Driver Licensing Laws and Insurance Collision Claim Frequencies of Teenage Drivers.* Insurance Institute for Highway Safety Report. 2009. Available at: http://www.iihs.org/research/topics/pdf/h0101.pdf.
9. National Highway Traffic Safety Agency. *Teen Driver Crashes: A Report to Congress.* 2008. Available at: https://www.nhtsa.gov/sites/nhtsa.dot.gov/files/811005.pdf.
10. Robertson LS, Zador PL. Driver education and crash involvement of teenaged drivers. *Am J Public Health.* 1978;68:959-965.
11. U.S. Department of Transportation Federal Highway Administration. *Rumble Strips and Rumble Stripes.* 2019. Available at: https://safety.fhwa.dot.gov/roadway_dept/pavement/rumble_strips/.
12. Cohn D, Taylor P, Lopez M, Gallagher C, Parker K, Maass KT. *Firearm Deaths.* Pew Research Center. 2013. Available at: https://www.pewsocialtrends.org/2013/05/07/chapter-2-firearm-deaths/.
13. Naghavi M, Marczak LB, Kutz M, et al. Global mortality from firearms, 1990-2016. *JAMA.* 2018;320:792-814. doi:10.1001/jama.2018.10060. (Erratum in: *JAMA* 2018;320:1288.)
14. Steinbrook R, Stern RJ, Redberg RF. Firearm violence: a JAMA internal medicine series. *JAMA Intern Med.* 2017;177:19-20. doi:10.1001/jamainternmed.2016.7180.
15. Tessler RA, Arbabi S, Bulger EM, Mills B, Rivara FP. Trends in firearm injury and motor vehicle crash case fatality by age group, 2003-2013. *JAMA Surg.* 2019;154(4):305-310. doi:10.1001/jamasurg.2018.4685.
16. Butkus R, Doherty R, Bornstein SS. Health and Public Policy Committee of the American College of Physicians. Reducing firearm injuries and deaths in the United States: a position paper from the American College of Physicians. *Ann Intern Med.* 2018;169(10):704-707.
17. Taichman D, Bornstein SS, Laine C. Firearm injury prevention: AFFIRMing that doctors are in our lane. *Ann Intern Med.* 2018;169:885-886, 2018. doi:10.7326/M18-3207.
18. Ault A. Physicians to NRA: this is our lane. *Medscape Medical News.* 2018. Available at: https://www.medscape.com/viewarticle/904730.
19. RAND Corporation. *The Science of Gun Policy: A Critical Synthesis of Research Evidence on the Effects of Gun Policies in the United States.* Santa Monica, CA: RAND Corporation; 2018. Available at: https://www.rand.org/pubs/research_reports/RR2088.html.
20. Chapman S, Alpers P, Agho K, Jones M. Australia's 1996 gun law reforms: faster falls in firearm deaths, firearm suicides, and a decade without mass shootings. *Inj Prev.* 2006;12:365-372.
21. Kaufman EJ, Morrison CN, Branas CC, Wiebe DJ. State firearm laws and interstate firearm deaths from homicide and suicide in the United States: a cross-sectional analysis of data by county. *JAMA Intern Med.* 2018;178:692-700.
22. Rubenstein LZ. Falls in older people: epidemiology, risk factors and strategies for prevention. *Age Ageing.* 2006;35(suppl 2):ii37-ii41. doi:10.1093/ageing/afl084.
23. Gillespie LD, Gillespie WJ, Robertson MC, Lamb SE, Cumming RG, Rowe BH. Interventions for preventing falls in elderly people. *Cochrane Database Syst Rev.* 2003;(4):CD000340.
24. National Highway Traffic Safety Administration. *Fatality Analysis Reporting System (FARS) Encyclopedia.* 2019. Available at: https://www-fars.nhtsa.dot.gov/Main/index.aspx.

REVIEW QUESTIONS

1. Specialists in the field of injury prevention differentiate *accidents* from *injuries* for the following reason:
   A. There is no difference and the two terms are used interchangeably by specialists.
   B. Specialists do not refer to injuries sustained from automobile crashes or incidents in the home or worksite as *accidents*, because the word carries the connotation that they are not predictable.
   C. Specialists use the term *intentional injury* instead of *accidents* to refer to injuries resulting from nonvolitional but preventable causes.

D. Accidents are not predictable, thus the two terms are used by specialists.

E. None of the answers A to D are correct.

2. Which of the following examples that illustrate the burden of injuries among individuals in the United States is true?

A. Injuries are the leading cause of years per life lost (YPLL) before age 65.

B. For people age 1 to 44, intentional injuries are the leading cause of death.

C. Injuries from sexual assault and domestic violence account for 35% of all injuries sustained by young people.

D. Suicide ranks outside of the top 10 leading causes of death for age group 25 to 34.

E. Among the deaths due to unintentional injuries in the United States in 2016 a small percentage (<2%) were related to falls.

3. Which of the following is one of Haddon's strategies to prevent an injury in the preevent phase?

A. Increase the resilience of the host

B. Control the pattern of release of the agent to minimize damage

C. Provide protection for the host

D. Minimize the amount of agent present

E. Control the interaction between the agent and host to minimize damage

4. Which of the following is one of Haddon's strategies to prevent an injury in the postevent phase?

A. Provide a treatment and rehabilitation for the host

B. Minimize the amount of agent present

C. Control the interaction between the agent and host to minimize damage

D. Separate the agent from the host

E. Provide protection for the host

5. Which of the following is *not* a human risk factor in motor vehicle crashes during the preinjury phase?

A. Fatigue

B. Inexperience

C. Immaturity

D. Use of protection devices

E. Driving while intoxicated

6. Which of the following vehicle factors may influence the risk of injuries in motor vehicle crashes during the postinjury phase?

A. The ability of the vehicle to brake appropriately

B. A taillight pattern that catches the attention of drivers and reduces the likelihood of rear-end collisions

C. Seat belts

D. Protection of gas tank that prevents postcrash fire

E. In-door side protection

7. Which of the following is *not* a common injury occurring in the home?

A. Falls

B. Drowning

C. Poisoning

D. Fires

E. Overexertion

8. Globally, the majority of firearm deaths in 2016 came from:

A. Suicides

B. Mass shootings

C. Homicide

D. Unintentional firearm incidents

E. Terrorists attacks

ANSWERS AND EXPLANATIONS

1. **B.** Specialists do not refer to injuries sustained from automobile crashes or incidents at home or worksites as *accidents* because the word carries the connotation that such injuries are not predictable. Instead, injuries are commonly classified by specialists based on whether they are *intentional* (resulting from purposeful human action) or *unintentional* (nonvolitional but preventable). Thus (C) is incorrect. Specialists differentiate the two terms, thus (A) is incorrect. Injuries sustained from motor vehicle accidents can be predicted and prevented, thus (D) is incorrect.

2. **A.** Injuries are the leading cause of years per life lost (YPLL) before age 65, thus (A) is the correct response. Unintentional injury (not intentional injury) is the leading cause of death for people age 1 to 44 (B). Injuries from sexual assault, domestic violence, and violence are not ranked in the top 10 leading causes of death among young people and do not account for 35% of all injuries sustained by young people (C). Suicide is an important cause of death among young adults, especially age 25 to 34 (E). Falls are a major public health problem and accounted for 34,673 of the 161,374 deaths due to unintentional injuries in 2016.

3. **C.** Provide protection for the host is Haddon's fourth strategy for preventing an injury in the preevent phase. Other strategies in the preevent phase include preventing the existence of the agent, preventing the release of the agent, and separating the agent from the host. Increase the resilience of the host (A), control the pattern of release of the agent to minimize damage (B), minimize the amount of agent present (D), and control the interaction between the agent and host to minimize damage (E) are Haddon's strategies during the event.

4. **A.** Provide treatment and rehabilitation for the host is one of Haddon's strategies to prevent injury in the postevent. Haddon's other postevent phase strategy is to provide a rapid treatment response for the host. Minimize the amount of agent present (B) and control the

interaction between the agent and host to minimize damage (C) are strategies during the event (not postevent). Separate the agent from the host (D) and provide protection for the host (E) are two of Haddon's preevent strategies.

5. **D.** Use of protection devices is the correct answer. Use of protection devices (D) is not a human risk factor in the injury phase. Fatigue (A), inexperience (B), immaturity (C), and driving while intoxicated (E) are all human risk factors associated with increased risk for crashes in the preinjury phase.

6. **D.** The construction of a vehicle, including the protection of the gas tank to prevent a postcrash fire, may determine whether passengers survive a crash in the postinjury phase. The ability of the vehicle to brake appropriately (A), seat belts (C), and in-door side protection (E) are vehicle risk factors in the injury phase. A taillight pattern that catches the attention of drivers and reduces the likelihood of rear-end collisions (B) is an example of a vehicle risk factor in the preinjury phase.

7. **E.** Many preventable injuries occur in the home, including falls (A), drowning (B), poisoning (C), and fires (D). Overexertion (E) is a consistent workplace-related injury.

8. **C.** Globally, the majority of firearm injury deaths in 2016 were homicides (64%), followed by suicide (27%) (A), and unintentional firearm (9%) (D) deaths. Mass shootings (B) and terrorist attacks (E) receive a lot of media attention but are less frequent causes of death.

Public Health

24

Introduction to Public Health

"Public health is what we, as a society, do collectively to assure the conditions in which people can be healthy."

> **Institute of Medicine (now renamed the National Academy of Medicine)**

Thus far in this book, the discussion has focused mostly on what individuals and their clinicians can do to evaluate and promote health and prevent disease and injury. Section 4 of this book focuses on public health.[1,2] To ensure better health, the responsibilities in public health are threefold: assessment, policy development, and assurance[1] (i.e., ensuring that appropriate services are available and accessible to meet the needs of the population). Chapter 2 provides tools for estimating the health of a population, and Chapter 14 discusses several definitions of health and their limitations. This chapter summarizes the current health of the US population and discusses data sources that public health practitioners can use to better understand the health issues in their communities. This chapter and Chapter 25 outline the US public health system and how communities can improve their health. Chapters 26 and 27 address the specific public health topics of preparing for

emergencies and ensuring the best quality of health care. Chapters 28 and 29 considers the complex and sometimes contradictory efforts of the medical care system to provide high-quality medical care, some of which can be considered preventive. Chapter 30 closes the section with an outlook of the main themes of the book and where we see public health going in the future.

1. DEFINITIONS OF PUBLIC HEALTH

The term *public health* has the following two meanings:
- Health status of the public (i.e., a defined population)
- Organized social efforts to preserve and improve the health of a defined population

The best-known definition of public health in terms of this second meaning was written in 1920 by Winslow[1] and is still remarkably current:

"Public health is the science and art of preventing disease, prolonging life, and promoting physical health and efficiency through organized community efforts for the sanitation of

the environment, the control of community infections, the education of the individual in principles of personal hygiene, the organization of medical and nursing service for the early diagnosis and preventive treatment of disease, and the development of the social machinery which will ensure to every individual in the community a standard of living adequate for the maintenance of health."

This definition is especially significant in the following three ways:

1. It states the central emphasis of all public health work—promoting health and preventing disease.
2. It emphasizes the diverse strategies required to promote health and prevent disease, including environmental sanitation, specific disease control efforts, health education, medical care, and an adequate standard of living.
3. It clarifies that for these goals to be achieved, organized social action is required. This action is largely expressed in the policies of the federal, state, and local governments and in the activities of the agencies designed to promote and protect the health of the public.

2. ASSESSING THE HEALTH OF A POPULATION

2.1 MAJOR SOURCES OF MORTALITY AND MORBIDITY

All efforts to improve public health start with an assessment. Table 24.1 shows major *metrics* of public health in the United States. The US population has transformed from the historic pyramid (many young people and much fewer older people) into a more oblong shape—a decreasing group of young individuals support more and more older people. Overall metrics of mortality have been steadily improving since 1950. Life expectancy at birth has improved to just below 79 years, and overall infant mortality has declined to less than 6 per 1000 newborns.[3] These mortality gains have slowed and even reversed for some populations since 2014. Especially among white men and women in rural areas, so-called diseases of despair—namely suicides, accidental poisoning, and liver disease—have been on the rise.[4] A similar effect was seen in Russia after the collapse of the former Soviet Union and economic crisis, where a significant increase in mortality came from cardiovascular disease and violent deaths (such as suicides, homicides, and traffic accidents), mainly among young and middle-aged adults.[5]

The three leading causes of death have changed over the last decades. Historically, heart disease has been the number-one killer (which it remains), followed by cancer and stroke. As the mortality of all these diseases has decreased, mortality from chronic lower respiratory diseases has increased and is now third on the list. Mortality from Alzheimer dementia has also increased, surpassing that from diabetes in 2009. The three leading causes of cancer-specific death have long been lung, breast/prostate, and colorectal cancer. The trends over time have shown a large increase in lung cancer after the widespread use of tobacco. This peak has leveled off for men, but not yet women.

While society has an interest in reducing *all* mortality, public health efforts generally focus on reducing *premature* deaths. One way to account for the impact of mortality causes on premature death is to calculate **years of potential life lost** (YPLL). Fig. 24.1 shows the 10 leading causes of YPLL before age 65 between 1999 and 2017. Analyzing the data in this way changes the order of conditions in the list. Cancer is now the second leading cause of premature death,

TABLE 24.1 Major Metrics and Sources of Mortality and Morbidity, United States

	1950	1980	2000	2006	2007	2009	2015
Life Expectancy in Years							
At birth	68.1	73.9	76.8	77.7	77.9	78.2	78.8
At age 65	13.8	16.4	17.6	18.5	18.6	18.8	19.4
Infant Deaths per 1000 Live Births							
All infants	29.2	12.6	6.91	6.69	6.75	6.42	5.9
Deaths per 100,000 Population, Age Adjusted							
All causes	1446.0	1039.1	869.0	776.5	760.2	741.0	733.1
Heart disease	586.8	412.1	257.6	200.2	190.9	179.8	168.5
Cancer	193.9	207.9	199.6	180.7	178.4	173.6	158.5
Stroke	180.7	96.2	60.9	43.6	42.2	38.9	37.6
Chronic lower respiratory diseases	—	28.3	44.2	40.5	40.8	42.2	41.6
Unintentional injuries	78.0	46.4	34.9	39.8	40.0	37.0	43.2
Motor vehicle	24.6	22.3	15.4	15.0	14.4	11.7	11.1
Diabetes	23.1	18.1	25.0	23.3	22.5	20.9	21.3

Data from Health, United States, 2005: Chartbook on trends in the health of Americans (www.cdc.gov/nchs/data/hus/hus05.pdf); At a glance table, Health, United States, 2010 (http://www.ncbi.nlm.nih.gov/books/NBK54373/#ataglance.s1); Deaths: preliminary data for 2009, *Natl Vital Stat Rep* 59:4, 2011 (http://www.cdc.gov/nchs/data/nvsr/nvsr59/nvsr59_04.pdf); Chartbook United States report 2016 (https://www.cdc.gov/nchs/data/hus/hus16.pdf).

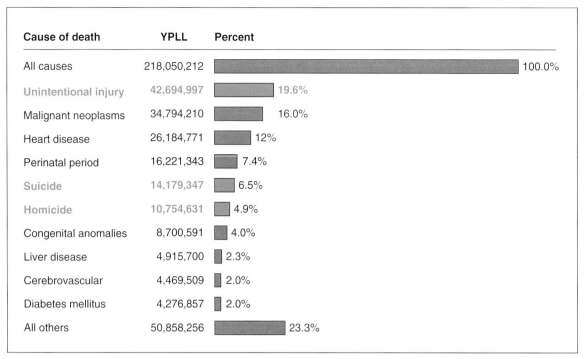

Cause of death	YPLL	Percent	
All causes	218,050,212		100.0%
Unintentional injury	42,694,997		19.6%
Malignant neoplasms	34,794,210		16.0%
Heart disease	26,184,771		12%
Perinatal period	16,221,343		7.4%
Suicide	14,179,347		6.5%
Homicide	10,754,631		4.9%
Congenital anomalies	8,700,591		4.0%
Liver disease	4,915,700		2.3%
Cerebrovascular	4,469,509		2.0%
Diabetes mellitus	4,276,857		2.0%
All others	50,858,256		23.3%

Fig. 24.1 Years of potential life lost (YPLL) before age 65, 1999–2017, United States; all races, both sexes, all deaths. (Produced by: National Center for Injury Prevention and Control, CDC. Data Source: National Center for Health Statistics (NCHS) Vital Statistics System. From: https://webappa.cdc.gov/sasweb/ncipc/ypll.html.)

and unintentional injuries is first because it affects more young people.

2.2 ACTUAL CAUSES OF DEATH

The previous death statistics are based on death certificates filled out by clinicians and do not account for the full causal pathway leading to death. One metric that attempts to account for this is the **actual causes of death.** This metric was outlined for the first time in a landmark paper by McGinnis and Foege and last updated in 2004.[6] This analysis showed that *smoking, poor diet,* and *lack of physical activity* were the main drivers of mortality (see also Chapter 19). However, analyzing actual causes of death should not be interpreted as a reduction of all mortality on individual behavior and an exoneration of structural determinants of health. As discussed in Chapters 14 and 30, social determinants of health such as poverty, food environments, and safe environments all play an important role in shaping or enabling behavior.

2.3 MATERNAL-CHILD HEALTH OUTCOMES

Outcomes of pregnant women and their children are of paramount importance to public health providers and policy makers for many reasons. The deaths of newborn babies and young women are often preventable and represent many years of potential life lost. Because of the high risk inherent in childbirth and the vulnerabilities of infants, maternal-child health outcomes function as "canaries in the mine" by serving as indicators of health care quality and equity. In addition, maternal-child health reflects "structures and resources of societies, (and) the function and responsiveness of health systems."[7] This underscores the importance of the rising maternal mortality rates in the United States in recent years, despite reductions in other developed countries.[8] The principal definitions of maternal-child metrics have been outlined in Chapter 2.

Fig. 24.2 illustrates how these different metrics fit together.

2.4 DISABILITY-ADJUSTED LIFE YEARS

With death rates falling, many persons live with serious illness and disability for many years. To assess this burden of disease, a metric called **disability-adjusted life years** (DALY) has been developed. This metric captures both the length of life lost from premature death and the time spent in poor health.[9] By this metric, the leading sources of premature death and disability were cardiovascular disease, low back and neck pain, drug use disorder, and cancer.[10] There were significant differences between genders and among ethnic groups. For example, for women, depression was the second leading cause of DALY (10 for males), whereas motor vehicle injuries and human immunodeficiency virus (HIV)–related deaths accounted for more DALY among ethnic minorities.

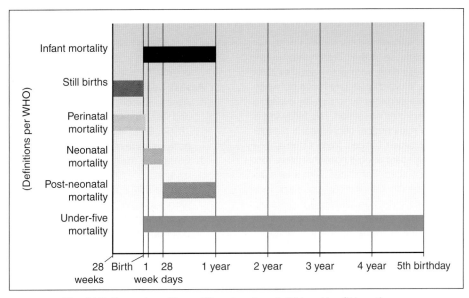

Fig. 24.2 Illustration of how different maternal-child metrics fit together.

2.5 HEALTH CARE DISPARITIES

The goal of public health is not just to decrease mortality and morbidity overall but also to decrease disparities. Historically, there has long been a gap between male and female life expectancy, as well as between whites and blacks. This gap has decreased somewhat but still exists; overall, white women live the longest, and black men are most likely to die early. In this analysis, race is likely not the causative agent but may be a correlate of proximate causes of decreased life expectancy, such as the social determinants of health (see Chapters 14 and 30). Many strategies to address health care disparities are being trialed at the state and local level (see Chapter 26).

Health care disparities occur in all age groups but are exacerbated in particular groups. Although mortality rates and infant and child mortality have improved significantly in the past five decades, this is not the case for young persons age 15 to 24.[11] The three leading causes of death in this age group include unintentional injuries (mainly motor vehicle crashes), homicide, and suicide.

Even among young people, injury rates vary by region and ethnicity. Non-Hispanic black and American Indians/Alaska Natives have much higher mortality rates than those of other races, largely because of higher rates of unintentional injuries (American Indian), homicides (non-Hispanic black), and suicide (American Indian).

Disparities in access to care, outcomes, and mortality persist, especially among poor and minority populations. The elimination of such disparities remains a public health priority and is the subject of dedicated institutes.

3. DATA SOURCES IN PUBLIC HEALTH

Public health data are used in research and community assessment to evaluate, plan, foster accountability, and spur change. To obtain and analyze **health indicator data,** epidemiologists rely on a variety of sources. Data for the rates used in epidemiologic studies can be discussed in terms of **numerator data,** which define the population experiencing events or conditions of concern, and **denominator data,** which define the population at risk. Statistics gathered from health, disease, birth, and death registries, as well as from other surveys, are used in the numerator. Census statistics are used in the denominator.

In clinical epidemiology, health-related data usually derive from patient examinations, clinical records, and studies of specific clinical populations. When monitoring the health of large populations, epidemiologists use existing databases as much as possible to reduce costs and accelerate results.

The increasing availability of **electronic medical records** and other digitized repositories constitutes an explosion of public health data. The main challenge is no longer to find data, but to find *useful* data in a sea of sources. Box 24.1 illustrates an example of pulling information together for assessing the burden of disease from asthma in a community.

Public health planning in the United States benefits from many high-quality, health-related periodic surveys. With the growth of the Internet, social media, and applications that pinpoint the location of multiple people, new sources for surveillance have become available.

The most important uses of the data remain to foster *accountability* and to spur *change.* In an ideal world, everyone would use a coherent set of population health metrics to drive such change. To date, however, no coherent and consistent set is available.[12] Health knowledge should not devolve into its converse, morbidity and mortality (Fig. 24.3).[13] In keeping with theories of health and its determinants, such a consistent set of health indicators should measure not only disease burden but also health equity, social determinants of health, environmental monitoring, quality of life, and aspects of health system performance.

BOX 24.1   Using Data From Multiple Sources to Assess Level of Asthma Morbidity in a New York County

In assessing the burden of disease in their community, public health planners need to access data from many sources. This involves an iterative process in which planners move between primary data collection in their community to publicly available data and back to more primary data collection. The following is a description of the steps a hypothetical public health planner might take to assess the disease burden from asthma in a county in New York State. Readers should note that New York has additional state-level resources. For states with a less active (or well-funded) state health department, planners may need to do more primary data collection. Because hospitalizations for asthma are considered preventable with optimal primary care, benchmark data are available from the Agency for Healthcare Research and Quality (AHRQ). This may not be true for other community health problems.

A. **Describe the asthma prevalence and mortality among adults and children in the state, and describe trends.**
1. Assess the prevalence rate of adult asthma in certain subgroups (age, gender, race/ethnicity). (BRFSS)
2. Compare the county adult asthma prevalence rate with the state. (BRFSS/EBRFSS)
3. Assess the county adult asthma prevalence in population subgroups (age, gender, race/ethnicity). (BRFSS/EBRFSS)
4. Compare the county population subgroup patterns to the state subgroups for adult asthma prevalence. (BRFSS/EBRFSS)
5. Assess current asthma prevalence among children in the state. (National Asthma Surveillance—NY)
6. Compare the state childhood asthma prevalence among population subgroups. (National Asthma Surveillance—NY)
7. Perform primary data collection for county childhood asthma prevalence.
8. Compare the county childhood asthma prevalence with the state prevalence.

9. Compare the asthma mortality rate for the state and county. (Vital Records—3 years)
B. **Assess health care utilization resulting from asthma.**
1. Assess current rate of hospital discharge from asthma, and describe trends in different age groups (total, 0–17, 18–64, 65+; likely need to obtain from hospitals directly or from state hospital association).
2. Compare the 3-year rates for state versus county by age.
3. Compare hospitalization rate by zip code for 3 years; where are the high-risk areas?
4. Assess emergency room data—1-year cross sectional; what percentage is asthma-related? Look at age, gender, race/ethnicity, and payment source distributions.
5. Calculate the risk ratio for someone who lives in the zip code being hospitalized/seen in the emergency room for asthma compared to other zip codes in the county.
6. Compare county asthma hospitalization rate to benchmark. (AHRQ)
C. **Describe overall health of the county.**
1. Assess median family income/per capita income by zip code (from census).
2. Assess county health ranking (countyhealthranking or American Community Survey).
3. Assess air quality (EPA).
4. Could also assess adult and adolescent smoking rates (BRFSS and YBRFSS).
D. **Perform primary data collection.**
1. Estimate sample size for sampling school asthma survey.
2. Compare prevalence rates from school asthma data of four schools (two high-risk areas, one moderate-risk area, and one low-risk area).
E. **Review primary data and determine if other data sources need to be accessed.**

Note: The primary data collection will likely bring up more issues that require comparison to state and county averages.
BRFSS, Behavioral Risk Factor Survey System (*E*, Expanded; *Y*, Youth); *EPA*, Environmental Protection Agency.
Modified from Epi Info Community Health Assessment Tutorial 2.0, 2005, Department of Health and Human Services, CDC, National Center for Public Health Informatics. https://ftp.cdc.gov/pub/software/epi_info/eihat_web/introductorymaterials.pdf

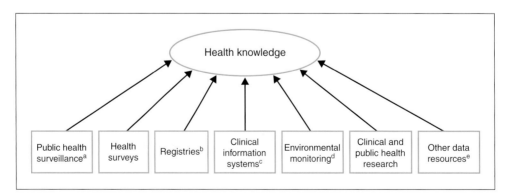

Fig. 24.3 Knowing about health. [a]The ongoing, systematic collection, analysis, and interpretation of health-related data with the a priori purpose of identifying unusual events of public health importance, or preventing or controlling disease or injury, followed by their dissemination for public health action. For example: [b]Vital registration, cancer registries, exposure registries. [c]Medical and laboratory records, pharmacy records. [d]Weather, climate change, pollution. [e]Criminal justice information, Lexis-Nexis, census. (From Lee LM, Thacker SB: Public health surveillance and knowing about health in the context of growing sources of health data. *Am J Prev Med* 41:636–640, 2011.)

3.1 SURVEILLANCE AND DATABASES

Public health surveillance is defined as the ongoing systematic collection, analysis, and dissemination of data regarding a health-related event for use in public health action to reduce morbidity and mortality and to improve health.[14] Many entities on the local, state, and federal level are engaged in collecting such data. The data are usually used descriptively to do the following[15]:

- Measure the burden of disease or trends in the burden of disease
- Educate the public
- Guide action and develop priorities for public health action
- Acquire resources (e.g., state grants)
- Develop policies
- Guide the planning, implementation, and evaluation of programs
- Provide a basis for research

Public health databases usually track health-related events that affect large segments of the population. Some events may be important, however, even if they affect a small number of people, such as an outbreak of a severe or highly infectious disease (e.g., active tuberculosis).

Data from public health databases differ from research data in a variety of ways. The data are usually reported based on regulatory requirements or by law. Public health data come from a patchwork of local and state sources. Data may be incomplete or of low quality, and changes in data definition or wording of questions make it difficult to compare data over time. When reviewing any metric, it is important to ask the following questions to understand data attributes[16]:

- Is the survey based on a sample, or is it population based?
- Are the data based on individual patients (e.g., mortality), events (e.g., hospitalizations), or local conditions (e.g., level of pollutants)?
- Do data points represent individual records or the aggregate?
- What are the criteria for reporting the location of the event?

For some events, such as motor vehicle deaths or hospitalization records, the database might report the location where an event was discovered (e.g., hospital where a foodborne illness was diagnosed). That county of discovery might be different from the county where the patient lives or where the exposure occurred.

3.2 SUMMARY MEASURES OF HEALTH

Summary measures of health are usually mortality data for the general population (e.g., measures of neonatal health) and data on morbidity and mortality. As people live longer and more often develop chronic diseases, the focus has moved from mortality to more useful metrics of **health-adjusted life expectancy,** such as quality-adjusted life years and DALY (see earlier). Since 1990, the WHO publishes Global Burden of Disease studies that summarize the impact of various diseases, injuries, and risk factors in causing premature death, morbidity, and disability in different countries.[17]

3.3 CENSUS DATA

Most countries conduct censuses periodically (e.g., every 10 years) to obtain data on the number and characteristics of their populations. They also use **continuous registration** (reporting) **systems** to collect data on the number and characteristics of births and deaths. Census data are the most fundamental data for a population. **Vital statistics registration systems** use recent census data for the denominators of birth and death rates. Access to recent statistics of various countries provides data for international comparisons of such data as infant mortality rates (see earlier).

Not all countries have effective disease-reporting systems (Box 24.2), however, and the accuracy of census and vital statistics data varies from country to country. The collection of these data is a national responsibility, and most countries report their data to the United Nations (population, social, and economic data) and the World Health Organization (vital statistics and disease data). The best place to find census data on a specific country is the website of the country of interest. In addition, several websites are dedicated to collecting addresses of epidemiologic websites of global interest.[18]

3.3.a US Census

In the United States, public data systems collect many types of health-related statistics, including birth and death data. Collecting such data frequently involves local, state, and national agencies. Data on births, deaths, causes of death, fetal deaths, marriages, and divorces are initially collected locally by the registrar of vital statistics for the municipality or county involved. Birth certificates are completed by a physician or other birth attendant, and death certificates are completed by a physician, medical examiner, or coroner. The local jurisdiction sends the original birth and death certificates to the state government, which is responsible for maintaining permanent records. The state governments (often state health departments) prepare summaries of these data. The states also send copies of the birth and death certificates to the **National Center for Health Statistics** (NCHS), a branch of the US Centers for Disease Control and Prevention (CDC), which prepares national summaries.

The federal government conducts the census. A complete population census, effective April 1, is performed in every

---

BOX 24.2 Making Everyone Count

"Most people in Africa and Asia are born and die without leaving a trace in any legal record or official statistic. Absence of reliable data for births, deaths, and causes of death are at the root of this scandal of invisibility, which renders most of the world's poor as unseen, uncountable, and hence uncounted."

From Setel PW, Macfarlane SB, Szreter S, et al: Monitoring of vital events (MoVE) writing group. A scandal of invisibility: making everyone count by counting everyone. *Lancet* 370:1569–1577, 2007.

year ending in 0. Census surveys are first distributed by mail; data collection is then supplemented by door-to-door interviews. Findings from the most recent census are available online (see Websites at the end of this chapter). Because the data are based on self-reporting, underestimates are likely, especially among certain population groups such as undocumented immigrants. Because some data are suppressed to maintain confidentiality, data may also be less reliable for some population groups.[19] States use projections to estimate the size of the population between censuses.

3.4 NUMERATOR DATA

3.4.a US Vital Statistics System

The federal government collates data on births, deaths, causes of death, fetal deaths, marriages, and divorces in the United States and its territories, as obtained by local and state officials. Because analyses are only as good as the data on which they are based, great care is taken to make the vital statistics system as accurate as possible. Nevertheless, there are many potential sources of error in these data, including unreported births and deaths, inaccurate death certificate diagnoses, and erroneous demographic and clinical data on birth and death certificates.

When the numbers of deaths in the United States are categorized by cause of death and reported in government publications, the cause provided is the **underlying cause of death,** not the **immediate cause of death.** The attending physician is responsible for completing the information on the cause of death. If a person dies without medical attention, or if foul play is suspected, a medical examiner or coroner must decide the cause of death for that individual, sometimes aided by an autopsy.

3.4.b Death Certificates

Death certificates usually do not suggest risk factors. For example, obesity is seldom mentioned on death certificates, despite its impact on mortality. There are fields to document tobacco use, but these may not be filled in consistently or correctly. Either way, death certificates are unlikely to represent the full causal pathways leading to death.

Fig. 24.4 shows the **cause-of-death** section of a death certificate. If a person dies of pneumonia after a cerebral hemorrhage, the physician probably would write "pneumonia" on

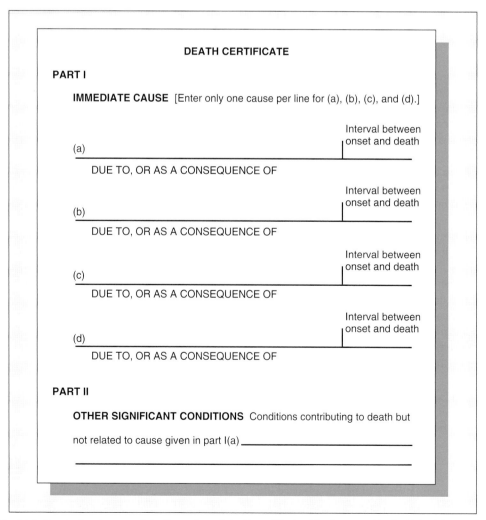

Fig. 24.4 Facsimile of cause-of-death portion of death certificates. The form used in the United States also requests information regarding autopsy, referral to a medical examiner or coroner, and homicide investigation.

line (a) in Part I and "cerebral hemorrhage" on line (b). The cerebral hemorrhage would be considered the underlying cause of death. If the physician decided that the person's co-existent hypertension caused the cerebral hemorrhage, however, "hypertension" would be recorded on line (c), and that would be considered the underlying cause of death. On the other hand, if the physician decided that the hypertension was too mild to cause the hemorrhage, he or she would enter "hypertension" under "Other Significant Conditions" in Part II. In that case, "spontaneous cerebral hemorrhage" would be the underlying cause of death.

Crafting an accurate cause-of-death narrative may become more difficult when a provider unfamiliar with the patient's full medical history is asked to perform this function. Another source of inaccuracy is the translation of the narrative opinion on the death certificate to numeric codes using a set of complex rules. Vital statistics staff are trained to do this, but the added layer of interpretation remains another potential source of error. Once a death certificate is completed, errors, omissions, or inaccuracies can be corrected only through a formal process of amendment.

Although death certificate data are sufficiently accurate for setting many national priorities in funding, research suggests that the data are not accurate enough for robust epidemiologic research. One study focusing on test cases found only 56% agreement among physicians on diagnoses of underlying cause of death, with significant questions remaining among the rest.[20]

3.5 LEADING HEALTH INDICATORS

Since a US Surgeon General's report in 1979, a group of federal agencies called the Healthy People Initiative collaborates with experts and other agencies to define and measure health objectives. Every decade, the Healthy People Initiative develops a new set of goals (and sometimes indicators) to improve the health of all Americans (see Websites at the end of this chapter). Currently, important health indicators come from the *Healthy People 2020* and *2030* process. The *Healthy People 2020* indicator selection process attempts to map out the interplay between ecologic factors, social determinants, and health outcomes (Fig. 24.5). In *Healthy People 2020,* indicators focus on the following **foundational health measures:**

- General health status
- Health-related quality of life and well-being
- Determinants of health
- Disparities

Progress on these metrics can be accessed from an interactive website.[21] *Healthy People 2020* metrics are laudably extensive and very helpful to guide community health assessment efforts and program planning. The metrics are also highly complex, so it is difficult to synthesize overall progress. A smaller, more comprehensive set of indicators has also been developed and is tracked on a dedicated website (www.stateoftheusa.org) (Table 24.2).[22]

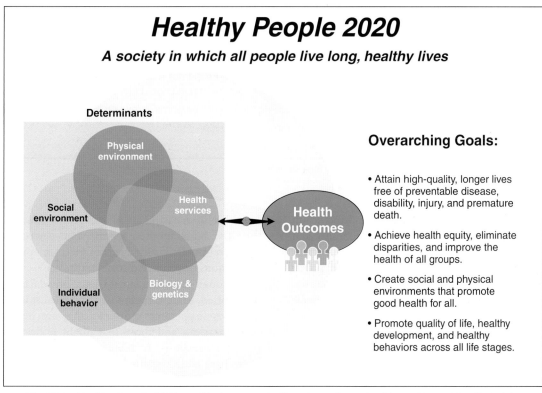

Fig. 24.5 *Healthy People 2020* graphic framework. (From https://www.healthypeople.gov/sites/default/files/HP2020Framework.pdf.)

TABLE 24.2 State of Health Indicators: Outcomes, Behaviors, Systems

Metric	Definition
Health Outcomes	
Life expectancy at birth	Number of years that a newborn is expected to live if current mortality rates apply.
Infant mortality	Deaths of infants age under 1 year per 1000 live births.
Life expectancy at age 65	Number of years of life remaining to a person at age 65 if current mortality rates continue to apply.
Injury-related mortality	Age-adjusted mortality rates from intentional or unintentional injuries; includes deaths caused by motor vehicle crashes, poisoning, firearms, and falls.
Self-reported health status	Percentage of adults reporting fair or poor health.
Unhealthy days, physical and mental	Mean number of physically or mentally unhealthy days in the past 30 days.
Chronic disease prevalence	Percentage of adults reporting one or more of six chronic diseases: diabetes, cardiovascular disease, chronic obstructive pulmonary disease, asthma, cancer, and arthritis.
Serious psychologic distress	Percentage of adults with serious psychologic distress, as indicated by score of 13 or more on K6 scale.
Health-Related Behaviors	
Smoking	Percentage of adults who have smoked more than 100 cigarettes in their lifetime and who currently smoke some days or every day.
Physical activity	Percentage of adults meeting the recommendation for moderate physical activity: at least 5 days a week for 30 minutes a day of moderate activity, or at least 3 days a week for 20 minutes a day of vigorous activity.
Excessive drinking	Percentage of adults consuming four drinks or more (women) or five drinks or more (men) on one occasion and/or consuming more than an average of one (women) or two (men) drinks per day during the past 30 days.
Nutrition	Percentage of adults with a good diet, as indicated by score of ≥80 on the Healthy Eating Index.
Obesity	Percentage of adults reporting a body mass index of ≥30.
Condom use	Proportion of youth in grades 9–12 who are sexually active and who do not use condoms, placing them at risk for sexually transmitted infections.
Health Systems	
Health care expenditures	Per capita health care spending.
Insurance coverage	Percentage of adults without health care coverage through insurance or entitlement.
Unmet medical, dental, and prescription drug needs	Percentage of (noninstitutionalized) people who did not receive or who faced delays in receiving needed medical services, dental services, or prescription drugs during the previous year.
Preventive services	Percentage of adults who are current with age-appropriate screening services and flu vaccination.
Preventable hospitalizations	Hospitalization rate for ambulatory care–sensitive conditions.
Childhood immunization	Percentage of children ages 19–35 months who are current with recommended immunizations.

Modified from Institute of Medicine: *State of the USA health indicators,* Washington, DC, 2009, State of the USA.

The United States is fortunate to have many large health surveys that regularly assess broad swaths of health and health behaviors. These surveys are large enough to have representative data on the state level. Researchers and public health activists can compare indicators over time. However, below the state level, these surveys usually only provide enough data for larger metropolitan areas.

3.5.a National Notifiable Disease Surveillance System

Physicians, hospitals, clinics, and laboratories in the United States are required to report to local and state health departments all cases of many infectious diseases and certain noninfectious diseases, such as elevated lead levels in children.

Local health departments in turn report this information to the CDC. Based on these reports, and as needed, local, state, or federal public health agencies perform epidemiologic investigations of possible disease outbreaks.

Although the states largely agree on which diseases must be reported, some variation persists. The list usually includes zoonoses (e.g., rabies), diseases that are highly infectious (e.g., measles), and those that might indicate an outbreak (e.g., salmonellosis) or bioterrorism (e.g., smallpox). Some states have added healthcare-associated infections to the list (see Chapter 20). Notifiable conditions are frequently updated if new diseases or disease entities (re-)appear (e.g., anthrax, dengue). Readers are encouraged to visit the CDC website and their state website for a current list.

Only a fraction of the actual disease cases is reported, largely depending on the seriousness of the disease. Most extremely serious diseases, such as paralytic poliomyelitis, tend to be reported if recognized. Even then, epidemiologists must be wary because numbers may be too low. In some cases the problem may be **underdiagnosis.** In others, clinicians may be hesitant to report a condition that could cause social stigma if discovered by others. Such illnesses include sexually transmitted diseases and tuberculosis.

Underreporting is even more likely for common and less serious diseases. This does not mean that epidemiologic statistics have no value, particularly if the diseases are preventable by a vaccine. As long as the proportion of reported cases remains constant, the pattern revealed by reporting probably will reflect actual trends in disease occurrence and distribution.

3.5.b National Center for Health Statistics

The National Center for Health Statistics (NCHS) runs the national vital statistics system. In addition, it performs many important studies on such topics as current levels of illness and disability, the practice of preventive health services, population use of preventive measures and medical care, and strategies to improve sampling methods and instrument design for health surveys. NCHS also carries out its own surveys on a variety of topics. In the past, these have included hospital discharges, ambulatory medical care, and long-term care services. Other surveys include information about family growth and use of preventive health measures. Ongoing surveys include the following:

- National Health Interview Survey (NHIS), to determine yearly changes in acute and chronic illness and disability in the United States
- National Health and Nutrition Examination Surveys (NHANES), in which a large, random sample of the US population participates in health interviews, physical examinations, and laboratory tests (see upcoming discussion)
- National Health Care Survey, which monitors the use of medical care in the United States

Data from most NCHS surveys can be found on the Internet. The NCHS also publishes a yearly chartbook of the nation's health.[23]

3.5.c Behavioral Risk Factor Surveillance System

State health departments cooperate with the CDC on ongoing surveys of behavioral risk factors in the US population. The largest example of this is the Behavioral Risk Factor Surveillance System (BRFSS). With over 400,000 interviews per year, this is the world's largest telephone-based survey and is the primary source that most states use to assess health behaviors. In this survey, a random sample of the population is interviewed by telephone regarding a variety of behaviors that affect health, including exercise, smoking, obesity, alcohol consumption, drinking and driving, use of automobile seat belts and child restraints, and use of medical care (see Websites at the end of this chapter). The BRFSS is highly respected but often of limited use below state level.

Also, its sampling depends on landlines and cell phones. The Youth Risk Behavior Surveillance System is a special BRFSS effort that monitors high-priority health risk behaviors and the prevalence of obesity and asthma among youth and young adults.

3.5.d National Health and Nutrition Examination Survey

The NHANES is a large survey by CDC that assesses the health and nutritional status of adults and children in the United States. NHANES is the only large survey that combines interviews and physical examinations. NHANES includes interview questions about demographics, socioeconomic, dietary, and health-related topics. The examination component consists of medical, dental, and physiologic measurements as well as laboratory tests. NHANES therefore provides cross-sectional data on the relationships among activity, diet, and various laboratory markers.

3.6 OTHER HEALTH-RELATED REGISTRIES

Many types of registries collect information about health and health care, including secondary data on patients who share a specific disease, symptom, medical regimen, or medical procedure. Depending on the registry, such reports can be used to assist individual patients, medical providers, insurance carriers, industry, and government. Many registries for chronic diseases (e.g., diabetes) allow public health managers to identify patients who need testing or who are not receiving a specified level of care. Measures tracked by these registries are often determined by panels of scientists and are defined by national organizations, such as the National Committee for Quality Assurance (see Chapter 28).

In some states and US regions, government agencies or other authorities have established special registries to record information on specific conditions such as cancer, tuberculosis, and birth defects. The oldest population-based cancer registry in the United States is the Connecticut Tumor Registry, which is maintained by the Connecticut State Department of Health. The name of every Connecticut resident with cancer since 1935 has been reported to the registry, along with information from patient records, including extensive clinical, pathologic, and risk factor data. This registry and other cancer registries conduct extensive surveillance efforts to ensure complete reporting of cancers.

The National Cancer Institute sponsors the **Surveillance, Epidemiology, and End Results** (SEER) program and supports a network of US cancer registries, including the Connecticut Tumor Registry and other regional population-based registries. SEER currently collects and publishes data on cancer incidence and survival from registries covering approximately 28% of the US population. Investigators involved in the SEER program study trends in the incidence and treatment of cancer and analyze treatment results over time.

Cancer registries are valuable aids for evaluating outcomes of cancer screening programs and determining whether certain risk factors are linked with cancer.

Many states supplement national surveys with additional questions or state-level surveys (e.g., California Health Interview Survey). Private foundations (e.g., Kaiser Family) also allow state-by-state comparisons (see Websites at end of this chapter). States that have active research organizations collaborating with statewide health foundations tend to have particularly rich databases. Because baseline data are needed to apply for grants and access other resources, disparities in available data will become exacerbated over time (data beget more data). Therefore, the best first step to address community health problems is often to collect data.

For public health professionals working at the *county* level, it can be difficult to obtain data with sufficient level of detail. Some health departments have taken the initiative to develop county-level surveys that focus on particular topics.[24] The Georgia State Health Department focuses on health disparities, quality of and access to care, and health

professional workforce. The New York City Health Department conducts surveys on health disparities based on social inequities. Seattle tracks living wage, affordable housing, homelessness, and other societal, environment, and art resources for health.

These surveys illustrate how collecting data is intertwined with community health action ("data begets data"). The data were obtained because a community coalition identified these areas as a special interest. In turn, obtaining the data leads to action and more data. With help from private foundations, the Public Health Institute publishes a summary ranking of all US counties by health factors and health outcomes.[25] For more help with county-level data, the Department of Health and Human Services (HHS) and CDC use the Community Health Data Initiative to pull data from various websites and provide a county's health status profile[26] (Table 24.3).

TABLE 24.3   Selected National Data Sources of Health Indicators*

Survey	Examples of Measures	GEOGRAPHIC AVAILABILITY			Approximate Sample Size	Administering Agency Source/Link
		Nation	State	County		
Health Outcomes						
National Vital Statistics System— Birth File	Birth data (infant mortality, low birth weight, educational attainment of parents)	X	X	X	Data for most jurisdictions, but might be limited events for single years/subgroups	Local vital registration systems and NCHS https://www.cdc.gov/nchs/ nvss/births.htm
National Vital Statistics System— Mortality	Cause-specific mortality, premature mortality (YPLL), life expectancy	X	X	X	Data for most jurisdictions; subgroup analysis and yearly data might be limited for some causes	Local vital registration systems and NCHS https://www.cdc.gov/nchs/ nvss/deaths.htm
Behavioral Risk Factor Survey System (BRFSS)	Health-related quality of life, health conditions, use of recommended health care services, behaviors, access to care; adults only	X	X	Some	Annual sample size about 350,000; has some data for large metropolitan statistic areas	States with Division of Adult and Community Health; national (CDC) https://www.cdc.gov/brfss/
Youth Risk Behavior Survey	Overweight, physical activity, diet, school foods	X	Some	Some large metro districts	>10,000 students	State, tribal, and local governments with CDC http://www.cdc.gov/ HealthyYouth/yrbs/ index.htm
Disease surveillance	Infectious diseases, Cancer	X	X Some	X	Variable completeness of reporting	CDC http://www.cdc.gov/ osels/ph_surveillance/ nndss/phs.htm#data National Cancer Institute http://seer.cancer.gov/data/
Monitoring the Future	Risky behavior among youth (tobacco, drug, alcohol in grades 8, 10, 12)	X			About 48,000 students in 2006	Institute for Social Research, University of Michigan http://monitoringthefu ture.org/

TABLE 24.3   Selected National Data Sources of Health Indicators—cont'd

Survey	Examples of Measures	GEOGRAPHIC AVAILABILITY			Approximate Sample Size	Administering Agency Source/Link
		Nation	State	County		
National Health Interview Survey (NHIS)	Illness, injuries, activity limitations, use of health services, vaccinations, screening	X			Adult and child data, about 35,000 households	CDC, U.S. Census Bureau https://www.cdc.gov/nchs/nhis/index.htm
National Health and Nutrition Examination Survey (NHANES)	Chronic diseases, mental health, oral health combined with physiologic measurements (BP, serum cholesterol)	X			Annual continuous sampling of about 10,000 participants	NCHS https://www.cdc.gov/nchs/nhanes/index.htm
National Immunization Survey	Childhood immunizations	X	X	Some	27,000 children age 19–35 months	NCHS https://www.cdc.gov/vaccines/imz-managers/nis/index.html
National Survey of Children's Health (NSCH)	Health and functional status; familial, social, and emotional environment; family function; neighborhood conditions	X	X		HRSA regions	NCHS http://www.cdc.gov/nchs/slaits/nsch.htm
National Survey on Drug Use and Health (NSDUH)	Use of illegal drugs, alcohol, and tobacco in people over age 12	X	X		Sample of about 70,000 noninstitutionalized Americans over age 12	Substance Abuse and Mental Health Service Administration https://nsduhweb.rti.org/respweb/homepage.cfm
Social and Environmental Health						
American Community Survey	Population and demographics (e.g., age, income, educational attainment)	X	X	X	65,000	U.S. Census Bureau https://www.census.gov/programs-surveys/acs/ https://www.childstats.gov/
Current Population Survey	Children's health insurance coverage, income, etc.	X	X		State-based sample of >50,000 households	U.S. Census Bureau https://www.census.gov/programs-surveys/acs/
National Assessment of Educational Progress	Educational achievement	X	X		Large urban districts	National Center for Education Statistics http://nces.ed.gov/nationsreportcard/
American Housing Survey	Housing		X	X	Large metropolitan areas	U.S. Census Bureau http://www.census.gov/housing/ahs/
Physical Environment						
Air quality system	Outdoor air quality, suspended particulates	X	X	Some	Data from air quality–monitoring agencies	EPA http://www.epa.gov/ttn/airs/airsaqs/
NHANES	Indoor air quality	X			See earlier in table	See earlier in table
Toxic release inventory	Toxic chemical releases to the environment	X	X	Some	Reported by facilities	EPA https://www.epa.gov/toxics-release-inventory-tri-program

BP, Blood pressure; *CDC*, Centers for Disease Control and Prevention; *EPA*, Environmental Protection Agency; *HRSA*, Health Resources and Services Administration; *NCHS*, National Center for Health Statistics; *YPLL*, years of potential life lost.

*All the surveys are cross sectional. It is therefore difficult to interpret causality and progress over time.

Modified from Wold C: *Health indicators: a review of reports currently in use*, Washington, DC, 2008, State of the USA.

3.7 OTHER DATA SOURCES

3.7.a Third-Party Payers and Insurance

Over the years, carriers of medical insurance and other third-party payers, such as Medicare, Medicaid, and the Veterans Administration, have collected increasing amounts of administrative and clinical data. These data often are used by clinical epidemiologists and health care researchers who are concerned with the patterns of health care utilization and the cost effectiveness of medical care. Hospital discharge records are often aggregated and sold by state hospital associations.

3.7.b Health of Special Populations

Population groups at both ends of life may experience health problems that are very different from the rest of the population. Because they can be underrepresented or not represented in national surveys, epidemiologists have designed dedicated data sets for children and elderly persons. For example, child health and development are highly dependent on safety, security, and social and emotional well-being, as well as developmental opportunities. Surveys dedicated to child health include the March of Dimes data on perinatal mortality and the America's Children and Kids Count surveys.[24] For the elderly population, who have problems with social support, ability to function independently, and availability of long-term care, the Older Americans survey provides this specialized data.[27] Dedicated websites list resources for particular diseases or topics of interest, such as HIV or genomics.[28]

3.7.c Environmental and Specialized Data

Environmental data are particularly challenging to interpret. Such data provide information on hazardous emissions into air, water, and soil and on the overall quality of the environment (see Chapter 22). Most environmental data are collected based on legislation. Not all regulations call for data on human health outcomes, or even data from human populations. Furthermore, data usually come from hourly or daily measurements at sampling stations, and results may not be reported unless they exceed a standard level. Levels are sometimes based on facility estimates rather than true samples.[29] Nevertheless, these sources provide rich data on the quality of the environment, emission of specific toxins (e.g., pesticides), weather data, and radiation levels. The information suggests areas of inquiry for the One Health approach (see Chapter 30), possible connections between hazard levels and poverty, and clustering of cancers. These databases are specialized and based on specific sampling methodologies, so readers should consult specialized literature.

Depending on the area of interest, public health planners can also access other databases. For example, the motor vehicle crash database from a state department of transportation shows crash frequencies by location; municipal data show clustering of emergency department (ED) visits or hospitalizations;[30] FBI crime databases assess an area's "walkable/bikable" status.[31] Other potential areas of interest may include legal databases listing international laws that protect vulnerable populations, animal health data for zoonotic diseases, US Department of Agriculture data on access to healthy food, school-based data for measuring educational attainment and high-school completion rates in a community, and economic data on community infrastructure and economic opportunities.

3.7.d Performance of Health Care Systems

Given rising health care costs, as well as more scrutiny on safety in health care, many researchers turn to databases identifying the performance variations in the health care system. For example, the Kaiser Family Foundation and *Dartmouth Atlas of Health Care* track unwarranted variations in spending (see upcoming discussion). Many organizations are involved in evaluating quality of health care (see Chapter 28). The following organizations are dedicated to tracking the progress on preventive health[24]:

* Trust for America's Health, a coalition of more than 130 organizations that publishes the 10 leading priorities for prevention
* Good Health Counts Report from the Prevention Institute
* Environmental Public Health Indicators project (CDC)
* National Center for Environmental Health
* Project Thrive (early childhood indicators)

3.7.e International Health

The World Health Organization (WHO) compares 193 countries in broad metrics of health and health care systems (Global Burden of Disease studies, see earlier discussion). The Commonwealth Fund publishes comparisons of health care systems across selected countries. In Europe, the Organization for Economic Cooperation and Development (OECD) provides data for member countries on quality of life, life expectancy, infant mortality, and obesity. The European Union (EU) also conducts surveys on health care expenditures and Self-Perceived Health. The Institute for Health Metrics and Evaluation also provides national and global health measurements on global health problems (see Websites at the end of this chapter).

4. FUTURE TRENDS

4.1 SELF-REPORTED HEALTH AND WELL-BEING

Most surveys tend to underreport physical and social environments that optimize health[24] and instead focus on objective morbidity data. To counteract this trend, some surveys have sought to collect self-reported health and well-being data from a representative sample of the population. For example, the Gallup-Healthways Index measures life evaluation, emotional health, work environment, and basic access to safe living in addition to physical health.[32]

4.2 CONFIDENTIALITY CONCERNS

In response to the Health Insurance Portability and Accountability Act (HIPAA; see Chapter 29), several public health agencies have worked together to make their systems more interchangeable. However, more data exchange increases the risk of accidental release of individually identifiable health data. In several cases, health care organizations have inadvertently released large amounts of patient data. For public health databases, confidentiality is at least as important.

4.3 BIG DATA

Data from different administrative or nontraditional data sources can also be combined to make connections. For example, **syndromic surveillance** in EDs measures the chief complaints of patients. A spike in patients with rashes or upper respiratory symptoms might signal the outbreak of smallpox or influenza, respectively. Other useful data sources for the detection of an outbreak might be work or school absentee rates, pharmaceutic sales of over-the-counter cold medicines, or calls to emergency hotlines. Search engine use for particular keywords such as *symptom clusters* or *emerging infectious diseases* (e.g., influenza, dengue) offer an interesting addition to traditional epidemiologic studies.[33]

Other studies have connected data within or between different surveys. Examples include estimating deaths from healthcare-associated infections,[34] integrating data on nutrition and alcohol use with mortality statistics to delineate the mortality effects of various dietary or lifestyle risk factors,[35] assessing the impact of different countries' policies on maternal leave on neonatal mortality,[36] and mapping geographic and racial disparities in premature mortality against economic and environmental variables.[37]

4.4 GENOMICS

Recent advances in the study of the genome (genomics) and pharmacogenomics are likely to affect public health databases. Already, genomic information has been integrated in NHANES.[38] One opportunity in the near-term is to explore the interaction of genetic and environmental factors influencing health in populations.

4.5 MAPS

Visualization of data can provide insights that might otherwise be missed. Clusters of disease outbreaks, unintentional injuries, or health care utilization may not become apparent until these are mapped. Mapping of clusters dates back to the beginning of public health investigations with John Snow's maps of water sources and cholera cases (see Chapter 3, Fig. 3.13). Fig. 24.6 shows a map of access to good nutrition in an Ohio neighborhood. More recently, however, the opportunities for such applications have increased exponentially. In an era of real-time data, when many citizens are equipped with mobile devices that can immediately upload pictures, it might become possible to shorten the time between surveillance and discovery and to *crowd-source* environmental monitoring.[39]

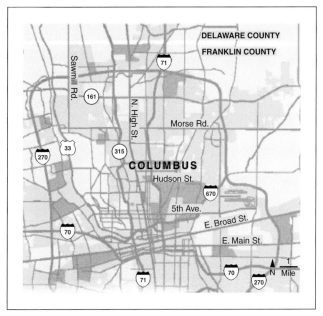

Fig. 24.6 Closer to fast food. Columbus Public Health of Ohio has identified neighborhoods where the proximity to fast-food restaurants far outweighs the proximity to a large, full-service grocery. At least half the census blocks in these neighborhoods *(gray areas)* had worse access than average. (From Crane M: Lack of access to nutritious fare in poor areas contributes to obesity, other problems, Columbus Public Health, Ohio, 2010, *Columbus Dispatch*. http://www.dispatch.com/content/stories/local/2010/08/01/food-deserts.html.)

The evolving field of **geographic information systems** provides powerful tools to mine such data. Several data sources provide innovative use of maps. Most prominent is the Dartmouth Atlas, which shows potentially unwarranted variation in measures of health services and outcomes by geographic areas. One particularly famous map of health care spending by enrollee showed large variations that were not associated with underlying costs, comorbidities, or measurable difference in health outcomes (Fig. 24.7) (see Websites at the end of this chapter).

4.6 ONE HEALTH

The health of people, animals, and the environment are interconnected. The One Health approach aims to characterize and improve health overall by working collaboratively across multiple disciplines. Examples of fruitful use of this approach include climate change, emerging diseases, and mental health, among others (see Chapter 30).

5. SUMMARY

Public health refers both to assessing the health status of a population and trying to improve this health. Important ways to view the health of a country come from census data, morbidity and mortality from major diseases, and years of potential life lost and disability-adjusted life years. Using measures of premature death and disability adjusting provides greater weight to the many lives lost to suicide and unintentional injuries. Significant disparities persist for all

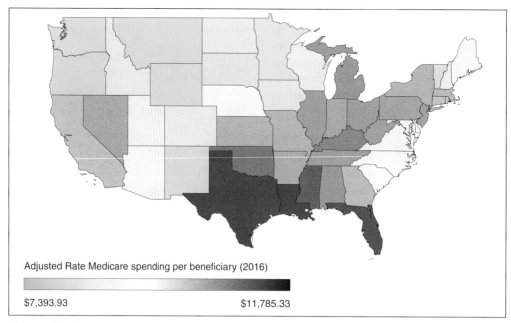

Fig. 24.7 Medicare healthcare spending per enrollee 2016. (Price-Adjusted Total Medicare Reimbursements per Enrollee (Parts A and B), by state (2016), from the Dartmouth Atlas Project: https://www.dartmouthatlas.org/interactive-apps/medicare-reimbursements/#state.)

these metrics. Epidemiologists rely on a variety of sources for obtaining data to analyze health-related rates and risks. Data for the rates used in epidemiologic studies can be discussed in terms of denominator data, which define the population at risk, and numerator data, which define the population experiencing events or conditions of concern. Denominator metrics come from census data. Large, ongoing databases that provide numerator data include the BRFSS (telephone survey of behavioral risk factors), NHANES (survey of nutrition that includes biometric data), and SEER data (for cancer disease registries). A variety of other data sources inform health planning on state and county levels. Mapping technology, One Health approaches, and connections between data and real-time reporting could transform the field.

REFERENCES

1. Winslow CE. The untilled field of public health. *Modern Medicine*. 1920;2:183-191.
2. Institute of Medicine. *The Future of Public Health*. Washington, DC: National Academy Press; 1988.
3. Centers for Disease Control and Prevention. *NCHS: Death Rates and Life Expectancy at Birth*. Available at: https://data.cdc.gov/NCHS/NCHS-Death-rates-and-life-expectancy-at-birth/w9j2-ggv5.
4. Stein EM, Gennuso KP, Ugboaja DC, Remington PL. The epidemic of despair among white Americans: trends in the leading causes of premature death, 1999–2015. *Am J Public Health*. 2017;107:1541-1547. doi:10.2105/AJPH.2017.303941.
5. Men T, Brennan P, Boffetta P, Zaridze D. Russian mortality trends for 1991-2001: analysis by cause and region. *BMJ*. 2003;327:964.
6. Mokdad AH, Marks JS, Stroup DF, Gerberding JL. Actual causes of death. *JAMA*. 2004;291:1238-1245.
7. Kruk ME, Kujawski S, Moyer CA, et al. Next generation maternal health: external shocks and health-system innovations. *Lancet*. 2016;388:2296-2306.
8. GBD 2015 Maternal Mortality Collaborators. Global, regional, and national levels of maternal mortality, 1990–2015: a systematic analysis for the Global Burden of Disease Study 2015. *Lancet*. 2016;388:1775-1812.
9. McKenna MT, Michaud CM, Murray CJ, Marks JS. Assessing the burden of disease in the United States using disability-adjusted life years. *Am J Prev Med*. 2005;28:415-423.
10. Institute for Health Metrics and Evaluation (IHME). *GBD Compare Data Visualization*. Seattle, WA: IHME, University of Washington; 2018. Available at: http://vizhub.healthdata.org/gbd-compare.
11. Singh GK. *Youth Mortality in the United States, 1935–2007: Large and Persistent Disparities in Injury and Violent Death*. A 75th Anniversary Publication, Health Resources and Services Administration, Maternal and Child Health Bureau. Rockville, MD: US Department of Health and Human Services; 2010. Available at: http://www.mchb.hrsa.gov/.
12. Institute of Medicine. *For the Public's Health: The Role of Measurement in Action and Accountability*. Washington, DC: National Academy Press; 2011.
13. Lee LM, Thacker SB. Public health surveillance and knowing about health in the context of growing sources of health data. *Am J Prev Med*. 2011;41:636-640.
14. Thacker SB, Berkelman RL. Public health surveillance in the United States. *Epidemiol Rev*. 1988;10:164-190.
15. CDC Guidelines Working Group, German RR, Lee LM, et al. Updated guidelines for evaluating public health surveillance systems. *MMWR*. 2001;50(RR-13):1-35.
16. Ballard J. *Concepts of Data Analysis for Community Health Assessment*. Available at: http://www.nwcphp.org/docs/bcda_series/data_analysis_mod1_transcript.pdf.
17. World Health Organization. *About the Global Burden of Disease Project*. Available at: http://www.who.int/healthinfo/global_burden_disease/about/en/.

18. The WWW Virtual Library. *Medicine and Health: Epidemiology*. Available at: http://www.vlib.org/Medicine.

19. Alexander JT, Davern B, Stevenson B. *Inaccurate Age and Sex Data in the Census PUMS Files: Evidence and Implications*. 2010. Available at: https://www.nber.org/papers/w15703.

20. Messite J, Stellman SD. Accuracy of death certificate completion: the need for formalized physician training. *JAMA*. 1996;275:794-796.

21. Office of Disease Prevention and Health Promotion. *Healthy People 2020: Foundation Health Measures*. Available at: https://www.healthypeople.gov/2020/About-Healthy-People/Foundation-Health-Measures.

22. Institute of Medicine. *State of the USA Health Indicators*. 2019. Available at: www.stateoftheusa.org.

23. National Center for Health Statistics. *Health, United States, 2010: With Special Feature on Death and Dying*. Hyattsville, MD: 2011.

24. Wold C. *Health Indicators: A Review of Reports Currently in Use*. Washington, DC: State of the USA; 2008. Available at: https://www.ncbi.nlm.nih.gov/books/NBK215070/.

25. *2019 County Health Rankings Key Findings Report*. 2019. Available at: https://www.countyhealthrankings.org/. Accessed October 6, 2019.

26. Centers for Disease Control and Prevention. *National Center for Health Statistics: Interactive Data Tools and Systems*. Available at: https://www.cdc.gov/nchs/tools/index.htm.

27. Federal Interagency Forum on Aging-Related Statistics. *Aging Stats*. Available at: https://agingstats.gov/.

28. Partners in Information Access for the Public Health Workforce. *Public Health Resources: Health Data, Tools & Statistics*. Available at: https://phpartners.org/ph_public/display_links/784.

29. Meyer R. How the US protects the environment, from Nixon to Trump: a curious person's guide to the laws that keep the air clean and the water pure. *The Atlantic*. March 29, 2017. Available at: https://www.theatlantic.com/science/archive/2017/03/how-the-epa-and-us-environmental-law-works-a-civics-guide-pruitt-trump/521001/.

30. Gawande A. The hot spotters: can we lower medical costs by giving the neediest patients better care? *New Yorker*. 2011:40-50.

31. Federal Bureau of Investigation. *Criminal Justice Information Services: Uniform Crime Reporting Program*. Available at: Available at: https://ucr.fbi.gov/ucr.

32. Gallup-Healthways. *Well-Being Index*. Available at: https://wellbeingindex.sharecare.com/.

33. Milinovich GJ, Williams GM, Clements AC, Hu W. Internet-based surveillance systems for monitoring emerging infectious diseases. *Lancet*. 2014;14:160-168.

34. Klevens RM, Edwards JR, Richards CL, et al. Estimating health care–associated infections and deaths in U.S. hospitals, 2002. *Public Health Rep*. 2007;122:160-166.

35. Danaei G, Ding EL, Mozaffarian D, et al. The preventable causes of death in the United States: comparative risk assessment of dietary, lifestyle and metabolic risk factors. *PLoS Med*. 2009;6:e1000058.

36. Heymann J, Raub A, Earle A. Creating and using new data sources to analyze the relationship between social policy and global health: the case of maternal leave. *Public Health Rep*. 2011;126:127-134.

37. Cullen MR, Cummins C, Fuchs VR. Geographic and racial variation in premature mortality in the US: analyzing the disparities. *PLoS ONE*. 2012;7:e32930. doi:10.1371/journal.pone.0032930.

38. Chang MH, Lindegren ML, Butler MA, et al. Prevalence in the United States of selected candidate gene variants. Third National Health and Nutrition Examination Survey, 1991–1994. *Am J Epidemiol*. 2009;169:54-66.

39. Hesse BW. Public health surveillance in the context of growing sources of health data: a commentary. *Am J Prev Med*. 2011;41:648-649.

SELECT READINGS

Boslaugh S. *Secondary Data Sources for Public Health*. St Louis, MO: Washington University; 2007.

Frieden TR. The future of public health. *N Engl J Med*. 2015;373:1748-1754. doi:10.1056/NEJMsa1511248.

Friis RH, Sellers TA. Sources of data for use in epidemiology. In *Epidemiology for Public Health Practice*. 4th ed. Boston, MA: Jones & Bartlett; 2009.

Institute of Medicine. *The Future of Public Health*. Washington, DC: National Academy Press; 1988.

Meyer R. How the US protects the environment, from Nixon to Trump: a curious person's guide to the laws that keep the air clean and the water pure. *The Atlantic*. March 29, 2017. Available at: https://www.theatlantic.com/science/archive/2017/03/how-the-epa-and-us-environmental-law-works-a-civics-guide-pruitt-trump/521001/.

Structure and function of the public health system in the United States. VII. Injury and violence. In: Wallace RB, ed. *Maxcy-Rosenau-Last: Public Health and Preventive Medicine*. 15th ed. New York, NY: McGraw-Hill Medical; 2008.

WEBSITES

Behavioral Risk Factor Surveillance System Survey Data: www.cdc.gov/brfss

Centers for Disease Control and Prevention Injury Factbook: https://www.cdc.gov/injury/publications/index.html

Centers for Disease Control and Prevention notifiable diseases: https://wwwn.cdc.gov/nndss/

County Health Rankings: www.countyhealthrankings.org

Dartmouth Atlas of Health Care: http://www.dartmouthatlas.org/

Fatal Accident Reporting System: http://www-fars.nhtsa.dot.gov/Main/index.aspx

Gateway for statistics from federal agencies: https://www.usa.gov/statistics

Information about state level: Trust for America: https://www.tfah.org/

Institute for Health Metrics and Evaluation: http://www.healthdata.org/

Kaiser Family Foundation: www.statehealthfacts.kff.org

March of Dimes: https://www.marchofdimes.org/peristats/Peristats.aspx

National Cancer Institute: www.nci.org

National Center for Health Statistics: www.cdc.gov/nchs/

National Highway Traffic and Safety Administration: www.nhtsa.gov

Partners in Information Access for Public Health Workforce: health data tools and statistics: https://phpartners.org/ph_public/display_links/784

Public Health Institute: www.phi.org

State of the USA: leading health indicators: www.stateoftheusa.org

United Health Foundation; America's Health Rankings: http://www.americashealthrankings.org

US Census Bureau: www.census.gov

World Health Organization Global burden of disease: http://www.who.int/healthinfo/global_burden_disease/about/en/

WWW Virtual Library: Medicine and Health: Epidemiology: http://www.vlib.org/

REVIEW QUESTIONS

1. Which of the following is *true* of mortality in the United States?
   A. Most mortality is caused by infectious diseases.
   B. Most cancer mortality among US women is caused by breast cancer.
   C. Because of increasingly earlier overall mortality, life expectancy in the United States is on the decline.
   D. The three leading causes of mortality remain heart disease, cancer, and stroke.
   E. Overall, metrics of mortality have been steadily improving.

2. Cancer is the second leading cause of death in the United States, but the leading contributor to years of potential life lost, whereas heart disease is the leading cause of death in the United States, but the second leading contributor to years of potential life lost. Which explanation best accounts for this discordance?
   A. Cancer is an infectious disease.
   B. Cancer is a chronic disease.
   C. Cancer more often is rapidly fatal.
   D. Cancer causes death in younger people.
   E. Cancer is curable less often than heart disease.

3. Which of the following metrics best captures the morbidity of suffering with severe illness?
   A. Life expectancy
   B. Mortality rate
   C. Age-adjusted mortality rate
   D. Disability-adjusted life years (DALY)
   E. Years of potential life lost (YPLL)

4. Which racial/ethnic group has the highest rate of mortality overall among youth?
   A. Non-Hispanic white
   B. Non-Hispanic black
   C. Hispanic
   D. American Indian/Alaskan Native
   E. Asian/Pacific Islander

5. Which racial/ethnic group has the highest rate of mortality among youth by self-injury (both intentional and unintentional)?
   A. Non-Hispanic white
   B. Non-Hispanic black
   C. Hispanic
   D. American Indian/Alaskan Native
   E. Asian/Pacific Islander

6. Which is *true* of US census data?
   A. Comes from the National Center for Health Statistics
   B. Includes birth and death data for each state
   C. Based largely on a mailed survey
   D. Collected every 5 years across the United States
   E. Overrepresents undocumented immigrants

7. A 63-year-old man with a bullet wound to the chest has a thoracotomy (open-chest surgery) to repair the damage. The operation is a success, and the man survives the procedure. He is a long-time smoker, however, with underlying cardiovascular (coronary artery) disease. Many days later, while still recovering from his trauma and surgical repair, he goes outside to smoke a cigarette, has cardiac arrest in front of the hospital, and ultimately cannot be resuscitated. He dies. On his death certificate, tobacco use would most likely be listed as which of the following?
   A. The immediate cause of death
   B. The underlying cause of death
   C. The actual cause of death
   D. Another significant condition
   E. A risk factor

8. Which population health survey is administered by state health departments in cooperation with the US Centers for Disease Control and Prevention (CDC)?
   A. Behavioral Risk Factors Surveillance System (BRFSS)
   B. National Health Interview Survey
   C. National Health and Nutrition Examination Survey (NHANES)
   D. National Health Care Survey
   E. Decennial census

9. Which population health survey includes actual physical exams and laboratory specimens from individuals in addition to self-report data?
   A. Behavioral Risk Factors Surveillance System (BRSS)
   B. National Health Interview Survey
   C. National Health and Nutrition Examination Survey (NHANES)
   D. National Health Care Survey
   E. Decennial census

10. A baby dies age 1 year 5 months. Her death will appear as part of
    A. Infant mortality
    B. Neonatal mortality
    C. Under-5 mortality
    D. Postneonatal mortality
    E. Perinatal mortality

ANSWERS AND EXPLANATIONS

1. **E.** Although metrics of mortality in the United States remain relatively poor compared to other industrialized nations, overall they have been slowly improving. Life expectancy (C) continues to rise, and most US deaths are not caused by infections (A). Rather, most deaths result from chronic degenerative diseases. Heart disease, cancer, and stroke (D) had long been the leading killers until recently, when stroke dropped to fourth place and was replaced by chronic lung diseases. This fact reminds us that smoking remains one of the leading actual causes of death in the United States, accounting for why lung cancer outpaces breast cancer (B) as the leading cause of cancer death among US women.

2. **D.** Cancer is a group of diseases, some of which affect the very young and cause death in early life. Heart disease is much more limited to later life, although this pattern

is subject to change as cardiac risk factors in younger people proliferate. Still, currently deaths from heart disease in young people are very unusual. As a whole, individuals with cancer often die much earlier (i.e., much further from life expectancy than those with heart disease). Cancer is sometimes curable (E) but is often discovered too late for any chance at cure. This, however, does not distinguish cancer from heart disease, which also tends not be to be curable but rather treatable. Cancer can be rapidly fatal (C), but heart disease can be rapidly fatal as well (e.g., by heart attack or sudden cardiac death). Both cancer and heart disease are chronic diseases (B), and infections (A) may contribute to both (e.g., hepatitis B virus in cancer, *Chlamydia pneumoniae* in heart disease).

3. **D.** DALY captures the burden of living with disease, considering both length of life lost from premature death and time spent in poor health. Years of potential life lost (E) only captures length of life lost. Life expectancy (A) is a forecast of potential life remaining from a given point, usually time of birth. Mortality rate (B) describes the frequency of death in a population. For specific causes of death, it is particularly important to adjust mortality rates for age (C), the most ubiquitous and important confounder.

4. **B.** Severe disparities persist in health outcomes for poor and minority US populations. Non-Hispanic blacks fare the worst overall of racial/ethnic groups, most notably with more than 10 times the mortality by homicide as non-Hispanic whites (A) or Asian/Pacific Islanders (E). American Indians/Alaskan Natives (D) do not fare much better overall.

5. **D.** American Indian/Alaskan Native youth commit suicide at almost twice the rate of any other group and also die more frequently by unintentional injury. Social factors, such as poverty and high-risk/demeaning employment, undoubtedly contribute to both.

6. **C.** Census surveys first go out by mail. Following the mailed survey, door-to-door interviews occur to supplement data collection. A complete population census is performed every 10 years (D) in years ending in 0. The census includes neither birth data nor death data (B). It is administered by the US Census Bureau, not the National Center for Health Statistics (A). Based on self-report, census data might underrepresent certain population groups, such as undocumented immigrants (E).

7. **D.** The immediate cause of death (A) is that the heart stopped beating (i.e., the patient had cardiac arrest). The underlying cause (B) was probably his coronary artery disease (CAD), although damage from the gunshot wound may have also contributed. An autopsy might clarify this, but even with a postmortem examination, the underlying cause will largely be based on physician judgment. Smoking may have triggered the incident, and although smoking can precipitate an acute coronary event (e.g., through platelet aggregation and blood vessel constriction and blockage), generally the detrimental effects of smoking are incremental and cumulative over years. Smoking is a risk factor (E) for CAD and cardiac arrest, but risk factors are not listed on death certificates. As a risk factor and likely contributor to the immediate and underlying causes of death, smoking may also be an actual cause of death (C) in this case. As with risk factors, however, actual causes are not listed on death certificates, and moreover, *actual cause* is not an accepted term but rather a way to view how risk behaviors lead to poor health outcomes. If included at all on the death certificate, tobacco use would most likely be another significant condition (D), or contributor, although the way that contributing conditions and circumstances are counted is highly subjective. Ultimately, the final common pathway of death is that the brain does not receive enough oxygenated blood to maintain its metabolic activities. This is equally true for deaths from asphyxiation by drowning, blood shunting by tumors, arrested circulation by bullet damage, or decapitation. However, coding cerebral anoxia as the immediate cause of death in every case is not productive and prevents pattern recognition of more upstream causes that may be beneficial to medicine and public health (from the bullet that ripped the aorta, to the drug deal that led to the shooting, to the poverty and exclusion from legitimate employment that led to drug dealing, etc.). This case illustrates the difficulties in completing death certificates accurately and highlights the problems of placing too much weight on population mortality data.

8. **A.** The BRFSS is administered by state health departments in cooperation with the CDC to assess behavioral risk factors in the US population. The BRFSS is the world's largest telephone-based survey and is the primary source that most states use to assess health behaviors. The decennial census (E) is administered by the US Census Bureau. All other surveys listed (B, C, and D) are conducted by the National Center for Health Statistics with other federal agencies.

9. **C.** NHANES is the only large survey that combines interviews, physical examinations, and biologic specimens for analysis. NHANES includes self-reported data on demographic, socioeconomic, dietary, and health-related topics. The examination component consists of medical, dental, and physiologic measurements. Biologic specimens include blood and urine for laboratory analyses. NHANES uniquely allows for correlations between reported activity and diet and various lab markers. All the other surveys (A, B, D, E) rely on subjective (self-report) data only, having no objective (e.g., physical exam or lab) components.

10. **C.** Only deaths up to 1 year are counted under infant mortality (A). Neonatal mortality is the period until 28 days (B), postneonatal mortality are deaths up to 1 year of age. Perinatal mortality covers deaths from 28 weeks pregnancy to 28 days after birth (E). Therefore, C is correct, as it covers all mortality from birth to 5 years.

25

The US Public Health System: Structure and Function

"The public health community is currently situated at the fulcrum of many of society's greatest challenges. Population health, chronic disease, emergency preparedness, and even the more familiar ground of infectious disease are all fraught with uncertainties to which public health will need to respond in the years to come. (....) [P]ublic health leaders have an opportunity to influence which future unfolds and how."

**Institute for Alternative Futures: Public Health 2030:
A Scenario Exploration.**

The US National Academy of Medicine (formerly the Institute of Medicine, IOM) describes the challenges inherent in organizing the public health system for the 21st century:

The systems and entities that protect and promote the public's health, already challenged by problems like obesity, toxic environments, a large uninsured population, and health disparities, must also confront emerging threats, such as antimicrobial resistance and bioterrorism. The social, cultural, and global contexts of the nation's health are also undergoing rapid and dramatic change. Scientific and technological advances, such as genomics and informatics, extend the limits of knowledge and human potential more rapidly than their implications can be absorbed and acted upon. At the same time, people, products, and germs migrate and the nation's demographics are shifting in ways that challenge public and private resources.[1]

The US public health system was designed at a time when most threats to health were infectious, before computer information systems, and when local autonomy prevailed. For historical reasons and in keeping with Americans' dislike of centralized structures, the US public health system is a complex network of many different public and private payers, who collaborate to varying degrees on local, state, and national levels. Surprisingly little research exists on which organizational form and public health practices provide for the best outcomes, particularly for small and rural populations.[2] This chapter describes the structure of the US health system and discusses how it must respond to contemporary challenges. Public health systems in other countries are often structured very differently but still need to adapt to the same challenges.

1. ADMINISTRATION OF US PUBLIC HEALTH

1.1 RESPONSIBILITIES OF THE FEDERAL GOVERNMENT

The public health responsibility of the US federal government is based on two clauses from Article 1, Section 8, of the US Constitution. First, the Interstate Commerce Clause gives the federal government the right "to regulate Commerce with foreign Nations, and among the several States, and with the Indian Tribes." Second, the General Welfare Clause states, "the Congress shall have Power to lay and collect Taxes . . . for the common Defense and general Welfare of the United States." Federal responsibility also is inferred from statements that Congress has the authority to create and support a military and the authority to negotiate with Indian tribes and other special groups.

1.1.a Regulation of Commerce

The regulation of commerce involves controlling the entry of people and products into the United States and regulating commercial relationships among the states. People may be excluded from entry to the United States if they have infectious health problems, such as active tuberculosis. Products may also be excluded from entry, such as fruits and vegetables if infested with certain organisms (e.g., Mediterranean fruit fly) or treated with prohibited insecticides or fungicides. As examples, similar prohibitions have been extended to the importation of animal products from cattle that might contain the prions of bovine spongiform encephalopathy and produce that might be contaminated with *Escherichia coli.*

The regulation of commercial relationships between states has increased over time. Contaminated food products that cross state lines are considered to be "interstate commerce." One example is the multistate *E. coli* O157:H7 outbreak in 2018 from contaminated romaine lettuce[3]; what crossed state lines in this case were harmful microorganisms. The federal government takes the responsibility for inspecting all milk, meat, and other food products at their site of production and processing. (In contrast, the state or local government is responsible for inspecting restaurants and food stores.) Likewise, polluted air and water flowing from state to state are deemed to be "interstate commerce" in pollution and come under federal regulation.

1.1.b Taxation for the General Welfare

The power to "tax for the general welfare" is the constitutional basis for the federal government's development and support of most of its public health programs and agencies, including the Centers for Disease Control and Prevention (CDC, part of the Department of Health and Human Services) and the Occupational Safety and Health Administration (OSHA, part of the Department of Labor); for research programs, such as those of the National Institutes of Health (NIH); and for the payment for medical care, such as Medicare and Medicaid (see Chapter 29).

1.1.c Provision of Care for Special Groups

The federal government has taken special responsibility for providing health services for special groups. Military hospitals serve active military personnel and their families; the Indian Health Service, a part of the US Public Health Service, cares for Native Americans and Alaska Natives. Lastly, veterans receive health care through the Veterans Administration medical system, the nation's largest integrated health care system.[4]

1.1.d Funding Federal Legislation

All federal medical services are funded through federal legislation. This requires a two-step process. The initial bill provides an **authorization** of funds. An authorization bill only sets an *upper limit* to the amount of funds that can be spent. No monies can be spent, however, until they have been specifically **appropriated** for that bill's purposes in a subsequent appropriations bill. The authorization is a political fiction for which members of Congress can claim political gain. In practice, the amount *appropriated* tends to be about *half* the amounts *authorized* in the bills, and the amounts are usually appropriated for only one fiscal year at a time. It is in the funding bills that fiscal (and political) reality must be faced. Because a funding bill covers many items, the voters usually are unaware that the amount actually appropriated is much smaller than the amount promised in the authorization bill.

1.1.e Coordination of Federal Agencies

In the United States the federal department most concerned with health is the Department of Health and Human Services (DHHS)[5] (Fig. 25.1). The department comprises many agencies, which administer programs, set standards, and advise on policies, such as:

- Administration on Aging
- Administration for Children and Families
- Centers for Medicare and Medicaid Services

The Centers for Medicare and Medicaid Services (CMS) is responsible for administering two major programs of the Social Security Act. **Medicare** is covered under **Title 18** of the Social Security Act and pays for medical care for the elderly population. **Medicaid** is covered under **Title 19** and pays for medical and nursing home care in cooperation with the states for low-income and needy people. Medicaid covers children, the aged, blind, and/or disabled and other people who are eligible to receive federally assisted income maintenance payments. CMS duties include setting standards for programs and institutions that provide medical care, developing payment policies, contracting for third-party payers to cover the bills, and monitoring the quality of care provided. CMS also supports graduate medical education, residency, and fellowship programs that provide care for individuals covered by Medicare or Medicaid.

Public Health Service. The US Public Health Service (PHS) comprises the following eight constituent agencies:

1. The **Agency for Healthcare Research and Quality** (AHRQ) is the main federal agency for research and policy development in the areas of medical care organization, financing, and quality assessment. Since 2000, the agency has placed increasing emphasis on medical care quality.

2. The **Agency for Toxic Substances and Disease Registry** (ATSDR) provides leadership and direction to programs designed to protect workers and the public from exposure to and adverse health effects of hazardous substances that are kept in storage sites or are released by fire, explosion, or accident.

3. The **Centers for Disease Control and Prevention** (CDC) has the responsibility for "protecting the public health of the [United States] by providing leadership and direction in the prevention and control of diseases and other preventable conditions and responding to public health emergencies." The CDC directs and enforces federal quarantine activities, works with states on disease surveillance and control activities, develops programs for prevention and immunization, is involved in research and training, makes recommendations on how to promote occupational health and safety through the *National Institute on*

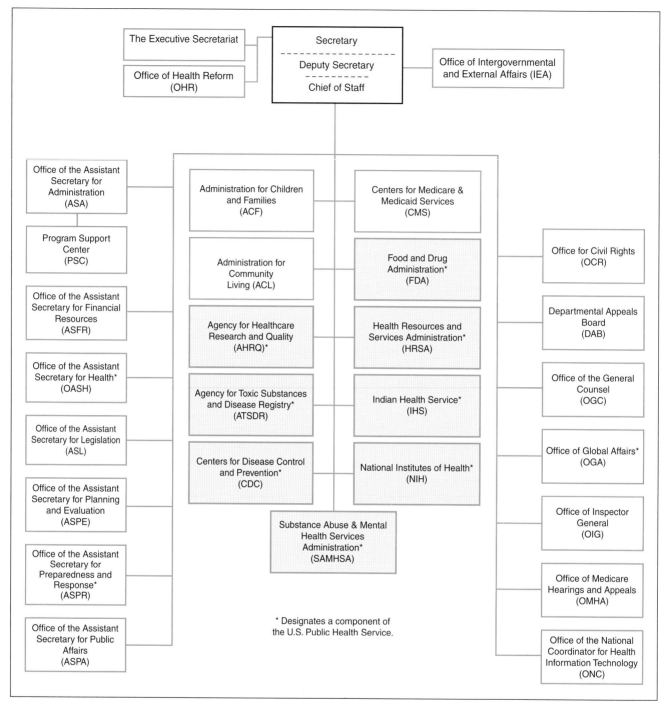

Fig. 25.1 US Department of Health and Human Services (DHHS) organizational chart. (From http://www.hhs.gov/about/orgchart.) *Office of Global Affairs operates under the Office of the secretary and is therefore not highlighted here as an agency within the public health service (see below)

Occupational Safety and Health (NIOSH), provides consultation to other nations in the control of preventable diseases, and participates with international agencies in the eradication and control of diseases around the world. The CDC has a complex organizational structure (Fig. 25.2).

4. The **Food and Drug Administration** (FDA) is the primary agency for regulating the safety and effectiveness of drugs for use in humans and animals, vaccines and other biologic products, diagnostic tests, and medical devices (including ionizing and nonionizing radiation–emitting electronic products). The FDA is also responsible for the safety, quality, and labeling of cosmetics, foods, and food additives and colorings.

5. The **Health Resources and Services Administration** (HRSA) is responsible for developing human resources and methods to improve health care access, equity, and quality, with an emphasis on promoting primary care. HRSA also supports training grants and training programs in preventive medicine and public health.

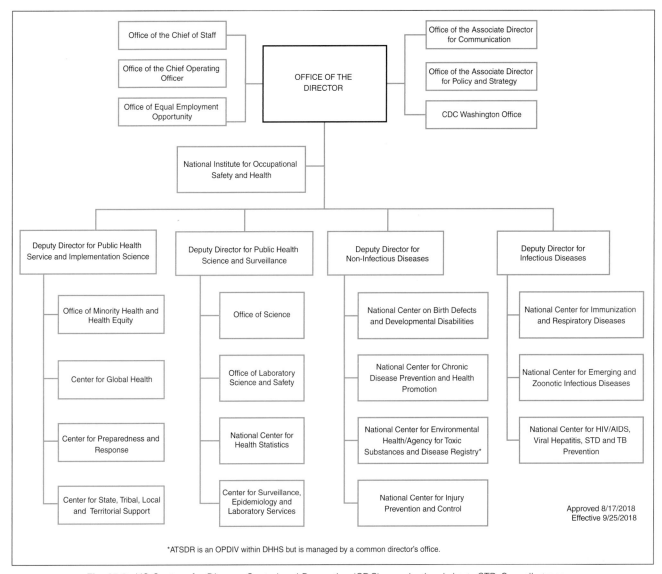

Fig. 25.2   US Centers for Disease Control and Prevention (CDC) organizational chart. *STD,* Sexually transmitted disease; *TB,* tuberculosis. (From https://www.cdc.gov/maso/pdf/CDC_Official.pdf.)

6. The **Indian Health Service** promotes the health of and provides medical care for Native Americans and Alaska Natives.

7. The **National Institutes of Health** (NIH) consists of 27 institutes and centers, which perform *intramural* (in-house) research on their particular diseases, organ systems, or topics (e.g., National Cancer Institute; National Heart, Lung, and Blood Institute; National Human Genome Research Institute; National Center for Advancing Translational Science). The institutes also review and sponsor *extramural* research at universities and research organizations through competitive grant programs. Some of the institutes also undertake disease control programs and public and professional education in their area (e.g., National Library of Medicine, National Institute for Neurological Disorders and Stroke).

8. The **Substance Abuse and Mental Health Services Administration** (SAMHSA) provides national leadership in preventing and treating addiction and other mental disorders, based on up-to-date science and practices, and has four major operating divisions: Center for Mental Health Services, Center for Substance Abuse Prevention, Center for Substance Abuse Treatment, and Center for Behavioral Health Statistics and Quality.

Furthermore, two staff offices within the Public Health Service also have public health impact: the **Office of the Assistant Secretary for Preparedness and Response** and the **Office of Global Affairs**. The Public Health Service is not the only important agency in public health. The other major federal organization is the Office of Public Health and Science (OPHS), which leads the Healthy People initiative through its Office of Disease Prevention and Promotion and leadership and coordination on many important public health topics, such as minority health, human immunodeficiency virus (HIV) and acquired immunodeficiency syndrome (AIDS) policy, vaccines programs, and many more. The US Surgeon General's office is also part of the OPHS (Fig. 25.3).

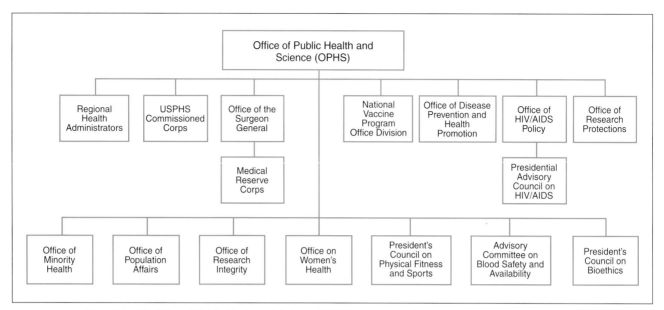

Fig. 25.3 US Office of Public Health and Science (OPHS) organizational structure. *HIV/AIDS,* Human immunodeficiency virus and acquired immunodeficiency syndrome. (From http://www.hhs.gov/about/orgchart/ophs.html.)

1.2 RESPONSIBILITIES OF STATES

In the United States the fundamental responsibility for the health of the public lies with the states. This authority derives from the 10th Amendment to the Constitution: "The powers not delegated to the United States by the Constitution, nor prohibited by it to the States, are reserved to the States respectively, or to the people."

As the mission of public health is to ensure conditions in which people can be healthy, the three core functions of public health agencies at all levels of government, including at the state level, are assessment, policy development, and assurance.[6]

1. The **assessment** role requires that the public health agency (a) systematically collects and analyzes data on the health status of individuals and the community, and (b) makes this information available.
2. The **policy development** role requires that the public health agency aids in developing comprehensive public health policies by promoting the use of the scientific knowledge base in decision making about public health, by leading in developing public health policy, and by taking a strategic approach.
3. The **assurance** role requires that public health agencies ensure that their constituents receive necessary services by (a) encouraging action by other entities (private or public sector), (b) requiring such action through regulation, or (c) providing services directly.

Within these three core functions, 10 essential public health services have been defined (Box 25.1). Administrators and others involved in public health have been struggling to define how the mission and three core functions can best be

BOX 25.1 Governmental Public Health Infrastructure: The 10 Essential Public Health Services

Assessment
1. Monitor health status to identify community health problems.
2. Diagnose and investigate health problems and health hazards in the community.

Public and Policy Development
3. Inform, educate, and empower people about health issues.
4. Mobilize community partnerships to identify and solve health problems.
5. Develop policies and plans that support individual and community health efforts.

Assurance
6. Enforce laws and regulations that protect health and ensure safety.
7. Link people to needed personal health services and assure the provision of health care when otherwise unavailable.
8. Ensure a competent public health and personal health care workforce.
9. Evaluate effectiveness, accessibility, and quality of personal and population-based health services.

Serving All Functions
10. Research for new insights and innovate solutions to health problems.

From US Centers for Disease Control and Prevention: https://www.cdc.gov/stltpublichealth/publichealthservices/essentialhealthservices.html

fulfilled. As indicated by the assurance role, public health agencies enjoy considerable latitude. Although not required to provide all (or even most of) the services themselves, the agencies are expected to use all their authority and resources to ensure that needed policies, laws, regulations, and services exist.

Each state has a health department to perform or oversee the performance of the 10 essential public health services. The state health department oversees the implementation of the **public health code,** a compilation of the state laws and regulations regarding public health and safety. (Laws are rules passed by a legislature. In contrast, **regulations** are technical rules added later by an empowered body with specific expertise, such as a state or local board of health.) In some states, responsibility for mental health services falls to the health department, whereas other states have separate departments of mental health services. Every state also licenses medical and other health-related practitioners and medical care institutions, such as hospitals, nursing homes, and home care programs.

1.3   RESPONSIBILITIES OF MUNICIPALITIES AND COUNTIES

Although the states hold the fundamental police power to protect health, they delegate much of this authority to chartered **municipalities,** such as cities, or other incorporated areas. These municipalities accept public health responsibilities in return for a considerable degree of independence from the state in running their affairs, including property ownership and tax levies. In this respect, the municipalities differ from **counties.** Counties are bureaucratic subdivisions of the state created to administer state responsibilities (with varying degrees of local control), such as health services, as well as courts of law, educational programs, highway construction and maintenance, and police and fire protection.

Local public health departments usually are administrative divisions of municipalities or counties, and their policies are established by a city or county **board of health.** These boards of health have the right to establish public health laws and regulations, provided that they are at least as strict as similar laws and regulations in the state public health code, and provided that they are *reasonable.* Anything that is too strict risks being overturned by the courts on the grounds that it is *unreasonable.*

The courts have generally upheld local and state health department laws and regulations when they pertain to the control of communicable diseases. The courts have also upheld laws relating to safe water and subsurface sewage disposal, immunization, regulation of restaurants and food stores, quarantine or treatment of persons with an infectious disease, investigation and control of acute disease outbreaks, and abatement of complaints relating to the spread of infectious disease (e.g., rabid animals).

Outside the area of communicable diseases, neither legislatures nor courts have been as supportive of laws and regulations. Laws requiring motorcyclists and bicyclists to wear helmets sometimes have not been enacted or have been repealed, despite abundant evidence of their benefits.[7] If an individual risk factor for disease can be shown to have a negative *public* impact, however, such as passive smoke inhalation, legislatures usually support controls, provided the direct fiscal impact is minimal.

1.4   RESPONSIBILITIES OF LOCAL PUBLIC HEALTH DEPARTMENTS

1.4.a   "Basic Six" to Winnable Battles

The best-known description of the responsibilities of local health departments defines six primary areas of responsibilities[8]:
1. Collecting vital statistics
2. Controlling communicable diseases
3. Protecting maternal and child health
4. Monitoring and protecting environmental health
5. Promoting health education
6. Maintaining public health laboratories

These functions of local health departments, known as the "basic six," influence the direction of local departments, despite the many changes in the nature of public health problems over time. However, these six functions are not fully adequate to deal with some more recent public health problems, such as environmental pollution crossing state lines and the increased incidence of chronic degenerative diseases. For a time, public health leaders debated the proper functions and responsibilities of health departments at the local and state levels.[9,10] To help health departments in evaluating their work, the CDC has created a National Public Health Performance Standards Program that creates a framework to identify areas for system improvement, to strengthen state and local partnerships, and to ensure that a strong system is in place for providing the 10 essential public health services (see "Accreditation in Public Health" later in the chapter).[11] These standards aim to:
- Improve communication and collaboration
- Educate participants about public health and the interconnectedness of public health activities
- Strengthen the network of partnering agencies within state and local public health systems
- Aid in quality improvement efforts
- Provide a benchmark for public health practice improvements.[11]

As part of the performance standards, the CDC provides self-assessment instruments for various public health agencies. These include questions such as, "At what level does the local health system conduct regular community health assessments?" and "At what level does the local health system use computer software to prepare charts, graphs, and maps to display complex public health data?"[12] Results of these self-assessments can be used in community health intervention models such as the MAP-IT tool (see Chapter 26). Public health agencies perennially struggle to garner enough popular and government support to promote health and prevent disease effectively. Nonetheless, Americans have benefited greatly from the many achievements of public health efforts, in conjunction with laboratory research, clinical medicine, and sanitary and safety engineering. Box 25.2 provides the CDC's list of the 10 leading public health achievements of the 20th century. For the 21st century, the following domains have been defined as "winnable battles"[13]:

- Food safety
- Global immunization against polio, measles, rubella, meningitis, pneumococci, and rotaviruses
- Healthcare-associated infections
- HIV infection
- Lymphatic filariasis
- Mother-to-child transmission of HIV and congenital syphilis
- Motor vehicle injuries
- Nutrition, physical activity, and obesity
- Teen pregnancy
- Tobacco use (especially smoking)

The CDC tracks progress on winnable battles on a dedicated website.[14] The winnable battles program signaled an effort to increase collaboration between the CDC and local agencies around issues which have the following[15]:

- A large-scale impact on health
- Evidence-based and feasible interventions
- Intensive focus and efforts that have a significant impact in a relatively short period of time

While progress on the winnable battles targets has been mixed, the strategy itself clearly has broader applicability in public health.

1.4.b Health Director's Duties

The programs run by a local health department vary by region or county and depend on available funding, state and local priorities, and availability of other providers and institutions. Some local health departments manage a complex set of services, including mental health and primary care for underserved populations, which involves managing teams and human resources, analyzing organizational performance, and overseeing budgeting analysis. Health directors must

adhere to applicable federal and state rules when they hire, evaluate, and fire employees. Directors must also ensure that employees are supervised appropriately, including regular performance evaluation, pay equity to comparable jobs, and compliance with grievance process. Particular challenges arise if different staff members with similar responsibilities are paid from different payrolls (e.g., county, city, state, grant funders).

In addition to running these services, the health director serves as the *chief health policy advisor* to local elected officials for public health, community assessment, access to medical care, and financing of health and medical care.[16] The director also serves as the *chief public health educator* for politicians and the public, to ensure ongoing funding, grassroots support, and collaboration with community groups and health care institutions. In the future, the health director's role is likely to shift further in the efforts to become the "chief health strategist" in a community (see upcoming discussion).

1.4.c Environmental Protection

Among the functions of local health departments, protecting the public from foodborne illness and inspecting septic systems are among the most important.

Restaurant inspection. Most contamination occurs through just a few breakdowns: unwashed hands, improper cooking, improper storage, unclean utensils, and contact between food and nonfood surfaces.[16] Local food regulations vary by county and district. However, most local health departments inspect restaurants episodically, assign points for violations of code depending on the gravity of violations, and provide grades to restaurants as a summary assessment (e.g., A–C or colors). Some health departments also provide certificates of excellence. Health inspectors particularly look at major violations that pose an immediate health hazard, as follows[17]:

- Improper hand hygiene or overall hygiene (i.e., employees working while sick)
- Food is not kept at temperatures high enough or low enough to inhibit bacterial growth
- Incorrect sanitizer concentrations of dishwasher or cleaning solutions
- Cross-contamination between raw and cooked products
- Plumbing hazards (e.g., no hot water, defective waste-water disposal)
- Presence of vermin

If an establishment is found to pose an immediate hazard, or if it has a history of persistent failure to comply with recommendations, health inspectors can shut it down. In those cases, the establishment usually cannot reopen until the health inspector has returned to confirm that the violations have been corrected. Some departments also perform compliance inspections for restaurants with borderline scores to document improvement.[18]

Wastewater disposal. Many rural areas have no central sewage system. Every new building needs a septic tank and a "drain field," the size of which varies with the drainage pattern and depth of the topsoil. Otherwise, raw sewage may contaminate an aquifer and pollute everybody's drinking water. Given the amount of money involved in developing land and the potential for damage, the health director and environmental staff need to coordinate closely with local and county officials in planning and zoning and the granting of building permits.[16]

In an age of vanishing rain forests, receding polar ice caps, and progressive climate change, environmental protection has taken on new meaning. Such issues as conservation and biopreservation intersect meaningfully with public health (see concept of One Health in Chapter 30).

1.4.d Accreditation in Public Health

In 2004, the CDC identified accreditation as a key strategy to strengthen the infrastructure and performance of public health. As a result, the public health accreditation board was formed, which published accreditation standards in 2009. These were further refined, with standards published in 2011.[19] While accreditation is voluntary, it is a powerful tool for continuous quality improvement in public health agencies through:

- The measurement of health department performance against a set of nationally recognized, practice-focused, and evidenced-based benchmarks.
- The issuance of recognition of achievement of accreditation within a specified time frame by a nationally recognized entity.
- The continuing development, revision, and distribution of public health standards.[20]

2. BROADER DEFINITIONS OF PUBLIC HEALTH POLICY

The current view of public health policy in the United States is narrower than that in the world public health scene. According to the **Ottawa Charter for Health Promotion,** which guides much of the international work in this area, health promotion requires that *all* policies be reviewed for their health impact and adjusted to strengthen, rather than hinder, the effort to achieve good health, as follows:

"Health promotion goes beyond health care. It puts health on the agenda of policy makers in all sectors and at all levels, directing them to be aware of the health consequences of their decisions and to accept their responsibilities for health.

Health promotion policy combines diverse but complementary approaches including legislation, fiscal measures, taxation and organizational change. Ideally, it should increase the health of vulnerable populations most to achieve greater health equity. Joint action contributes to ensuring safer and healthier goods and services, healthier public services, and cleaner, more enjoyable environments.

Health promotion policy requires identification of obstacles to the adoption of healthy public policies in non-health sectors, and ways of removing them. The aim must be to make the healthier choice the easier choice for policy makers as well."[21]

The switch from *public health policy* to *healthy public policies* is subtle but important. The point of this approach was that *all* public policies must be evaluated and, if necessary, modified for their impact on public health.

3. INTERSECTORAL APPROACH TO PUBLIC HEALTH

So far, this chapter has emphasized the role of specific US public health agencies at the federal, state, and local levels. However, as the Ottawa Charter emphasizes, many duties with public health implications are carried out by government agencies that are not usually considered "health agencies." Departments of **agriculture** are responsible for monitoring the safety of milk, meat, and other agricultural products and controlling zoonoses (animal diseases that can be spread to humans). The US Department of Agriculture (USDA) also administers the program for **Women, Infants, and Children** (WIC), which supports low-income women and children up to age 5 who are at nutritional risk by providing foods to supplement diets and financial support. This program has a substantial impact on food choices, childhood obesity, and oral health. Departments of **parks and recreation** must monitor the safety of water and sewage disposal in their facilities. **Highway** departments are responsible for the safe design and maintenance of roads and highways. **Education** departments are charged with overseeing health education and providing a safe and healthful environment in which to learn. Government departments that promote a **healthy economy** are crucial as well, because when an economy falters, the people's health suffers as well.

Because health is the result of the entire fabric of the environment and life of a population, a true public health approach must be **intersectoral;** that is, it must consider the health impact of policies in every sector of a society and government, not just in the health sector or medical care sector. Intriguingly, countries that spend relatively more on social priorities such as housing and social services than health care services may have better health outcomes.[22] The perspectives of the Ottawa Charter and **intersectoral policy analysis** are foundations for the broader, more community action–oriented approach to public health currently emphasized in Europe and elsewhere. This approach is sometimes called the "healthy communities" approach[23].

The United States is fortunate to be home to many voluntary health agencies and other **nongovernmental organizations (NGOs)** whose focus is to prevent or control diseases and promote health. Some focus on certain diseases (e.g., American Heart Association [AHA], American Lung Association [ALA]), and others confront a related group of diseases (e.g., American Cancer Society [ACS]). Sometimes groups join forces; cigarette smoking is a major risk factor for heart disease, lung disease, and cancer, so the AHA, ALA, and ACS have worked together to curtail smoking. These organizations raise money for research, public education, and preventive programs. Some NGOs even provide direct patient care, such as Planned Parenthood, which strives for a comprehensive approach to reproductive health. These agencies strive to fill the gaps left by the public health system. At the same time, these agencies form important stakeholders that can substantially influence the success or failure of public health initiatives.

4. ORGANIZATIONS IN PREVENTIVE MEDICINE AND PUBLIC HEALTH

Many organizations in the United States emphasize public health and preventive medicine; the largest is the **American Public Health Association** (APHA), with annual meetings typically bringing together 12,000 to 15,000 people. APHA has gradually changed from an organization focusing on science and the practice of public health to one emphasizing national public health and medical care policy, although some sections still emphasize science or practice. It publishes the *American Journal of Public Health* and welcomes as members anyone who is trained in, working in, or just interested in public health.

The Public Health Accreditation Board (PHAB) is a nonprofit organization dedicated to improving and protecting the health of the public by advancing and ultimately transforming the quality and performance of state, local, tribal, and territorial public health departments through accreditation (see earlier discussion).

Other organizations that promote the health of communities include **American College of Preventive Medicine** (ACPM) and **Association of Teachers of Preventive Medicine** (ATPM). With ATPM, ACPM copublishes the *American Journal of Preventive Medicine* and cosponsors a yearly conference on prevention science and policy. ATPM members include university faculty, preventive medicine residency program directors and faculty, and others interested in teaching health promotion and disease prevention in schools of medicine, public health, and other health professions. The goal of ATPM is to improve research, training, and practice in preventive medicine and to support the funding for training programs. Chapter 14 provides more details on training for physicians. A newer organization, the American College of Lifestyle Medicine, focuses more on providing individuals with the knowledge and tools to protect their health (see Websites at the end of the chapter).

5. ASSESSMENT AND FUTURE TRENDS

A 2002 IOM report on the status of the US public health system remains relevant[1]:

> *"The governmental public health infrastructure has suffered from political neglect and from the pressure of political agendas and public opinion that frequently override empirical evidence. Under the glare of a national crisis [attacks of 9/11/2001, Hurricane Katrina], policy makers and the public became aware of vulnerable and outdated health information systems and technologies, an insufficient and inadequately trained public health workforce, antiquated laboratory capacity, a lack of real-time surveillance and epidemiological systems, ineffective and fragmented communications networks, incomplete domestic preparedness and emergency response capabilities, and communities without access to essential public health services. These problems leave the nation's health vulnerable—and not only to exotic germs and bioterrorism."*

In response to this report and other voices, DHHS has disseminated sample policies, established grant programs to upgrade and integrate information systems, and developed an accreditation system for public health providers and local health departments. However, much remains to be done so that the public health system can maintain the gains made in the 20th century and prepare for the challenges of the 21st century.

To do so, public health practitioners need to address factors outside the traditional purview of public health, such as education, safe environments, housing, transportation, economic development, and access to healthy foods.[24] To facilitate providing such services, the CDC has developed a "three buckets of prevention" model for Public Health 3.0 (Fig. 25.4).[23]

To achieve such community-wide prevention, five major recommendations have been made[24]:

1. Public health leaders should think of themselves as chief health strategists, and work with all relevant partners to address "upstream" social determinants of health.
2. Public health departments should collaborate with community stakeholders to form cross-sector partnerships.
3. Public Health Accreditation Board criteria and processes for department accreditation should be enhanced and supported, so that every person in the United States is served by nationally accredited health departments.
4. Timely, reliable, local-level, and actionable data should be made accessible to communities throughout the country, and clear metrics to document success in public health practice should be developed to guide, focus, and assess the impact of prevention initiatives.
5. Funding for public health should be enhanced and substantially modified, by allowing blending and braiding of funds from multiple sources, and the recapturing and reinvesting of generated revenue.

Public health is indeed at the "fulcrum of many of society's greatest challenges."[25] Big data, climate change, rapid dissemination of knowledge, and widespread use of social media all have the capacity of hindering or helping a future in which public health integrates with clinical care and best data to achieve a "health system" rather than a "health care system." How public health infrastructure responds to the challenges will determine which future we will live in.[25]

6. SUMMARY

Public health services in the United States are provided by the federal, state, and local levels of government, although the primary authority for health lies with the states. The federal government becomes involved in health mostly by regulating international and interstate commerce and by its power to tax for the general welfare. Local governments become involved

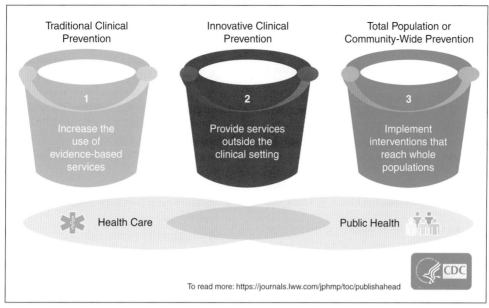

Fig. 25.4 CDC's "three buckets of prevention" model. (From https://nam.edu/public-health-3-0-call-action-public-health-meet-challenges-21st-century.)

in health as the states delegate authority for health to them. The fundamental health responsibilities have expanded greatly from the "basic six" minimum functions, when infectious diseases were the greatest concern, to a large and diverse set of functions that now include the control of chronic diseases, injuries, and environmental toxins. In the intersectoral approach to public health, all public policies are scrutinized for their impact on health. In the future, Public Health 3.0 will hopefully address "upstream" social determinants of health in an integrated way.

REFERENCES

1. Institute of Medicine. *The Future of the Public's Health in the 21st Century.* Washington, DC: National Academies Press; 2002. http://www.nationalacademies.org/hmd/Reports/2002/The-Future-of-the-Publics-Health-in-the-21st-Century.aspx, Accessed September 10, 2019.
2. Hyde JK, Shortell SM. The structure and organization of local and state public health agencies in the U.S.: a systematic review. *Am J Prev Med.* 2012;42:S29-S41.
3. Centers for Disease Control and Prevention. *Multistate Outbreak of E. Coli O157:H7 Infections Linked to Romaine Lettuce (Final Update).* June 28, 2018. Available at: https://www.cdc.gov/ecoli/2018/o157h7-04-18/index.html.
4. U.S. Department of Veterans Affairs. *Veterans Health Administration.* Available at: https://www.va.gov/health/. Accessed September 10, 2019.
5. U.S. Department of Health and Human Services. Available at: http://www.hhs.gov. Accessed September 10, 2019
6. Institute of Medicine. *The Future of Public Health.* Washington, DC: National Academies Press; 1988.
7. Centers for Disease Control and Prevention. Injury-control recommendations: bicycle helmets. *MMWR.* 1995;44:1-17.
8. Jekel JF. Health departments in the U.S. 1920-1988: statements of mission with special reference to the role of C.-E.A. Winslow. *Yale J Biol Med.* 1991;64:467-479.
9. Hanlon JJ. Is there a future for local health departments? *Health Serv Rep.* 1973;88:898-901.
10. Terris M. The epidemiologic revolution, national health insurance, and the role of health departments. *Am J Public Health.* 1976;66:1155-1164.
11. Centers for Disease Control and Prevention. *National Public Health Performance Standards.* Available at: https://www.cdc.gov/stltpublichealth/nphps/index.html. Accessed September 10, 2019.
12. Association of State and Territorial Health Officials. *National Public Health Performance Standards Version 3: Score Sheet and Report.* 2019. Available at: http://www.astho.org/Programs/Accreditation-and-Performance/National-Public-Health-Performance-Standards/Scoresheet-and-Report/Version-3/Overview-Slides/.
13. Centers for Disease Control and Prevention. *Winnable Battles.* Available at: http://www.cdc.gov/winnablebattles/FocusAreas.html. Accessed September 10, 2019.
14. Centers for Disease Control and Prevention. *Winnable Battles:* Progress Reports. 2017. Available at: https://www.cdc.gov/winnablebattles/report/progress-targets.html.
15. Centers for Disease Control and Prevention. *Winnable Battles: Final Report.* 2017. Available at: https://www.cdc.gov/winnablebattles/report/docs/winnable-battles-final-report.pdf.
16. Buttery CMG. *The Local Health Department.* Chapter 1. 2012. Available at: http://www.commed.vcu.edu/LOCAL/2012/Ch1_local_health_director_12.pdf.
17. San Francisco Department of Public Health. *Environmental Health: Food Safety Program: Violation Types.* Available at: https://www.sfdph.org/dph/EH/Food/Score/Violation.asp. Accessed September 10, 2019.
18. New York City Department of Health and Mental Hygiene. *Letter Grading for Restaurants.* 2012. Available at: https://www1.nyc.gov/assets/doh/downloads/pdf/rii/how-we-score-grade.pdf. Accessed September 10, 2019.

19. Public Health Accreditation Board. *Accreditation Background.* Available at: https://phaboard.org/accreditation-background/. Accessed September 10, 2019.

20. Public Health Accreditation Board. *What is Public Health Department Accreditation: Overview.* Available at: http://www.phaboard.org/what-is-public-health-department-accreditation/.

21. Ottawa Charter for Health Promotion. Report of an International Conference on Health Promotion, sponsored by the World Health Organization, Health and Welfare Canada, and the Canadian Public Health Association, Ottawa, 1986.

22. Bradley EH, Canavan M, Rogan E, et al. Variation in health outcomes: the role of spending on social services, public health, and health care, 2000-09. *Health Aff (Millwood).* 2016;35:760-768.

23. Ashton J. *The New Public Health.* Buckingham, UK: Open University Press; 1988.

24. National Academy of Medicine. *Public Health 3.0: A Call to Action for Public Health to Meet the Challenges of the 21st Century.* Discussion Paper September 7, 2017. Available at: https://nam.edu/public-health-3-0-call-action-public-health-meet-challenges-21st-century/.

25. Institute for Alternative Futures. *Public Health 2030: A Scenario Exploration.* Alexandria, VA: 2014. Available at: www.altfutures.org/pubs/PH2030/IAF-PublicHealth2030Scenarios.pdf.

SELECT READINGS

Douglas FD, Keck CW. Structure and function of the public health system in the United States. In: Wallace RB, ed. *Maxcy-Rosenau-Last: Public Health and Preventive Medicine.* 15th ed. New York, NY: McGraw-Hill Medical; 2008.

Institute for Alternative Futures. *Public Health 2030: A Scenario Exploration.* Alexandria, VA: 2014. Available at: www.altfutures.org/pubs/PH2030/IAF-PublicHealth2030Scenarios.pdf.

Institute of Medicine. *For the Public's Health: Revitalizing Law and Policy to Meet New Challenges.* Washington, DC: National Academies Press; 2011.

Lewenson SB, ed. *Public Health Nursing: Practicing Population-Based Care.* Cambridge, MA: Jones & Bartlett Learning; 2017.

Novick LF, Morrow CB, Mays GP. *Public Health Administration. Principles for Population-Based Management.* 2nd ed. Boston Toronto London Singapore: Jones & Bartlett; 2008.

WEBSITES

American College of Preventive Medicine: www.acpm.org

American Public Health Organization: www.apha.org

Lifestyle Medicine: https://www.lifestylemedicine.org/

Public Health Accreditation Board: http://www.phaboard.org/

Robert Wood Johnson Program for leaders of health who want to promote health and equity: http://cultureofhealth-leaders.org/about-the-program/

Winnable Battles: https://www.cdc.gov/winnablebattles/index.html

REVIEW QUESTIONS

1. The authority of the US federal government to inspect food and regulate air pollutants derives from the:
   A. Department of Agriculture
   B. Environmental Protection Agency
   C. Food and Drug Administration (FDA)
   D. Interstate commerce clause in US Constitution
   E. Centers for Disease Control and Prevention (CDC)

2. The FDA and the CDC are appropriately categorized as:
   A. Constituent agencies of the Public Health Service
   B. Agencies that are subject to state law
   C. Agencies that are independent of the federal government
   D. Major operating units of the Department of Health and Human Services
   E. Major operating units of the Environmental Protection Agency

3. Public health laws established by city or county boards of health must be:
   A. Approved by referendum
   B. Approved by the state
   C. At least as strict as regulations in the state public health code
   D. Revised annually
   E. Free of control on human behavior (nonchallenging of free will)

4. Which is *true* of funding of federal legislation, including legislation for policies and programs related to health?
   A. This two-stage process requires an approval bill and then an appropriations bill
   B. This two-stage process requires an appropriations bill and then an authorization bill
   C. This two-stage process requires an authorization bill and then an appropriations bill
   D. This three-stage process requires an authorization bill, an appropriations bill, and then an approval bill
   E. This three-stage process requires an authorization bill, an appropriations bill, and then approval by a congressional committee

5. A health inspector from a local health department identifies a significant plumbing hazard in a restaurant: The main prep sink is not properly piped, allowing kitchen waste materials to potentially contact food that might be served. Given this immediate hazard, what would be the correct next step?
   A. Forgive this one problem given the restaurant's stellar performance on all other measures in the inspection
   B. Issue a written warning and suggest that a licensed plumbing contractor be consulted
   C. Assess a fine for the violation, with additional penalties to be assessed if the issue is not promptly addressed
   D. Close the restaurant and disallow reopening until the sink is properly piped
   E. Issue a summons to appear in court for willful endangerment of the public's health

6. The USDA administers a program to improve nutrition for low-income individuals that specifically excludes, among others, adult men. The program is called:
   A. Medicaid
   B. Food Stamps
   C. SNAP

D. WIC
E. EBT

7. Match the administrative body (A–P) with the corresponding definition or description provided (not all agencies will be identified).
Oversees Medicare and Medicaid
A. Administration on Aging
B. Administration for Children and Families
C. Centers for Disease Control and Prevention
D. Department of Health and Human Services
E. Environmental Protection Agency
F. Food and Drug Administration
G. Centers for Medicare and Medicaid Services
H. Health Resources and Services Administration
I. National Academy of Medicine
J. National Center for Health Statistics
K. National Institute of Environmental Health Sciences
L. National Institute for Occupational Safety and Health
M. National Institutes of Health
N. Occupational Safety and Health Administration
O. Social Security Administration
P. US Preventive Services Task Force

8. Match the administrative body (A–P) with the corresponding definition or description provided (not all agencies will be identified).
Responsible for infectious disease surveillance
A. Administration on Aging
B. Administration for Children and Families
C. Centers for Disease Control and Prevention
D. Department of Health and Human Services
E. Environmental Protection Agency
F. Food and Drug Administration
G. Centers for Medicare and Medicaid Services
H. Health Resources and Services Administration
I. National Academy of Medicine
J. National Center for Health Statistics
K. National Institute of Environmental Health Sciences
L. National Institute for Occupational Safety and Health
M. National Institutes of Health
N. Occupational Safety and Health Administration
O. Social Security Administration
P. US Preventive Services Task Force

9. Match the administrative body (A–P) with the corresponding definition or description provided (not all agencies will be identified).
Responsible for the funding of biomedical research
A. Administration on Aging
B. Administration for Children and Families
C. Centers for Disease Control and Prevention
D. Department of Health and Human Services
E. Environmental Protection Agency
F. Food and Drug Administration
G. Centers for Medicare and Medicaid Services
H. Health Resources and Services Administration

I. National Academy of Medicine
J. National Center for Health Statistics
K. National Institute of Environmental Health Sciences
L. National Institute for Occupational Safety and Health
M. National Institutes of Health
N. Occupational Safety and Health Administration
O. Social Security Administration
P. US Preventive Services Task Force

10. Match the administrative body (A–P) with the corresponding definition or description provided (not all agencies will be identified).
Generates and provides numerator data for US population statistics
A. Administration on Aging
B. Administration for Children and Families
C. Centers for Disease Control and Prevention
D. Department of Health and Human Services
E. Environmental Protection Agency
F. Food and Drug Administration
G. Centers for Medicare and Medicaid Services
H. Health Resources and Services Administration
I. National Academy of Medicine
J. National Center for Health Statistics
K. National Institute of Environmental Health Sciences
L. National Institute for Occupational Safety and Health
M. National Institutes of Health
N. Occupational Safety and Health Administration
O. Social Security Administration
P. US Preventive Services Task Force

11. Match the administrative body (A–P) with the corresponding definition or description provided (not all agencies will be identified).
Enforces workplace standards
A. Administration on Aging
B. Administration for Children and Families
C. Centers for Disease Control and Prevention
D. Department of Health and Human Services
E. Environmental Protection Agency
F. Food and Drug Administration
G. Centers for Medicare and Medicaid Services
H. Health Resources and Services Administration
I. National Academy of Medicine
J. National Center for Health Statistics
K. National Institute of Environmental Health Sciences
L. National Institute for Occupational Safety and Health
M. National Institutes of Health
N. Occupational Safety and Health Administration
O. Social Security Administration
P. US Preventive Services Task Force

12. Match the administrative body (A–P) with the corresponding definition or description provided (not all agencies will be identified).
Oversees the Behavioral Risk Factor Surveillance System
A. Administration on Aging

B. Administration for Children and Families
C. Centers for Disease Control and Prevention
D. Department of Health and Human Services
E. Environmental Protection Agency
F. Food and Drug Administration
G. Centers for Medicare and Medicaid Services
H. Health Resources and Services Administration
I. National Academy of Medicine
J. National Center for Health Statistics
K. National Institute of Environmental Health Sciences
L. National Institute for Occupational Safety and Health
M. National Institutes of Health
N. Occupational Safety and Health Administration
O. Social Security Administration
P. US Preventive Services Task Force

13. Match the administrative body (A–P) with the corresponding definition or description provided (not all agencies will be identified).
Responsible for promoting access and equity in health care
A. Administration on Aging
B. Administration for Children and Families
C. Centers for Disease Control and Prevention
D. Department of Health and Human Services
E. Environmental Protection Agency
F. Food and Drug Administration
G. Centers for Medicare and Medicaid Services
H. Health Resources and Services Administration
I. National Academy of Medicine
J. National Center for Health Statistics
K. National Institute of Environmental Health Sciences
L. National Institute for Occupational Safety and Health
M. National Institutes of Health
N. Occupational Safety and Health Administration
O. Social Security Administration
P. US Preventive Services Task Force

14. Match the administrative body (A–P) with the corresponding definition or description provided (not all agencies will be identified).
Responsible for regulating the safety and effectiveness of vaccines
A. Administration on Aging
B. Administration for Children and Families
C. Centers for Disease Control and Prevention
D. Department of Health and Human Services
E. Environmental Protection Agency
F. Food and Drug Administration
G. Centers for Medicare and Medicaid Services
H. Health Resources and Services Administration
I. National Academy of Medicine
J. National Center for Health Statistics
K. National Institute of Environmental Health Sciences
L. National Institute for Occupational Safety and Health
M. National Institutes of Health
N. Occupational Safety and Health Administration
O. Social Security Administration
P. US Preventive Services Task Force

ANSWERS AND EXPLANATIONS

1. **D.** Most of the responsibility for protecting the public health resides with the states. Factors that influence health but cross state lines often fall under federal jurisdiction. Contaminated food products and air pollutants are apt to cross state lines and are considered a form of (undesirable) interstate commerce. As such, their regulation is a federal responsibility under the interstate commerce clause of the US Constitution. Another clause allows for taxation for the common defense and general welfare and the creation of most public health programs, offices, and agencies, including the Department of Agriculture (A), Environmental Protection Agency (B), Food and Drug Administration (C), and Centers for Disease Control and Prevention (E).

2. **A.** The Centers for Disease Control and Prevention (CDC) is responsible for the investigation and control of communicable diseases and other public health threats. The Food and Drug Administration (FDA) is responsible for regulating the safety and effectiveness of drugs, vaccines, and additives to the food supply. The CDC and FDA, along with six other agencies, are incorporated within the Public Health Service, a major operating unit of the Department of Health and Human Services (D). The CDC and FDA are part of the federal government (vs C), not subject to state law (vs B), and not part of the Environmental Protection Agency (vs E), which does not fall under DHHS.

3. **C.** City and county boards of health receive their authority by the state government, which has the fundamental responsibility for protecting the public health. These boards may generate local policy regulations that comply with statewide standards. In other words, any adopted law must be at least as strict as the state public health code. However, laws that are too strict may be deemed "unreasonable" and challenged in court. Laws need not be free of control of human behavior (E); indeed, most public health laws will compromise individual autonomy to some degree for the greater public good. Such compromise is generally considered reasonable where cases of communicable diseases are concerned, but are often challenged as unreasonable in other cases. Public health laws established by city or county boards of health do not need to be approved by referendum (A), revised annually (D), or approved by the state (B), although as noted, must comply with state public health code.

4. **C.** The funding of federal legislation is a two-step process. An initial bill provides an authorization of funds, which is really only setting an upper limit to the amount of funds that can be spent. No monies can be spent under a bill, however, until they are specifically appropriated for that bill's purposes in a subsequent appropriations bill. There is no "approval bill" (A and D); the appropriations bill approves how monies will be appropriated. There is no subsequent approval

required by any congressional committee (E) once an appropriations bill passes. Appropriation never precedes authorization (B).

5. **D.** If an establishment is found to pose an immediate hazard or has a history of persistent failure to comply with recommendations, health inspectors may close it. In these cases, the restaurant usually cannot reopen until a reinspection documents resolution of the offense(s). A health inspector should not overlook a potentially serious immediate health hazard, even if isolated (A). Neither a warning (B) nor a fine (C) would be sufficient in this case to protect public health. However, it is not an inspector's job to issue court summons (E), and it is unlikely the restaurant, scoring high on all other inspection measures, is intentionally and willfully placing their customers at risk.

6. **D.** As the name implies, WIC (Women, Infants, and Children) provides nutritional assistance exclusively for women and young children. Specifically, the program is for pregnant women and new mothers (up to 6 months postpartum or up to 12 months postpartum if breastfeeding) and for children up to 5 years of age. SNAP (C) is the Supplemental Nutrition Assistance Program for all low-income citizens, irrespective of age, gender, or pregnancy status. SNAP was formerly called "Food Stamps" (B). However, in its latest iteration, rather than relying on "stamps" or paper coupons, the program makes use of EBT (E), or electronic benefits transfer cards, that can be used for food purchases at stores in much the same way as debit cards. Medicaid (A) is the federal program that pays for medical and nursing home care for poor people in cooperation with the states.

7. **G.** Medicare pays for medical care for elderly persons, and Medicaid provides health care coverage for indigent people and certain other groups. Although these programs were created under Title 18 and Title 19 of the Social Security Act, they are overseen by CMS. The Social Security Administration does not oversee health care programs; it administers retirement payments for Social Security recipients and disability payments.

8. **C.** Although much infectious disease surveillance is conducted at the level of local health departments, responsibility for nationwide surveillance in the United States rests with the CDC.

9. **M.** The NIH is largely responsible for the funding of biomedical research.

10. **J.** The National Center for Health Statistics generates and provides numerator data for population statistics in the United States.

11. **N.** Workplace standards may be recommended by the National Institute for Occupational Safety and Health (NIOSH) but are enforced by OSHA.

12. **C.** The Behavioral Risk Factor Surveillance System (BRFSS) is an ongoing survey of behavioral risk factors for chronic disease. The assessment of these risk factors falls within the purview of the CDC, which is charged with disease surveillance.

13. **H.** The HRSA is responsible for the oversight of health system resource allocations and for the promotion of access and equity in health care.

14. **F.** The FDA is the primary agency for regulating the safety and effectiveness of drugs, vaccines and other biologic products, diagnostic tests, and medical devices. It also is responsible for the safety and labeling of cosmetics, foods, and food additives and colorings.

26

Improving Public Health in Communities

With Thiruvengadam Muniraj

"Think globally, act locally."

No attribution, origin disputed, circa 1969-1979.

CASE INTRODUCTION

Joe is a 28-year-old man with type 1 diabetes. He lives in a friend's condemned, boarded-up house, which he enters through the marshlands. His shoes are full of holes and his diet is often poor, both because he cannot afford better. After a lifetime of inadequate insulin control, he is losing feeling and circulation in his feet. His doctor keeps emphasizing the need for keeping the feet dry, taking insulin, and eating healthy, which Joe finds hard to do for various reasons. In the course of the next several years, Joe has several toes removed from his feet and requires repeated emergency room treatment at a cost of more than $20,000, paid for by a state medical assistance program. Meanwhile, a decent pair of shoes costs $50.[1]

While the previous chapters discuss the organization of the public health system overall, this chapter discusses the theory and practice of improving community health. Theories are important because a theory-based program is more likely to be effective (see Chapter 15). The technical term for attempts to improve community health is *community program planning.*

Community planning is defined as an organized process to design, implement, and evaluate a clinic or community-based project to address the needs of a defined population. Community planning is often the province of personnel in a public health agency, such as the commissioner of health or agency staff. However, the principles of community planning and evaluation pertain to any person who has a stake in improving the community, including an employee of a foundation, school, mayor's office, or political party and any interested citizen. Moreover, almost any successful public health effort is built on a coalition of community stakeholders, not just executed by one agency. Although there are plenty of ideas on how to improve the health of a community, many good ideas fail. Reasons include insufficient data, lack of community or organizational support, lack of coordination, "turf battles," inefficient and duplicative efforts, and failure to use evidence-based interventions.

Careful planning before a project begins can make a significant impact on the success of the project.[2] A shining example of a successful public health program is the **North Karelia Project.** The Finnish province of North Karelia, a rural area of 180,000 inhabitants, had high rates of cardiovascular disease and deaths. In a quasi-experimental design, a comprehensive program with participation of health services, media, industry, public policy and nongovernmental organizations addressed primary and secondary risk factors for cardiovascular disease in the 1970s. Through careful evaluation, the program authors were able to show significant declines in risky behavior rates, disease rates, and deaths from cardiovascular disease[3] (see Select Readings at the end of the chapter).

BOX 26.1   Prevention Efforts: Tobacco Use (Cigarette Smoking)

The decrease in tobacco use has been called one of the 10 great public health achievements in the 20th century. This success illustrates what is required to change community health practices. Several historic factors came together to enable significant improvements in this important public health problem.

A. **Credible evidence and effective interventions led to medical consensus:**

1. Changes in understanding of the genesis of tobacco addiction reframed the problem as not one of individual control and choice, but of addiction. Evidence for harm to nonsmokers (secondary tobacco exposure) strengthened the case for regulation.
2. Behavioral and pharmacologic treatments became available, making it easier to support smokers desiring to quit.

B. **Trusted experts and grassroots groups provided effective advocacy:**

3. The American Cancer Society, American Lung Association, and American Heart Association were each advocating against tobacco independent from each other. In 1981 they formed a coalition on smoking, which was later joined by the American Medical Association. This broad coalition led legitimacy to the argument against smoking.
4. Grassroots efforts in many communities and from many sources changed cultural norms about smoking. Examples include flight attendants advocating for their right for a smoke-free workplace and the *Reader's Digest* series educating its readers. These grassroots groups framed their issues as part of the broader environmental protection movement and increased consumer health consciousness.

C. **Political will on many levels and available funds led to effective tobacco control.**

5. On a federal level, Congress passed several laws addressing tobacco labeling, advertising on television and radio,

smoking bans on airlines and buses, and changes to Food and Drug Administration (FDA) rules for more oversight over tobacco production and marketing.

6. On a state level, states use excise tax on tobacco to fund smoking control programs, which led to the development and evaluation of community-level approaches to tobacco control.
7. New litigation strategies opened up even more monies and created willingness in industry to agree to changes.

Because of this high level of attention at all levels and significant funding for community prevention programs, multiple effective interventions to reduce smoking were developed, evaluated, and disseminated. The US Community Preventive Services recommends a three-pronged approach combining strategies to:

- Reduce exposure to environmental tobacco smoke
- Reduce tobacco use initiation, especially among adolescents
- Increase tobacco use cessation

Recommended interventions include:

- Smoking bans and restrictions in public areas, workplaces, and areas where people congregate
- Increasing the unit price for tobacco products
- Mass media campaigns of extended duration using brief, recurring messages to motivate children and adolescents to remain tobacco free
- Provider reminders to counsel patients about tobacco cessation
- Provider education combined with such reminders
- Reducing out-of-pocket expenses for effective cessation therapies
- Multicomponent patient telephone support through a state quit line

Modified from Institute of Medicine: Ending the tobacco problem: a blueprint for the nation, 2007; Task Force on Community Preventive Services (TFCPS): Recommendations regarding interventions to reduce tobacco use and exposure to environmental tobacco smoke. *Am J Prev Med* 20:10–15, 2001; Tobacco. In Zaza S, Briss PA, Harris KW, editors: *The guide to community preventive services: what works to promote health?* Atlanta, 2005, Oxford University Press, http://www.thecommunityguide.org/tobacco/Tobacco.pdf.

This chapter discusses the steps involved in planning and evaluating a program, highlighting two special applications of community planning: (1) tobacco prevention, as an example of multiple successful community interventions (Box 26.1), and (2) health equity, one of the greatest public health challenges (Box 26.2). While many models and acronyms describe the steps of community planning they all have their strengths and weaknesses. We follow mainly the steps outlined in the Centers for Disease Control and Prevention (CDC) model, Community Health Assessment and Group Evaluation (CHANGE).[4] (Many other models exist, but space does not allow us to describe them all. Interested readers should consult the websites or readings at the end of the chapter.) Any model of community planning likely works equally well as long as planners follow these basic principles:

- Assemble community stakeholders and collaboratively create strategy and define the agenda, values, and priorities
- Perform a needs assessment to identify primary issues
- Design measurable objectives and interventions

- Choose effective multilevel approaches rather than single interventions
- Implement the selected interventions
- Build evaluation into the entire process

Table 26.1 provides an overview of the process and possible resources for each step.

1. THEORIES OF COMMUNITY CHANGE

Improving health almost always requires behavior change. Unhealthy behaviors (e.g., sedentariness) need to be replaced by healthy ones (e.g., exercise). Individual behavior, however, does not occur in a vacuum; it is strongly influenced by group norms and environmental cues. Practitioners aiming to change group norms and environmental cues should be aware of theories of community changes, so that their interventions have a higher chance of success (see Chapter 15 for theories of individual behavior change). A number of

---

BOX 26.2 Addressing Health Equity

Health in the US population is characterized by pervasive and persistent health care disparities, sometimes also called *health inequities*. Despite the deeply rooted and intractable nature of many health care disparities, many states and communities have successfully implemented interventions to reduce them. Characteristics of successful programs include:

- Strong data skills with geographic mapping of premature death clusters and other determinants of health
- Strong coalitions among agencies, community leaders, and other stakeholders
- Assessment of the community environment as a whole and addressing the social determinants at the root of health inequities (e.g., poverty, low rates for high school graduation, violence)

- Empowering communities to a sense of increased ownership and leadership
- Emphasizing community participation
- Addressing environmental factors such as safe walkability, bikeability of environment, and access to high-quality food
- Making health equity a component of all policies, including housing, youth violence, transportation, and agriculture

Interventions against health inequities can be successful even on a very small scale. Examples for such successful interventions include librarians who visit schools to give each child a library card, public housing directors who address lead and mold, and safe route to school initiatives with "human school buses" (group of parents who take turns in walking children to school).

Modified from Centers for Disease Control and Prevention: Health disparities and inequalities report (CHDIR), 2011, http://www.cdc.gov/minorityhealth/CHDIReport.html#ExecSummary; Institute of Medicine (IOM) reports on unequal treatment and reducing healthcare disparities, https://www.nap.edu/catalog/13103/state-and-local-policy-initiatives-to-reduce-health-disparities-workshop.

TABLE 26.1 Overview of Steps for Community Program Design, Implementation, and Evaluation

Step/Description	Suggested Resources[a]
1. Create strategy and elicit community input.	Community Health Assessment and Group Evaluation (CHANGE): http://www.cdc.gov/healthycommunitiesprogram/tools/change.htm
2. Identify primary health issues in your community.	Community Health Assessment and Group Evaluation County Health Rankings: http://www.countyhealthrankings.org/ National Public Health Performance Standards: http://www.cdc.gov/nphpsp/ Mobilizing for Action through Planning and Partnerships (MAPP): http://www.naccho.org/topics/infrastructure/MAPP/index.cfm
3. Develop measurable process and outcome objectives to assess progress in addressing these health issues.	*Healthy People 2020* leading health indicators: http://www.healthypeople.gov/2020/default.aspx Healthcare Effectiveness Data and Information Set (HEDIS) performance measures: http://www.ncqa.org/tabid/59/default.aspx National Committee for Quality Assurance (NCQA)
4. Select effective interventions to help achieve these objectives.	*Guide to Community Preventive Services* *Guide to Clinical Preventive Services*: http://www.uspreventiveservicestaskforce.org National Guideline Clearinghouse: http://guidelines.gov/ Research-Tested Intervention Programs: http://rtips.cancer.gov/rtips/index.do
5. Implement selected interventions.	Partnership for Prevention: http://preventioninfo.org/ CDCynergy: http://www.cdc.gov/healthcommunication/CDCynergy/ http://rtips.cancer.gov/rtips/index.do
6. Evaluate selected interventions based on objectives; use this information to improve program.	Framework for program evaluation in public health: http://www.cdc.gov/mmwr/preview/mmwrhtml/rr4811a1.htm CDCynergy: www.re-aim.org

[a]For all steps (1–6): *Community health promotion handbook: action guides to improve community health,* http://www.prevent.org/Action-Guides/The-Community-Health-Promotion-Handbook.aspx; Cancer Control Plan, Link, Act, Network with Evidence-based Tools (P.L.A.N.E.T.), http://cancercontrolplanet.cancer.gov/; Community tool box, http://ctb.ku.edu/en/default.aspx; Diffusion of Effective Behavioral Interventions (DEBI), http://www.effectiveinterventions.org/en/Home.aspx.
Modified from Centers for Disease Control and Prevention: *The community guide*, Atlanta, 2011, CDC, http://www.thecommunityguide.org/uses/program_planning.html.

---

theories have been developed to describe how individual change is brought about through interpersonal interactions and community interventions. These theories can be broadly characterized as **cognitive-behavioral theories** and share the following key concepts:

- Knowledge is necessary but is not in itself sufficient to produce behavior changes

- Perceptions, motivations, skills, and social environment are key influences on behavior

Some well-known theories governing social change are social cognitive theory, community organization and other participatory approaches, diffusion of innovations, and communication theory. Taken together, these theories can be used to influence factors within a social-ecological framework, as follows:

Interpersonal: Family, friends, and peers provide role models, social identity, and support.

Organizations: Groups influence behavior through organizational change, diffusion of innovation, and social marketing strategies.

Community: Social marketing and community organizing can change community norms on behavior.

Public policy: Public opinion process and policy changes can change the incentives for certain behaviors and make them easier or more difficult (e.g., taxes on high-sugar beverages).

Physical environment: The availability of food, walkability of a neighborhood, presence of mold in housing with asthmatic children are all examples for the profound impact of the physical environment on behavior.

1.1 SOCIAL COGNITIVE THEORY

Social cognitive theory is one of the most frequently used and robust health behavior theories.[5] It explores the reciprocal interactions of people and their environments and the psychosocial determinants of health behavior (see Chapter 15). Its most important tenet is that environment, people, and their behavior constantly influence each other (**reciprocal determinism**).[6]

1.2 COMMUNITY ORGANIZATION THEORIES

A heterogeneous mix of various theories covers community organization. The **social action theory** describes how to increase the *problem-solving ability* of entire communities through achieving concrete changes toward social cause. The theory includes several key concepts. **Empowerment** is a social action process that improves community's confidence and life skills beyond the topic addressed. For example, individuals in a community may feel more empowered as they work together to strengthen their cultural identity and their community assets. Empowerment builds community capacity.

Community capacity is the unique ability of a community to mobilize, identify, and solve social problems. It requires the presence of leadership, participation, skills, and sense of community. Community capacity can be enhanced in many ways, such as through skill-building workshops that allow members of the community to become more effective leaders.

Critical consciousness is a mental state by which members in a community recognize the need for social change and are ready to work to achieve those changes. Critical consciousness can be built by engaging individuals in dialogues, forums, and meaningful discussions.

Social capital refers to social resources such as trust, reciprocity, and civic engagement that exist because of the network between community members. Increasing the social cohesion and support are vital methods that build social capital.[7]

Media advocacy is an essential component of community organizing. It aims to change the way community members look at various problems and to motivate community members and policy makers to become involved. *Social media* and games can generate extensive publicity with minimal investment but are much less under the control of the message sender. Table 26.2 summarizes how social marketing, public relations, and media advocacy complement each other.

1.3 DIFFUSION OF INNOVATIONS THEORY

To be successful, a community strategy needs to be disseminated (**diffusion into the community**). Diffusion of innovations theory is characterized by four elements: innovations, communication channels, social systems (i.e., the individuals who adopt the innovation), and diffusion time. Many health behaviors and programs have been publicized successfully, including condom use, smoking cessation, and use of new tests and technologies by health practitioners.[8] Although the diffusion of innovations theory can be applied to behaviors, it is most closely associated with medical devices or tangible technology.

Groups are segmented by the speed with which they will adopt innovations. *Innovators* are eager to embrace new concepts. Next, *early adopters* will try out innovations, followed by members of the *early majority* and *late majority*. *Laggards* are the last to accept an innovation. Consequently, innovations need to be marketed initially to innovators and early

TABLE 26.2	Relationship of Social Marketing, Public Relations, and Media Advocacy		
	Social Marketing	**Public Relations**	**Media Advocacy**
Message focus	"Look at you" Know about risk Change your behavior	"Look at me" Enhance image and relationship with public	"Look at us" Sets agenda Shapes debate Advances policy
Target audience	Individuals at risk General public	Funders Clients	Stakeholders Policy makers
Effect	Individuals	Individuals	Social environment
Benefits	Motivates individual behavioral change	Develops strategic relationships Generates support for cause	Community change through policy

Modified from Media Advocacy to Advance Public Health Policy, UCLA Center for Health Policy Research, 2002, http://www.healthpolicy.ucla.edu/healthdata/tw_media2.pdf.

adopters, then marketing needs to address each segment in sequence. The relevant population segments are generally referred to as innovators (2.5% of the overall population), early adopters (13.5%), early majority (34%), late majority (34%), and laggards (16%).[9]

The speed of adoption by any group depends on *the perceived positive characteristics* of the innovations themselves (relative advantage). **Relative advantage** comes from:

- *Compatibility,* the degree to which an innovation is consistent with the existing values, current processes, past experiences, and needs of potential adopters
- *Low complexity,* the degree to which an innovation is perceived as easy to use
- *Trialability,* the opportunity to experiment with the innovation on a limited basis
- *Observability,* the degree to which the results of an innovation are visible to others

1.3.a Social Marketing in Public Health

Social marketing is typically defined as a program-planning process that applies commercial marketing concepts and techniques to promote behavior change in a **target audience.** Social marketing has also been used to analyze the social consequences of commercial marketing policies and activities, such as monitoring the effects of the tobacco and food industries' marketing practices.[10] As in commercial marketing, social marketing depends on the following:

Audience segmentation. Dividing markets into small segments based on sociodemographic, cultural, or behavioral characteristics.[11]

Tailoring messages to individuals. Tailored messages address specific cognitive and behavioral patterns as well as individual demographic characteristics. For example, the CDC's VERB campaign specially promoted the benefits of daily physical activity to children age 9 to 13 years. (VERB is not an acronym, but a program emphasizing *verb* as a part of speech, meaning an *action* word: "It's what you do.")[12]

Branding. Public health branding is the application of commercial branding strategies to promote health behavior change[13]; for example, a study recruited highly regarded peers to make condom use "cool" among a group of men at risk for human immunodeficiency virus (HIV) infection.[10,14]

Marketing mix. Marketing mix is commonly executed by addressing the four *P*s:

- Product (the desired type of behavioral change and its benefits)
- Price (barriers and costs in money, time, and effort)
- Place (accessibility and convenience of adopting the new behavior)
- Promotion (informing the target market of product, benefits, convenience)

Social marketing techniques have been used successfully in many communities that seemed impervious to traditional health promotion messages. Examples include HIV, malaria, influenza, diarrheal and other communicable diseases, as well as antismoking, alcohol dangers, and healthy eating.[15]

1.4 COMMUNICATION THEORY

Communication theory describes the use of communication to effect change at the community level and in society as well. Communication influences community and societal change in areas such as building a community agenda of important public health issues, changing public health policy, allocating resources to make behavior change easier, and legitimizing new norms of health behavior. Within communication theory, the **Delphi technique** highlights the importance of organizing a discussion so that all participants have a chance to be heard.[16] In **media communication,** particular emphasis is placed on how media *frame* a problem. Framing influences how the public understands it, how much attention people will pay, and which actions individuals or communities are likely to take. For example, the Harvard School of Public Health mounted a successful campaign to persuade television producers to include messages about designated drivers with their ads.[17]

Table 26.3 summarizes key concepts and potential change strategies for communication. Table 26.4 outlines theories related to community organization.

1.5 ENVIRONMENTAL INFLUENCES ON BEHAVIOR

Many health promotion campaigns seek to reduce high-risk behaviors such as unhealthy eating, alcohol and drug abuse, and smoking. Such programs should not ignore the material, social, and psychological conditions in which the targeted behaviors occur (see Chapters 14 and 30 regarding social determinants of health). Modifications of the regulatory environment (e.g., taxes on tobacco products) and "built" environment (e.g., impact of an environment that is conducive to exercise or obesity) seem to be at least as effective as interventions directly aimed at behaviors.

2. AIMING FOR HEALTH EQUITY

Health equity has been defined as "the state in which everyone has the opportunity to attain full health potential and no one is disadvantaged from achieving this potential because of social position."[18] Currently, the United States is far from this state. Fairness alone would suggest that the deep and enduring disparities in health outcomes in the United States[19] and elsewhere should be a primary focus of public health efforts. There is a staggering cost to unequal care. So-called high-need, high-cost patients often face combined medical, cultural, social, economic, or other challenges in getting the right care at the right time. Collectively, they account for more than $120 billion in health care spending per

TABLE 26.3 Concepts in Communication: Agenda Setting

Concept	Definition	Potential Change Strategies	Example
Media agenda setting	Institutional factors and processes influencing how the media define, select, and emphasize issues	Understand media professionals' needs and routines for gathering and reporting news	Have updated information on food safety available when current outbreak is covered by media
Public agenda setting	The link between issues covered in the media and the public's priorities	Use media advocacy or partnerships to raise public awareness of key health issues	Establish secondary tobacco smoke as public health concern
Policy agenda setting	The link between issues covered in the media and the legislative priorities of policy makers	Advocate for media coverage to educate and pressure policy makers about changes to the physical and social environment needed to promote health	Former first lady Michelle Obama taking on healthy eating and advocating for community gardens
Problem definition	Factors and process leading to identification of an issue as a "problem" by social institutions	Community leaders, advocacy groups, and organizations define an issue for the media and offer solutions	Definition of "gaming addiction" as a disease with guidelines for parents, therapy options
Framing	Selecting and emphasizing certain aspects of a story and excluding others	Advocacy groups "package" an important health issue for the media and the public	Telling personalized stories about communities and families affected by drug overdoses to raise awareness and build sympathy

Adapted from Glanz K, Rimer BK, Viswanath K: *Health behavior and health education: theory, research, and practice*, Bethesda, MD, 2008, National Cancer Institute at National Institutes of Health, http://www.cancer.gov/cancertopics/cancerlibrary/theory.pdf.

TABLE 26.4 Overview of Community-Level Theories of Behavior Change

Theory	Description	Key Factors
Community organization	Community-driven approaches to assessing and solving health and social problems	Empowerment Community capacity Participation Relevance Issue selection Critical consciousness
Diffusion of innovations	How new ideas, products, and practices spread within a society or from one society to another	Relative advantage Compatibility Complexity Trialability Observability
Communication theory	How different types of communication affect health behavior	Media agenda setting Public agenda setting Policy agenda setting Problem identification and definition Framing

From Glanz K, Rimer BK, Viswanath K: *Health behavior and health education: theory, research, and practice*, Bethesda, MD, 2008, National Cancer Institute at National Institutes of Health, http://www.cancer.gov/cancertopics/cancerlibrary/theory.pdf.

year,[20] the foundation of a very solid business core for improving their care and decreasing the disparities underlying their problems. Strategic practices to improve health equity include the following:

- Building capacity (mobilizing data, building organizational capacity, aligning internal processes, working toward upstream policy change, and allocating resources to advance equity)
- Working across government agencies (by building alliances with other agencies, developing a shared analysis, and integrating equity concerns)
- Building community partnerships (fostering relationships and meaningful participation)
- Aiming for transformative change (confronting root causes, developing leadership and supporting innovation, changing the conversation to include health equity)[21]

Examples of county-level efforts to improve health equity include recruiting and developing your leadership from diverse communities, creating cross-divisional health equity teams,[21] addressing access to healthy food, and redirecting at-risk school children.[22]

3. STEPS IN DEVELOPING A HEALTH PROMOTION PROGRAM

One model of program planning comes from the CDC's **Community Health Assessment and Group Evaluation (CHANGE).** The CHANGE program is a comprehensive data collection tool and resource for community program planning with the following steps (see Table 26.1):

1. Define a strategy and assemble a team.
2. Identify primary health issues.
3. Develop objectives to measure progress.
4. Select effective interventions.
5. Implement innovations.
6. Evaluate.

Some of the specific programs relevant to each of these steps are explained in detail next. Again, other planning resources/programs are described under those headings where they have a strong emphasis.

3.1 DEFINE STRATEGY AND ASSEMBLE A TEAM

Broad-based participation in the planning process from the start is critical to the success of a project.[23] Possible coalition participants include physicians, nurses, social workers, teachers, emergency medical services (EMS) personnel, health educators, parents, and police. However, partners can also come from churches, businesses, dental clinics, and unions. It is important to stress that building a coalition should come *before* gathering any data. There is no reason to gather data on problems nobody is willing or able to change. Primary care providers[24] and emergency room staff can be very helpful partners, since they often have unique knowledge of and relationships with vulnerable populations.

3.2 IDENTIFY PRIMARY HEALTH ISSUES

The second step in program planning is to identify the primary health issues concerning the community. This involves a **needs assessment** (areas for improvement) as well as **asset mapping** (identifying the people, institutions, available funds, and capacity to solve problems). Examples for a needs assessment that emphasizes the environmental factors of diet, exercise, and smoking include the following questions[25]:

Do sidewalks make walking (walkability) and biking (bikeability) easy and safe? Are they connected, continuous, free from barriers, and safe from traffic and crime?

Are healthier food options in grocery stores available and affordable? Are they of good quality?

How many homes, parks, hospitals, and schools have easy access to tobacco and are exposed to tobacco advertising?

Are there tobacco-free campus policies in hospitals, on college campuses, and in multiunit housing?

Tools used in screening and identifying overall problems in the community include the following:
- PRECEDE-PROCEED model
- Planned Approach to Community Health (PATCH)
- Mobilizing for Action through Planning and Partnerships (MAPP)
- National Public Health Performance Standards Program (NPHPSP)
- Data sources (see Chapter 25)
- Tools within the CHANGE process

For reasons of space, we describe only a few models.

3.2.a PRECEDE-PROCEED Model

The PRECEDE-PROCEED tool provides a comprehensive structure for (1) assessing health and quality-of-life needs and (2) designing, implementing, and evaluating. The PRECEDE part—**Predisposing, Reinforcing, and Enabling Constructs in Educational Diagnosis and Evaluation**—outlines a diagnostic planning process. The second part, PROCEED, provides an implementation and evaluation program—**Policy, Regulatory, and Organizational Constructs in Educational and Environmental Development**—for the program designed using PRECEDE. The process starts with desired outcomes and works backward to identify a mix of strategies for achieving objectives[6] (Fig. 26.1).

PRECEDE comprises the following steps[26]:

Step 1: **Social assessment.** Determining the quality of life or social problems and needs of a given population through multiple data collection activities (e.g., key informant interviews, focus groups, participant observation, surveys.)

Step 2: **Epidemiologic assessment.** Identifying the health determinants of these problems and needs through secondary data analysis or original data collection to prioritize the community's health needs and establish program goals and objectives

Step 3: **Behavioral and environmental assessment.** Analyzing the behavioral and environmental determinants of the health problems through reviewing the literature and applying theory

Step 4: **Educational and ecological assessment.** Identifying the factors that predispose to, reinforce, and enable the behaviors and lifestyles; distinguishing individual, interpersonal, or community-level factors

Step 5: **Administrative and policy assessment.** Identifying the best-suited health promotion, health education, and policy-related interventions

PROCEED comprises four additional steps[27]:

Step 6: **Implementation.** Carrying out the interventions from step 5

Step 7: **Process evaluation.** Evaluating the process for implementing the interventions

Step 8: **Impact evaluation.** Evaluating the impact of the interventions on the factors supporting behavior and on behavior itself

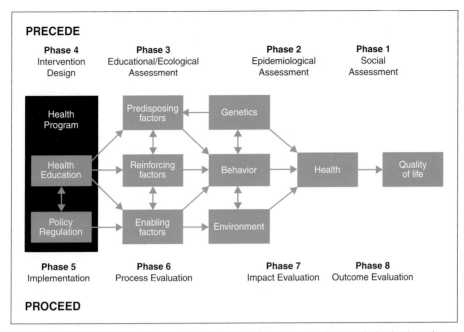

PRECEDE

Phase 4	Phase 3	Phase 2	Phase 1
Intervention Design	Educational/Ecological Assessment	Epidemiological Assessment	Social Assessment

Phase 5	Phase 6	Phase 7	Phase 8
Implementation	Process Evaluation	Impact Evaluation	Outcome Evaluation

PROCEED

Fig. 26.1 The PRECEDE-PROCEED model. (In this graph, in contrast to the text, behavioral, environmental as well as administrative and policy assessment are left out, and the intervention design is listed as its own phase. From: http://brightsmileshawaii.org/wp-content/uploads/2017/01/BSH-Precede-Proceed-Model.png.)

Step 9: **Outcome evaluation.** Determining the ultimate effects of the interventions on the health and quality of life of the population

3.3 DEVELOP OBJECTIVES TO MEASURE PROGRESS

One of the most important parts in planning change is to define objectives. **Objectives** are defined as specific measurable parameters; each objective should be specific, relevant, measurable, and associated with a time frame. One source of helpful objectives is the *Healthy People* database.[28]

3.3.a *Healthy People 2020*

During the 1970s, representatives from many public health and scientific organizations began to develop national health promotion and disease prevention objectives. Their efforts resulted in the publication of science-based, national 10-year objectives to improve the health of all Americans. The most recent version of these is *Healthy People 2020,* but the next set of indicators for *Healthy People 2030* is already being discussed. The *Healthy People* objectives represent a national consensus strategy of the government, public health organizations, and public-spirited citizens and have a major impact on the way government and other institutions direct their resources in public health. For example, most federal grants require possible grantees to describe how proposals will advance *Healthy People 2020* goals.

Healthy People 2020 proposed the following four overarching goals (Table 26.5):
1. Attain high-quality, longer lives free of preventable disease, disability, injury, and premature death.
2. Achieve health equity, eliminate disparities, and improve the health of all groups.
3. Create social and physical environments that promote good health for all.

4. Promote quality of life, healthy development, and healthy behaviors across all life stages.

Four **foundational health measures** serve as an indicator of progress: (1) general health status, (2) health-related quality of life and well-being, (3) determinants of health, and (4) disparities. Each foundational health measure is further divided into submeasures. A subset of objectives, called **leading health indicators,** has been selected to communicate high-priority health issues and actions that can be taken to address them (Table 26.6).

The document includes measurable indicators of progress, which are helpful in tracking progress or documenting the lack of progress. For each leading indicator, an objective is described and appropriate background information provided. Each focus area objective is broken into many subobjectives, each of which has baseline values and target values for subgroups of the population (age, gender, ethnic, and other subgroups).[29]

Mobilize, assess, plan, implement, track (MAP-IT) is a framework that can be used to plan and evaluate public health interventions in a community using the *Healthy People 2020* objectives (Fig. 26.2). Using MAP-IT, a step-by-step, structured plan can be developed by a coalition and tailored to a specific community's needs. The phases of mobilize-assess-plan-implement-track provide a logical structure for communities to address and resolve local health problems and to build healthy communities.

3.4 SELECT EFFECTIVE INTERVENTIONS

3.4.a Community Preventive Services

The US Preventive Services Task Force (USPSTF) *Guides to Clinical Preventive Services* championed a rigorous, evidence-based approach to **clinical** preventive services.

TABLE 26.5 Healthy People 2020: Goals, Foundational Health Measures, and Progress

Overarching Goals	Foundational Health Measures Category	Measures of Progress
Attain high-quality, longer lives free of preventable disease, disability, injury, and premature death	General health status	Life expectancy Healthy life expectancy Physically, mentally unhealthy days Self-assessed health status Limitation of activity Chronic disease prevalence International comparisons (where available)
Achieve health equity, eliminate disparities, and improve the health of all groups	Disparities and inequity	*Disparities/inequity to be assessed by:* Race/ethnicity Gender Socioeconomic status Disability status Lesbian, gay, bisexual, and transgender status Geography
Create social and physical environments that promote good health for all	Social determinants of health	*Determinants can include:* Social and economic factors Natural and built environments Policies and programs
Promote quality of life, healthy development, and healthy behaviors across all life stages	Health-related quality of life and well-being	Well-being/satisfaction Physical, mental, and social health-related quality of life Participation in common activities

From *Healthy People 2020*, US Department of Health and Human Services, http://healthypeople.gov/2020/TopicsObjectives2020/pdfs/HP2020_brochure_with_LHI_508.pdf.

TABLE 26.6 Healthy People 2020: Leading Health Indicators

12 Topic Areas	26 Leading Health Indicators
Access to health services	Persons with medical insurance Persons with a usual primary care provider
Clinical preventive services	Adults who receive colorectal cancer screening based on most recent guidelines Adults with hypertension whose blood pressure is under control Adult diabetic population with HbA_{1c} value >9% Children age 19–35 months who receive recommended doses of diphtheria, tetanus, and pertussis; polio; measles, mumps, and rubella; *Haemophilus influenzae* type b; hepatitis B; varicella; and pneumococcal conjugate vaccines
Environmental quality	Air Quality Index >100 Children age 3–11 years exposed to secondhand smoke
Injury and violence	Fatal injuries Homicides
Maternal, infant, and child health	Infant deaths Preterm births
Mental health	Suicides Adolescents who experience major depressive episodes
Nutrition, physical activity, and obesity	Adults who meet current federal physical activity guidelines for aerobic physical activity and muscle-strengthening activity Adults who are obese Children and adolescents who are considered obese Total vegetable intake for persons age 2 years and older
Oral health	Persons age 2 years and older who used oral health care system in past 12 months
Reproductive and sexual health	Sexually active females age 15–44 who received reproductive health services in past 12 months Persons living with HIV infection who know their serologic status
Social determinants	Students who graduate with a regular diploma 4 years after starting ninth grade

TABLE 26.6	**Healthy People 2020: Leading Health Indicators—cont'd**
12 Topic Areas	**26 Leading Health Indicators**
Substance abuse	Adolescents using alcohol or any illicit drugs during past 30 days
	Adults engaging in binge drinking during past 30 days
Tobacco	Adults who are current cigarette smokers
	Adolescents who smoked cigarettes in past 30 days

Modified from *Healthy People 2020*, US Department of Health and Human Services, http://healthypeople.gov/2020/TopicsObjectives2020/pdfs/ HP2020_brochure_with_LHI_508.pdf.

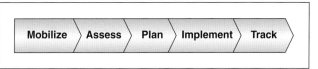

Fig. 26.2   MAP-IT. This framework to help set objectives for the health of the US population is from *Healthy People 2020*, a joint effort between the US Department of Health and Human Services with representatives from the Department of Agriculture, Department of Education, Department of Housing and Urban Development, Department of Justice, Department of the Interior, and Department of Veterans Affairs, as well as the Environmental Protection Agency.

Modeled on this process, the Department of Health and Human Services (DHHS) tasked the CDC to develop a parallel guide to **community preventive services (CPS)**.[30] The Community Preventive Services Task Force provides an annual report to Congress outlining gaps in the evidence, new recommendations, and how communities use task force recommendations. *Guide to Community Preventive Services* is a free, online resource to help choose programs and policies to improve health and prevent disease in the community.[31] The guide identifies effective interventions through a rigorous evidence-based process (see Chapters 13 and 18).

Recommendations address a wide variety of topics, such as the following:

- Worksite health promotion (e.g., tobacco policy, physical inactivity, health risk appraisal)
- Supporting local community health (e.g., community water fluoridation, school vaccination program, school-based physical education)
- Improving chronic disease self-care
- Emergency preparedness
- Health communication and health information technology
- Decreasing violence
- Addressing health equity[32]

After balancing the evidence and cost-effectiveness of recommendations, the guide provides the following ratings: *recommended, recommended against,* and *insufficient evidence.*

Recommendations

Changing risk behaviors. Commensurate with policy successes, data are abundant to rate tobacco interventions (see Box 26.1), but much less for other less-funded topics, such as high-calorie foods and firearms. There are also sometimes heterogeneous results for identical interventions on various diseases, such as patient reminders for breast cancer screenings versus other cancers. Examples for community interventions aimed at changing risk behaviors[33] include community-wide campaigns to promote the intake of folic acid among women of childbearing age and restricted hours for teenage drivers.

Addressing the environment. Many community guide recommendations address the importance of the environment. Examples include laws mandating seat belt use, community-level urban redesign to make neighborhoods more walkable and bikeable, and community water fluoridation to decrease caries. Other agencies have also published numerous strategies to improve diet and exercise (e.g., improving school food policies to make healthy choices available for lunches and snacks), adopting worksite wellness policies that promote healthy lifestyle choices for staff and the community, establishing smoke-free environments in parks, and establishing farmers' markets and community gardens.

Reducing disease, injury, and impairment. Community guide recommendations addressing the reduction of disease, injury, and impairment include early childhood home visitation programs for violence and injury prevention, influenza vaccination programs for health care workers, and partner notification for HIV-positive individuals.

3.4.b Cultural Congruence of Interventions

It is important to balance evidence-based interventions with those that are culturally congruent with the community. Health program evaluators have long known that a particular program may be an outstanding success in one community, place, and time, yet fail miserably in another community or even in the same community at another time. Evidence supports that interventions with community support and perceived as culturally congruent are more effective.[34] Lastly, any intervention needs to be tailored to individual patients' needs for maximum engagement, especially for hard-to-reach populations.[35]

3.4.c Frequent Evidence Gaps

A number of evidence gaps in regard to the USPSTF recommendations surface repeatedly. These might be of interest to researchers and include:

- Which components of interventions are essential, and which increase effectiveness?
- How are programs sustained to gain maximum benefit?
- Does effectiveness differ by race, ethnicity, age, disability, education, income, etc.?

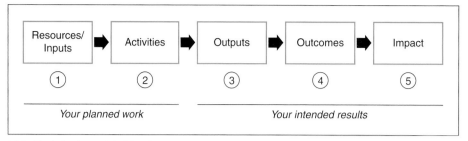

Fig. 26.3 Basic logic model. (Modified from the 1998 WK Kellogg Foundation's *The Logic Model Development Guide,* http://www.wkkf.org/knowledge-center/resources/2006/02/WK-Kellogg-Foundation-Logic-Model-Development-Guide.aspx.)

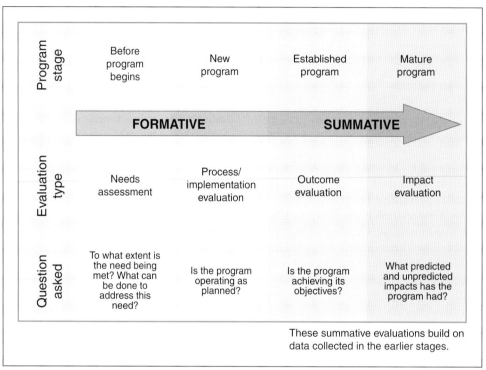

Fig. 26.4 Summary of evaluation procedures. (Modifed from Norland E: From education theory...to conservation practices. Annual Meeting of the International Association for Fish & Wildlife Agencies, Atlantic City, NJ, 2004; Pancer SM, Westhues A: A developmental stage approach to program planning and evaluation. *Eval Rev* 13:56–77, 1989; Rossi PH, Lipsey MW, Freeman HE: *Evaluation: a systematic approach,* Thousand Oaks, CA, 2004, Sage.)

- What are the long-term benefits in term of health, economic, and other outcomes?
- What are the main drivers of intervention economic costs and benefits?[36]

3.5 IMPLEMENT INNOVATIONS

Implementation of interventions poses its own challenges, mainly managing people's reaction to change. The role of the environment and community capacity should not be underestimated. The *Guide to Community Preventive Services* evaluates the effectiveness of types of interventions (vs. individual programs) by conducting systematic reviews of all available research in collaboration with partners. One such innovation is the **Research Tested Intervention Program,** a searchable database of cancer control interventions with detailed program materials.

3.6 EVALUATE

Evaluation should be built into the entire process of any project. The evaluation must be planned at the start of the planning process and cover all aspects of the project, such as **reach, efficacy, adoption, implementation, maintenance (RE-AIM).**[37]

For evaluating, it can sometimes be helpful to structure evaluation of a project in the logic model. The **basic logic model** distinguishes resources, input, output, outcomes, and impact (Fig. 26.3).

Evaluations can be done using qualitative or quantitative methods and can be of formative or summative type. Questions for a **formative** evaluation include: Was the process implemented? Which activities, meetings, or training sessions were implemented, and when? A **summative** evaluation attempts to assess if the program had the expected impact/outcome (Fig. 26.4).

4. FUTURE CHALLENGES

Multiple challenges are inherent in the program planning process and are likely to become worse with decreasing resources and an environment less and less conducive to healthy lifestyles. A few of these challenges are outlined here.

4.1 INTEGRATING CLINICAL CARE AND PREVENTION

Interventions that address multiple levels simultaneously are much more effective than interventions aimed at one group (e.g., tobacco quit rates among adolescents are higher if parents and adolescents are targeted at the same time).[38] Although some health problems might be best addressed by either a clinical prevention approach *or* a community approach, the theories listed at the beginning of this chapter teach us that an integrated and combined approach is usually most effective.[39] Interventions on both levels usually reinforce each other and also leverage existing resources for maximum impact.

4.2 E-HEALTH AND SOCIAL MEDIA

With information technology advancing rapidly, health informatics and social media impact public health care as much as clinical care. Electronic health information (e-health) includes the use of traditional media for new uses (e.g., TV series to promote healthy eating among Hispanic viewers)[40] as well as new media. Newer communication strategies include, but are not limited to, health information on the Internet, online support groups, online collaborative communities, information tailored by computer technologies, educational computer games, computer-controlled in-home telephone counseling, personalized smartphone apps, and patient-provider email contact. Major benefits of e-health strategies follow:

- Increased reach (ability to communicate to broad, geographically dispersed audiences).
- Asynchronous communication (interaction not bounded by having to communicate at the same time).
- Ability to integrate multiple communication modes and formats (e.g., audio, video, text, graphics).
- Ability to track, preserve, and analyze communication (computer records of interaction, analysis of interaction trends).
- User control of the communication system (ability to customize programs to user specifications).
- Interactivity (e.g., increased capacity for feedback).

Examples for such successful use of social media include a video game series to improve children's and adolescents' self-care behaviors for asthma[41]; texting adolescents with sexual health test messages[42]; text messaging to improve medication adherence,[43] the use of Internet tools to increase diagnosis of hepatitis C,[44] and combining social media campaign with health-related products (e.g., pedometers).[45]

Social media and emerging technologies will likely blur the line between expert and peer health information. Monitoring and assessing the impact of these new media (e.g., mobile health) on public health will be challenging. Further challenges arise with changes in health care quality and efficiency resulting from the creative use of health communication and **information technology (IT)**. Capturing the scope and impact of these changes—and the role of health communication and health IT in facilitating them—will require multidisciplinary models and data systems. Such systems will be critical to expanding the collection of data to better understand the effects of health communication and health IT on population health outcomes, health care quality, and health disparities.[28] E-health also assigns newer roles for stakeholders, government, health care providers, health authorities, community, patients, and others. The Center for Connected Health Policy (CCHP) is a not-for-profit public interest organization that develops and advances telehealth policy solutions to promote methods for enhancing health care, public health, and health education delivery and support using telecommunications technologies (see Websites at the end of the chapter).

CASE RESOLUTION

A new program is implemented in Joe's neighborhood that supports housing counselors and social workers in close proximity of the emergency room with extended working hours. Joe is referred to this program and receives a clothing allowance, which allows him to purchase new shoes. A community outreach worker visits him regularly and goes grocery shopping with him. While Joe is still struggling with his health and good eating, his feet seem much improved. The program is cofinanced by the Department of Health and Human Services (HHS) and the hospital. A rigorous evaluation of the program following the PRECEDE-PROCEED model determines that it is improving health outcomes while decreasing outlays for emergency care.

---

5. SUMMARY

Community program planning is defined as an organized process to design, implement, and evaluate a community-based project to address the needs of a defined population. Community planning should be guided by theories (social cognitive, diffusion, communication). Changing the structural, social, and political environment to be more conducive to healthy behavior is crucial. Multiple models to guide community planning are available, including the PRECEDE-PROCEED model. Community planning includes these steps: assemble a team, assess community health status, define objectives, select effective intervention, implement the intervention, and evaluate. The *Healthy People 2020* objectives provide science-based objectives for 26 leading health indicators. The *Guide to Community Preventive Services* evaluates community interventions in a rigorous, science-driven process, providing science-based recommendations on interventions proved effective. Evaluations can be formative or summative, and the evaluation process should be built into the entire program process rather than appended at the end. Future trends in community prevention may include integrating clinical and community preventive services as well as integrating preventive services with other community activities.

REFERENCES

1. Bradley EH, Taylor LA, Fineberg HV. *The American Healthcare Paradox.* New York, NY: Public Affairs; 2015.

2. Frazier PJ, Horowitz AM. Priorities in planning and evaluating oral health programs. *Fam Community Health.* 1980;3:103-113.

3. Puska P. Successful prevention of non-communicable diseases: 25 year experiences with North Karelia Project in Finland. *Pub Health Med.* 2002;4:5-7.

4. Centers for Disease Control and Prevention. *Community Health Assessment and Group Evaluation: Building a Foundation of Knowledge to Prioritize Community Needs.* Available at: www.cdc.gov/healthycommunitiesprogram/tools/change.htm. Accessed October 10, 2019.

5. Bandura A. *Self-Efficacy: The Exercise of Control.* New York, NY: W H Freeman; 1997.

6. Glanz K, Rimer BK, Lewis FM. *Health Behavior and Health Education: Theory, Research, and Practice.* San Francisco, CA: Wiley & Sons; 2002.

7. Minkler M, Wallerstein N, Wilson N. Improving health through community organization and community building. In: Glanz K, Rimer BK, Viswanath K, eds. *Health Behavior and Health Education: Theory, Research, and Practice.* San Francisco, CA: Wiley & Sons; 2008.

8. Jacobs G. Conflicting demands and the power of defensive routines in participatory action research. *Action Res.* 2010;8:367.

9. Rogers EM. *Diffusion of Innovations.* 5th ed. New York, NY: Free Press; 2003.

10. Hastings G, Saren M. The critical contribution of social marketing: theory and application. *Mark Theory.* 2003;3:305-322.

11. Forthofer MS, Bryant CA. Using audience-segmentation techniques to tailor health behavior change strategies. *Am J Health Behav.* 2000;24:36-43.

12. Huhman M, Berkowitz JM, Wong FL, et al. The VERB campaign's strategy for reaching African-American, Hispanic, Asian, and American Indian children and parents. *Am J Prev Med.* 2008;34:S194-S209.

13. Evans WD, Hastings G. Public health branding: recognition, promise, and delivery of healthy lifestyles. In: Evans WD, Hastings G, eds. *Public Health Branding: Applying Marketing for Social Change.* London, UK: Oxford University Press; 2008.

14. Kelly JA, St Lawrence JS, Diaz YE, et al. HIV risk behavior reduction following intervention with key opinion leaders of population: an experimental analysis. *Am J Public Health.* 1991;81:168-171.

15. Darnton A, Elster-Jones J, Lucas K, Brooks M. *Promoting Pro-Environmental Behaviour: Existing Evidence to Inform Better Policy Making.* London, UK: The Centre for Sustainable Development, University of Westminster, The Department for Environment, Food and Rural Affairs (DEFRA); 2006.

16. Linstone HA, Turoff M. *The Delphic Methods: Techniques and Applications.* Boston, MA: Addison-Wesley; 1975/2002. Available at: http://is.njit.edu/pubs/delphibook.

17. Harvard TH. *Chan School of Public Health: Center for Health communication: Harvard Alcohol Project.* Available at: http://www.hsph.harvard.edu/research/chc/harvard-alcohol-project/.

18. National Academies of Sciences, Engineering, and Medicine. *Communities in Action: Pathways to Health Equity.* Washington, DC: National Academies Press; 2017.

19. Commonwealth Fund Report. *Rising to the Challenge. The Commonwealth Fund Scorecard on Local Health System Performance.* 2016. Available at: http://www.commonwealthfund.org/~/media/files/publications/fund-report/2016/jul/1885_radley_rising_to_the_challenge_local_scorecard_2016.pdf.

20. Commonwealth Fund Report. *Can Building Relationships Help Engage High-Need Patients?* 2017. Available at: http://www.commonwealthfund.org/publications/newsletters/headlines-in-health-policy/2017/apr/april-3-2017/high-need-feature-tanya.

21. Health Equity Guide. *Strategic Practices.* 2017. Available at: https://healthequityguide.org/strategic-practices/.

22. Robert Wood Johnson Foundation. *RWJF Culture of Health Prize Winners.* Kansas City, MO: Culture of Health Prize Winner; 2015. Available at: https://www.rwjf.org/en/library/articles-and-news/2015/10/coh-prize-kansas-city-mo.html.

23. Hanlon JJ, Pickett GE. *Public Health Administration and Practice.* St. Louis, MO: Mosby; 1984.

24. National Academy of Medicine. *Primary Care and Public Health: Exploring Integration to Improve Population Health.* March 28, 2012. Available at: http://nationalacademies.org/hmd/~/media/Files/Report%20Files/2012/Primary-Care-and-Public-Health/Primary%20Care%20and%20Public%20Health_Revised%20RB_FINAL.pdf.

25. Washington State Department of Health. *Cowlitz County Healthy Communities Assessment Workbook,* Pub No 345–296. 2018. Available at: https://www.co.cowlitz.wa.us/1549/Healthy-Workforce-Forms

26. Washington State Department of Health. *Washington State Health Assessment.* 2018. Available at: https://www.doh.wa.gov/DataandStatisticalReports/StateHealthAssessment.

27. Gold R, Green LW, Kreuter MW. *EMPOWER: Enabling Methods of Planning and Organizing within Everyone's Research.* Sudbury, MA: Jones & Bartlett; 1997.

28. Office of Disease Prevention and Health Promotion. *Healthy People 2020 Topics and Objectives.* Available at: http://healthypeople.gov/2020/topicsobjectives2020/overview.aspx?topicid=18.

29. Office of Disease Prevention and Health Promotion. *Healthy People 2020: Leading Indicators.* Available at: https://www.healthypeople.gov/2020/leading-health-indicators/Healthy-People-2020-Leading-Health-Indicators%3A-Progress-Update.

30. Truman BI, Smith-Akin CK, Hinman AR, et al. Developing the guide to community preventive services—overview and rationale. The Task Force on Community Preventive Services. *Am J Prev Med.* 2000;18:18-26.

31. Community Preventive Services. *The Community Guide.* Available at: www.thecommunityguide.org.

32. The Community Guide. *CPS Active Findings at a Glance.* 2019. Available at: https://oemmndcbldboiebfnladdacbdfmadadm/https://www.thecommunityguide.org/sites/default/files/assets/All-Task-Force-Findings.pdf.

33. Natioanl Recreation and Parks Association. Available at: https://www.nrpa.org/About-National-Recreation-and-Park-Association/pressroom/new-parks-and-recreation-risk-assessment-tool-now-available/.

34. Plescia M, Herrick H, Chavis L. Improving health behaviors in an African American community: the Charlotte racial and ethnic approaches to community health project. *Am J Public Health.* 2008;98:1678-1684.

35. Lee E, Mitchell-Herzfeld SD, Lowenfels AA, Greene R, Dorabawila V, DuMont KA. Reducing low birth weight through home visitation: a randomized controlled trial. *Am J Prev Med.* 2009;36:154-160.

36. Community Preventive Services. *Annual Report to Congress 2016.* Available at: https://www.thecommunityguide.org/content/2016-annual-report-congress.

37. National cancer Institute. *Division of Cancer Control and Population Sciences: Implementation Science at a Glance, p. 26.* Available at: https://cancercontrol.cancer.gov/IS/docs/NCI-ISaaG-Workbook.pdf.

38. Guilamo-Ramos V, Jaccard J, Dittus P, Gonzalez B, Bouris A, Banspach S. The linking lives health education program: a randomized clinical trial of a parent-based tobacco use prevention

program for African American and Latino youths. *Am J Public Health*. 2010;100:1641-1647.

39. Ockene JK, Edgerton EA, Teutsch SM, et al. Integrating evidence-based clinical and community strategies to improve health. *Am J Prev Med*. 2007;32:244-252.

40. Hinojosa MS, Nelson D, Hinojosa R, et al. Using fotonovelas to promote healthy eating in a Latino community. *Am J Public Health*. 2011;101:258-259.

41. Lieberman DA. Management of chronic pediatric diseases with interactive health games: theory and research findings. *J Ambul Care Manage*. 2001;24:26-38.

42. Levine D, McCright J, Dobkin L, Woodruff AJ, Klausner JD. Sexinfo: a sexual health text messaging service for San Francisco youth. *Am J Public Health*. 2008;98:393-395.

43. Community Preventive Services Guide. *Health Information Technology: Text Messaging Interventions for Medication Adherence Among Patients with Chronic Diseases*. Available at: https://www.thecommunityguide.org/findings/health-information-technology-text-messaging-medication-adherence-chronic-disease.

44. Zuure FR, Davidovich U, Coutinho RA, et al. Using mass media and the internet as tools to diagnose hepatitis C infections in the general population. *Am J Prev Med*. 2011;40:345-352.

45. Community Preventive Serivces Guide. *The Community Guide: Health Communication and Social Marketing: Campaigns that Include Mass Media and Health-Related Product Distribution*. 2019. Available at: https://www.thecommunityguide.org/findings/health-communication-and-social-marketing-campaigns-include-mass-media-and-health-related.

SELECT READINGS

National Academies of Sciences, Engineering, and Medicine: *Communities in Action: Pathways to Health Equity*. Washington, DC, 2017, The National Academies Press.

National Cancer Institute: *Making Health Communication Programs Work*. 2004. https://www.cancer.gov/publications/health-communication/pink-book.pdf.

Rundall TG: Public Health Management Tools. In Wallace RB, editor, *Maxcy-Rosenau-Last: Public Health and Preventive Medicine*, ed 15, New York, 2008, McGraw-Hill Medical.

Puska P, Vartiainen E, Laatikainen T, et al: The North Karelia project: from North Karelia to national action. Helsinki, 2009, National Institute for Health and Welfare, Helsinki University Printing House. https://www.julkari.fi/bitstream/handle/10024/80109/731beafd-b544-42b2-b853-baa87db6a046.pdf

Yarbrough DB, Shulha LM, Hopson RK: *The Program Evaluation Standards: A Guide for Evaluators and Evaluation Users*, ed 3, Thousand Oaks, CA, 2011, Sage, American Evaluation Association.

WEBSITES

Agency for Healthcare Research and Quality: http://www.ahrq.gov

Center for Connected Health Policy: http://www.cchpca.org/

Centers for Disease Control and Prevention: http://www.effectiveinterventions.org

County Health Rankings: http://www.countyhealthrankings.org/

Health People: http://www.healthypeople.gov

Interventions for Health Equity: https://healthequityguide.org/

National Association of County and Health Officials: http://www.naccho.org/

Partnership for Prevention: http://www.prevent.org

The Community Guide: http://www.thecommunityguide.org

REVIEW QUESTIONS

1. Cognitive-behavioral theories share which of the following key concepts?
   A. Individual knowledge is necessary and sufficient to produce most behavior changes
   B. Perceptions, motivations, and skills are key influences on behavior
   C. Family, friends, and peers get in the way of individual behavior change
   D. Organizational changes and individual behavior are independent of each other
   E. Public opinion process and policy changes have little influence on individuals

2. When individuals are influenced by witnessing other people's behaviors and society's norms in action, this is known as:
   A. Social capital
   B. Community capacity
   C. Reciprocal determinism
   D. Observational learning
   E. Critical consciousness

3. Which is *true* of media advocacy?
   A. Influencing policy makers is a secondary aim
   B. It motivates individual behavior change
   C. The thrust of its message is about knowing personal risks
   D. Its primary audience is people at risk
   E. It is an essential component of community organizing

4. Innovations need to be marketed initially to which of the following groups on the innovativeness continuum?
   A. Early adopters
   B. Early majority
   C. Late majority
   D. Laggards
   E. Recalcitrants

5. The degree to which an innovation reflects existing values is known as:
   A. Relative advantage
   B. Compatibility
   C. Low complexity
   D. Trialability
   E. Observability

6. Which of the following is one of the four *P*s of marketing redefined for social marketing?
   A. Person
   B. Purchasing
   C. Perishability
   D. Place
   E. Possibility

7. Consistent with the CDC's Community Health Assessment and Group Evaluation (CHANGE) model, the first

step in community planning is defining a strategy and assembling a team. Which of the following might be used for this step?

A. Delphi technique
B. Needs assessment
C. Asset mapping
D. PRECEDE-PROCEED
E. Impact evaluation

8. PRECEDE-PROCEED is an acronym for a comprehensive structure to assess health and quality-of-life needs and to design, implement, and evaluate health promotion and other public health programs to meet those needs. One of the five *E*s in this acronym stands for:

A. Empathizing
B. Empowering
C. Enlisting
D. Emboldening
E. Evaluation

9. For *Healthy People 2020,* two of the foundational health measures that serve as indicators of progress are:

A. Tobacco use and health-related quality of life
B. Chronic disease prevalence and determinants of health
C. Obesity rates and vaccinations
D. General health status and disparities
E. Community engagement and social capital

ANSWERS AND EXPLANATIONS

1. **B.** A number of theories have been developed to describe how individual change is brought about through interpersonal interactions and community interventions. These theories are broadly characterized as *cognitive-behavioral theories* and share the concept that perceptions, motivations, skills, and social environment are key influences on behavior. These theories also share the concept that individual knowledge (A) is necessary but insufficient to produce most behavior changes. Family, friends, and peers (C) can provide role models, social identity, and support for change. Organizations (D) can influence individual behavior change through organizational change and social marketing strategies, and individuals can influence organizations through reciprocal determinism. Public opinion process and policy changes (E) can change the incentives for certain individual behaviors and can facilitate or complicate them.

2. **D.** People learn from watching other people; this is observational learning. Bidirectional influence between individuals and their social environments is called reciprocal determinism (C). Social capital (A) refers to resources (e.g., trust, reciprocity, civic engagement) that result from the network between community members. Community capacity (B) is the ability of a community to mobilize þund identify and solve social problems. Critical consciousness (E) is a mental state

by which members in a community recognize the need for social change and are ready to work to achieve those changes.

3. **E.** Advocacy is used to promote an issue to encourage social change. Influencing policy makers (A) is a primary aim. Media advocacy campaigns are not about personal risks (C and D) and are not designed to motivate individual behavior change (B). Such campaigns are directed at setting agendas, shaping debate, and advancing policy through a reliable, consistent stream of publicity for an organization's issues and activities. The goal is to change the social environment.

4. **A.** Innovations need to be marketed initially to innovators and early adopters. The strategies then need to change to attract the early majority (B), late majority (C), and laggards (D). Recalcitrants (E) is not a recognized category of innovativeness.

5. **B.** The degree to which an innovation is perceived to be consistent with the existing values, current processes, past experiences, and needs of potential adopters is termed *compatibility*. Relative advantage (A) is the degree to which an innovation is perceived as being better than the idea it supersedes. Low complexity (C) is the degree to which an innovation is perceived as easy to use. Trialability (D) is the opportunity to experiment with the innovation on a limited basis. Observability (E) is the degree to which the results of an innovation are visible to others.

6. **D.** The four *P*s of marketing redefined for social marketing are *product* (the right kind of behavioral change), *price* (an exchange of benefits and costs in terms of money, time, effort, etc.), *place* (making the product accessible and convenient), and *promotion* (delivering the message in a compelling way to the target audience). Person (A), purchasing (B), perishability (C), and possibility (E) are not part of this established framework.

7. **A.** The Delphi technique is a method for structuring a group communication process so that the process is effective in allowing a group of individuals (as a whole) to deal with a complex problem. Assembling a team and building a coalition should come before gathering any data. It is important to match data gathering to what the community wants to talk about; there is no sense in gathering data on problems nobody is willing or able to change. Needs assessment (B), asset mapping (C), and PRECEDE-PROCEED (D) are involved in data gathering and introduce the next step in community planning: identifying the primary health issue. Impact evaluation (E) describes the last stage of community planning once a developed program is running.

8. **E.** PRECEDE stands for Predisposing, Reinforcing, and Enabling Constructs in Educational Diagnosis and Evaluation, outlining a diagnostic planning process to assist in the development of targeted and focused public

health programs. PROCEED stands for Policy, Regulatory, and Organizational Constructs in Educational and Environmental Development, guiding the implementation and evaluation of the programs designed using PRECEDE. Empathizing (A), empowering (B), enlisting (C), and emboldening (D) may be elements of work in the PRECED-PROCEED construct but are not expressly part of the system.

9. **D.** *Healthy People 2020* includes four foundational health measures that serve as indicators of progress: (1) general health status, (2) health-related quality of life and well-being, (3) determinants of health, and (4) disparities. Targets for tobacco use (A), chronic diseases (B), and such issues as obesity and vaccinations (C) are expressly addressed in *Healthy People 2020* under 12 topic areas, but these are not foundational health measures. Issues of community engagement and social capital (E) are not explicitly addressed.

27

Disaster Epidemiology and Surveillance

Linda C. Degutis

CHAPTER OUTLINE

"We have had the lesson before us over and over again— nations that were not ready and unable to get ready found themselves overrun by the enemy."

Franklin D. Roosevelt

1. OVERVIEW

Before discussing disaster epidemiology and surveillance, it is important to define what is meant by disaster. A **disaster** is generally considered to be an event that puts an overwhelming stress on a system such that the resources used on a daily basis are inadequate for dealing with the impact of the event. The resources may be inadequate because of the number of people affected by the event, or because the resources themselves have been damaged or limited as a result of the event. Disasters may be further categorized by *intent* or *cause*. Whereas **natural disasters** are events such as tsunamis, hurricanes, tornadoes, earthquakes, and floods, **human-made disasters** are related to human-developed technology and may be *unintentional,* such as a train crash, building collapse, or fire, or *intentional,* such as a terrorist attack, mass shooting, or the intentional distribution of a toxic agent (e.g., 1995 sarin gas release in Tokyo subway, 2011 anthrax letters sent in United States, 2017 Las Vegas concert killings, 2018 Parkland, Florida school killings). In either case, the epidemiology and surveillance needs in a disaster may be impacted by the type of event that has occurred.

Disaster epidemiology and surveillance are rooted in epidemiologic principles that apply to other diseases, but unique challenges and concerns need to be considered in the context of disaster epidemiology. Investigators use disaster epidemiology to assess the short-term and long-term health effects (both physical and mental) of disasters. In addition, disaster epidemiology is important in allowing epidemiologists and public health practitioners to understand how to prevent deaths, injuries, and disease spread in disaster situations. Despite advances in disaster epidemiology, however, there is still a need to refine the approaches to surveillance and epidemiology in disaster situations.[1]

Unlike in other types of events, when we perform epidemiologic studies and surveillance in disasters, we focus on not only the inhabitants of a community affected by the disaster but also the workers and volunteers who respond to a disaster. These responders are often at risk for injury or disease because of their involvement in the response (e.g., a New York City Fire Department chaplain responding on 9/11 was killed by a falling object). In other situations, workers may be exposed to infectious diseases or injury risks. In addition, while we routinely do not perform surveillance and epidemiology of the impact of disasters on communities and populations that are not directly affected by an event, there may be both short-term and long-term impacts on both nearby and distant communities and populations, some of which may perceive risks similar to the people and communities affected by the disaster.

1.1 BURDEN OF DISASTER

The World Health Organization (WHO) estimates that 2.6 billion people have been affected by natural disaster phenomena in the past decade.[2] In the United States, there has been a steady increase in the number of official disaster "declarations" with more than 100 declarations in 2017. The Global Disaster Alert and Coordination System (GDACS) provides real-time information on disaster alerts around the globe and includes maps and other information about types of disasters that are current or past.[3]

2. DEFINITIONS AND OBJECTIVES IN THE STUDY OF DISASTERS

To have a basis for understanding the issues associated with disaster epidemiology and surveillance, it is important to understand the definitions commonly used in the study of disasters. First, a disaster could be considered an event that places a strain on the health or public health system such that additional resources are needed to respond. Disasters may occur within an institution, in a community, or on a broader scale. Disasters can be classified in a number of ways, but are usually described as natural or human-made, as previously noted. Natural disasters encompass a range of situations that put people at risk for significant health effects.

Disaster epidemiology is defined as the use of epidemiology to assess the short-term and long-term adverse health effects of disasters and to predict and prevent consequences of future disasters. It brings together various topic areas of epidemiology, including acute and communicable disease, environmental health, occupational health, chronic disease, injury, mental health, and behavioral health. Disaster epidemiology provides *situational awareness*—that is, it provides information that helps responders understand what the needs are, plan the response, and gather the appropriate resources.

The main objectives of disaster epidemiology are as follows:
- Prevent or reduce the number of deaths, illnesses, and injuries caused by disasters
- Provide timely and accurate health information for decision makers
- Improve prevention and mitigation strategies for future disasters by collecting information for future response preparation

As with other types of epidemiology, disaster epidemiology focuses on identifying disease and injury patterns and risk factors to the population and community affected by the disaster. This information serves as the basis for developing prevention and mitigation strategies that are driven by three contexts of disasters: *time, place,* and *person.* For example, hurricane season on the US East Coast, as well as in the Caribbean, is June 1 through November 30, whereas the Eastern Pacific season runs from May 15 to November 30.[4] In addition, the geographic area generally at risk is defined. Although people who live on or near the coast are at increased risk of injury or death during a hurricane, evacuation from the hurricane zone minimizes or eliminates this risk.

In contrast to the disaster epidemiology of hurricanes, the usual season for flu occurrence is over the late fall and winter months in the United States. Flu risk is related to exposure, immunization status, and other factors such as age; generally, elderly and very young populations, people with chronic illness or immunocompromised, and pregnant women are at increased risks for complications and mortality, depending on the flu strain that is active in a given year.[5] Prevention strategies would focus on prioritizing immunization of highest risk populations but incorporating immunization strategies to cover as much of the population as possible, and depending on the severity of an outbreak, isolation and possible medical treatment of people who have contracted flu or who have been exposed and are likely to expose others to risk.

In a disaster situation, three types of epidemiology generally are used: descriptive, analytic, and evaluative. Each contributes to the understanding of the disaster event, as well as the prevention and mitigation of harm of future events.

2.1 DESCRIPTIVE EPIDEMIOLOGY

Epidemiologists use descriptive epidemiology to identify the distribution of disease or injury among the population groups affected by the disaster. This includes identifying the health-related issues that occur among people who are responding to the event.

After the 9/11 World Trade Center disaster, responders to the scene were exposed to various types of particulate matter, as well as larger pieces of debris, some of which fell from the collapsing towers. Other responders complained of resulting respiratory problems. The epidemiology of the health aftermath of the disaster continues to emerge; longitudinal surveys are providing information on various health outcomes. A study of 2960 nonrescue disaster workers deployed to the World Trade Center following 9/11 found that at 6 years after the event, 4.2% still exhibited symptoms of posttraumatic stress disorder (PTSD). Risk factors for ongoing PTSD included major depressive disorder 1 to 2 years after the event, history of trauma, and extent of occupational exposure.[6] Asthma rates are increased in the 9/11 disaster responders as well, with a lifetime prevalence 6 years later that was almost twice (19% vs 10%) that of the general population.[7] On a larger scale, the World Trade Center Health Registry at the New York City Department of Health and Mental Hygiene will provide a 20-year follow-up through periodic contact with the enrollees.[8] To date, several research studies have provided information about the long-term effects of the disaster, including hospitalizations for asthma,[9] heart disease and lung disease,[10] parent physical and mental health,[11] among other topics.[12] This large disaster registry is continuing to provide information that may be helpful in planning prevention and intervention strategies (Box 27.1). The development of registries to monitor long-term effects of disasters has not been generalized to all disaster events but has the potential to inform efforts at prevention and mitigation strategies.

2.2 ANALYTIC EPIDEMIOLOGY

Analytic epidemiology can provide information about differences between people who were injured or became ill during an event and those who did not. The benefit is that analytic

BOX 27.1   World Trade Center Health Registry Projects

The current survey includes over 36,000 respondents as of October 2016 and is split between survivors (>37,000) and responders (>29,000). Through the overall survey and special surveys, the registry is being used to investigate the following:

- Cardiovascular disease
- Skin rash
- Alcohol use
- Posttraumatic stress disorder (PTSD) among police
- Unmet mental health care needs
- Cancer rates among enrollees
- Health of Staten Island landfill and barge recovery workers
- Respiratory and behavioral health of children
- Impact of 9/11 injuries on long-term enrollee health
- Coexistence, or comorbidity, of respiratory and mental health conditions experienced by many enrollees

Data from New York City Department of Health and Mental Hygiene, World Trade Center Registry, Survey response rate: https://www1.nyc.gov/assets/911health/downloads/pdf/wtc/wtc-datafile-manual15.pdf.

epidemiology gives information about the **risk and protective factors** related to a disaster event. For example, an investigation of deaths and injuries after a tornado outbreak can provide data about where people were when they were killed or injured, the types of injuries sustained, and whether protective factors had an impact on the occurrence of injuries. These may be environmental or behavioral factors. This type of study allows informed recommendations for interventions to help protect people from injury caused by tornadoes. It is easy to imagine how information about and descriptions of risk and protective factors in disaster events can be useful to preparedness and response planners.

2.3 EVALUATIVE EPIDEMIOLOGY

In using evaluative epidemiology, investigators can determine the effectiveness of specific interventions that have been implemented and identify factors that have resulted in their success or failure. It allows them to modify strategies and develop new interventions. This allows epidemiologists to determine, for example, if specific immunization strategies are effective in preventing spread of flu, or whether environmental changes (e.g., building standards) are effective in decreasing building collapses, and therefore deaths and injuries, in earthquakes.

Consider the example of mass shooting in schools in the United States (e.g., Parkland, Florida, in February 2018). There have been numerous suggestions about how to prevent similar incidents, ranging from arming teachers or placing armed guards in all schools, to continuing to hold active shooter drills to prepare school children for possible events. Evaluative epidemiology can provide information about the use of these interventions, as well as the risk and protective factors associated with them if an event occurs. Evaluative epidemiology may add to the data needed for research across events in addition to research related to a specific event.

3. PURPOSE OF DISASTER EPIDEMIOLOGY

Disaster epidemiology allows investigators to identify the priority health problems in the community affected by a disaster. Although the primary focus is on health problems related to the disaster itself, epidemiologists can also learn about preexisting health problems that impact a community's resilience and create needs for specific services during a disaster. In a disaster or public health emergency, it is also important to identify the causes of disease and injury and associated risk factors in the context of the event. This may include examining the results of laboratory testing of biologic and other specimens to identify specific disease agents or toxic substances involved in the event.

Various methods of classifying severity of injury or illness can aid in determining priorities for health interventions. The epidemiologic assessment of health problems allows for a rapid needs assessment that leads to planning for interventions, identification of the need for additional help, and modifications as well as additional support for the infrastructure. As an event evolves, continued surveillance and epidemiology allow tracking of the course of diseases, as well as identification of emerging issues. For example, although many people were killed and injured in the 7.0 earthquake in Haiti on January 12, 2010, it took several days to identify the emergence of cholera, which presented a significant risk to the survivors. Epidemiology was used to identify cases and limit the spread of the disease. In January 2011 the Pan American Health Organization[13] released a report on the health impact of the earthquake, highlighting lessons that could be applied to the next major disaster event. In this way, the epidemiology and surveillance from one disaster can be used to inform planning and response for future events.

3.1 FORENSIC EPIDEMIOLOGY

Forensic epidemiology is not discussed as often as it might be with respect to disaster epidemiology. The field of forensic epidemiology brings together public health and a legal investigative approach to examining a disaster or emergency situation. This is especially important in cases of suspected bioterrorism and other intentionally created events. Forensic epidemiology explores the intent, persons involved, degree of harm, and risk factors, to form a complete picture of an intentional disaster. As an example, the 1985 investigation of intentional contamination of salad bars in Oregon led to the prosecution of the religious group responsible.[14] In the case of mass shootings, a forensic epidemiology approach can provide critical information to identifying commonalities and differences between the mass shooting events.

4. DISASTER SURVEILLANCE

As with other parts of epidemiologic practice, surveillance plays a critical role in epidemiologic investigations during and after a disaster. One of the major challenges of surveillance in disasters is that many routine surveillance systems may not provide the information necessary to assess needs or identify disease or injury patterns. This occurs in both natural and human-made disasters and creates difficulty for all types of disaster epidemiology. Disasters present special circumstances in which surveillance may be difficult, and during which routine surveillance systems may not be functional or accessible because of the circumstances of the disaster. As technologies continue to emerge, the potential for using new data collection systems can increase our ability to initiate and maintain surveillance systems early in the course of a disaster.

4.1 SYNDROMIC SURVEILLANCE

Syndromic surveillance uses indicators of population and individual health that may appear before widespread disease is confirmed through clinical or laboratory diagnosis. This type of surveillance is often set up as a routine surveillance mechanism that is in place to monitor for specific diseases. For example, a sharp increase in sales of over-the-counter cold remedies might indicate the emergence of a new respiratory virus. Across the United States, emergency departments participate in syndromic surveillance systems designed to detect clusters of events in the early phases of an outbreak, such as gastrointestinal illness caused by food poisoning or disaster. Syndromic surveillance systems may be based on existing data systems, particularly when electronic health records are available in real time. If the focus is looking for a specific disease, case criteria for surveillance are identified, whereas in a more general syndromic surveillance strategy, data may be monitored for unusual patterns that could indicate emerging disease. The Centers for Disease Control and Prevention (CDC) has developed definitions for diseases associated with critical bioterrorism agents.[15] In addition, syndromic surveillance may be implemented on a short-term basis during specific events when there is a possibility of either disease transmission or an intentional act that results in illness. For example, during the 2002 Kentucky Derby Festival, 12 hospitals successfully participated in the surveillance system that was set up to quickly interpret emergency department patients' chief complaints to serve as a disease sentinel for the community.[16] Syndromic surveillance is being integrated into practice in health care settings, and entire countries are now using this approach. The CDC has established a committee, Syndromic Surveillance and Public Health Emergency Preparedness, Response and Recovery (SPHERR), that helps integrate syndromic surveillance data and information into preparedness and emergency response.[17]

4.2 CHALLENGES IN DISASTER SURVEILLANCE AND EPIDEMIOLOGY

To perform disaster surveillance activities, it is important to predefine the variables and data points that would be of interest during a particular type of disaster. Although a core set of variables is important in any disaster event, each type of event has unique circumstances that need to be documented to understand fully the impact of the event. For example, the spread of a newly emerging strain of flu would necessitate identification of the strain causing infections in the population of interest, at least to the extent that one can assume the cases beyond a

certain point in time could be attributable to the agent that has already been identified. In the case of a tornado or earthquake, the specific location of victims, with details about the type of building, the force of the tornado or earthquake, the injuries sustained and their severity, and the outcome for each person injured are all important data to collect. In an infectious disease outbreak, the trajectory of the impact on the population is very different, and there may be more time to collect data to plan for the resources and interventions that will be needed. These are data points in addition to demographic data.

Surveillance is also important after the disaster, particularly if there are risks for the development and increased transmission of infectious diseases due to the nature of the event or other known or potential long-term health impacts. Events that disrupt water supplies and sanitation place the communities affected at risk for the spread of infectious disease from contaminated water sources. Other postdisaster outcomes of interest include recovery status of injured disaster victims. An understanding of the severity of injuries sustained, as well as long-term rehabilitation and support needs, will aid in community planning.

4.3 DESIGNING A DISASTER SURVEILLANCE SYSTEM

As much as possible, a disaster surveillance system should not require a large amount of additional resources or personnel during a disaster event. Because personnel will be consumed with responding to the disaster and implementing interventions, requirements for collecting large amounts of additional data are likely to create difficulties for the personnel involved. The number of skilled staff may be insufficient to collect the data needed, or the staff responding may not have a good understanding of basic epidemiologic principles and measurement. There may be limited access to the population of interest. If a sample of the population is surveyed, it may not be representative of the overall population affected by the disaster. Cultural and language barriers pose additional problems, along with the difficulty in investigating the long-term needs of the affected population.

A core set of data points can be used in surveillance in most disaster events. Demographic data as well as simple outcome data for both victims and responders are useful in tracking the impact of the disaster as well as identifying the need for resources. A data system design that allows for a *modular* approach, which adapts the data to be collected depending on the type of event as well as the phase of the event, may be useful. System design requires consideration of the data collection methods that are routinely available and that may be available after the disaster. In addition, it is important to consider the burden that data collection will present to an already-stressed system. When possible, it is important to use existing data systems rather than creating new systems that have not been tested or accepted by those involved in a disaster response; the simpler the data collection, the better. It is also possible to collect postdisaster data and interview people who were at the scene, but this is not always optimal because of the potential for *recall bias* and for data to be missing from patient records. Data collection during and after a disaster must take into account existing data sets and information; the size, demographics, and baseline health status of the population affected; and available resources. Geographic mapping can be useful in examining the impact of environmental factors in a disaster. Consideration should be given to collecting data that will be, or are likely to be, used.

When there is an urgent need for information or acquisition of resources, a rapid survey may be done. In this scenario, only the minimum information necessary to meet the surveillance goals is collected. Only information that is not already available or cannot be collected in another way is obtained, and the goal becomes to collect as representative a sample as possible to ensure generalizability to the population affected. This type of survey is sometimes repeated and refined over the course of the event and postevent period.

In the postdisaster period, surveys of persons who were present during the event may be helpful, as may surveys of those who were injured or who became ill during the event. Key informant interviews can provide information about risks and mitigating factors experienced in the community and can help identify approaches to planning for future events. As previously described, longitudinal surveys of survivors and responders provide information about long-term health and social impacts.

5. ROLE OF GOVERNMENT AGENCIES AND NONGOVERNMENTAL ORGANIZATIONS

Preparedness for and response to disasters and pandemics require a coordinated effort from multiple agencies and organizations. Although an in-depth discussion is beyond

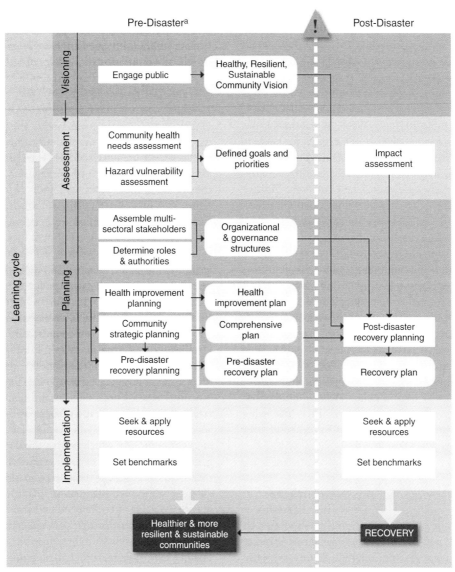

a Although the committee strongly encourages communities to undertake these activities in the pre-disaster period to maximize the opportunities to leverage the post-event recovery process for the purpose of creating healthier, more resilient and sustainable communities, in the event that they have not been undertaken beforehand, there is still benefit to incorporating them into post-disaster recovery planning.

Fig. 27.1 Building healthy, resilient, and sustainable communities before and after disasters. (From National Academies: http://nap.edu/resource/18996/Post-Disaster-Report-Brief-Insert.pdf

the scope of this chapter, a brief summary of the role of federal agencies and nongovernmental organizations (NGOs) is helpful in understanding the multifaceted nature of preparedness and response.

Public health focuses on overall population health and ensuring that population-based measures are in place for disaster preparedness and response. Surveillance activities are in the realm of public health, as is disease reporting and investigation of disease and injury occurrence. **Emergency management** agencies, which exist at various governmental levels, focus on the overall management of a disaster response and coordination of recovery services, and may be responsible for allocation of resources. The US Federal Emergency Management Agency (FEMA), now in the Department of Homeland Security, works to plan for disasters and terrorism, makes recommendations to the public on how to prepare for events, provides education for responders, and reviews disaster declaration requests from governors to ensure that resources are appropriately allocated and distributed.[18]

Various other agencies are involved in preparing for and responding to disasters at the local, state, and federal levels. The private sector and NGOs, such as the American Red Cross,[19] have an important role as well, providing services such as shelter, food, and clothing. NGOs also respond to disasters that occur around the world, providing emergency and long-term shelter, health care, food, clothing, and other services.

6. SUMMARY

Disaster epidemiology and surveillance are critical components of a disaster response and can contribute to understanding the nature of an event as well as the implications for planning for future events. There are unique challenges presented in performing surveillance during disasters, but the efforts made at surveillance using epidemiology principles provide valuable contributions to our understanding of disasters and planning for future events. Efforts to build healthy, resilient and sustainable communities after disasters can be addressed both predisaster and postdisaster (Fig. 27.1).

REFERENCES

1. Noji EK. Disaster epidemiology: challenges for public health action. *J Public Health Policy.* 1992;13:332-340.
2. World Health Organization. *Emergency and Essential Surgical Care.* Available at: http://www.who.int/surgery/challenges/esc_disasters_emergencies/en/.
3. Global Disaster Alert and Coordination System. Available at: http://www.gdacs.org.
4. National Oceanographic and Atmospheric Administration: *National Hurricane Center.* Available at: https://www.nhc.noaa.gov/climo/.
5. Centers for Disease Control and Prevention. *People at High Risk of Developing Flu-Related Complication.* Available at: https://www.cdc.gov/flu/about/disease/high_risk.htm.
6. Cukor J, Wyka K, Mello B, et al. The longitudinal course of PTSD among disaster workers deployed to the World Trade Center following the attacks of September 11th. *J Trauma Stress.* 2011;24:506-514.
7. Kim H, Herbert R, Landrigan P, et al. Increased rates of asthma among World Trade Center disaster responders. *Am J Ind Med.* 2012;55:44-53.
8. New York City Department of Health and Mental Hygiene. *9/11 Health, WTC Health Registry.* Available at: http://www1.nyc.gov/site/911health/about/wtc-health-registry.page.
9. Miller-Archie SA, Jordan HT, Alper H, et al. Hospitalizations for asthma among adults exposed to the September 11, 2001 World Trade Center terrorist attack. *J Asthma.* 2018;55(4): 354-363.
10. Alper HE, Yu S, Stellman SD, Brackbill RM. Injury, intense dust exposure, and chronic disease among survivors of the World Trade Center terrorist attacks of September 11, 2001. *Inj Epidemiol.* 2017;4:17.
11. Gargano L, Locke S, Brackbill RM. Parent physical and mental health comorbidity and adolescent behavior. *Int J Emerg Ment Health.* 2017;19:358-365.
12. New York City Government. *NYC 911 Health.* Available at: https://www1.nyc.gov/site/911health/researchers/published-research-publications.page.
13. Pan American Health Organization. *Health Response to The Earthquake in Haiti*: January 2010. Washington, DC: PAHO; 2011.
14. Török TJ, Tauxe RV, Wise PR, et al. A large community outbreak of salmonellosis caused by intentional contamination of restaurant salad bars. *JAMA.* 1997;278:389-395.
15. Centers for Disease Control and Prevention. *Syndrome Definitions for Diseases Associated With Critical Bioterrorism-Associated Agents.* Available at: https://www.cdc.gov/mmwr/preview/mmwrhtml/su5301a3.htm.
16. Carrico R, Goss L. Syndromic surveillance: hospital emergency department participation during the Kentucky Derby Festival. *Disaster Manage Response.* 2005;3:73-79.
17. Centers for Disease Control and Prevention. *Syndromic Surveillance and Public Health Emergency Preparedness Response and Recovery Committee (SPHERR).* Available at: https://www.healthsurveillance.org/page/SPHERR/Public-Health-Emergency-Preparation-Group.htm.
18. Federal Emergency Management Agency. *FEMA's Role in Winter Weather.* Available at: https://www.fema.gov/blog/2010-12-28/femas-role-winter-weather.
19. American Red Cross. Available at: https://www.redcross.org.

REVIEW QUESTIONS

1. Which of the following is an objective of disaster epidemiology?
   A. Prevent or reduce the number of deaths, illnesses, and injuries caused by disasters
   B. Provide timely and accurate information for decision makers
   C. Improve prevention and mitigation strategies for future disasters by collecting information for future response preparation
   D. Identify disease and injury patterns and risk factors to the population and community affected by the disaster
   E. All of these

2. Which contexts of disasters must be taken into consideration to develop prevention and mitigation strategies to prevent disasters?
   A. Costs, time, place
   B. Time, place, person
   C. Person, costs, time
   D. Costs, place, person
   E. None of these

3. Forensic epidemiology refers to the:
   A. Identification of the distribution of diseases or injury among the population groups affected by a disaster
   B. Analysis of risk factors associated with a disaster
   C. Evaluation of the effectiveness of an intervention to prevent disasters
   D. Analysis of the protective factors associated with a disaster
   E. Assessment of intent, persons involved, degree of harm, and risk factors associated with an intentional disaster

4. Emergency management agencies function to:
   A. Make recommendations on how to prepare for disaster events
   B. Provide short-term shelter, health care, food, clothing, and other services
   C. Review disaster declaration requests
   D. Provides education for responders
   E. Perform all of these

5. Which of the following is *not* a challenge associated with designing a disaster surveillance system?
   A. Limited access to the population of interest
   B. Cultural and language barriers
   C. Difficulty in assessing the long-term needs of the affected population
   D. Lack of public interest in identifying disaster trends
   E. Insufficient number of staff available to collect the data needed

6. An investigation of death and injuries after a hurricane identifies the environmental and behavioral factors that affected the occurrence of injuries. This is an example of:
   A. Analytic epidemiology
   B. Descriptive epidemiology
   C. Evaluative epidemiology
   D. Forensic epidemiology
   E. None of these

7. The 1972 investigation of intentional *Salmonella typhi* contamination of Chicago's municipal water system led to the arrest of two college students involved. This is an example of:
   A. Ecologic epidemiology
   B. Descriptive epidemiology
   C. Analytic epidemiology
   D. Forensic epidemiology
   E. Evaluative epidemiology

ANSWERS AND EXPLANATIONS

1. **E.** Disaster epidemiology assesses the short-term and long-term adverse health effects of disasters to predict and prevent consequences of future disasters. It brings together various topic areas of epidemiology, including acute and communicable disease, environmental health, occupational health, chronic disease, injury, mental health, and behavioral health. Disaster epidemiology focuses on identifying disease and injury patterns and risk factors to the population and community affected by the disaster.

2. **B.** Three contexts—time, place, and person—drive the development of prevention and mitigation strategies. Cost (A, C, and D) is not a contextual factor that drives how prevention and mitigation strategies are implemented.

3. **E.** Forensic epidemiology integrates public health and a legal investigative approach to examining a disaster situation. Identification of the distribution of diseases or injury among the population groups affected by a disaster (A) characterizes descriptive epidemiology. Analysis of the risk (B) and protective factors (D) is conducted under analytic epidemiology. Evaluation of the effectiveness of an intervention to prevent disasters (C) is the primary purpose of evaluative epidemiology.

4. **E.** The US Federal Emergency Management Agency (FEMA) makes recommendations on how to prepare for disasters (A), reviews disaster declaration requests from governors to ensure proper allocation of resources (C), and provides education for responders (D). NGOs respond to disasters by providing both short-term and long-term shelter, health care, food, clothing, and other services (B).

5. **D.** Limited access to the population of interest (A), cultural and language barriers (B), difficulty in assessing the long-term needs of the affected population (C), and insufficient number of staff available (E) are factors that are likely to create difficulties for personnel involved.

6. **A.** Analytic epidemiology involves the assessment of risk and protective factors associated with a disaster event. Descriptive epidemiology (A) is used to identify the distribution of disease or injury among the population groups affected by a disaster. Evaluative epidemiology (C) allows investigators to determine the effectiveness of interventions that have been implemented; forensic epidemiology (D) explores the intent, persons involved, degree of harm, and risk factors to form a complete picture of an intentional disaster.

7. **D.** Forensic epidemiology brings together public health and a legal investigative approach to examining a disaster situation. This is especially important in bioterrorism cases, such as the one described here, to identify the intent, persons involved, degree of harm, and risk factors of the intentionally created event.

28

Health Services Organization, Financing, and Quality Improvement

With Haq Nawaz

CHAPTER OUTLINE

"Management's job is to create an environment where everybody may take joy in his work."

W.E. Deming

Health care systems are complex organizations developed for the provision of care that include multiple players, such as hospitals, government, doctors, pharmaceutic companies, private practices, and public health departments. The main mission of a given health care system is to keep the population healthy and to treat disease. In the United States, outlays for medical care have steadily risen and are currently taking up close to 18% of the gross domestic product (GDP).[1,2] Health systems management exists to measure and improve how well our health care system meets its stated goals.

Improving an organization's performance first requires understanding its mission, core functions, inputs, and outputs. Health managers also must understand the environment in which they operate, and be able to assess organizational performance in regard to finances, clients or patients, and other stakeholders. Health care managers also need to know how to manage change, supervise employees, and lead teams to improve quality of care. This chapter will provide a broad overview of organizational structure of American health care institutions, financing of health care organizations, and key managerial skills required to run health care organizations. The basic functions of management include planning, organizing, controlling, and leading. Often the first three functions are called management or **operational skills,** summarized as "doing things right." The tools for operational analysis are covered under measuring organizational performance and quality improvement. In contrast, leadership or **strategic skills** are defined as "doing the right things." This is covered toward the end of the chapter. To thrive, an organization needs both. Some of the facts discussed here are unique to the US health care system. However, international readers should be able to apply most of the content of quality improvement to their own systems. Readers who want to

391

know more should consult the specialized literature (see Select Readings at the end of the chapter).

1. ORGANIZATION AND STRUCTURE OF THE US HEALTH SYSTEM

1.1 HEALTH CARE DELIVERY SYSTEMS

In contrast to many other developed nations, the health system in the United States is a hybrid of private and governmental health systems. State governments establish policies and laws, which govern the conduct of health care providers and institutions. Traditionally there has been a dichotomy of functions between the public health departments and health care institutions, such as hospitals. Many public health departments do not engage in the direct provision of health care, although some function as provider of last resort to special populations. On the other hand, hospitals and private clinics traditionally deal only with direct patient care and often expend little effort to engage in health promotion in the community. Laypersons usually think of the health care system consisting only of a hospital and affiliated practices where they usually get care. However, there are many other entities that are integral to the health system, such as pharmacies, visiting nurses, nursing homes, and rehabilitation centers. The government has a direct role in financing of health care services through Medicare, Medicaid, and the Children's Health Insurance Program (see Chapter 29). Because these programs are funded through taxpayer money, there is a great deal of interest in ensuring that health care consumers are getting the best health outcomes for their tax payments.

1.2 MANAGEMENT OF HEALTH CARE ORGANIZATIONS

In the United States, most hospitals are designated as nonprofit under the Internal Revenue Service code 501(c)(3). The majority of private practices, in contrast, are for-profit entities. Nonprofit health organizations are exempt from paying income taxes. Some believe that, if an organization is nonprofit, it cannot or need not make profit. However, despite their name, even nonprofit organizations need to make a profit to be financially viable. If they do not, they cannot invest in infrastructure, new technology, or personnel development; consequently, they will eventually close or become obsolete ("no (profit) margin, no mission").

To qualify as a **nonprofit,** an organization's purpose must meet one of the *exempt purposes* in the federal tax code, which include charitable, religious, educational, and scientific endeavors.[3] Nonprofit hospitals, for instance, must demonstrate that they provide charity care to poor patients to remain exempt from income taxes.

1.3 GOVERNANCE OF HEALTH CARE INSTITUTIONS

The governance and hierarchic structure of each health care organization vary tremendously. In private clinics, the owner of the practice also functions as its manager. In hospitals and larger health care institutions, governance structure can become quite bureaucratic with multiple layers of leadership. Nonprofit organizations are governed by a **board of trustees;** in for-profits, such an oversight committee is called the **board of directors.** These boards are ultimately responsible for setting the organization's policies and strategies. One of the board's most important jobs is to hire and fire the **chief executive officer** (CEO). The board also approves budgets, oversees the organizational performance, and sets the overall mission of the organization. The CEO is assisted by vice presidents or chiefs of service, such as a **chief financial officer** (CFO) in charge of finances and the **chief operational officer** (COO), who oversees day-to-day operations. Most organizations have additional chief officers, depending on their mission and size, such as **chief nursing officer** (CNO), **chief medical officer** (CMO), and **chief information officer** (CIO). In other organizations, such positions might be called **vice president** (VP), such as VP of nursing or VP of medical affairs.

Organizations also have **stakeholders.** A stakeholder is someone who has a vested interest in or is affected by the organization's operations. Stakeholders can include patients, community members, employees, local governments, churches, charitable organizations, vendors, visiting nurses, and unions. Most organizations cannot reach major public health goals by themselves; they need to build coalitions with stakeholders to leverage resources and build political will.

Lastly, public health and health care delivery are moral pursuits. This requires that the management and conduct of a public health agency or health care organization be *ethical,* and that the organization's mission should be reflected in its management methods.

2. FINANCING OF HEALTH CARE FACILTIES AND PUBLIC HEALTH

2.1 FINANCING MECHANISMS

Health care organizations are financed and supported through various sources. Out of 6210 registered hospitals in the United States in 2019, about 21% are for-profit, 16% are owned by the state or county government, while federally owned hospitals constitute only about 3.3% of the total.[4] An overwhelming majority (51%) are community-based nonprofit hospitals. While federal, state, and county hospitals are supported by government funding, the community-based hospitals are not. Hospitals bill for their services and receive contracted payments (revenues). Payment from Medicare forms a substantial revenue stream for hospital services, whereas Medicaid is a major payer for nursing home care (see Chapter 29). State and federal governments lack direct control over most health care institutions, but they utilize payment and financial incentives to hold organizations to certain performance standards.

2.2 BUDGETING AND FINANCIAL MANAGEMENT OF HEALTH CARE ORGANIZATIONS

Public funds are limited, which means that health care leaders must allocate existing resources wisely. There are always competing demands for available funds (e.g., salaries and benefits for employees, upgrading infrastructure, or supporting new services or initiatives). Budgeting is a way to allocate available dollars based on priorities set by leadership and is a tool to evaluate and control expenditures. The **capital budgeting process** is used to evaluate and fund major infrastructure projects, such as building a new hospital wing or expanding operating rooms. While most budgets are formulated for one fiscal year, capital budgeting is used to purchase equipment or upgrades, which are expected to last more than a year. However, all budgeting is based on assumptions and therefore represent a "best guess."

Different budgeting strategies are available. In **incremental budgeting,** budgets are built based on last year's expenses. For example, a department with five salaried employees the previous year would budget for the same five employees the following year, possibly with their salaries adjusted for any cost-of-living increases. The alternative to this is **zero-based budgeting** in which an organization pretends it starts from zero. All expenditures must be justified not based on precedent, but by current need. Incremental budgets are easy to generate, but they may not serve an organization well if its conditions and environment have changed significantly. Zero-based budgeting allows optimal matching of resources to current needs, although it can be disruptive to employees, stakeholders, and clients.

2.3 FIXED AND VARIABLE COSTS IN HEALTH CARE

Financial forecasts are improved by distinguishing between fixed and variable costs. **Fixed costs** are those that do not change over a given time span, including buildings, offices, computers, beds, and monitors. If a hospital has 200 beds, its fixed cost of doing business (such as heating the building or maintaining the office space) is the same whether all beds are occupied or not. **Variable costs** are those costs that vary with activity (e.g., use of antibiotics, dressing gauze or intravenous needles, hours of staff time). Variable costs will increase for each patient if more tests or services are offered to a patient. Both fixed and variable costs contribute to the average cost of care. The average cost of care is a useful concept in health care for budgeting and planning purposes. For example, a hospital needs to know its fixed costs and variable costs of care for particular types of patients when negotiating contracts with health insurances companies.

2.4 VARIANCE ANALYSIS

The act of comparing actual performance to budgets is called *variance analysis*. This is an extremely important step because

TABLE 28.1 Variance Analysis, Unadjusted		
	Budget	**Actual**
Sales volume	100	90
	═══	═══
Sales value	1000	990
Variable costs	500	495
Fixed costs	200	210
Profit	300	285
	═══	═══

From Palmer DA: Financial management development, No 213. © David A. Palmer 2012. http://www.financialmanagementdevelopment.com/Slides/handouts/213.pdf

TABLE 28.2 Variance Analysis, With Adjusted Variance			
	Original Budget	**Revised Budget**	**Actual**	**Variances**
Sales volume	100	90	90	
	═══	═══	═══	
Sales value	1000	900	990	90
Variable costs	500	450	495	[45]
Fixed costs	200	200	210	[10]
Profit	300	250	285	35
	═══	═══	═══	

From Palmer DA: Financial management development, No 213. © David A. Palmer 2012. http://www.financialmanagementdevelopment.com/Slides/handouts/213.pdf

it allows managers to decide if they need to take action now to spend more or less in the future.[5] Budget variances are traditionally categorized as *favorable* and *unfavorable,* and as *expected* and *unexpected.*

Tables 28.1 and 28.2 provide examples of a budget variance analysis. Budget variance can be caused by unexpected changes in clients, client mix, reimbursements, or expenses. Other types of variance include the following:

- **Volume variance.** There were fewer or more people served (e.g., more homeowners requested water safety assessment).
- **Quantity** (use) **variance.** It took more of a certain resource to deliver a certain service (e.g., restaurant inspector needed double the number of test strips per restaurant inspection than anticipated).
- **Price** (spending, or rate) **variance.** This variance occurs if the price of an input is different from the budgeted price, such as the price of a radiology machine.[6]

2.5 BREAK-EVEN ANALYSIS

Before buying new equipment or starting a new service line, it is important to model if and how the new equipment or

---

BOX 28.1 Break-Even Calculations for Buying a Piece of Medical Equipment

Estimate the number of procedures you will perform with the new medical equipment:

How many of your current patients go to another physician to have the procedure done?

How many of your current patients who otherwise would not have had the procedure done at all will now have you perform the procedure?

How many new patients will you attract by offering the procedure?

On average, how many procedures will each of these patients have per year?

What growth percentage do you expect each year in the number of procedures performed?

Estimate the additional net revenue you expect to receive from the new procedure:

How much will you charge for the procedure?

What percentage of your practice is Medicare?

What is your discount rate for Medicare?

What percentage of your practice is Medicaid?

What is your discount rate for Medicaid?

What percentage of your practice is capitated managed care?

What is your discount rate for capitated managed care?

What percentage of your practice is discounted fee-for-service?

What is your discount rate for fee-for-service?

What percentage of your practice is self-pay?

What is your discount rate for self-pay?

What percentage of your practice is some other payer?

What is your discount rate for those payers on average?

Estimate the lost revenue per year:

What is the amount of revenue you will lose by doing this procedure instead of what you normally do?

Estimate the acquisition costs of the equipment:

What is the purchase price of the equipment (including any interest paid)?

What is the transportation cost of obtaining the equipment?

What are the remodeling costs associated with installation of the equipment?

Estimate the fixed costs of the equipment:

What is the cost of additional salaried personnel you will hire to use the equipment?

What is the cost of additional space you will acquire to use the equipment (including rent and property tax)?

What is the additional cost of insurance associated with the equipment (i.e., malpractice insurance, property insurance for the equipment, business hazard/loss of use insurance)?

Estimate the variable costs of the equipment:

What is the additional wage and benefit cost for hourly personnel associated with each procedure?

What is the per-procedure cost of additional supplies you will use to perform this procedure?

Estimate the rate of return on your alternative investments:

What percent return do you expect to make on your other investments during the duration of the analysis?

Modified from Willis DR: How to decide whether to buy new medical equipment. Fam Pract Manage 11:53-58, 2004. http://www.aafp.org/fpm/2004/0300/p53.html

---

service would become profitable under various assumptions. Given that most people are (too) optimistic, it is important to have break-even calculations that examine if you will recoup money under all or most realistic scenarios.[7] The simplest way to view break-even calculations is to calculate the **break-even point.** For this calculation, one sums up the costs of the equipment and the fixed costs associated with it, then divides it by the expected volume times the profit margin of the procedure (i.e., the charge minus the costs):

$$\text{Break-even point} = \frac{\text{Costs of equipment} + \text{Other fixed costs (staff)}}{\text{Volume} \times \text{Profit margin}}$$

In reality the calculation needs to consider many other factors. The most important other economic consideration would be the economic **opportunity cost** of this investment. Opportunity cost describes the next best use of the money and resources. Any investment needs to be better than doing nothing, but also better than the next best use. Box 28.1 outlines the process for buying a new piece of equipment for a physician's office.

3. ASSESSING AND MEASURING ORGANIZATIONAL PERFORMANCE

3.1 PROGRAM ASSESSMENT AND EVALUATION

If an organization is to survive, it must periodically assess various dimensions of its performance: finances, processes, people, and mission. Usually the assessment begins with the organization's mission as the basis for goals and measurable objectives.

3.2 MEASUREMENT TOOLS

An important way to assess operational organizational performance is **benchmarking.** To benchmark, an organization conducts a self-assessment and then compares itself to similar organizations to gauge its relative performance. For public health agencies, the National Public Health Performance Standards program has developed such standards for both state and local health agencies[8]. The Joint Commission provides similar guidance for health care providers.

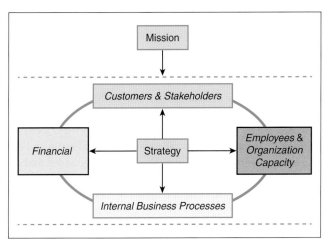

Fig. 28.1 Example of a balanced scorecard for a local government. (From Rohm H: A balancing act. *Perform* 2.)

Instruments to report performance include dashboards and balanced scorecards. **Dashboards** are operational management tools that track many indicators together. For each indicator, there are benchmarks; indicators outside acceptable benchmarks may be shaded red or yellow, whereas acceptable ones may be green. This allows managers and personnel to see immediately which domains are working well and which are not. **Balanced scorecards** provide similar feedback but present a more holistic picture of an organization to link strategic and operational domains (Fig. 28.1).[9,10]

4. QUALITY IMPROVEMENT IN HEALTH CARE

4.1 OVERVIEW OF HEALTH CARE QUALITY

While everybody likes to talk about quality in health care, it is not always clear what they mean. There are several definitions of quality. The World Health Organization (WHO) defines health care quality as "the extent to which health care services provided to individuals and patient populations improve desired health outcomes. To achieve this, health care must be safe, effective, timely, efficient, equitable and people-centered."[11] In another definition, quality is defined as "the degree to which health care services for individuals and populations increase the likelihood of desired health outcomes and are consistent with current professional knowledge."[12] According to the National Academy of Medicine (formerly the Institute of Medicine), health care quality has six dimensions: it must be safe, effective, patient-centered, timely, efficient, and equitable[13] (Table 28.3).

While these domains describe the quality of the care provided, a different model is needed to describe the quality of the health care system providing this care. In this regard, a widely used framework for health system improvement called the **Triple Aim**[14] includes (Fig. 28.2):

- Improving the patient experience of care
- Improving the health of populations
- Reducing the per capita cost of health care.

Some have advocated to add a fourth aim of *care team well-being*, thus making it a **Quadruple Aim.**[15] Others have proposed to use *equity* as an additional aim, thus making it a Quintuple Aim.[16] The Triple Aim has been widely adapted by many health care organizations and countries as a guiding principle to improve the health system.

With the increasing importance of chronic diseases (see Chapter 19), special care models have been developed to describe how best to organize care for chronically ill patients. The **Chronic Care Model**[17] in the early 1990s called for improved care of chronic illness through enhanced coordination of care at the community, organization, provider, and patient levels. Successfully treating chronic diseases requires that an *activated* patient be treated by an *activated* team who provides engagement, coaching, and links to community resources.[18] The chronic care model aims to empower, prepare, and train patients to manage their own health. This requires a collaborative

TABLE 28.3	**The Six Dimensions of Quality According to the Institute of Medicine**	
Domain	**Description**	**Examples**
Safe	Avoiding harm to patients from the care that is intended to help them	Not giving the wrong medication to a patient
Effective	Providing services based on scientific knowledge to all who could benefit and refraining from providing services to those not likely to benefit (avoiding underuse and misuse, respectively)	Giving aspirin to a patient with myocardial infarction
Patient-centered	Providing care that is respectful of and responsive to individual patient preferences, needs, and values and ensuring that patient values guide all clinical decisions	Involving patients in medical decision making; providing treatment options for patients
Timely	Reducing waits and sometimes harmful delays for both those who receive and those who give care	Giving clot-dissolving medicine to a patient with a stroke within 3 hours
Efficient	Avoiding waste, including waste of equipment, supplies, ideas, and energy	Avoiding unnecessary radiologic testing for benign and self-limited back pain
Equitable	Providing care that does not vary in quality because of personal characteristics such as gender, ethnicity, geographic location, and socioeconomic status	Providing the same level of care to patients with and without insurance

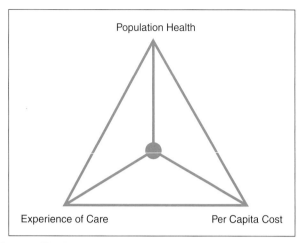

Fig. 28.2 The Triple Aim according to the Institute for Healthcare Improvement. (From http://www.ihi.org/Engage/Initiatives/TripleAim/Pages/default.aspx.)

approach between the care team and patient to define goals and establish treatment plans.

4.2 ASSESSING THE QUALITY OF CARE

The quality of medical practice has been a major concern since the early 20th century. In 1969, Donabedian pioneered the framework of assessing health care quality by proposing that quality should be examined in terms of **structure** (the physical resources and human resources that a hospital or health maintenance organization [HMO] possesses for providing care), **process** (the way in which the physical and human resources were joined in the activities of physicians and other health care providers), and **outcome** (the end results of care, such as whether the patients actually do as well as would be expected, given the severity of their problems).

Box 28.2 lists common health administration organizations and related terms by their acronym.

Several institutions and programs evaluate the quality of health institutions. **The Joint Commission** (TJC) is an independent, nonprofit organization that evaluates the quality and safety of most health care institutions in the United States and abroad. Quality review programs of the past, including the programs of **professional review organizations** (PROs),[19] tended to focus on particular aspects of process called *procedural end points* and offered a detailed review of the methods of care provided and an analysis of how well certain disease-specific treatment criteria were met. In contrast, current quality improvement efforts emphasize *quality monitoring* and focus increasingly on outcomes.

One of the primary national data sets on quality of care focuses on the services provided by **managed care organizations** (MCOs), with particular attention to prevention and health maintenance aspects of their health plans. Called the **Healthcare Effectiveness Data and Information Set** **(HEDIS),**[20] this includes several areas of prevention, such as screening for various diseases, providing immunizations, and counseling patients to quit smoking.

Several federal agencies play an important role in defining and fostering high-quality health care. The **Centers for Medicare and Medicaid Services** (CMS) requires that hospitals, nursing homes, and medical practices submit data on key metrics relating to various domains of health care quality. As the largest payer in health care, CMS makes decisions on how to pay for healthcare services (diagnosis-related groups [DRGs]; see Chapter 29), which preventive services to pay for (Chapter 18), and which quality initiatives to pursue, and thus CMS has significant impact on health care organizations. Increasingly, performance on quality of care is being tied by the CMS to reimbursement under its initiative called *value-based purchasing*. CMS reduces the payments to hospitals by a few percentage points (as of 2019, 2%), which hospitals can "earn

BOX 28.2	**Common Acronyms**			
ACO	Accountable care organization		IHI	Institute for Healthcare Improvement
AHRQ	Agency for Healthcare Research and Quality		IOM	Institute of Medicine (now the National Academy of Medicine)
CEO	Chief executive officer			
CFO	Chief financial officer		MCO	Managed care organization
CIO	Chief information officer		MEPS	Medical Expenditure Panel Survey
CMO	Chief medical officer		NCQA	National Committee for Quality Assurance
CMS	Centers for Medicare and Medicaid Services		NGC	National Guideline Clearinghouse
CNO	Chief nursing officer		NGO	Nongovernmental organization
COO	Chief operational officer		NQF	National Quality Forum
DRG	Diagnosis-related group		PCMH	Patient-centered medical home
EEOC	Equal Employment Opportunity Commission		PDSA	Plan-do-study-act
FMEA	Failure mode and effects analysis		PRO	Professional review organization
FMLA	Family and Medical Leave Act		QI	Quality improvement
HCAHPS	Hospital Consumer Assessment of Healthcare Providers and Systems		RCA	Root cause analysis
			SPC	Statistical process control
HCUP	Healthcare Cost & Utilization Project		TJC	The Joint Commission[a]
HEDIS	Healthcare Effectiveness Data and Information Set		USPSTF	US Preventive Services Task Force
HMO	Health maintenance organization		VP	Vice president
HRSA	Health Resources and Services Administration			

[a]Formerly Joint Commission on Accreditation of Healthcare Organizations (JCAHO).

back" by meeting quality requirements.[21] The increasing importance of quality of care is demonstrated by the fact that CMS plans to apply equal weights (25%) to quality domains of safety, efficiency/cost reduction, clinical care, and care experience. Therefore, it is imperative that leaders of health care organizations understand that their economic survival may depend on managing and improving quality of care.

The following **organizations** play an important role in defining and promoting high-quality health care:

The **Agency for Healthcare Research and Quality** (AHRQ) is the lead federal agency to improve the quality, efficiency, safety, and effectiveness of US health care. The AHRQ website hosts the US Preventive Services Task Force (USPSTF) (see Chapter 18) recommendations and the National Guideline Clearinghouse (NGC), as well as survey data on the Medical Expenditure Panel Survey (MEPS) and the Healthcare Cost and Utilization Project (HCUP). The AHRQ also finances projects to study the comparative effectiveness of various interventions and publishes technology reports that synthesize the status of the evidence on various health care topics.

The **National Quality Forum** (NQF) convenes expert panels to study and endorse quality and performance metrics. In the prevention area, NQF collaborates with the Department of Health and Human Services (DHHS) to promote homogeneous reporting of adverse events and to align with other organizations in improving the care of people with chronic conditions.

The **Institute for Healthcare Improvement** (IHI) is an independent nonprofit organization. It focuses on motivating and building the will for change by setting concrete goals and deadlines, identifying and testing new models of care in partnership with both patients and health care professionals, and ensuring the broadest possible adoption of best practices and effective innovations. IHI's highly publicized "5 Million Lives" campaign involved recruiting 4050 hospitals to implement bundles of proven improvement tools between December 12, 2006 and December 9, 2008. This initiative focused on reducing preventable diseases, such as adverse drug reactions, central line infections, and surgical infections.

The **National Committee for Quality Assurance** (NCQA, www.ncqa.org) recognizes and accredits health care institutions and providers for implementing programs such as the patient-centered medical home (PCMH),[22] accountable care organizations (ACOs) (see Chapter 29), and various disease management programs.

4.3 METHODOLOGIC ISSUES IN MEASURING QUALITY OF CARE

Efforts to fairly measure the quality of medical outcomes pose significant methodologic problems. Unless outcomes are adjusted for the severity of patients' illnesses, hospitals treating the sickest patients will be at an unfair disadvantage. The process of adjusting for the severity of illness usually is referred to as **case mix adjustment.**[23] The question arises as

to whose judgment of outcome—the judgment of patients or that of professionals—should be used to evaluate outcomes and how to account for patient compliance.

The federal government now rates hospitals by calculating a **case mix–adjusted mortality** rate for each hospital. In addition, the federal government has put increased pressure on hospitals to improve the quality of their care by mandating that they report certain indicators about care of patients with pneumonia, heart failure, and acute myocardial infarction to the Centers for Medicare and Medicaid Services (**CMS quality indicators**)[24] and by tying part of reimbursement to good performance.

One major concern about current efforts to reduce costs is whether reducing cost would reduce quality of care as well. Clinicians and epidemiologists continue to address this question in ongoing studies.

4.4 QUALITY IMPROVEMENT IN HEALTH CARE: THE SCIENCE OF IMPROVEMENT

Many concepts used in the medical care quality improvement come from the business world. The theory of quality improvement consists of four components:

1. *Appreciation of a system.* Health care delivery is accomplished through the complicated interactions among the many components of a health care system (e.g., health care providers, hospitals, drugs, equipment, and patients).
2. *Understanding variation.* Variation in a given system's structure, process, and outcomes is common. Just like patients' symptoms may differ for the same disease, patients' outcomes also may vary even with similar treatment. In addition, regional or geographic variation in approach to treatment is common.
3. *Theory of knowledge.* Knowledge is built by making incremental changes and observing the results (see cycle of improvement, to come).
4. *Psychology of workers.* Because health care delivery is complex and relies heavily on humans, we must understand the interactions between the health system and workers and the impact of any changes in the system on health care workers.

Borrowing techniques from the business world, nine key **organizational performance approaches** have been recommended, as depicted in Table 28.4.

4.5 HEALTH CARE QUALITY VARIATION AND DISPARITIES

The current state of health care quality in the United States continues to show large variability, unequal improvement, and continued disparities. Particularly striking are the disparities in **social determinants of health,** such as high school noncompletion and poverty, which have not narrowed in the last decades in spite of overall improvements in health[25] (see Chapters 14 and 30).

Part of the problem is the emphasis on research. Many interventions could improve outcomes, but they remain

TABLE 28.4	Strategies for Organizational Performance Improvement[a]
1. Eliminate waste	Remove redundancies that do not enhance patient care or care quality.
2. Improve workflow	Streamline steps in care delivery to make it more efficient.
3. Optimize inventory	Excess inventory, whether it is medical products or personnel input, may be a waste. Inventory should be adjusted to meet the demand.
4. Change work environment	Improving work environment can enhance worker's productivity and patient safety.
5. Improve provider/patient relationship	Both patients and health care workers benefit from better relationships to reduce stress and increase job satisfaction.
6. Manage time effectively	Health care workers can have best productivity if their time is managed well. Wasteful activities do not benefit patients. Patients appreciate timely service.
7. Manage variation	Variation in delivery in health care is a major source of less than optimal health outcomes. Make efforts to standardize care when possible.
8. Redesign system to avoid errors	Systems and components should be designed or redesigned in a way to avoid errors. Predict common human errors and use technology to avoid or guard against those errors.
9. Focus on service	Improve services to patients, seek input from patients, and figure out ways to enhance patient satisfaction.

[a]Adapted from Langley GL, Moen R, Nolan KM, et al: *The improvement guide: a practical approach to enhancing organizational performance,* ed 2, San Francisco, CA, 2009, Jossey-Bass Publishers.

underused. Yet most research energy in the United States goes toward finding still more *new* solutions. If just a fraction of this energy were instead focused on consistently implementing *established* effective care, the gains in averted mortality and morbidity would be breathtaking (see also Chapter 19).

Another source of variation in health care quality involves provider preferences and local customs. This is illustrated by the significant geographic variation that exists in health services delivery, often in counterintuitive ways. Health care spending rises significantly if more physicians and hospitals practice in a given area, and some regions have much higher rates of performing certain invasive procedures than others.[26] John Wennberg at Dartmouth pioneered the concept of analyzing such variation through **small area variation analysis** in the Dartmouth Atlas of Health Care.[27] For example, unadjusted per capita spending on Medicare beneficiaries averaged $9415 in 2013, but was as high as $13,149 in some counties compared to $6726 in other counties. Even after adjustment for demographics, incomes, and comorbidities, the spending difference remains,[28] with no difference in patient outcomes.[29] This variability is driven in part by a payment system in which physicians and hospitals make money by seeing more patients because payments are tied to episodes of care. Fortunately, new payment systems are emerging (e.g., accountable care organizations; see Chapter 29) that reward organizations for improving overall health outcomes. Hopefully such models will contribute to hospitals and providers focusing their efforts on prevention of disease and health promotion rather than on maximizing the volume of care.

4.6 MEDICAL ERRORS AND PATIENT SAFETY

Medical errors are a serious concern in health care. The Institute of Medicine (IOM) report, "To Err Is Human," first highlighted the pervasive existence of medical errors.[30] Based on this report, the IOM estimated that about 44,000 to 98,000 preventable deaths occur each year as a result of medical error. Newer estimates put the number at close to 250,000 per year.[31] A medical error is defined as the failure of a planned action to be completed as intended or the use of a wrong plan to achieve an aim.

Not all medical errors result in deaths. Many, however, harm patients and can lead to costly treatment. Most errors result from a chain of events in faulty systems of care or care processes rather than from individual oversights. Based on analysis of catastrophic failures in the aviation industry, the **Swiss cheese model** was developed to describe this phenomenon as the failure of multiple layers of safety (Fig. 28.3).

4.7 METHODS AND TOOLS TO IMPROVE QUALITY OF CARE

4.7.a Method of Improvement

Health care organizations use various methods to maintain and improve quality of care. Once a quality problem has been identified, hospitals may use specialized tools, such as a root-cause analysis (see upcoming discussion), to understand what led to medical error. The next challenge is how to make improvements in health care delivery systems to avoid such errors in the future.[32]

4.7.b The Plan-Do-Study-Act (PDSA) Cycle

The basic model of improvement is shown in Fig. 28.4. It consists of three preparatory questions and repeated cycles of improvements, with the repeated cycle steps of plan, do, check (or study), and act.

The first preparatory question is to ask what the goal is: "What are we trying to accomplish?" Examples include *reduce* patient complaints, *reduce* waiting time, and *decrease* expenses from overtime.

Second, and most importantly, managers must ask, "How will we know that a change is an improvement?" In simple systems, it is easy to see if a change is an improvement. But in

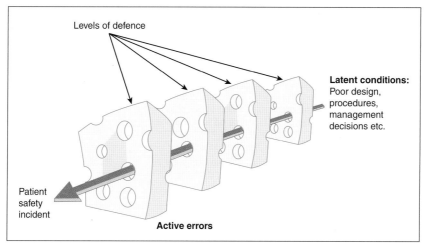

Fig. 28.3 The Swiss cheese model of errors. (From Carthey J: Understanding safety in health care: the system evolution, erosion, and enhancement model. *J Pub Health Res* 2, 2013.)

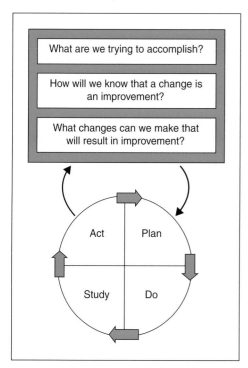

Fig. 28.4 The plan-do-study-act (PDSA) worksheet is a useful tool for documenting a test of change. (From http://www.ihi.org/resources/Pages/HowtoImprove/default.aspx.)

health care, most problems are complex, and change is not easy to detect. Measures of improvement should be balanced and include metrics of efficiency, staff engagement, and patient satisfaction.

In the third preparatory question, the manager must ask, "What change can we make that will result in improvement?" For most problem categories, certain changes have a good chance of succeeding. For example, for workflow issues with bottlenecks, tasks can be moved to be done in parallel, staffing can be matched to demand spikes, or multiple data entry can be simplified.[33]

In the fourth step of repeated cycles of improvement, each possible solution is then evaluated in a **plan-do-study-act** (PDSA) **cycle** (or **rapid cycle improvement**).[34] The *plan* part describes exactly who will do what, where, and when, and how data will be collected. In the plan part, it is also important to make predictions for how any changes are expected to impact the problem. In the *do* part, the plan is carried out, problems and unexpected developments are documented, and data analysis is begun. In the *study* stage, data analysis is completed and compared to predictions, and learning points are summarized. These learning points lead to new changes to be made in the next cycle. This process is repeated until an intervention has been tried out in different environments and circumstances, and the change seems robust enough to be broadly implemented.

Most projects are best improved by *small increments* of change with **rapid cycle improvement,** which means that any possible interventions are tested and retested with repeated improvements within a small setting (e.g., with one nurse or on one floor). It is much better to test and tweak solutions to a problem than to roll out a grand strategy throughout the organization and then realize it does not work as intended.

Several other tools have been developed to analyze complex problems. Specific tools to increase safety include **failure mode and effects analysis** (FMEA)[35] and **root cause analysis** (RCA),[36] which are described next.

4.7.c Failure Mode and Effect Analysis (FMEA)

FMEA was originally developed by the US military as a tool to predict the effect of system and equipment failures. It has since been successfully used in health care to identify vulnerabilities proactively and deal with them effectively.[37] It asks the question, "What can go wrong?" In this step, a team tries to think of all possibilities how a failure can occur. Every failure possibility is assigned a **severity rating** (How grave would this failure be?), an **occurrence rating** (How likely is this failure to occur?), and a **detection rating** (How likely is

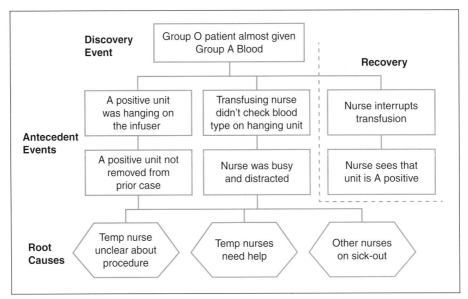

Fig. 28.5 Root cause analysis example. (From https://www.ahrq.gov/professionals/education/curriculum-tools/cusptoolkit/modules/identify/identify.html#sl15.)

this failure to be detected?). Severity, occurrence, and detection ratings are multiplied for a **risk priority number.** This risk priority number ensures that those failure modes are first addressed that are most likely, most harmful if they occur, and hardest to detect.

4.7.d Root Cause Analysis (RCA)

RCA, as the name implies, is a tool or exercise used to retrospectively review medical errors to understand what happened. In a root cause analysis, a safety team drills into the system issues behind mistakes by asking "what" and "why" multiple times until all aspects of the process are reviewed and the contributing factors considered.[38] A variation of RCA often used in medical practice is **clinical debrief.** In a clinical debrief, all staff members who were involved in an incident sit together and analyze the event step by step. Together the group determines in a blame-free environment what happened and which policies are needed to prevent a similar error from happening again. A sample of RCA is shown in Fig. 28.5.

4.7.e Lean and Six Sigma

The **Lean** approach was developed by the Japanese automobile manufacturer Toyota. Its central aims are to avoid waste and to concentrate on activities that bring value to the customer. Important concepts in Lean include defining value from the consumer perspective, identifying value streams, smoothing out the flow of steps, and removing waste and activities that do not add value.[39] The **Six Sigma** methodology concentrates on decreasing variation.[40] The first steps are defining the project goals and requirements of internal and external customers, measuring and determining customers' needs and specifications, and then setting benchmarks to meet industry standards. The next steps include analyzing if the process meets customer needs, then redesigning it if

necessary. Lastly, the process is standardized until it shows only minimal variability.

4.7.f Statistical Process Control

A **statistical process control** (SPC) chart is a way to analyze data over time, taking into account random fluctuation. SPC charts have been successfully used to improve processes in public health[41] (Fig. 28.6). An SPC chart helps to distinguish random fluctuation from change caused by interventions.

4.7.g High Reliability Organizations

High reliability organizations (HROs) have unwavering focus on patient safety. The concept of HRO is modeled after studying other high-risk industries such as airlines, navy aircraft carriers, and nuclear power plants.[42] Accidents and bad outcomes are exceedingly rare in these industries. The HRO model uses this construct to improve patient safety in health care organizations by empowering employees, especially frontline staff, to act in real time to safety concerns.[43] The HRO model is a proactive model in which health care leaders anticipate medical errors, prepare for them, and respond in a timely manner. There are five key elements of HRO: preoccupation with failure, reluctance to simplify explanations for failures, situational awareness, relying on frontline staff, and commitment to resilience after failures.

4.8 CHANGE MANAGEMENT

Most changes will not succeed without the support of people, and most improvement efforts require teamwork.[44] Anyone engaged in improvement efforts will have to deal with staff reacting to change, also called the human side to change. Change often results in some people losing control, power, or

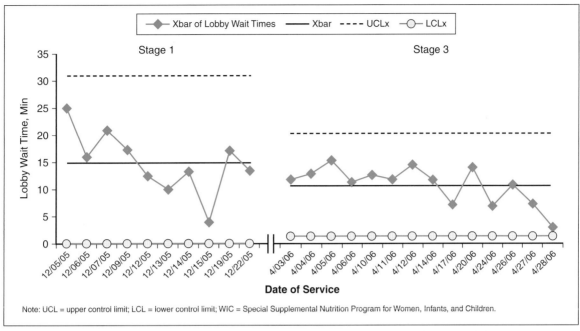

Fig. 28.6 Example of statistical process control (SPC) chart for wait times in WIC clinic. *WIC,* Special Supplemental Nutrition Program for Women, Infants, and Children. Cbar, Average. (From Boe DT, Riley W, Parsons H: Improving service delivery in a county health department WIC clinic: an application of statistical process control techniques. *Am J Public Health* 99, 2009.)

privileges. Concerns regarding such losses should be elicited and addressed. Machiavelli deftly described the difficulties this entails: "There is nothing more difficult to carry out, nor more doubtful of success, nor more dangerous to handle, than to initiate a new order of things. For the reformer has enemies in all those who profit by the old order, and only lukewarm defenders in all those who would profit by the new." Managers must distinguish among subtly different reactions to change, as follows:

- Hostility ("I don't like it, and I will say so")
- Apathy ("I don't care and will neither fight nor hinder")
- Compliance ("I won't fight but will disagree privately")
- Conformance ("It's a good idea, but not my fight")
- Commitment ("I will implement and advocate a change")

People are not really allies until they reach the last stage, and they do this in the same way as patients change behavior, that is, in steps.

Initial hesitation should not be viewed as resistance. However, ambivalence can easily become resistance. The main pitfall is to underestimate the resistance that does emerge and to think of changes as only technical in nature. How this can be overcome is covered next.

4.8.a Implementation of Change and Overcoming Resistance to Change

Many successful solutions have been set aside because managers underestimate the energy and persistence necessary to hardwire a process. The following strategies can help:

1. Communicating persistently why the change is needed and why the status quo is no longer an option. Such communication is most powerful if it relates back to the organization's mission and speaks with the voice of the patient, client, or consumer.
2. Gathering input about the ideas from those affected by the change. Those most affected often understand best what will or will not work.
3. Informing everyone about progress made during testing.
4. Allowing for longer improvement cycles during the implementation phase so that kinks can be worked out and doubters have time to come onboard.
5. Sharing specific information as early as possible about how the change will affect people.
6. Designing the system so that making the correct choices is easy.

The implementation process of a change needs copious amounts of managerial support so it is monitored, adjusted, and sustained for a significant time before it can be trusted to be permanent.

5. STRATEGIC PLANNING AND LEADERSHIP IN ORGANIZATIONS

The competitive nature of the health care market forces leaders of health care organizations to develop strategies about how they will compete. Strategy can be defined as "basic long term goals and objectives of a firm and the adoption of a particular course of action and allocation of resources to achieve these objectives."[45] Strategy is central to future survival of health care organizations and provides a vision on how a particular organization will compete in the market.

For example, hospitals may promote a particular line of service such as a childbirth center or introduce robotic surgery as a way to attract patients.

5.1 STRENGTHS, WEAKNESSES, OPPORTUNITIES, AND THREATS (SWOT) ANALYSIS

In devising a strategic vision, organizations need to understand their business environment in a formal industry analysis. Two commonly used methods are SWOT[46] (Fig. 28.7) and Porter's Five Forces analyses.

5.2 ANALYZING MARKETS-PORTER'S FIVE FORCES ANALYSIS

Health care providers compete with one another for patients and market share. Therefore a market analysis should be done to analyze market forces whenever new lines of service are considered or when the future of the organization is considered. **Porter's Five Forces Analysis**[47] provides a framework to analyze market forces:

- Internal Rivalry. Do other providers in the same area already offer similar services?
- Threat of Entry. How are other hospitals positioned in regard to services? Could they start to offer similar services?
- Substitute and Complementary Products. What are the alternatives to the services offered? Could patients get similar outcomes from different providers or other procedures?
- Supplier Power. Suppliers may have a monopoly and charge higher prices. Has the supplier market changed? Are price increases likely?
- Buyer Power. Patients may have multiple choices of facilities to get elective surgery done.

5.3 FUTURE TRENDS: INTEGRATING CLINICAL CARE AND COMMUNITY HEALTH

Traditionally, clinical care providers have concentrated on treating sick patients that came to them, and public health providers have aimed to promote health in the communities. With the advent of the chronic care model, the responsibility of the health care system to help patients stay healthy has come into focus. Currently an even bigger shift is occurring. Many health care organizations are taking on financial risk for the health of a defined population through accountable care organizations (see Chapter 29). With this shift, hospitals have become much more interested in the upstream causes of poor health and how to improve them, for example by partnering with community agencies, schools, or public health departments.[48] Another model of integration involves **community-centered health homes.**[49] In these, community-based clinics, such as an Indian health center or a federally qualified health center, team up with housing agencies, hospitals, or other community agencies to address social determinants of health. Many such programs identify patients who would benefit from referrals to housing support or transportation services and provide in-house referrals. Others ensure that data collected in clinical care settings (e.g., the areas in which patients live who present to the emergency room for asthma) is shared with housing authorities to see what improvements can be made.[49] In all likelihood it will take such integration to achieve the triple aim of increasing health outcomes for individuals and populations while also providing low-cost care.

6. SUMMARY

There is a growing awareness that the quality and efficiency of the US health care system in general is a public health concern. Many higher level public health jobs also require a

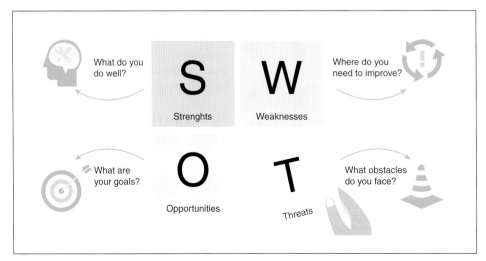

Fig. 28.7 SWOT analysis. (From Gregory A: How to conduct a SWOT analysis for your small business. The Balance Small Business. www.thebalancesmb.com/swot-analysis-for-small-business-2951706.)

degree of managerial skills and understanding of organizational decision making. Organizations are accountable to their boards, employees, clients, and community stakeholders. In a well-managed organization, the operational details (doing things right) flow from the overall strategic goals (doing the right things). Responsibility for nonprofit organizations is vested in a board of trustees, which hires and fires the chief executives and oversees day-to-day operations.

Tools to measure organizational performance include identifying relevant standards, benchmarking, dashboards, and balanced scorecards. The main tools to assess financial performance are budget planning and variance analysis. Budgets can be planned in an incremental or zero-based manner. For budget variance analysis, actual revenue and expenses are compared to the budget, and favorable and unfavorable variances are identified. Sources for variance include volume, sale, and price variances.

Quality of care can be measured for structure, processes, and outcomes. Aims for high-quality health care include safe, effective, patient-centered, timely, efficient, and equitable outcomes. The Triple Aim, a standard for considering health system improvement, consists of the care experience, the population health, and the cost of care. The basis of a quality improvement process is the basic plan-do-study-act cycle. Changes should be tested in small increments with rapid improvement cycles before implementation. When planning an implementation process, managers should plan for and address staff resistance. Specialized tools to address quality problems in health care include failure mode and effects analysis, root cause analysis, Six Sigma, and Lean methodology. Strategies to decrease resistance include constant communication regarding the need for change, involvement of frontline staff, and high-level support.

Tools for strategic planning include SWOT analysis as well as Porter's tools for market analysis. In the future, clinical care organizations and public health agencies may team up more than in the past to address upstream causes of poor health and the social determinants of health together.

REFERENCES

1. Centers for Medicare and Medicaid Services. *NHE Fact Sheet.* 2018. Available at: www.cms.gov/research-statistics-data-and-systems/statistics-trends-and-reports/nationalhealthexpenddata/nhe-fact-sheet.html.

2. Martin AB, Hartman M, Benson J, Catlin A. National health spending in 2014: faster growth driven by coverage expansion and prescription drug spending. *Health Aff (Millwood).* 2016;35:150-160.

3. Internal Revenue Service. *Exemption Requirements Section 501(c)(3) Organizations.* 2018. Available at: www.irs.gov/charities-non-profits/charitable-organizations/exemption-requirements-section-501c3-organizations.

4. American Hospital Association. *Fast Facts on US Hospitals.* 2019. Available at: www.aha.org/statistics/fast-facts-us-hospitals.

5. Kavanagh S, Swanson CJ. *Tactical Financial Management: Cash Flow and Budgetary Variance Analysis.* 2018. Available at: www.gfoa.org/sites/default/files/GFR_OCT_09_8.pdf.

6. Variance Analysis and Sensitvity Analysis. In *Tools to Plan, Monitor, and Manage Financial Status.* Boston, MA: Jones & Barlett Publishers. Available at http://samples.jbpub.com/9780763778941/78941_18_CH17_189_204.pdf.

7. Gallo A. A quick guide to breakeven analysis. *Harvard Business Review.* 2014. Available at: https://hbr.org/2014/07/a-quick-guide-to-breakeven-analysis.

8. Centers for Disease Control and Prevention. *National Public Health Performance Standards—STLT Gateway.* 2017. Available at: www.cdc.gov/stltpublichealth/nphps/index.html.

9. Kaplan RS, Norton DP. Using the balanced scorecard as a strategic management system. *Harvard Business Review.* 2007. Available at: https://hbr.org/2007/07/using-the-balanced-scorecard-as-a-strategic-management-system.

10. Rohm H. *Performance Measurement in Action—a Balancing Act.* Available at: www.balancedscorecard.org/Portals/0/PDF/perform.pdf.

11. World Health Organization. *What is Quality of Care and Why is it Important?* 2017. Available at: www.who.int/maternal_child_adolescent/topics/quality-of-care/definition/en/.

12. Agency for Healthcare Research and Quality. *Understanding Quality Measurement.* 2018. Available at: www.ahrq.gov/professionals/quality-patient-safety/quality-resources/tools/chtoolbx/understand/index.html.

13. Agency for Healthcare Research and Quality. *The Six Domains of Health Care Quality.* 2018. Available at: www.ahrq.gov/professionals/quality-patient-safety/talkingquality/create/sixdomains.html.

14. Institute for Healthcare Improvement. *The IHI Triple Aim.* 2018. Available at: www.ihi.org/Engage/Initiatives/TripleAim/Pages/default.aspx.

15. Bodenheimer T, Sinsky C. From triple to quadruple aim: care of the patient requires care of the provider. *Ann Fam Med.* 2014;12:573-576.

16. Agency for Healthcare Research and Quality. *Redefining Primary Care for the 21st Century.* Rockville, MD: Agency for Healthcare Research and Quality; October 2016.

17. Improving Chronic Illness Care. *The Chronic Care Model.* 2018. Available at: www.improvingchroniccare.org/index.php?p=the_chronic_caremodel&s=2.

18. Improving Chronic Illness Care. *Model Elements.* 2018. Available at: www.improvingchroniccare.org/index.php?p=Model_Elements&s=18.

19. Social Security Administration—Program Operations Manual System (SSA-POMS). *HI 00208.080—Role of Professional Standards Review Organizations (PSRO).* 2018.

20. National Committee for Quality Assurance. *HEDIS & Quality Measurement.* 2018. Available at: www.ncqa.org/hedis-quality-measurement.

21. Centers for Medicare and Medicaid Services. *CMS Hospital Value-Based Purchasing Program Results for Fiscal Year 2019.* December 3, 2018. Available at: www.cms.gov/Newsroom/fact-sheets/CMS-Hospital-value-based-program-results-for-fiscal-year-2019.

22. Agency for Healthcare Research and Quality/PCMH Resource Center. *Defining the PCMH.* 2018. Available at: https://pcmh.ahrq.gov/page/defining-pcmh.

23. Mendez CM, Harrington DW, Christenson P, Spellberg B. Impact of hospital variables on case mix index as a marker of disease severity. *Popul Health Manag.* 2014;17:28-34.

24. Centers for Medicare and Medicaid Services. *Core Measures*. 2017. Available at: www.cms.gov/Medicare/Quality-Initiatives-Patient-Assessment-Instruments/QualityMeasures/Core-Measures.html.

25. Singh GK, Daus GP, Allender M, et al. Social determinants of health in the United States: addressing major health inequality trends for the nation, 1935-2016. *Int J MCH AIDS.* 2017;6: 139-164.

26. Ko DT, Wang Y, Alter DA, et al. Regional variation in cardiac catheterization appropriateness and baseline risk after acute myocardial infarction. *J Am Coll Cardiol.* 2008;51:716-723.

27. Fisher ES, Wennberg DE, Stukel TA, Gottlieb DJ, Lucas FL, Pinder EL. The implications of regional variations in Medicare spending. Part 1: The content, quality, and accessibility of care. *Ann Intern Med.* 2003;138:273-287.

28. Kaiser Family Foundation. *The Latest on Geographic Variation in Medicare Spending: A Demographic Divide Persists But Variation Has Narrowed.* 2015. Available at: www.kff.org/medicare/report/the-latest-on-geographic-variation-in-medicare-spending-a-demographic-divide-persists-but-variation-has-narrowed/.

29. Gawande A. The cost conundrum. *New Yorker.* 2009. Available at: www.newyorker.com/magazine/2009/06/01/the-cost-conundrum.

30. Institute of Medicine. In: Kohn LT, Corrigan JM, Donaldson MS, eds. *To Err is Human: Building a Safer Health System.* Washington, DC: The National Academies Press; 2000:312.

31. Makary MA, Daniel M. Medical error—the third leading cause of death in the US. *BMJ.* 353:i2139, 2016.

32. Hughes RG, ed. Advances in patient safety tools and strategies for quality improvement and patient safety. In *Patient Safety and Quality: An Evidence-Based Handbook for Nurses.* Rockville, MD: Agency for Healthcare Research and Quality; 2008.

33. Langley GJ, Moen RD, Nolan RD, Nolan TW, Norman CL, Provost LP. *The Improvement Guide: A Practical Approach to Enhancing Organizational Performance.* 2nd ed. San Francisco, CA: Jossey-Bass; 2009.

34. Institute for Healthcare Improvement. *Science of Improvement: Testing Changes.* 2018. Available at: www.ihi.org/resources/Pages/HowtoImprove/ScienceofImprovementTestingChanges.aspx.

35. Institute for Healthcare Improvement. *Failure Modes and Effects Analysis (FMEA) Tool.* 2018. Available at: www.ihi.org/resources/Pages/Tools/FailureModesandEffectsAnalysisTool.aspx.

36. Parker J. *Root Cause Analysis in Health Care: Tools and Techniques.* 5th ed. Oak Brook: The Joint Commission; 2015. Illinois.

37. U.S. Department of Veterans Affairs. *VA National Center for Patient Safety. Healthcare Failure Mode and Effect Analysis.* 2015. Available at: www.patientsafety.va.gov/professionals/onthejob/hfmea.asp.

38. Neily J, Ogrinc G, Mills P, et al. Using aggregate root cause analysis to improve patient safety. *Jt Comm J Qual Saf.* 2003;29:434-439.

39. Lawal AK, Rotter T, Kinsman L, et al. Lean management in health care: definition, concepts, methodology and effects reported (systematic review protocol). *Syst Rev.* 2014;3:103.

40. American Society for Quality. *Six Sigma Definition—What is Lean Six Sigma?* 2018. Available at: http://asq.org/learn-about-quality/six-sigma/overview/overview.html.

41. Thor J, Lundberg J, Ask J, et al. Application of statistical process control in healthcare improvement: systematic review. *Qual Saf Health Care.* 2007;16:387-399.

42. Chassin MR, Loeb JM. High-reliability health care: getting there from here. *Milbank Q.* 2013;91:459-490.

43. High Reliability in Health Care is Possible. Joint Commission Center for Transforming Healthcare; 2019. Available at: https://www.centerfortransforminghealthcare.org/en/high-reliability-in-health-care. Accessed October 7, 2019.

44. Kotter JP. Leading change, Why transformation efforts fail. *Harv Bus Rev.* 1995:73:59–67. Available at: https://hbr.org/1995/05/leading-change-why-transformation-efforts-fail-2. Accessed October 7, 2019.

45. Dranove D, Besanko D, Shanley M, et al. *Economics of Strategy.* 7th ed. Hoboken, NJ: Wiley; 2018.

46. Gregory A. *How to Conduct a SWOT Analysis for Your Small Business.* 2019. Available at: www.thebalancesmb.com/swot-analysis-for-small-business-2951706.

47. Mind Tools. Porter's Five Forces. *Understanding Competitive Forces to Maximize Profitability.* 2018. Available at: www.mindtools.com/pages/article/newTMC_08.htm.

48. American Hospital Association. *Trends in Hospital-Based Population Health Infrastructure.* 2017. Available at: www.hpoe.org/resources/ahahret-guides/1467.

49. Pañares R, Mikkelsen L, Do R. *The Community-Centered Health Homes Model: Updates & Learnings.* 2016. Available at: www.preventioninstitute.org/publications/community-centered-health-homes-model-updates-learnings.

SELECTED READINGS

Adams K, Corrigan JM. *Priority Areas for National Action: Transforming Health Care Quality.* Washington, DC: National Academies Press; 2003.

Committee on Quality of Health Care in America and Institute of Medicine. *Crossing the Quality Chasm: A New Health System for the 21st Century.* Washington DC: National Academies Press; 2001.

Deming WE. *Out of The Crisis.* Cambridge, MA: MIT Press; 1986.

Donabedian A. A guide to medical care administration. In: *Medical Care Appraisal.* Vol 2. New York, NY: American Public Health Association; 1969.

Fallon LF, McDonnell CR. *Human Resource Management in Health Care: Principles and Practice.* Sudbury, MA: Jones & Bartlett; 2007.

Fallon LF, Zgodzinksi EJ. *Essentials of Public Health Management.* 2nd ed. Sudbury, MA: Jones & Bartlett; 2008.

Institute of Medicine. *Priority Areas for National Action: Transforming Health Care Quality.* Washington, DC: National Academies Press; 2003.

Institute of Medicine. The state of quality improvement and implementation research. 2007. http://www.nap.edu/catalog/11986.html.

Pañares R, Mikkelsen L, Do R. *The Community-Centered Health Home Model: Updates and Learnings.* Oakland, CA: Prevention Institute; 2016.

Penner SJ: *Introduction to Health Care Economics & Financial Management: Fundamental Concepts With Practical Applications.* Philadelphia, PA: Lippincott Williams & Wilkins; 2004.

Pham JC, Aswani MS, Rosen M, et al. Reducing medical errors and adverse events. *Ann Rev Med.* 2012;63:447-463. doi:10.1146/annurev-med-061410-121352.

Swartzmann RH, Sewell RH. *Principles of Public Health Management.* New York, NY: Wiley; 2010.

WEBSITES

Agency for Healthcare Research and Quality: http://www.ahrq.gov

Baldrige Program: http://www.nist.gov/baldrige/about/what_we_do.cfm

Centers for Medicare and Medicaid Services: http://www.cms.gov

Centers for Medicare and Medicaid Services—Hospital Compare: https://www.medicare.gov/hospitalcompare/search.html?

Commonwealth Fund: data center and health systems rankings: http://www.commonwealthfund.org/

Dartmouth Atlas of Health Care: http://www.dartmouthatlas.org

Health Resources and Services Administration: http://www.hrsa.gov

Institute for Healthcare Improvement: www.ihi.org

The Joint Commission: http://www.jointcommission.org

National Committee for Quality Assurance: http://www.ncqa.org

National Guideline Clearinghouse: http://www.ncqa.org/tabid/1415/Default.aspx

National Quality Forum: http://www.qualityforum.org

Organization for Economic Cooperation and Development: http://stats.oecd.org/

Veterans Administration: Safety topics: http://www.patientsafety.gov

REVIEW QUESTIONS

1. Nonprofits are sometimes called tax-exempt organizations, or referred to by the section of the tax code that designates them (a code that should be remembered as it is part of the accepted parlance):
   A. 501(c)(3)
   B. 501(c)(4)
   C. 105(c)(3)
   D. 105(c)(4)
   E. 105(b)(4)

2. The final responsibility in a nonprofit health organization rests with the:
   A. Chief executive officer (CEO)
   B. Chief financial officer (CFO)
   C. Chief medical officer (CMO)
   D. Board of directors
   E. Board of trustees

3. In a nonprofit organization, any profits go to:
   A. The chief executive officer
   B. Stakeholders
   C. Shareholders
   D. The organization
   E. Nonprofit organizations do not make profits

4. The act of comparing actual performance to budgets is called:
   A. Variable costing
   B. Variance analysis
   C. Volume variance
   D. Quantity variance
   E. Price variance

5. Before purchasing new equipment or starting a new budgetary line to provide health-related services, what is the most important economic question that must be asked?
   A. What are the fixed costs of the equipment or service?
   B. What are the variable costs of the equipment or service?
   C. What is the expected volume of procedures or services to be provided with the new equipment or service line?
   D. What will be the expected lost revenue with the new equipment or service line?
   E. What is the expected net revenue compared with the alternatives of not moving forward or doing something else?

6. The Joint Commission (TJC, formerly JCAHO) is an independent, nonprofit organization that evaluates the quality and safety of most US health care institutions. In TJC assessment, how institutions screen and treat patients for tobacco use is an example of what type of measure?
   A. Structure
   B. Process
   C. Outcome
   D. Small area
   E. HEDIS

7. Which of the following is a governmental organization involved in defining and fostering high-quality health care?
   A. JCAHO
   B. IHI
   C. AHRQ
   D. NCQA
   E. NQF

8. Two hospitals have comparable facilities, staff, polices, and procedures. However, when an independent group measured quality based on outcomes only, Hospital A performed much better than Hospital B. In response, leadership at Hospital B put procedures in place to stop accepting the sickest patients, knowing that these most severe cases were driving the institution's poor quality score. The next year, Hospital B performed just as well as Hospital A, receiving an excellent quality score. In this ironic case, measuring quality likely led to poorer quality for the patients most in need; the sickest patients were effectively abandoned. The moral fabric of Hospital B's leadership aside, this unfortunate result might have been avoided if Hospitals A and B were compared using:
   A. Failure mode and effects analysis (FMEA)
   B. Root cause analysis (RCA)
   C. Six Sigma
   D. Case-mix adjustment
   E. Rapid cycle improvement

9. In general, regarding health care at present, the largest and most expedient improvements in quality might come from:
   A. Studying novel health care delivery approaches
   B. Proposing innovative community programs
   C. Developing new service delivery systems
   D. Finding fresh solutions to quality problems
   E. Implementing existing interventions

ANSWERS AND EXPLANATIONS

1. **A.** The term *501(c)(3)* is often used as a synonym for nonprofit organization. Under the US tax code, organizations that qualify for tax-exempt status under section 501(c)(3) include religious, educational, charitable, scientific, and literary organizations, and organizations that do testing for public safety, that foster national or international amateur sports competition, or that prevent cruelty to children or animals. For the other answer choices, (B) 501(c)(4) concerns civic leagues, social welfare organizations, and local associations of employees; (C) to (E) are nonsense distracters.

2. **E.** The final responsible body in a nonprofit organization is the board of trustees; the board of directors (D) is the analogous body in a for-profit organization. The board of trustees hires and fires the CEO, who then hires the various officers representing the other answer choices. The board also approves the budget and oversees the overall organizational performance. The chief executive officer (A) is the highest ranking officer under the board, and similarly approves budgets and oversees overall organizational performance. Underneath the CEO is a vice presidential suite that usually includes the chief financial officer (B). Organizations engaged in direct patient care will also have a chief medical officer (C).

3. **D.** Even nonprofit organizations need to have revenues exceed expenses. In other words, they hope to have profit (not E), although this profit is then reinvested into the organization. Profits go to infrastructure, new technology, or personnel development, as opposed to being distributed to shareholders (C), the case with for-profit organizations. Because the aim is to operate successfully without generating net losses (i.e., to generate profit), there has been a shift away from the term *nonprofit* to the term *not for profit,* which helps clarify that organizations definitely want to do more than break even, even though the ultimate goal is not to produce financial return for investors. The profits do not go directly to stakeholders (B) but may indirectly affect them through organizational improvements and enhanced service delivery. The chief executive officer (A) is paid a salary, and although there may be financial incentives for high performance determined by the board of trustees, the CEO is not the direct recipient of organizational profits.

4. **B.** The act of comparing actual performance to budgets is called variance analysis. In conducting variance analysis, both fixed and variable costs need to be considered, but variable costing (A) is not a legitimate term. Types of variance that might be discovered in conducting a variance analysis are volume variance (C), quantity or use variance (D), and price (spending or rate) variance (E).

5. **E.** While fixed (A) and variable (B) costs are important considerations, as well as expected utilization (C) and possible losses of revenue (D), from an economic perspective, the most fundamental question is, *Will moving forward with new equipment or a new service line result in greater net revenue?* In other words, will making the change produce greater profit than the alternatives of making no change, or doing something else (e.g., purchasing different equipment, starting different service line). Economics is not the only consideration in plans for change, however, and the organization might be willing to accept less of a profit margin if a change will result in greater care delivery or improved client services. As long as the organization will confidently break even and maintain some revenue over cost for safety, a relative decrease in profit might be acceptable given humanitarian, service, or other concerns related to the organization's mission.

6. **B.** Assessing the procedures in place to identify and treat smoking patients would be an example of a process measure. Process measures are not as common as outcome measures; current quality improvement efforts focus increasingly on outcomes (C). With smoking patients, the number counseled to quit would be a related outcome measure, an example of a HEDIS (E) measure. A related measure pertaining to structure (A) might be whether a health care facility has an established smoking cessation program or substance abuse counselors available. Small area (D) is a term referring to a type of geographic analysis, looking at variation in quality measures by different geographic regions.

7. **C.** The Agency for Healthcare Research and Quality is the lead federal agency to improve the quality, efficiency, safety, and effectiveness of US health care. The Joint Commission, formerly known as JCAHO (A), the Institute for Healthcare Improvement (B), the National Committee for Quality Assurance (D), and the National Quality Forum (E) are independent, nonprofit, nongovernmental groups involved in defining and fostering quality health care.

8. **D.** Case-mix adjustment describes the process of adjusting quality analyses for the severity of illness. Unless outcomes are adjusted for the severity of patient illnesses, organizations treating the sickest patients (e.g., Hospital B) would be at an unfair disadvantage. The case in the question demonstrates one means of dealing with this unfair disadvantage and illustrates the limitations of relying on outcome measures only for quality assessment. Outcome assessments inherently

create incentives to "cherry pick" or (to use terminology of the insurance industry) to avoid "adverse selection," such that only the healthiest people remain patients, and outcomes naturally improve as a result. Although scores are better and quality improves for the organization, quality actually can worsen for a community, or at least its most vulnerable segments. What you may achieve with nonadjusted outcome scoring is institutions gaming the system rather than actually improving care. Failure mode and effects analysis (A), root cause analysis (B), and Six Sigma (C) are different quality improvement methodologies, and rapid cycle improvement (E) is about making system improvements in small, incremental steps.

9. **E.** Although there are many established, effective interventions, substantial energy goes into finding still more new solutions. If just a fraction of energy pursuing new ideas were instead focused on implementing established, effective care consistently (giving every patient the right interventions the right way at the right time), the gains in mortality and morbidity would be great. Quests to develop new, novel, fresh, and innovative approaches (A–D) might ultimately be helpful, but also might be completely fruitless. Regardless, they would not be as expedient as implementing existing interventions now.

29

Health Care Organization, Policy, and Financing

With Casey Covarrubias

CHAPTER OUTLINE

"America's health care system is neither healthy, caring, nor a system."

Walter Cronkite

1. OVERVIEW

In an ideal world, health care would meet three goals: universal access, high quality, and limited costs. In the real world, there are tradeoffs; at best, systems can attain only two of these three goals at any one time[1] (Fig. 29.1). The United States spends approximately 18% of its gross domestic product (GDP) on health care. Prices of services and goods, including administrative costs in particular, contribute to this high spending.[2] The United States, among other countries, faces the challenge of effectively allocating limited resources to ensure the best health outcomes. In the United Kingdom, for example, the National Institute for Health and Care Excellence (NICE) uses clinical and cost-effectiveness measures to provide guidance to the National Health System on which health care services and technologies to cover.

In 1968, Garrett Hardin[3] wrote about "the tragedy of the commons," perhaps the most famous contribution to the population-control debates of the 1960s. He noted that individuals and groups tend to maximize their own gains and use more than their fair share of any common good (known as **moral hazard**). Because the shared resources of the earth (the "commons") are limited, the attempt by one individual or group to maximize its own welfare would necessarily diminish the good that others can derive from the commons. This logic can be applied to the use of medical resources in the United States. Unless Americans are able and willing to organize, finance, and regulate medical care in light of the needs of the entire population, various individual groups (e.g., industries, hospitals, hospital chains, health maintenance organizations [HMOs], insurance companies, nursing homes, home care programs) will continue to seek to maximize their benefits (their share of the commons) at the expense of others.

This chapter examines the fundamental legal, social, and political framework underlying health care in the United States, how it is organized, and how it can provide the greatest value given limited resources. Although the legal and organizational framework of the health care delivery system is different in other countries, the challenges and need to distribute scarce resources are universal.

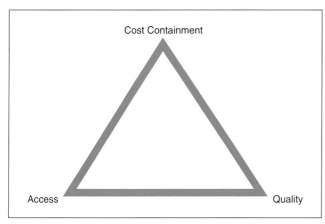

Fig. 29.1 The "iron triangle" of health care. (From Kissick W: *Medicine's dilemmas: infinite need versus finite resources,* New Haven, CT, 1994, Yale University Press.)

1.1 TERMINOLOGY IN HEALTH POLICY

Health care policy and financing require the use of economic terminology, including concepts such as needs and demand, utilization, and elasticity, often with an array of acronyms (Box 29.1). Although the term "felt need" is sometimes used to describe a patient's judgment about the need for care, more frequently the **demand for health care** is actually studied. Demand in the medical context is the quantity of care that is purchased at a given price. For this economic definition to work, there must be an assumption of **price elasticity** (i.e., an assumption that as prices increase, the demand for a given service will decrease).

This assumption was tested in one of the largest social science experiments, the **Health Insurance Experiment** conducted by the RAND Corporation in the 1970s. It randomized

---

BOX 29.1   Frequently Used Acronyms in Health Care Organization, Policy and Financing, With Descriptions

ACO   **Accountable Care Organization**
New care model that includes providers and hospitals cooperating together for better outcomes and taking financial risk for outcomes.

ADA   **Americans with Disabilities Act**
Forbids discrimination based on disabilities and requires employers to make reasonable accommodations for disabled workers.

CAA   **Clean Air Act**
Regulates emissions from area, stationary, and mobile sources.

CERCLA   **Comprehensive Environmental Response, Compensation, and Liability Act**
Also called **Superfund Act,** established a trust fund for cleanup of abandoned and uncontrolled hazardous waste sites.

CMS   **Centers for Medicare and Medicaid Services**
US federal agency that administers Medicare, Medicaid, and the Children's Health Insurance Program.

COBRA   **Consolidated Omnibus Budget Reconciliation Act of 1985**
Allows employees to continue their insurance after job termination.

EMR   **Electronic Medical Record**

EMTALA   **Emergency Medical Treatment and Active Labor Act**
Law that requires emergency departments to provide initial evaluation and stabilization of all patients regardless of their ability to pay.

EPA   **Environmental Protection Agency**

ERISA   **Employee Retirement Income Security Act**
Regulates the content of established employee health plans.

FIFRA   **Federal Insecticide, Fungicide, & Rodenticide Act**
Enacted in 1996, controls the distribution, use, and sale of pesticides.

FQHC   **Federally Qualified Health Centers**
Community health centers that qualify for special federal grants to treat Medicare and Medicaid patients.

HIPAA   **Health Insurance Portability and Accountability Act**
Calls for standards in implementing a national health information infrastructure and for regulation of the protection of individual health information in such a system.

HSA   **Health Savings Account**
Individual tax-preferred savings account for health expenses, usually coupled with a high-deductible insurance plan.

MCO   **Managed Care Organization**

PCMH   **Patient-Centered Medical Home**
Care model in which patients are cared for by a physician-directed team that provides comprehensive care with enhanced access and responsibilities for patient engagement, coordination, and population management.

PPACA   **Patient Protection and Affordable Care Act**
Health care reform bill passed in 2010 under President Obama in an effort to enact universal health care; Supreme Court ruled it constitutional in 2012. The Affordable Care Act (ACA) remains a law as of this edition (2019).

Continued

BOX 29.1   **Frequently Used Acronyms in Health Care Organization, Policy and Financing, With Descriptions—cont'd**

PRO	**Peer Review Organization**
	Also formerly called *professional review organization;* group of medical professionals or a health care company that contracts with CMS to ensure that services covered by Medicare meet professional standards.
RCRA	**Resource Conservation and Recovery Act**
	Established that the Environmental Protection Agency should control hazardous waste "from cradle to grave."
SARA	**Superfund Amendments and Reauthorization Act**
	Expanded CERCLA and established a community's right to obtain information about hazards.
TRI	**Toxic Release Inventory**
	Publicly available database on toxic chemical releases and other waste management activities.

almost 6000 enrollees to insurance plans of different levels of coverage, deductibles, and copayments. The study found that patients *did* change their utilization of health care in response to different insurance levels (i.e., there was elasticity of health care to price). However, this elasticity was small compared with that of demand for nonmedical goods and services. Furthermore, health care spending was reduced for *both* necessary care and unnecessary care, which led to worse blood pressure control, vision, and oral health.[4]

Because of the difficulties of measuring demand, what is usually studied is the effective (realized) demand, called **utilization.** Utilization is usually less than need, so the concept of unmet need was developed. **Unmet need** can be defined by the following equation:

$$\text{Unmet need} = \text{Need} - \text{Utilization}$$

1.2 FACTORS INFLUENCING NEED AND DEMAND

Demographic factors are among the most important influences on the need and demand for medical care. Foremost is the age of the population, as well as mortality rates and fertility patterns. In the United States, a rather sudden decline in birth rates occurred in the 1970s with the wide availability of oral contraceptives and legalization of abortion. Fertility levels have remained low, leading to an extended period in which the proportion of employment-aged individuals in the US population will be the smallest in history. A major concern is whether the smaller number of workers will be able to support the large, older population with such benefits as Medicare and Social Security retirement payments. The expected shortage of workers will put upward pressure on wages, making care more expensive. The aging population has also become a global phenomenon. By 2050, the global population of individuals aged 65 or older is predicted to be 1.6 billion, up 17% from 2015.[5]

Other factors that influence medical needs and demands include advances in medical technology, especially pharmaceutical and medical devices. As new methods of prevention, diagnosis, and treatment become available, more providers and more patients will use them.

One might expect that the unmet need for medical care would be greatest among the poorest members of society, but that is not always true. People with income below some percentage of the poverty line are eligible for Medicaid (see later). The **medically indigent** are people whose incomes are too high to be eligible for Medicaid and those who do not receive medical insurance in their jobs. These individuals may be able to support themselves, but usually cannot afford to pay all of their medical bills. Many of the **medically uninsured** (those who have no health insurance) and **medically underinsured** (those whose health insurance is inadequate) are medically indigent. They are not on welfare, but they cannot financially tolerate major medical bills. In 2015, the medically uninsured population in the United States numbered about 29 million people, about 9% of the US population.[6]

1.3 INTERNATIONAL COMPARISON

The United States spends more on health care than other countries; it spends around two times as much as other high-income countries, despite reporting similar utilization rates and a higher uninsured population[7] (Fig. 29.2). However, these higher expenditures do not lead to uniformly superior outcomes.[8] Even worse, the United States has made much less progress than other industrialized countries in improving overall life expectancy in the past 40 year,[9] and has actually seen a decline in health expectancy in some groups.

The United States ranks last in health care system performance and last or next to last on four dimensions of a high-performance health care system: access, equity, health care outcomes, and administrative efficiency.[10] The mismatch between health expenditures and health and the inexorable rise of health cost are driving a push to control (i.e., reduce) health care spending.

To understand why we pay so much for so little health and how that could change, it is important to understand the underlying laws and functions of health care delivery in the United States. Laws build the underpinnings of health care delivery and the complex environment that generates the conditions for health.[11]

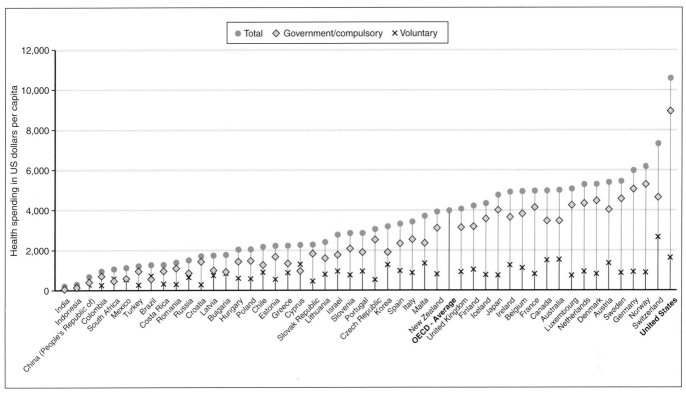

Fig. 29.2 Comparison of health spending in US dollars per capita among countries (2014–2017). (Organization for Economic Co-operation and Development: Health spending. https://data.oecd.org/healthres/health-spending.htm.)

2. LEGAL FRAMEWORK OF HEALTH

2.1 US PUBLIC HEALTH SYSTEM

Government's public health responsibilities exist at three levels: federal, state/tribal, and local/municipal.[11] The responsibility for public health below the federal level is usually scattered through multiple agencies, and each state and locality have a framework of laws and regulations. For all states, surveillance and required reporting are exercises of state police powers. Most of the existing legislation was enacted at a time when infectious diseases were the main threat to public health. Frequently these laws have not been meaningfully updated to account for new threats, such as chronic diseases, bioterrorism, or emerging epidemics, nor has the ability to share data kept pace with technologic innovations.[11]

2.2 ENVIRONMENTAL LAWS

The US Congress passed most important environmental regulations that impact health in the 1970s[12] (Box 29.2). In 2015, a landmark global effort resulted in the **Paris Agreement,** an international pact negotiated within the United Nations Framework Convention on Climate Change. The Paris Agreement aims to mitigate global climate change by keeping the global temperature rise below 2°C this century. Each country establishes nationally determined contributions (NDCs) and is accountable through regular reports on

---

BOX 29.2 Example US Environmental Laws

Clean Air Act (CAA)
Passed in 1970, amended in 1990. Regulates emissions from area, stationary, and mobile sources; also established National Ambient Air Quality Standards.

Clean Water Act (CWA)
Established in 1972 as the Federal Water Pollution Control Act, amended in 1977 to become the Clean Water Act. Instituted pollution control standards for discharges into US waterways.

Safe Drinking Water Act (SDWA)
Passed in 1974. Regulates water and underground injection of waste, protecting groundwater.

Resource Conservation and Recovery Act (RCRA)
Gives the Environmental Protection Agency (EPA) control over hazardous waste "from cradle to grave," on active and future facilities.

Comprehensive Environmental Response, Compensation, and Liability Act (CERCLA)
Created a tax on industries and established a trust for cleanup of abandoned and uncontrolled waste sites; also called the Superfund Act.

Superfund Amendments and Reauthorization Act (SARA)
Established the community's right to obtain information about hazards and the Toxic Release Inventory (TRI).

Federal Insecticide, Fungicide, & Rodenticide Act (FIFRA)
Enacted in 1996; controls the distribution, use, and sale of pesticides.

emissions and implementation efforts (see Chapter 22 for more on environmental health).

2.3 DUTIES OF HEALTH CARE PROVIDERS AND HOSPITALS

Title VI of the Civil Rights Act of 1964 states, "No person in the United States shall, on the ground of race, color, or national origin, be excluded from participation in, be denied the benefits of, or be subjected to discrimination under any program or activity receiving Federal financial assistance." This act has been interpreted to mean that facilities must provide qualified interpreter services. Similarly, the **Americans with Disabilities Act** (ADA) forbids discrimination based on disabilities. The **Hill-Burton Act** financed construction of public and not-for-profit community hospitals. It established a "community services obligation" in exchange for receiving funds that requires hospitals to demonstrate how they serve their communities. The **Emergency Medical Treatment and Active Labor Act** (EMTALA) requires emergency departments to evaluate and treat patients regardless of their ability to pay.

The **Patient Protection and Affordable Care Act** prohibits discrimination on the basis of race, color, national origin, sex, age, or disability in any health program that receives federal funding. This is the first federal civil rights law to prohibit discrimination in federally funded health programs on the basis of sex. The provision also extends to individuals receiving coverage through the Health Insurance Marketplaces and health programs provided by the US Department of Health and Human Services (DHHS). [13]

The **Health Insurance Portability and Accountability Act** (HIPAA) was enacted in 1996 to develop national standards for an information system and for the protection of health information in such a system. The HIPAA Privacy Rule mandates that all entities that handle identifiable health information implement standards to protect against the misuse of such information.

2.4 HEALTH CARE FINANCING AND INSURANCE

The **Employee Retirement Income Security Act** (ERISA) from 1974 regulates the content of established employee health plans. It was later amended by the **Consolidated Omnibus Budget Reconciliation Act** of 1985 (COBRA), which enables employees to purchase employer-sponsored health insurance for a limited time after termination.

2.4.a Patient Protection and Affordable Care Act

The **Patient Protection and Affordable Care Act** (PPACA) became law in 2010 and may be the most comprehensive health care legislation since Medicare in 1965. The act offers a mix of regulations covering a wide swath of topics.[14] In broad strokes, the PPACA does the following:

- Requires most US citizens and legal residents to have health insurance *(individual mandate),* and provides tax penalties if they do not. The federal tax penalty for violating the individual mandate was subsequently cancelled, starting in 2019.
- Expands Medicaid, provider payments in Medicaid, and Children's Health Insurance Program coverage.
- Provides subsidies to individuals at certain income levels to obtain insurance.
- Establishes **state-based insurance exchanges** for employers and individuals to obtain coverage
- Imposes rules on insurance plans, requiring them to provide basic preventive services at no cost and insurance coverage for dependent children up to age 26, and forbidding them to exclude patients because of preexisting conditions.
- Provides funds for various initiatives to explore innovative care approaches, such as accountable care organizations, comparative effectiveness research, and other attempts to reduce health care costs without jeopardizing quality.
- Established an **Independent Payment Advisory Board** to provide recommendations to reduce Medicare costs; these recommendations would become binding unless Congress found similar cost reductions elsewhere. In 2018, the Bipartisan Budget Act of 2018 repealed this component of the PPACA.
- Decreases expenses by penalizing readmissions, taxing high-end plans, cutting provider payments, and establishing a value-based purchasing program that penalizes hospitals for low rates on established quality metrics.
- Increases funds for employer-based wellness programs and preventive services with an A or B rating from the US Preventive Services Task Force (USPSTF), and recommendations from Bright Futures (children), the Women's Preventive Services Initiative (WPSI), and the CDC Advisory Committee on Immunization Practices (ACIP).

The PPACA closely mirrors the health reform law passed in Massachusetts in the early 2000s. Not surprisingly, given the political stakes, opinions differ about what the Massachusetts and PPACA experience has shown. Most analysts agree that the health care reform has expanded the insured pool and increased access to providers, perhaps more so for disadvantaged citizens.[15] Views on the impact on costs are more mixed. The reform has resulted in a net cost rather than net savings and has led to an influx of more newly insured patients without expanding the provider pool, which may have increased wait times. Also, the reform has not changed patient behavior or convincingly slowed the growth of health care costs.[16] In June 2012 the US Supreme Court ruled to enforce the individual mandate. The Court held that the individual mandate exceeded congressional power to regulate commerce but was constitutional under the power to levy taxes.[17] In December 2017, however, Congress enacted legislation that would remove the tax penalty associated with the individual mandate.

3. THE MEDICAL CARE SYSTEM

3.1 HISTORIC OVERVIEW

Until the late 1800s, most medical care was ambulatory. Patients paid local practitioners on a **fee-for-service** (see later) basis. The hospital tended to be viewed as a "death house" and a place for the sick poor, often supported by the church or other benevolent organizations. In the early 1900s, as medicine became more scientific and more surgical procedures available, the hospital came to be seen as the "doctors' workshop." The technology and ancillary personnel and services were usually provided at no charge to the physicians, which helped them practice their craft. In turn, physicians kept the hospitals in business by bringing in patients. With the founding of the National Institutes of Health (NIH) in 1948 came a push for improved biomedical technology. The research done since then has made the practice of medicine not only much more effective for some diseases, but also far more complex and costly. This increased complexity has resulted in increasing specialization of physicians and other health care workers.

3.2 LEVELS OF MEDICAL CARE

In an effort to maximize the effectiveness and efficiency of the process, health care professionals have proposed an integrated system of graded levels of care. The levels range from treatment in the patient's home, the least complex level, to treatment in a tertiary medical center, the most complex level of care (Box 29.3). Although the movement from one level to another should be easy, rapid, and smooth, often this is not the case. Transitions in care are risky, and transfers require particular care to accurately communicate medication changes, treatment plans, and follow-up tests.

Many medical care decisions are not made by professionals but instead by patients for themselves, or with input from friends or family members. In keeping with other trends in US society, patients increasingly are expected to take control over their own health care. The tremendous amount of health information now available has been a major force for empowering people regarding their own health. However, this information available on the Internet can often be incorrect or misleading. Also, to make informed decisions, patients need to be able to read and understand medical information, a capability called **health literacy.** Some patients may be overwhelmed by providers' expectations that they share or make important decisions about their health care.

BOX 29.3 Levels of the Medical Care System[a]

1. Acute, general hospital facilities	**Tertiary medical center** Most or all of the latest technology, usually participates in medical education and clinical research. Offers different levels of care, including intensive care units, special units, and standard units. **Intermediate hospital** Medium to large community hospital. Considerable amount of the latest technology. Less research and investigational activity. **Local community hospital** Services such as routine diagnosis, treatment, and surgery. Lacks the personnel and facilities for many complex procedures.
2. Rehabilitation, convalescent care facilities	**Special unit** Housed in a regular hospital. **Rehabilitation hospital** Patients recovering from trauma or from neurologic diseases or surgery may benefit from physical therapy, occupational therapy, and other methods of tertiary prevention (see Chapter 17).
3. Extended care facilities	**Skilled nursing facility (SNF)** Also called a nursing home. Provides 24-hour nursing care and special forms of care, such as intravenous fluids, medicines, and rehabilitation. **Intermediate care facility (ICF)** Suitable if the patient's primary need is for help with the activities of daily living (eating, bathing, grooming, transferring, toileting). Unlike an SNF, an ICF is not required to have a registered (skilled) nurse on duty at all times. **Hospice** A nursing home that specializes in providing *palliative* (comfort) *care* for terminally ill patients, such as patients with cancer.
4. Organized home care	**Public agencies** (local health departments or visiting nurse association) **Private organizations** May be necessary for patients discharged from the hospital to their homes, where they continue to receive treatment or follow-up procedures that require specialized skills (e.g., placing and monitoring intravenous lines for therapy, drawing blood for tests).
5. Self-care in the home	Treatment in the patient's home. Examples include home diagnostic tools such as blood pressure cuffs and blood glucose testing equipment.

[a]1 indicates most complex; 5 indicates least complex.

4. HEALTH CARE INSTITUTIONS

4.1 HOSPITALS

Although the term *hospital* is generally thought to refer to an institution providing acute, general care to persons with a wide range of health problems, there are various types of hospitals. Some focus on a special group of patients (e.g., children's hospital), whereas others focus on a special type of medical problem (e.g., psychiatric hospital) or a particular type of service (e.g., rehabilitation hospital).

Hospitals may be for-profit or not-for-profit. A for-profit hospital may be independent or part of a for-profit chain of hospitals. Not-for-profit hospitals may be sponsored by various institutions, such as the local community churches; the city, county, or state government; or a university (see Chapter 28). The Affordable Care Act included an additional requirement that not-for-profit hospitals must provide a "community benefit" to be eligible for their nonprofit tax status.[18]

4.2 PHYSICIAN PRACTICES

Historically, most US physicians were in **solo medical practice,** although they might share night and weekend coverage with other solo practitioners. Gradually, they began to develop **practice partnerships** to achieve efficiencies and economies by sharing the cost of office space, equipment, and staff. In a partnership, physicians still work only for themselves.

A logical extension of the partnership was the formation of a **group practice** consisting of three or more (often many more) physicians. This increased the efficiencies of sharing office space and staff, and had the advantage of providing availability of built-in consultation with other physicians concerning complex cases. In a group practice, physicians are employees of the practice. Group practices could be of the single-specialty or the multispecialty type. Although most group practices initially operated on a fee-for-service basis, some began to develop the concept of **prepaid group practice,** in which the practice collects money from patients or employers and commits to providing all the care needed for these patients. On the West Coast, the Kaiser Corporation set up its own multispecialty group practice before World War II to care for its workers. Membership has since been opened to the general public, and it is now known as Kaiser Permanente. This was the first example of a large, prepaid group practice in the United States.

4.3 HEALTH MAINTENANCE ORGANIZATIONS

During the mid-1970s, prepaid group practices that met certain standards and contractual arrangements were named **health maintenance organizations** (HMOs). People who enrolled in an HMO were usually part of some economic group, such as workers in a company or industry, but their enrollment had to be voluntary. They paid a fixed monthly fee, which varied depending on the size of the group. In return, the HMO had the contractual obligation to *provide* the types of medical care specified in the contract (rather than to provide *financial reimbursement*, as in the case of an insurance company), or at least to ensure that the stipulated care was provided. The HMO assumed some of the risk when income was less than expenses and made a profit when income was greater than expenses.

The HMO collects prepaid capitation premiums for medical services provided to its enrollees, monitors the service pattern, and approves and pays bills for services from physicians, hospitals, and others.

Health maintenance organizations can be organized in three different models: staff, group, and network. In the **staff model** HMO, most of the physicians are salaried, full-time employees who either work exclusively in the health plan or (as is typical in Kaiser Permanente) belong to a physician group that contracts to provide all the medical services in the health plan. A staff model HMO may own its hospitals; however, in most cases, the HMO contracts with one or more local hospitals for all hospital care. In the staff model, the physicians' time and effort are directed mainly or exclusively toward care of the HMO patients. These physicians coordinate patient care and refer patients to specialists. A **group model HMO** provides the physician services through contracts with one or more organized groups of physicians. The HMO also contracts with one or more area hospitals for hospital services at predetermined rates. A **network model HMO** is similar to a group model HMO but is looser in structure. The network model HMO has contracts with many physician groups (single-specialty and multispecialty groups) and sometimes with individual physicians. It may have a contract with one or more hospitals. The more providers an HMO has in a geographic area, the more attractive it is to patients because they are usually able to choose their preferred physicians and hospitals.

An **independent practice association** (IPA) is a legal entity, usually an organization of physicians, that solicits enrollees and their premiums (from HMO payers or companies) and contracts with office-based fee-for-service physicians in private practice to provide the required care, at a discounted rate. In addition, the IPA contracts with hospitals to provide inpatient care (the **physician-hospital organization** is a variant of IPA that is associated with a single hospital, which usually does the administrative work). In IPAs the practitioners are supposed to perform the gatekeeper function (although they are usually less effective in controlling costs than are practitioners in other HMOs), and the IPA monitors utilization for appropriateness. Enrollees must receive their care from an IPA-affiliated hospital and from members of the IPA's **physician panel** (primary care physicians and specialists who have a contractual arrangement with the IPA). A physician may be a member of the panel of several IPAs, which makes the referral process quite confusing.

Currently, the most dominant model is the **preferred provider organization** (PPO). A PPO is a variation on the IPA theme; it is not usually approved as a federally qualified

HMO because it lacks tight cost-control procedures. A PPO is formed when a third-party payer (e.g., insurance plan or company) establishes a network of contracts with independent practitioners. As with the standard IPA, the PPO has a panel of physicians who have contracted to provide services at agreed-on (reduced) rates. A major difference between the standard IPA and a PPO, however, is that the patients in a PPO can see physicians who are not on the PPO panel, although they will have to pay extra to do so (**point-of-service [POS] plan**).

In the past, many HMOs have used financial incentives for providers to shape their behavior and reduce unnecessary costs. Important ethical problems can arise, however, if the compensation plan puts physicians' financial incentives in conflict with their patients' interests, such as when primary care physicians receive a bonus if they keep referral rates to specialists low. In response to these ethical dilemmas, the American College of Physicians has published an **Ethics in Practice Statement** advocating for transparency in managed care, open and participatory processes in resource allocation policy, and an obligation for individual providers to enter into agreement only if they can ensure that these agreements do not violate professionalism and ethical standards.[19]

4.4 AMBULATORY CARE

Outside of physicians' offices, ambulatory care can be through hospital outpatient clinics, surgicenters (freestanding surgical centers), walk-in clinics inside pharmacies, or retail clinics, and urgent care clinics. Of particular importance for underserved patients are **community health centers.** Federal health programs in the 1960s and 1970s encouraged the development of community health centers. Many of these centers were supported partly through federal and state grants, and most were placed in underserved areas in big cities or rural locations. These **federally qualified health centers** (FQHCs) are eligible for federal grant support and enhanced reimbursement for Medicare and Medicaid patients and can provide free immunizations for uninsured children and reduced fees to other patients.

Starting in the early 2000s, **retail clinics** began to emerge as possible substitutes for costly visits to the emergency department. Retail clinics are ambulatory clinics housed within large retail stores, with care often delivered by nurse practitioners or physician assistants, and limited services provided. Many retail clinics accept commercial insurance, Medicare, and Medicaid coverage. Despite the cost-saving potential, early evidence shows that the rapid increase of retail clinic locations has not led to a decline in emergency department visits but has increased health care use and spending.[20]

4.5 TELEMEDICINE AND E-HEALTH

Telemedicine is an emerging area of alternative care delivery. Telemedicine can be broadly defined as the delivery of health services by telecommunications and can range from a virtual visit with a care provider to a health-related app on a smartphone. Early studies have found that the introduction of telemedicine may improve three major areas of health care—access, cost, and outcomes.[21]

5. PAYMENT FOR HEALTH CARE

A century ago, physicians were paid directly by patients for their services. As the cost of care became more expensive, the out-of-pocket payment method became inadequate. One solution to the cost problem was to create a third-party payer, such as an insurance company. The third-party payer collected money regularly from a large population in the form of medical insurance premiums and paid the hospitals and physicians when care was required.

5.1 PHYSICIAN PAYMENTS

Physicians are usually paid in one of three ways: fee-for-service, capitation, or salary. In the fee-for-service method, physicians are paid for each major item of service provided. Charges are established on the basis of the type and complexity of service (complete workup, follow-up visit, hospital visit, major surgical procedure). The amount charged by a physician may exceed the amount that a third-party payer is willing to reimburse, in which case the patient is expected to pay the difference. This payment system provides an incentive to provide more services than might be necessary, because each service brings in a fee.

Sometimes primary care physicians are paid on a **capitation** ("per head") basis. Regardless of the number of services needed by their patients, providers receive the same amount of money per period of time. This method of payment has much lower administrative costs than the fee-for-service method and is thought to promote physicians' efforts in preventive care, although it provides an incentive to do as little as possible. It also may lead to poor gatekeeping, because clinicians may find it easier to refer a patient to a specialist than to provide a service themselves. The capitation method is sometimes used in the United States to pay practitioners working in HMOs; it is commonly used in Great Britain to pay general practitioners.

The third method of payment is a **salary.** Physicians who work full-time for HMOs, hospitals, universities, companies, or some group practices may be paid a *flat salary.* Although this method does not provide an incentive to provide either too little or too much care, it also does not provide incentives for productivity or high-quality care. Providers receive the same amount of money regardless of the amount or quality of care they provide. **Pay-for-performance** methods and paying for quality outcomes have been explored. However, designing payment systems to reward quality also has drawbacks. It requires systems to measure quality of care and complex adjustments for comorbidities, which divert money and energy to measurement or documentation of care and away from the care itself (see "Cost Containment" later).

5.2 INSURANCE AND THIRD-PARTY PAYERS

Modern US medical insurance had its foundation in 1929 in Dallas, when a group of schoolteachers entered into a contract with Baylor University Hospital. Each teacher paid the hospital 50 cents per month. In turn, the hospital promised to cover the cost of any hospital stay. This scheme led to the development of **Blue Cross,** which is a form of insurance that covers only hospital care. Later, in response to recommendations from physicians and others, **Blue Shield** was developed as a parallel organization that allowed members to pay in advance for physician services.

To understand how insurance companies work, it is necessary to review a few concepts concerning benefits. If an insurance policy covers **indemnity benefits,** this means that the insurance company (carrier) will reimburse the insured patient a fixed number of dollars per service, regardless of the actual charges incurred; the patient must pay the difference. In contrast, if an insurance policy covers **service benefits,** the carrier must pay the full amount of the contracted payment for the needed services, regardless of their costs.

Actuaries, the statisticians who estimate risks and establish premiums for insurance companies, have a standard set of *actuarial principles* that guide the process of **underwriting** (insuring) medical risks and other risks such as fire and flood. Actuaries make sure that an insurance carrier does not collapse financially. Originally, insurance was designed to pool the risk from large groups to protect individuals from rare but devastating losses, such as fires in their homes or businesses. However, the actuarial principles developed to accomplish this objective do not adapt well to all medical care, for three reasons. First, medical care involves both frequent and fairly predictable costs as well as rare, catastrophic costs. Second, those at greatest risk of ill health and hospitalization can least afford the cost of insurance, although according to actuarial principles, they should be charged the most. Third, although homeowners may not be able to prevent fires and floods, many factors that affect health can be greatly influenced by personal behavior. Therefore medical insurance requires adaptations to achieve a just and equitable system for financing medical care.

So far, one of the primary solutions for this dilemma in health care has been **pooling risk**. If all of the people in a large, natural community (i.e., a community consisting of people of various ages and degrees of health) were to be insured by the same carrier and were to pay the same monthly premium rate, the law of averages would work so as to protect the carrier from excessive loss. In effect, the low-risk people in the population would help pay the premiums for the high-risk people; the risk would be averaged according to the *community rating* or *experience rating* of the entire group. This is not a complete solution, because low-income persons still might not be able to pay the established premium.

Initially, Blue Cross plans began to cover large segments of communities, and the community pooling of risk appeared to work. However, problems emerged as many insurance carriers sought to selectively attract the business of low-risk individuals. As the people with low risks were lured away from the community pool ("cream skimming" or "cherry picking"), those remaining in the pool were, on average, at higher risk. Consequently, they had to be charged a higher premium, making the community pool still less attractive. This phenomenon by which the highest-risk, highest cost people are most attracted to purchasing health insurance is called **adverse selection** and occurs in any insurance system.

5.2.a Benefit Design

All benefit plans offered by a third-party payer, including HMOs of various types, seek provisions to attract the patients they want to recruit to the plan, while at the same time limiting the financial exposure of the insurer. First, the plan may try to reduce premiums and costs by enlisting the patients themselves in reducing costs through such traditional methods as deductibles and copayments. Second, a common practice is to exclude or at least limit the amount of certain benefits. For instance, as previously mentioned, plans frequently limit or exclude benefits for mental health and dental health. A serious problem for many patients forced to change insurers is that the insurer may refuse to cover the cost of certain **preexisting conditions,** thus limiting the company's financial exposure for many chronic diseases and disorders. Legislation to control these loopholes is part of the Affordable Care Act (see earlier).

5.3 SOCIAL INSURANCE: MEDICARE AND RETIREMENT BENEFITS

Compulsory insurance for a population group is often called **social insurance** or **public insurance.** Most people employed in the United States must make payments into the Social Security Trust Fund for two national social insurance programs: Medicare and retirement benefits.

Medicare is authorized under Title 18 of the Social Security Act and is administered by the federal government (although it uses insurance carriers as fiscal intermediaries for managed Medicare plans, discussed later). The people eligible for Medicare include most individuals 65 years or older and most individuals who receive Social Security benefits because of disability. Part A and Part B of Medicare provide partial coverage for hospital and medical fees, respectively. Part A is paid by the Medicare Trust Fund, a separate government account funded by payroll taxes. Parts B and D (prescription drug coverage) are financed through premiums from enrollees and from general tax revenues. Part C of Medicare established managed care plans for Medicare enrollees (**Managed Medicare** or **Medicare Advantage**). In essence, Medicare pays an HMO to manage the Medicare recipient. Although Social Security beneficiaries do not pay premiums for Part A coverage after age 65, they do pay premiums if they elect to have Part B coverage. Medicare also will pay for a certain amount of home care or nursing home care for a medical problem that follows directly from a Medicare-covered hospitalization. However, Medicare does not pay for long-term nursing home care. Because Medicare does not cover all hospital expenses, patients are billed for the portion of charges not covered by Medicare.

5.4 SOCIAL WELFARE: MEDICAID

Medicaid is authorized under Title 19 of the Social Security Act. Unlike Medicare recipients, Medicaid recipients have not previously paid money into a trust fund. Medicaid is paid from general tax revenues of the federal and state governments. Therefore the benefits of Medicaid are considered to be social welfare instead of social insurance.

The people covered by Medicaid are low-income and usually receive additional assistance, such as **Aid to Families with Dependent Children** (AFDC). Unlike Medicare, which is entirely federally administered, Medicaid is administered by the states, which share the costs of the program with the federal government. Although the federal government usually reimburses a state for approximately half its Medicaid costs for a given year, poorer states receive slightly more. The federal government stipulates a minimum set of standards for Medicaid; beyond this, the eligibility criteria and covered services vary from state to state.

Medicaid basically covers two areas. First, it pays for medical care expenses, including both hospital and physician bills. The amount of reimbursement is often far below the customary charges of physicians, making the program unpopular with many providers and making it difficult for many patients to find physicians, especially specialists who accept Medicaid patients. Second, Medicaid pays for long-term nursing home care, but only after people have largely exhausted their personal resources, a process called "spend-down."

Under Title 21 of the Social Security Act, states have established **Children's Health Insurance Programs** (CHIP) to provide health insurance to families whose income is too high to qualify for Medicaid. As with Medicaid, these programs are funded jointly by the US DHHS and the states and have various eligibility requirements and benefits.

6. COST CONTAINMENT

The cost of medical care has long been a topic of concern. The first US Committee on the Costs of Medical Care was established in 1929 and published its landmark report in 1932 that recommended the development of prepaid group practices (the forerunners of HMOs) as the most effective and efficient means to provide and finance medical care.[22] Below we describe reasons for the high cost of medical care and strategies to reduce costs.

6.1 REASONS FOR RAPID INCREASE IN COST OF MEDICAL CARE

Medical costs have been increasing much faster than the general inflation rate; in 2016, health care spending represented about 18% of GDP. Although managed care was able to reduce the rate of medical care inflation for a time in the 1980s, rates have steadily increased since the 1990s. Among the reasons for this increase in costs were the following:

- Rapid innovation and implementation of costly new technologies, driven by a health care financing system that rewards using them
- Increases in wages for health care personnel
- Increases in the demand for care due to population changes and consumer expectations
- Inefficiencies in the delivery of care, stemming from such factors as underuse of facilities, fragmented care, inadequate insurance, and misuse of emergency rooms.

The fee-for-service payment system, which was the norm in the United States through the 1970s, provided no incentive to providers to decrease costs. In fact, it rewarded *overuse* of services because revenues could be generated simply by performing more procedures. It also encouraged use of complex technologies and specialists and had no mechanism to ensure that new, more expensive technologies were cost effective.[23]

6.1.a Inefficiencies in Health Care Delivery

Not providing medical insurance may be more costly than providing it. In some cases, lack of insurance may lead to delayed care and result in increased expenses if disease is found at a later, and less treatable, stage in a more costly setting. The costs of this care eventually must be borne by society. Historically, hospitals shifted the costs of providing care for uninsured persons by charging insured persons more. However, new requirements limit cost shifting as a strategy to pay for indigent health care.

Planning failures have also contributed to increasing costs of medical care. Beginning in the mid-1960s and continuing for almost 20 years, the federal government supported official health planning strategies, largely to control costs. Among the primary strategies it supported were the appointment of rate-setting authorities within states and the issuance of a **certificate of need** for the construction of new hospitals or purchase of expensive equipment. Planning efforts were often ineffective in preventing the duplication of facilities and expensive equipment. In some areas, however, the regulatory efforts were reasonably effective. For example, the number of beds per 1000 population varies considerably in the United States, with no related changes in outcomes correlated to the amount of beds. Similar inefficiencies in care have been amply documented by the Dartmouth Atlas Project (see Websites at the end of this chapter).

6.1.b Decreasing Ability of Employers to Fund Health Care

In the United States, most workers receive their health insurance as an earned benefit through their employers. However, more recently, costs are being shifted to employees, whether through high deductibles or in the so-called tax-preferred health savings accounts, which hand over almost all the responsibility for financing health care to individuals, as discussed next.

6.2 STRATEGIES TARGETED AT CONSUMERS OR SERVICES

The first and most basic method of discouraging the use of health care is to create **deductibles,** which are out-of-pocket payments made by the patient, often at the beginning of the care process. Medical deductibles work in much the same way as automobile or home insurance deductibles: they discourage the use of insurance and reduce the amount of paperwork for the insurance companies. Deductibles are usually applied for an entire year (e.g., the patient might have to pay the first $5000 of yearly medical costs) or to each physician visit (e.g., the patient might have to pay $25 for each visit), with the insurance company paying the remainder of the eligible charges after the deductible is met. In general, physicians have worried that deductibles might discourage patients from coming in for early symptoms of serious disease. Deductibles may range between $5000 and $10,000. At that rate, the deductible is so high that many patients basically pay for their entire health care costs (i.e., have **high-deductible plans**). Even though, in theory, the high-deductible plan covers expenses once the deductible is met, many patients may not exhaust their deductible unless they have a catastrophic illness.

The second basic cost-control method is **copayments.** In copayments, patients pay a given percentage of medical expenses. This provides an incentive for patients to contribute to keeping expenses low because copayments apply linearly to all costs. In contrast to deductibles, copayments are thought to *discourage* patients from staying in hospitals longer than necessary. **Coinsurance** refers to payments that vary with the underlying cost of the service. As with deductibles, this cost-containment method discourages overutilization. In addition, and unlike deductibles, it also encourages patients to seek out low-cost settings because the patient pays a fixed percentage of the entire cost of care.

The third common method is **exclusions** in insurance. Some insurance policies have excluded psychiatric care and dental care from coverage, whereas others have restricted the reimbursement for these types of care.

Policy makers have experimented with market-based health care policy solutions. Examples include private long-term care insurance for nursing home care and **health savings accounts** (HSAs), also called "consumer-driven health care." HSAs consist of a high-deductible health plan and an individual, "tax-preferred" savings account from which individuals would directly finance their health care without a third-party payer. Monies not used in 1 year roll over to the next year. In effect, such an account delegates the responsibility of dealing with foreseeable health care expenses to the individual consumer and limits health insurance for catastrophic events. In order to work, such a model requires sophistication and much decision making by patients. Therefore most proponents of market-based health policy solutions advocate for sponsors (employers or health care purchasing cooperatives) to act for a large group of subscribers to establish equity, manage risk selection, and create price-elastic demand.[24]

6.3 STRATEGIES TARGETED AT PROVIDERS AND SYSTEMS

If resources for medical care are inadequate to meet demand, there are three basic responses: increase resources, decrease demand (or at least utilization), and increase efficiency. Given the many resources already devoted to financing health care, emphasis is on *decreasing demand* and *increasing efficiency* through "bundling." One of the oldest bundling methods and the blueprint for newer versions is the **prospective payment system,** based on diagnosis-related groups, and the ambulatory payment classification system for the outpatient setting (see later). Bundling efforts include episode-based payments, accountable care organizations, and the patient-centered medical home.

6.3.a Prospective Payment System Based on Diagnosis-Related Groups

Developed in the 1970s, **diagnosis-related groups** (DRGs) have changed the way hospitals provide care. Each hospital admission is classified into major diagnostic categories based on organ systems, as outlined in the *International Classification of Diseases* (ICD), and then these diagnostic categories are further subdivided into DRGs. A DRG may consist of a single diagnosis or procedure, or it may consist of several diagnoses or procedures that, on average, have similar hospital costs per admission. An uncomplicated delivery of an infant, for example, is coded as DRG 775, and a percutaneous cardiovascular procedure with a non–drug-eluting stent without complications is coded as DRG 249.[25]

The federal government began to use DRGs in the treatment of Medicare patients in October 1983. Note that the hospital is actually reimbursed *after* a specific type of care is given; however, the amount of payment for the specific care is decided in advance. If a hospital can find a way to reduce the costs and provide the care for less than the amount reimbursed, it can retain the excess amount. If a hospital is inefficient and has higher-than-average costs, it loses money on that admission. The average cost for each of the more than 700 DRGs is set prospectively for each region of the country and is adjusted for region, comorbidities, severity of illness, and risk of mortality.[25] Although extra amounts are added for tertiary hospitals and for hospitals engaged in medical education, these adjustments do not always fully cover the costs of providing care to indigent persons and paying for hospital-based medical education. Because hospitals with the strongest administrative teams and data systems are best able to keep costs below reimbursements, the strong hospitals tend to become stronger and the weak hospitals weaker under this system.

The **prospective payment system** (PPS) added urgency to an already-growing trend to move as much medical care as possible out of acute, expensive, and poorly reimbursed general hospitals and into ambulatory surgery and diagnostic centers. Many hospitals and staff model HMOs began to develop infirmaries, where patients who did not need acute, intensive care could be given moderate supervision and some treatment at a much lower cost than in hospitals.

US government demonstrations such as **bundled payment programs** work to target the rising spending in acute care settings. In bundled payment programs, DRGs are "bundled" with post–acute care services at a set price. The goal is to incentivize physicians and systems to coordinate with post–acute providers in providing higher quality care at a lower cost. The government has implemented both voluntary (e.g., **Bundled Payments for Care Improvement**) and mandatory (e.g., **Comprehensive Care for Joint Replacement**) bundled programs.

6.3.b Ambulatory Care Financing

The US government has supported research to develop an improved system to pay for ambulatory care, particularly to reduce the tendency to overpay for procedures and underpay for primary care. The first result of this research was the **resource-based relative value scale** (RBRVS), which sought to reimburse providers more equitably for outpatient care, based on their time spent, their years of training, their level of skill, and their office equipment costs. At the same time, the government has been supporting research to determine how the general method used to develop DRGs could be applied to outpatient care. The result was the development of **ambulatory patient groups** (APGs) of conditions that require similar resources, based on the RBRVS. Thus the two lines of research were combined with elements from the inpatient and outpatient care classification systems to produce the current **ambulatory payment classification** (APC) system. This federally mandated outpatient PPS is now being used by the federal government to reimburse for ambulatory care under Medicare.

6.3.c Managed Care

Managed care is part of a complex balancing act created by society's struggles with two important questions.[26] First, how do we ensure that people receive needed health care without spending so much that we compromise other important social objectives? Second, how do we discourage unnecessary and inappropriate medical services without jeopardizing necessary high-quality care?

One answer to this dilemma was to develop standards of care to decide which patients can be admitted to the hospital, how long they may remain there, and what care must be done for them while they are hospitalized (**utilization management**). These determinations are variously referred to as **clinical pathways, medical protocols, best practices, practice guidelines,** or **clinical algorithms**. Another strategy to encourage high-quality care is to give providers financial incentives if they meet certain performance criteria (**pay-for-performance** method). Techniques used by managed care companies to keep utilization down include **preadmission reviews and certification** (a reviewer, often a specially trained nurse, must approve a nonemergent hospital admission before it occurs), **concurrent review** (care is reviewed every day to determine if patient still needs to remain an inpatient),

second opinions before expensive surgeries (second surgeon must agree service is indicated), and **gatekeeping** (referrals to specialists must be authorized by primary care provider).

6.3.d Sharing Risk

In the first decade of the 21st century, policy makers have experimented with sharing the risk of medical care with providers. This trend takes various forms. Primary care providers can receive additional payments by providing expanded access and care. A **patient-centered medical home** (PCMH) is defined by the following principles[27]:

- *Personal physician.* Each patient has a personal physician who provides continuous and comprehensive care
- *Physician-directed medical practice.* The personal physician leads a team that collectively takes responsibility for the ongoing care of the patient
- *Whole-person orientation.* The practice addresses emotional, psychologic, and medical needs of the patient
- Care is *coordinated/integrated across systems* and facilitated by the use of registries
- The practice engages in *continuous improvements* of quality and safety
- *Enhanced access to care* is available through such systems as open scheduling, expanded hours, and new options for communication
- *Payment appropriately recognizes* the added value

Hospitals and providers can organize together to form **accountable care organizations** (ACOs). ACOs essentially function as traditional HMOs; hospitals, providers, and other institutions form a system to provide care and control costs. The difference is in the stress on patient engagement and that patients are free to choose their location and provider of care. The ACO is *accountable* to the patients and the third-party payer for the quality, appropriateness, and efficiency of the health care provided. The system provides and coordinates care, distributes payments, and shares in any cost savings.[28]

7. SUMMARY

In the United States the medical care system has developed without strong and consistent direction from the local, state, or federal government. The result is a confusing mix of ways in which services are paid for and organized. The per capita cost of medical care and the proportion of the GDP used for medical care are higher in the United States than anywhere in the world, yet approximately 9% of Americans still have no financial protection from the costs of medical care. The outcomes purchased for the enormous amount of money spent on health care are not consistently better than those of other countries.

Because of the high costs of US medical care, cost-containment strategies are used extensively. In the prospective payment system, third-party payers reimburse hospitals for care at a predetermined rate, depending on the average duration and complexity of the medical care provided for each condition. Frequently used prospective payment systems include diagnosis-related groups and bundled payments for episodes of care. In managed care, hospitalizations are reimbursed by a third-party payer only if the payer has approved the admission (preadmission review and certification). If a patient is admitted through the emergency department, the admission is reviewed the next day and if not approved by the third-party payer, reimbursement may not be paid (emergency department admission review). Once a patient is in the hospital, the length of stay is closely monitored, and the patient may be denied full coverage if the patient is deemed stable enough to be discharged from the hospital as soon as possible (concurrent review and discharge planning). Other aspects of managed care include second opinions before elective surgery, use of primary care physicians as gatekeepers, benefit design, and the provision of financial incentives for physicians to practice economically.

The main government-funded health care financing mechanisms include social insurance (Medicare) and social welfare (Medicaid and state Children's Health Insurance Programs). The US medical care system has many costly inefficiencies, and correcting these may require major changes. New care models aimed at improving these inefficiencies include the patient-centered medical home and the accountable care organization.

REFERENCES

1. Kissick WL. *Medicine's Dilemmas: Infinite Needs Versus Finite Resources.* New Haven, CT: Yale University Press; 1994.
2. Papanicolas I, Woskie LR, Jha AK. Health care spending in the United States and other high-income countries. *JAMA.* 2018;319:1024-1039.
3. Hardin G. The tragedy of the commons. *Science.*1968;162: 1243-1248.
4. Keeler EB. Effects of cost sharing on use of medical services and health. *J Med Pract Manage.* 1992;8:317-321.
5. Wan H, Goodkind D, Kowal P. *An Aging World: 2015.* United States Census Bureau; 2016. Available at: https://www.census.gov/content/dam/Census/library/publications/2016/demo/p95-16-1.pdf.
6. Collins SR, Gunja MZ, Beutel S. New U.S. Census Data Show the Number of Uninsured Americans Dropped by 4 Million, with Young Adults Making Big Gains. *The Commonwealth Fund.* September 13, 2016. Available at: https://www.commonwealthfund.org/blog/2016/new-us-census-data-show-number-uninsured-americans-dropped-4-million-young-adults-making.
7. Organisation for Economic Cooperation and Development (OECD). *Health spending (indicator).* 2019. Available at: data.oecd.org/healthres/health-spending.htm.
8. Thompson D. OECD: U.S. outspends average developed country 141% in health care. *The Atlantic.* April 12, 2011. Available at: http://www.theatlantic.com/business/archive/2011/04/oecd-us-outspends-average-developed-country-141-in-health-care/237171.
9. Fineberg HV. A successful and sustainable health system—how to get there from here. *N Engl J Med.*2012;366:1020-1027.
10. Schneider E, Sarnak D, Squires D, et al. *Mirror, Mirror 2017: International Comparison Reflects Flaws and Opportunities for Better U.S. Health Care.* 2017. Available at: https://interactives.commonwealthfund.org/2017/july/mirror-mirror/.
11. Institute of Medicine. *For the Public's Health: Revitalizing Law and Policy to Meet New Challenges.* 2011. Available at: https://www.ncbi.nlm.nih.gov/books/NBK201023/pdf/Bookshelf_NBK201023.pdf.
12. Meyer R. How the U.S. protects the environment, from Nixon to Trump: a curious person's guide to the laws that keep the air clean and the water pure. *The Atlantic.* March 29, 2017. Available at: https://www.theatlantic.com/science/archive/2017/03/how-the-epa-and-us-environmental-law-works-a-civics-guide-pruitt-trump/521001/.
13. U.S. Department of Health and Human Services. *Section 1557 of the Patient Protection and Affordable Care Act.* 2016. Available at: https://www.hhs.gov/civil-rights/for-individuals/section-1557/index.html.
14. Summary of the Affordable Care Act. *Kaiser Family Foundation.* April 25, 2013. Available at: https://www.kff.org/health-reform/fact-sheet/summary-of-the-affordable-care-act/.
15. Pande AH, Ross-Degnan D, Zaslavsky AM, Salomon JA. Effects of healthcare reforms on coverage, access, and disparities: quasi-experimental analysis of evidence from Massachusetts. *Am J Prev Med.* 2011;41:1-8.
16. Joyce TJ, Holtz-Eakin D, Gruber J, eds. Point/counterpoint: what can Massachusetts teach us about national health insurance reform? *J Policy Anal Manage.* 2011;30:177-195.
17. Musumeci MB. *A guide to the Supreme Court's Affordable Care Act Decision.* Policy brief 8332. 2012. Available at: https://www.kff.org/health-reform/issue-brief/a-guide-to-the-supreme-courts-affordable/.
18. Internal Revenue Service. *New Requirements for 501(c)(3) Hospitals Under the Affordable Care Act – Section 501(r).* 2019. Available at: https://www.irs.gov/charities-non-profits/charitable-organizations/requirements-for-501c3-hospitals-under-the-affordable-care-act-section-501r.
19. American College of Physicians. *A Shared Statement of Ethical Principles for Those Who Shape and Give Health Care: A Working Draft.* 1999. Available at: http://ecp.acponline.org/mayjun99/tavistock.pdf.
20. RAND Research Brief. *The Evolving Role of Retail Clinics.* Available at: https://www.rand.org/pubs/research_briefs/RB9491-2.html.
21. RAND. *Organizing Care: In Depth.* Available at: https://www.rand.org/health/key-topics/organizing-care/in-depth.html.
22. Committee on the Costs of Medical Care. *Medical Care for the American People.* Chicago, IL: University of Chicago Press; 1932.
23. Povar GJ, Blumen H, Daniel J, et al. Ethics in practice: managed care and the changing health care environment: medicine as a profession managed care ethics working group statement. *Ann Intern Med.* 2004;141:131-136.
24. Enthoven AC. The history and principles of managed competition. *Health Aff (Millwood).* 1993;(suppl 12):24-48.
25. Garry C, Kruse M, Taillon H. *The Clinical Documentation Improvement Specialist's Handbook.* 2nd ed. Danvers, MA: HCPro; 2011. Available at: https://bit.ly/2TcKYaF.
26. Gray BH, Field MJ, eds. *Controlling Costs and Changing Patient Care? The Role of Utilization Management.* Washington, DC: National Academies Press; 1989.
27. Defining the Medical Home. *Patient-Centered Primary Care Collaborative.* Available at: pcpcc.org/about/medical-home.
28. Health policy brief. *Accountable Care Organizations.* January 31, 2012. Available at: https://www.healthaffairs.org/do/10.1377/hpb20120131.782919/full/.

SELECT READINGS

Fuchs VR, Emanuel EJ. Health care reform. Why? What? When? *Health Aff.* 2005;24:1399-1414.

Gostin LO. *Public Health Law: Power, Duty, Restraint.* 2nd ed. Los Angeles, CA: University of California Press; 2008.

Kazmier JL. *Health Care Law.* Clifton Park, NY: Delmar Cengage Learning; 2008.

Kovner AR, Jonas S. *Health Care Delivery in the United States.* 10th ed. New York, NY: Springer; 2011.

Rognehaugh R. *The Managed Health Care Dictionary.* 2nd ed. Gaithersburg, MD: Aspen; 1998.

Stone D. *Policy Paradox: The Art of Political Decision Making.* New York, NY: W. W. Norton; 2002.

WEBSITES

Center for Medicare and Medicaid Services: https://www.cms.gov/

Dartmouth Atlas Project: Supply-sensitive care: http://www.dartmouthatlas.org/downloads/reports/supply_sensitive.pdf

Environmental Protection Agency: Laws and regulations: https://www.epa.gov/laws-regulations

Health Resources and Services Administration: http://www.hrsa.gov/

Henry J. Kaiser Family Foundation: http://www.kff.org/

Institute of Medicine: http://www.iom.edu

REVIEW QUESTIONS

1. Approximately what percentage of the gross domestic product as of 2016 does the United States spend on health care?
   A. 4%
   B. 10%
   C. 18%
   D. 25%
   E. 38%

2. Which of the following is a strategy targeted at consumers to combat overutilization of health care?
   A. Deductibles
   B. Social insurance
   C. Accountable care organizations
   D. Universal health insurance
   E. Individual mandate

3. Most individuals 65 years or older are eligible for this social insurance program.
   A. Medicaid
   B. CHIP
   C. Patient Protection and Affordable Care Act
   D. Medicare
   E. EMTALA

4. What is the definition of the insurance term *adverse selection*?
   A. The tendency of insurance agencies to select against insuring sicker patients
   B. The tendency of people who are sicker to select the wrong insurance company to meet their needs
   C. The tendency of people who are sicker to be more interested in obtaining health insurance
   D. The tendency of insured people to use health insurance, even if they do not need it
   E. The tendency of insured people to use health insurance, even if they cannot afford it

5. Diagnosis-related groups (DRGs) are used to:
   A. Assess the quality of subspecialty care in hospitals
   B. Assign patients to appropriate hospital wards
   C. Provide support for patients after hospital discharge
   D. Review interobserver agreement in radiology
   E. Stipulate prospective payment to hospitals

6. This law developed national standards for an information system and for the protection of health information in such a system.
   A. HIPAA
   B. EMR
   C. ACO
   D. PPACA
   E. HSA

7. Which of the following is not a technique used by managed care companies to keep utilization down?
   A. Preadmission reviews
   B. Fee-for-service method
   C. Concurrent review
   D. Second opinions
   E. Gatekeeping

8. Which of the following acronyms refers to an organization of hospitals and providers accountable to the patients and the third-party payer for the quality, appropriateness, and efficiency of the health care provided?
   A. HMO
   B. ACO
   C. HIPAA
   D. FQHC
   E. EMTALA

9. In 2012 the US Supreme Court ruled which of the following components of the Patient Protection and Affordable Care Act to be constitutional?
   A. The individual mandate
   B. The establishment of the Independent Payment Advisory Board
   C. Increased funds for employer-based wellness programs
   D. State-based insurance exchanges
   E. Subsidies provided to individuals at certain income levels

ANSWERS AND EXPLANATIONS

1. **C.** In 2016 the United States spent 18% of its gross domestic product (GDP) on health care. The United States spends approximately two times the amount that other high-income countries spend on health care, while maintaining similar utilization rates. Prices of services and goods, and administrative costs in particular, contribute to this high spending.

2. **A.** Deductibles, which are out-of-pocket payments made by the patient, are used to discourage overutilization of services. Deductibles are usually applied for an entire

year (e.g., the patient might have to pay the first $5000 of yearly medical costs) or to each physician visit (e.g., the patient might have to pay $25 for each visit), with the insurance company paying the remainder of the eligible charges after the deductible is met. In general, physicians have worried that deductibles might discourage patients from coming in for early symptoms of serious disease.

3. **D.** Medicare is authorized under Title 18 of the Social Security Act and is administered by the federal government. The people eligible for Medicare include most individuals 65 years or older and most individuals who receive Social Security benefits because of disability. Medicare, Medicaid, and CHIP are all administered by the Centers for Medicare and Medicaid Services.

4. **C.** Adverse selection can occur when insurance agencies recruit the people they insure. People with poorer health have a higher interest in obtaining insurance and flock to insurance programs. Payouts for these sicker enrollees increase costs of the plan. The higher costs are passed on to all enrollees, including healthier people. At the higher cost, insurance is no longer a good deal for healthy enrollees, so they leave the plan. When this happens, the higher costs have to be redistributed over a smaller number of people, which increases costs for the individual even more, which cause more people to leave, costs to increase, and so on, known in the insurance industry as a "death spiral." The phenomenon of people using more medical care when they have insurance is called *moral hazard*.

5. **E.** Diagnosis-related groups (DRGs) represent categories of diagnosis for which a standard hospital stay and resultant cost of care are anticipated in the United States. Hospitals are paid by insurers such as Medicare on the basis of the diagnostic group, rather than the actual care delivered. Efficient care results in a profit for the hospital. Complications that cause hospital costs to exceed the DRG reimbursement will result in a financial loss for the hospital.

6. **A.** The Health Insurance Portability and Accountability Act (HIPAA), enacted in 1996, instructed the US Department of Health and Human Services to develop standards that would aid in the development of a national health information infrastructure and would guide providers and institutions in how to safeguard and protect individually identifiable health information. DHHS issued these guidelines in 2001.

7. **B.** Managed care companies use several techniques to keep utilization down, including preadmission reviews (A) and certification (a reviewer, often a specially trained nurse, must approve a nonemergent hospital admission before it occurs), concurrent review (C) (care is reviewed every day to determine if the patient still needs to remain an inpatient), second opinions (D) before expensive surgeries (second surgeon must agree service is indicated), and gatekeeping (E) (referrals to specialists must be authorized by primary care provider). In the fee-for-service method (B), physicians are paid for each major item of service provided. Charges are established on the basis of the type and complexity of service (complete workup, follow-up visit, hospital visit, major surgical procedure). The amount charged by a physician may exceed the amount that a third-party payer is willing to reimburse, in which case the patient is expected to pay the difference. This payment system provides an incentive to provide more services than might be necessary, because each service brings in a fee.

8. **B.** An accountable care organization (ACO) essentially functions as an HMO; hospitals, providers, and other institutions form a system together. The difference is in the stress on patient engagement and that patients are free to choose their location and provider of care. The system provides and coordinates care, distributes payments, and shares in any cost savings.

9. **A.** In June 2012 the US Supreme Court ruled to enforce the individual mandate. The Court held that the individual mandate exceeded congressional power to regulate commerce, but it was constitutional under the power to levy taxes. In December 2017, however, Congress enacted legislation that would remove the federal tax penalty associated with the individual mandate.

30

Integrating Efforts for Clinical Care, Research, and Public Health Action—One Science, One Planet, One Health

CHAPTER OUTLINE

"The health of soil, plant, animal, and man is one and indivisible."

Sir Albert Howard

CASE INTRODUCTION

Case 1

Consider a low-income mother with children who receive support from the US Supplemental Nutrition Assistance Program (SNAP). Because of their socioeconomic circumstances, the family lives in a *food desert*, defined as an area without access to fresh fruit, vegetables, and other healthful whole foods, usually found in impoverished communities. Food deserts result from the lack of grocery stores, farmers' markets, and healthy food providers, and lead to reliance on local convenience stores with processed, high-sugar, and high-fat content foods that contribute to obesity. In addition, the mother smokes heavily, and two of her children suffer from asthma. They have trouble purchasing and using their inhalers, and commonly experience asthma symptoms exacerbated by environmental exposure to mold and pest infestation in their home. Consequently, the family frequently visits the emergency room of the community hospital for acute care. The children's school attendance and grades have been affected by their frequent health problems. Meanwhile, the palm oil that is added to many of their processed foods is grown half a globe away on fields that have taken the place of native tropical rain forests through burning of timber and forest undergrowth. The warming climate that results from vanishing rain forests through deforestation and related smoke emissions in turn has been associated with higher allergen load and more respiratory disease such as asthma.[1]

Case 2

After several years of record drought and high temperatures reflecting climate change trends across the globe, on November 8, 2018, a fire broke out in a heavily forested area of northern California. Within hours, the fire raced through nearby communities killing at least 88 people; burning 153,336 acres; destroying 14,000 homes, schools, hospitals, and businesses; and displacing 50,000 residents. Evacuations, while heroic, were complicated by the fire's rapid spread and lack of planning for such a catastrophic event. Many survivors barely escaped the fire, evacuating without time to pack or prepare. These survivors faced additional challenges of securing adequate food and water, bathroom and sleeping facilities, and medical care. Norovirus infections in makeshift evacuation centers led to widespread illness with some evacuees requiring hospitalization. The fires affected air quality, adversely impacting individuals with pulmonary disease. Thousands of people were initially unaccounted for, leading to extensive searches, often guided by DNA samples from relatives. The psychological impact was immense, but difficult to measure and manage. When evacuation orders were finally lifted several weeks later, the county health officer warned residents not to inhabit their property until it was cleared of heavy metals, lead, mercury, dioxin, arsenic, and other carcinogens.[2] Masks, gloves, and protective suits were provided to residents and they were warned of possible future flash flooding from winter rain storms. Additional health outcomes from these experiences are yet to be known, and rebuilding these communities without considering future events may simply set the stage for similar disasters.

1. INTEGRATING EPIDEMIOLOGY, BIOSTATISTICS, PREVENTIVE MEDICINE, AND PUBLIC HEALTH

Seemingly separate actions across the world relate to or affect one another. By understanding the interrelationships between many of the factors affecting human health, including those outside the usual scope of medicine, we are better positioned to reduce morbidity and mortality and improve public health. While the majority of the readers of this textbook may ultimately care for individual patients, the health of individuals is directly related to their common experiences and environments.

This final brief chapter discusses how topics in this book interrelate to each other and in turn relate to an even broader set of issues, including environment, culture, policy, politics, commerce, and education. In outlining these connections, we hope to make a case for integrated efforts for improving health and health care.

The practice of clinical medicine is an exercise in integration. A clinician may treat one patient with diarrhea, then another, then several more before recognizing an outbreak. A patient's question about medication costs related to their cancer treatment may prompt evaluation of how decisions about insurance coverage are made. A discussion with one woman who experienced a stressful false-positive mammogram could prompt a study to quantify the rates of false-positive mammograms over the lifetime of women in the United States. Discussing healthy exercise with a group of school children may lead to a study on improving walkability and safety of a neighborhood. Our experience with patients should inform our research, and vice versa.

Clinician-researchers often have a micro and a macro view as they go between treating individual patients and their immediate environment, while also being able to see and affect change on a larger scientific and at times social and world level. The specific lens of preventive medicine and public health has additional lessons to teach that are important in placing human health within the context of global health (see upcoming discussion), in considering the impact of social determinants on health and health care (see "Social Determinants of Health"), and to our efforts to help both individual patients and larger populations (see "Lessons from HIV Prevention and Use of Big Data Going Forward").

2. ONE HEALTH

World population growth, the globalization of economic networks, and the food chain have resulted in a highly interconnected world. The human population is expected to reach 9.8 billion by 2050.[3] The resulting demands for living space, land, food, water, and energy are an increasing challenge and affect environmental sustainability and the health of humans and animals. To broaden our perspective on the scope and magnitude of these global trends, it is important to recognize the interrelationships of the environment and climate, human behavior and society, food and agriculture, and economics and development. All of these issues ultimately also impact human health (Fig. 30.1).

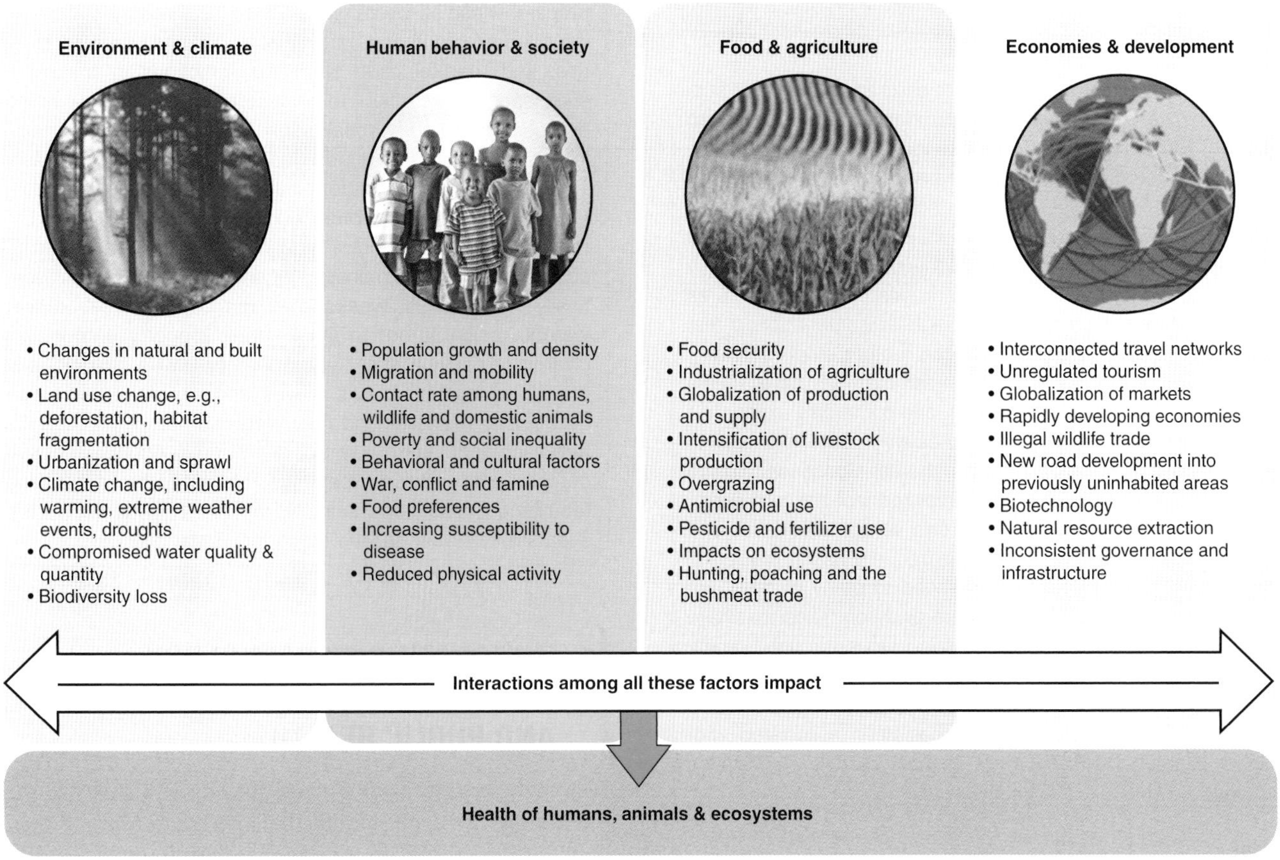

Environment & climate

- Changes in natural and built environments
- Land use change, e.g., deforestation, habitat fragmentation
- Urbanization and sprawl
- Climate change, including warming, extreme weather events, droughts
- Compromised water quality & quantity
- Biodiversity loss

Human behavior & society

- Population growth and density
- Migration and mobility
- Contact rate among humans, wildlife and domestic animals
- Poverty and social inequality
- Behavioral and cultural factors
- War, conflict and famine
- Food preferences
- Increasing susceptibility to disease
- Reduced physical activity

Food & agriculture

- Food security
- Industrialization of agriculture
- Globalization of production and supply
- Intensification of livestock production
- Overgrazing
- Antimicrobial use
- Pesticide and fertilizer use
- Impacts on ecosystems
- Hunting, poaching and the bushmeat trade

Economies & development

- Interconnected travel networks
- Unregulated tourism
- Globalization of markets
- Rapidly developing economies
- Illegal wildlife trade
- New road development into previously uninhabited areas
- Biotechnology
- Natural resource extraction
- Inconsistent governance and infrastructure

Interactions among all these factors impact

Health of humans, animals & ecosystems

Fig. 30.1 Rapid shifts in our environment and climate, human behavior and society, food and agriculture, and economic development interact to impact the health of humans, animals, and the environment. (Modified from World Bank: *People, pathogens and our planet: towards a One Health approach for controlling zoonotic diseases*, vol 1, Washington, DC, 2010; Institute of Medicine, National Research Council: *Sustaining global surveillance and response to emerging zoonotic diseases*, Washington, DC, 2009, National Academies Press.)

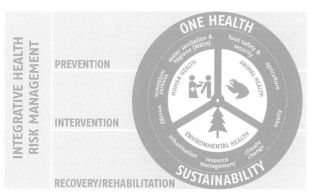

Fig. 30.2 The One Health model of integrative health risk management. (Image from: http://onehealth.grforum.org/about/about-one-health/.)

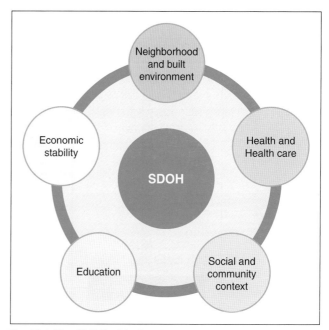

Fig. 30.3 The CDC *Healthy People* 2020 approach to social determinants of health (SDOH). (From: https://www.healthypeople.gov/2020/topics-objectives/topic/social-determinants-of-health.)

Connecting the dots in our clinical examples, the fires in California added to air pollution and increased asthma risk; processed foods contribute to obesity, and many related health risks; meanwhile, every step in the process from cutting down rain forests to eating highly processed foods adds to resource depletion and climate change—which threatens the health of us all, no matter whether or not we smoke, are obese, or eat highly processed food. We are truly all part of "One Health."

The term "One Health" serves as a comprehensive framework for public health that is characterized by the collaborative efforts of multiple disciplines working locally, nationally and globally to attain optimal health for people, animals, and our environment.[4-8] The One Health approach calls for a paradigm shift in developing, implementing, and sustaining health policies that more proactively engage human medicine, veterinary medicine, public health, environmental sciences, and a number of other disciplines that relate to health, land use, and the sustainability of human interactions with the natural world (Fig. 30.2).[5] This multifaceted perspective can be applied to diverse topics such as climate change, biodiversity loss, emerging diseases, and even chronic diseases and mental health.

The One Health concept is synergistic as it aims to shift the focus from single diseases to strengthening public and animal health systems, while also recognizing the environmental and social drivers of health.[6] Ideally, a One Health approach improves reach and efficiency in logistics, enhances provisioning of services globally, and strengthens health systems.[7,8] One Health offers a logical path forward by recognizing the interconnected nature of human, animal, and ecosystem health in an attempt to inform health and environmental policy, expand scientific knowledge, improve health care training and delivery, improve conservation outcomes, identify upstream solutions, and address sustainability challenges.

3. SOCIAL DETERMINANTS OF HEALTH

Our social and physical environment can impact health in positive and negative ways. The circumstances in which people are born, grow, live, work, and age, and the health care systems put in place to deal with illness, influence health and

health status. Health and health care systems are shaped by a wide set of forces, including economics, culture, social policies, and politics. Health is influenced by eating well, staying active, not smoking, getting the recommended immunizations and screening tests, and obtaining health care when we are sick. But our health is also (and maybe even more) determined by access to social and economic opportunities, the quality of our schools and educational systems, the safety of our workplaces, the cleanliness of our food and water and air, and the nature of our social interactions and relationships. These conditions in which we live explain in part why some individuals are healthier than others (see also Chapter 14 regarding social determinants of health). To ensure that all have the same opportunity for good health, advances are needed not only in our health care system, but also in fields such as education, child care, housing, business, law, media, community planning, transportation, and agriculture.

There are many underlying factors in the arena of social determinants of health (Fig. 30.3)[9,10]: economic stability (employment, food insecurity, housing instability, poverty), education (early childhood education and development, language and literacy), social and community context (discrimination, social cohesion), health and health care (access, health literacy), and the neighborhood and built environment (crime and violence, environmental conditions, quality of housing).

Health is more than what happens within a health system. Factors that might influence how long and how well we live are shown in Fig. 30.4. For some individuals, the essential elements for a healthy life are readily available, yet for others, their opportunities are significantly limited. Gaps still need to be closed between those with the most and least opportunities for good health. Health equity is defined by *Healthy People*

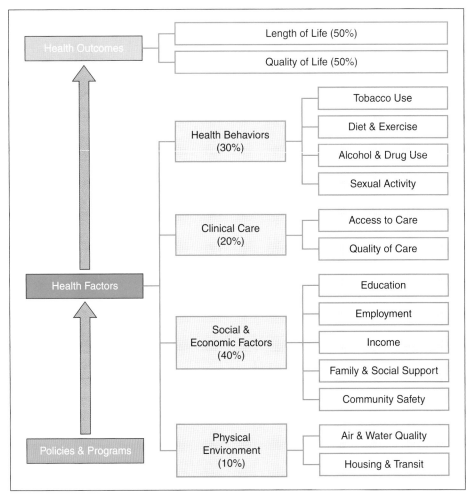

Fig. 30.4 Conceptual model of factors influencing health and health care. (From: http://www.countyhealthrankings. org/what-is-health.)

2020 as the "attainment of the highest level of health for all people. Achieving health equity requires valuing everyone equally with focus and ongoing societal efforts to address avoidable inequalities, historical and contemporary injustices, and the elimination of health and health care disparities."[11] Everyone should have the opportunity to be as healthy as possible, regardless of race, ethnicity, gender, income, location, or any other factor. Unfortunately, significant differences in health outcomes, from one country to the next and among racial/ethnic groups, for example continue. Health equity requires removing obstacles to health such as poverty and discrimination and lack of access to quality education and housing, a safe environment, and health care.

Action is needed at many different steps to improve health and health care. Key activities and suggested tools to guide progress in your efforts to change the health of your community are listed in Box 30.1. We encourage you to take action.

BOX 30.1   Steps to Move Your Actions and Community Forward to Improved Health and Health Care[a]

1. **Assess Needs and Resources**

   Start by taking stock of your current community strengths, resources, needs, and gaps to help you decide where and how to focus your efforts. Consider the challenges you face. Ask if there are some who face challenges that others do not. Review your county health rankings data or collect your own data. Analyze the data to move to action.

2. **Focus on What's Important**

   Decide which problems(s) to tackle. Without focus, all issues seem equally important. Taking time to set priorities will ensure that you direct your community's resources to the most important issues. Finalize priorities and resources to determine your guiding question.

BOX 30.1   Steps to Move Your Actions and Community Forward to Improved Health and Health Care[a]—cont'd

3. **Choose Effective Policies and Programs**

   Evidence matters. Selecting and implementing policies and programs that have been shown to work in real life and are a fit for your community will maximize success. Explore policies and programs while considering the impact and best strategy for your community.

4. **Act on What's Important**

   Move to action. There are no one-size-fits-all blueprints for success; therefore communities must build on strengths, leverage available resources, and respond to unique needs. Develop a strategy to take action, create resource plans, build your message, and mobilize public and political will.

5. **Evaluate Actions**

   Ongoing evaluation of your efforts helps to know if what you're doing is working the way you intended and achieving the results you desire. Build an evaluation plan and collect

credible data that you can use to analyze results and adjust your policy implementation or program(s).

6. **Work Together**

   Working together is the heart of making meaningful change. Every community is different, and as a result, efforts to improve health will vary. When people work together with a shared vision and commitment to improve health, it can yield better results than working alone. Recruit diverse stakeholders from multiple sectors and build organizational structure and relationships. Develop the group's vision, values, and mission statement to reinforce healthy partnership practices.

7. **Communicate**

   Effective communication throughout each step is essential. What you say and how you say it can motivate the right people to take the right action at the right time. Start the conversation, but know your audience, use a proper communications strategy, and deliver your message using the power of story.

[a]Modified from County Health Rankings, www.countyhealthrankings.org/take-action-improve-health/action-center.

---

4. LESSONS FROM HIV PREVENTION AND USE OF BIG DATA GOING FORWARD

Human immunodeficiency virus (HIV)/acquired immunodeficiency syndrome (AIDS) is a global problem being addressed by using carefully collected and analyzed data from epidemiologists and biostatisticians, as well as through the actions of individual clinicians and preventive medicine and public health experts and patient advocates. While the fight against HIV/AIDS continues, enormous gains in saving lives have also been made over the past 30 years.[12] The success in slowing the spread of HIV highlights lessons about prevention and disease control in general:

1. Knowledge is essential to successful prevention, but it is not effective without changes in attitudes, motivation, and behaviors. The most successful way to impact behavior is to change attitudes and social norms.

2. Successful prevention targets clusters of behavioral indicators, not just one. In the case of HIV, efforts to simultaneously target condom use, delayed initiation of sexual activity, and reducing multiple sexual partnerships resulted in marked reductions in HIV prevalence.

3. Target high-risk populations. In most communities, a minority of the population is high risk, including having multiple sexual partners or commercial or *transactional* sex (i.e., sex for drugs, food, or shelter). The same is true for other health problems: a smaller high-risk population accounts for a larger utilization of health care resources. Targeting prevention efforts to these groups has more impact on population health than general prevention.

4. Empowerment is part of prevention. Many high-risk individuals come from vulnerable and disempowered populations. Prevention programs combining outreach,

empowerment, and behavior modification have much better results than any of these interventions alone.[13]

Harnessing data is often key to understanding diseases and their effect on health, as well as designing and implementing more effective prevention programs and interventions. By understanding and using the increasing amounts of "big data" now available to us, we can gain a better understanding of how to help our patients and our communities.

As an example, the Centers for Disease Control and Prevention (CDC) offers AtlasPlus,[13] which provides quick access to more than 15 years of CDC's surveillance data on HIV. AtlasPlus is an interactive tool that gives users the ability to create customized tables, maps, and charts and to view social and economic data in conjunction with surveillance data for each disease. The AtlasPlus now has indicators on social determinants of health (AtlasPlus also provides data on viral hepatitis, sexually transmitted diseases [STDs], and tuberculosis [TB]). AtlasPlus is an interactive tool that gives users the ability to create customized tables, maps, and charts and to view social and economic data in conjunction with surveillance data for each disease.

AtlasPlus provides data on estimated incidence, estimated diagnosed AIDS among all persons living with HIV infection and estimated persons living with HIV infection nationally and by state, and linkage to care, receipt of HIV medical care, and viral suppression by state. The AtlasPlus data on social determinants of health includes five indicators: (1) poverty; (2) uninsured; (3) less than a high school education; (4) vacant housing nationally, by state, and by county; and (5) percentage of population living in rural areas nationally, by state, and by county urbanization level.

With the current generation of big data in medicine and health, we now have the ability to look at the complex, integrated, and overlapping social structures and economic systems that influence most health inequities. Using these new data, we can gain a deeper understanding of the intersection of our global world, the social determinants of health, and specific diseases.

CASE 1 AND 2 RESOLUTION

Fires in one place can add to air pollution and increased asthma risk far away; processed foods contribute to obesity, and many related health risks; meanwhile, every step in the process from cutting down rain forests to eating highly processed foods adds to resource depletion and climate change—which threatens the health of us all, no matter whether or not we smoke, are obese, or eat highly processed food. We are truly all part of "One Health." Hopefully, a comprehensive look at all the components that make up health and new data sources will give us the ability to understand and take action.

---

5. SUMMARY

Public health and preventive medicine should be the purview of all clinicians, not just specialists. We hope that a view on the interconnections of individual health, behavior, society, our environment, and global health will make our readers more efficient consumers of the relevant literature, more skilled in counseling their patients, and more humble, realistic, and empathic with their patients and themselves.

Thank you for reading our text. Please take great care of the patients and populations you serve and consider the interconnectedness of our patients' lives and the world we live in. We wish you all the best in your careers.

REFERENCES

1. D'Amato G, Vitale C, Rosario N, et al. Climate change, allergy and asthma, and the role of tropical forests. *World Allergy Organ J.* 2017;10:11.

2. Camp fire evacuees allowed to return home. *CBS News.* December 15, 2018. Available at: https://www.cbsnews.com/news/camp-fire-paradise-california-all-evacuation-orders-today-lifted-deadly-wildfire-2018-12-15.

3. United Nations, Department of Economic and Social Affairs, Population Division. *World Population Prospects: The 2017 Revision, Key Findings and Advance Tables.* Available at: https://esa.un.org/unpd/wpp/publications/files/wpp2017_keyfindings.pdf.

4. World Health Organization. *Adelaide Statement on Health in All Policies: Moving Towards a Shared Governance for Health and Well-Being.* Adelaide: WHO and Government of South Australia; 2010.

5. American Veterinary Medical Association. *One Health: A New Professional Imperative, One Health Initiative Task Force Final Report.* Washington, DC: AVMA; 2008.

6. Zinsstag J, Schelling E, Waltner-Toews D, et al, eds. One health: the theory and practice of integrated health approaches. *CABI.* 2015.

7. Leboeuf A. *Making Sense of One Health: Cooperating at the Human-Animal-Ecosystem Health Interface.* Health and Environment Reports No 7. Paris: 2011, Institute Francais des Relations Internationales.

8. Alliance for Health Policy and Systems Research. *Strengthening Health Systems: The Role and Promise of Policy and Systems Research.* Geneva, Switzerland: Global Forum for Health Research; 2004.

9. Secretary's Advisory Committee on Health Promotion and Disease Prevention Objectives for 2020. *Healthy People 2020: An Opportunity to Address the Societal Determinants of Health in the United States.* Available at: http://www.healthypeople.gov/2010/hp2020/advisory/SocietalDeterminantsHealth.htm.

10. World Health Organization, Commission on Social Determinants of Health. *Closing the Gap in a Generation: Health Equity Through Action on the Social Determinants of Health.* Available at: http://www.who.int/social_determinants/en.

11. Healthy People. *Disparities.* 2019. Available at: https://www.healthypeople.gov/2020/about/foundation-health-measures/Disparities#5.

12. Piot P, Abdool Karim SS, Hecht R, et al. Defeating AIDS—advancing global health. *The Lancet.* 2015;386:171-218.

13. Centers for Disease Control and Prevention. *NCHHSTP AtlasPlus.* Available at: https://www.cdc.gov/nchhstp/atlas/index.htm. Accessed November 25, 2019.